THE WRIST
AND ITS DISORDERS

1988

DAVID M. LICHTMAN, M.D., F.A.C.S.

Chairman, Department of Orthopaedic Surgery
Naval Hospital
Bethesda, Maryland

Professor of Surgery and Head
Division of Orthopaedic Surgery
Uniformed Services
University of the Health Sciences
Bethesda, Maryland

1988
W. B. SAUNDERS COMPANY
Harcourt Brace Jovanovich, Inc.
Philadelphia ☐ London ☐ Toronto ☐ Montreal ☐ Sydney ☐ Tokyo

W. B. SAUNDERS COMPANY
Harcourt Brace Jovanovich, Inc.

The Curtis Center
Independence Square West
Philadelphia, PA 19106

Library of Congress Cataloging-in-Publication Data

Lichtman, David M.

The wrist and its disorders.

1. Wrist—Wounds and injuries.   I. Title.   [DNLM: 1. Wrist
   Injuries. WE 830 L699w]

RD559.L53 1988   617'.574   87–16555

ISBN 0–03–011842–5

The opinions and assertions contained in the chapters contributed by employees of the United States Navy are the private views of the authors and are not to be construed as official or reflecting the views of the United States Navy.

Editor: Edward Wickland
Developmental Editor: David Kilmer
Designer: Karen Giacomucci
Production Manager: Peter Faber
Manuscript Editor: Diane Zuckerman
Illustrators: Risa Clow, Glenn Edelmayer, and Philip Ashley
Illustration Coordinator: Peg Shaw
Indexer: Phyllis Manner

The Wrist and Its Disorders   ISBN 0–03–011842–5

Last digit is the print number: 9   8   7   6   5   4   3   2

To my father, Harry S. Lichtman, a physician who hasn't stopped learning, caring, and teaching; and to my mother, Frances Lichtman, a wonderful woman who knows how to treat physicians.

Contributors

A. Herbert Alexander, M.D., F.A.C.S.
Clinical Associate Professor, Uniformed Services University of the Health Sciences, Bethesda, Maryland; Chairman, Department of Orthopaedic Surgery, Naval Hospital, Oakland, California
Kienböck's Disease

Charlotte E. Alexander, M.D.
Hand Surgeon, Naval Hospital, Oakland, California
Triquetrolunate and Midcarpal Instability

Robert D. Beckenbaugh, M.D.
Associate Professor, Mayo Medical School; Consultant, Orthopedic Surgery, Rochester Methodist Hospital and Rochester Saint Mary's Hospital, Rochester, Minnesota
Total Wrist Arthroplasty: Review of Current Concepts

Gerald Blatt, M.D.
Associate Clinical Professor, Orthopedic Surgery, UCLA; Hand Surgery Service, Harbor-UCLA Medical Center; Consultant, Hand Surgery Arthritis Center, Memorial Hospital Medical Center of Long Beach, Long Beach, California
Scapholunate Instability

George P. Bogumill, Ph.D., M.D.
Professor of Orthopaedic Surgery, Georgetown University; Clinical Professor of Orthopaedic Surgery, Uniformed Services University of the Health Sciences, Bethesda, Maryland; Adjunct Associate Professor of Orthopaedics, George Washington University; Staff, Georgetown University Hospital; Consultant, Veterans Administration Hospital and Walter Reed Army Medical Center, Washington, D.C.
Anatomy of the Wrist; Tumors of the Wrist

Michael J. Botte, M.D.
Assistant Professor of Surgery, Division of Orthopaedics and Rehabilitation; Chief, Hand and Microvascular Surgery, University of California, San Diego; Assistant Chief, Rehabilitation Medicine, Veterans Administration Hospital, San Diego, California
Vascularity of the Carpus

William H. Bowers, M.S., M.D.
Private Practice of Hand Surgery, Hand Center of Greensboro; Attending Surgeon, Hand Service, Moses Cone Hospital and Wesley Long Hospital, Greensboro, North Carolina
Surgical Procedures for the Distal Radioulnar Joint

Richard M. Braun, M.D.
Associate Clinical Professor of Orthopaedic Surgery, University of California, San Diego; Clinical Instructor in Orthopaedic Surgery, Ranchos Los Amigos Hospital and USC Medical Center, Los Angeles; Vice Chief of Staff and Director, Upper Extremity Rehabilitation, Donald Sharp Rehabilitation Center, San Diego, California
The Trapeziometacarpal Joint: Basic Principles of Surgical Treatment

Laurence H. Brenner, M.D.
Chief Resident in Plastic and Reconstructive Surgery, Downstate Medical Center, Brooklyn, New York
Degenerative Disorders of the Carpus

David E. Brown, M.D.
Assistant Professor of Surgery, Uniformed Services University of the

Health Sciences, Bethesda; Staff Orthopaedic Surgeon, United States Naval Academy and Anne Arundel General Hospital, Annapolis, Maryland
Physical Examination of the Wrist

Alvin H. Crawford, M.D., F.A.C.S.
Director of Orthopaedic Surgery, Cincinnati Childrens Hospital Medical Center; Professor of Pediatrics and Orthopaedic Surgery, University of Cincinnati College of Medicine; Director of Orthopaedics, Children's Hospital Medical Center; Consultant, Spinal Deformity Center, Good Samaritan Hospital; Attending Staff, University Hospital, Holmes Hospital, The Christ Hospital, and Jewish Hospital, Cincinnati, Ohio
Wrist Disorders in Children

David J. Curtis, M.D., F.A.C.R.
Professor of Radiology, George Washington University Medical Center; Head, General Radiology Section, George Washington University Medical Center, Washington, D.C.
Soft Tissue Radiography of the Wrist

Judy M. Destouet, M.D.
Associate Professor of Radiology, Mallinckrodt Institute of Radiology and Washington University School of Medicine, St. Louis, Missouri; Associate Professor of Radiology, Barnes Hospital and Children's Hospital, St. Louis, Missouri
Roentgenographic Diagnosis of Wrist Pain and Instability

Edward F. Downey, Jr., D.O.
Clinical Assistant Professor, West Virginia University Medical Center, Department of Radiology, Morgantown, West Virginia; Assistant Chief of Radiology, Monongalia General Hospital, Morgantown, West Virginia; Staff Radiologist, Fairmont General Hospital, Fairmont, West Virginia
Soft Tissue Radiography of the Wrist

Paul W. Esposito, M.D.
Assistant Professor of Surgery, Uniformed Services University of the Health Sciences; Head, Pediatric Orthopaedic Service, Department of Or-

thopaedic Surgery, Naval Hospital, Bethesda, Maryland
Wrist Disorders in Children

John F. Fatti, M.D.
Clinical Faculty, State University of New York, Upstate Medical Center, Crouse Irving Memorial Hospital, Veterans Administration Medical Center, Syracuse, New York
Arthrodesis of the Rheumatoid Wrist: Indications and Surgical Technique

Paul Feldon, M.D.
Clinical Assistant Professor of Orthopaedic Surgery, Tufts University School of Medicine, Boston; Chief, Hand Surgery Service, St. Elizabeth's Hospital of Boston; Attending Hand Surgeon, Newton-Wellesley Hospital, Newton, Massachusetts
Wrist Fusions: Intercarpal and Radiocarpal

Donald C. Ferlic, M.D.
Assistant Clinical Professor, University of Colorado Health Science Center; Staff Physician, St. Joseph Hospital, Presbyterian Denver Hospital, and Rose Memorial Hospital, Denver, Colorado
Inflammatory and Rheumatoid Arthritis

Geoffrey R. Fisk, M.B., B.S., F.R.C.S.Eng., F.R.C.S.Edin.
Hunterian Professor, Royal College of Surgeons, London; Honorary Orthopaedic Surgeon, Princess Alexandra Hospital, Harlow and St. Margaret's Hospital, Epping, England
The Development of Wrist Surgery: An Historical Review

Richard H. Gelberman, M.D.
Professor, Orthopaedic Surgery, Harvard Medical School; Chief, Upper Extremity Surgery, Massachusetts General Hospital, Boston, Massachusetts
Vascularity of the Carpus

Louis A. Gilula, M.D.
Professor of Radiology and Co-Director, Musculoskeletal Section, Mallinckrodt Institute of Radiology,

Washington University School of Medicine, St. Louis, Missouri; Professor of Radiology, Barnes Hospital and St. Louis Children's Hospital, St. Louis, Missouri
Roentgenographic Diagnosis of Wrist Pain and Instability

Stephen Flack Gunther, M.D.
Professor of Orthopaedic Surgery, George Washington University School of Medicine; Chairman, Department of Orthopaedic Surgery, Washington Hospital Center, Washington, D.C.; Consultant Surgeon, National Naval Medical Center, Bethesda, Maryland and Clinical Center, National Institutes of Health, Bethesda, Maryland
The Carpometacarpal Joint of the Thumb: Practical Considerations; The Medial Four Carpometacarpal Joints

Gregory R. Mack, M.D.
Chairman, Department of Orthopaedics and Chief, Hand Surgery Service, Naval Hospital, San Diego, California
Scaphoid Nonunion

Robert C. Martin, D.O.
Assistant Professor of Surgery, Department of Surgery, F. Edward Hebert School of Medicine, Uniformed Services University of the Health Sciences; Chief Resident, Department of Orthopaedics, Naval Hospital Bethesda, Maryland Capitol Region, Bethesda, Maryland
Introduction to the Carpal Instabilities

Jack K. Mayfield, M.D., M.S., F.A.C.S.
Clinical Faculty, Phoenix Combined Orthopedic Residency Program; Chairman, Section of Orthopaedics, Phoenix Children's Hospital, Phoenix, Arizona
Pathogenesis of Wrist Ligament Instability

H. Relton McCarroll, Jr., M.D.
Assistant Professor of Clinical Orthopaedic Surgery, University of California, San Francisco; Chairman, Depart-

ment of Hand Surgery, Presbyterian Hospital, Pacific Presbyterian Medical Center; Consultant in Hand Surgery, Shriners Hospital for Crippled Children, San Francisco, California
Nerve Injuries Associated with Wrist Trauma

Charles P. Melone, Jr., M.D., F.A.C.S.
Clinical Associate Professor of Orthopaedic Surgery, New York University Medical Center, New York, New York; Director of Hand Surgery, Cabrini Medical Center; Attending Orthopaedic Surgeon, St. Vincent's Hospital, and Medical Center, New York, New York
Unstable Fractures of the Distal Radius

Edward A. Nalebuff, M.D.
Clinical Professor of Orthopedic Surgery, Tufts University School of Medicine; Chief, Hand Surgery Service, New England Baptist Hospital, Boston, Massachusetts
Arthrodesis of the Rheumatoid Wrist: Indications and Surgical Technique

Eugene T. O'Brien, M.D.
Clinical Professor, Department of Orthopaedic Surgery, University of Texas Health Science Center, San Antonio, Texas
Acute Fractures and Dislocations of the Carpus

Andrew K. Palmer, M.D.
Professor of Orthopedics, Heath Science Center at Syracuse; Professor of Orthopedics, Health Science Center at Syracuse, and University Hospital, Syracuse, New York
The Distal Radioulnar Joint

William R. Reinus, M.D.
Attending, St. Joseph's Hospital, St. Louis, Missouri
Roentgenographic Diagnosis of Wrist Pain and Instability

James H. Roth, M.D., F.R.C.S.(C)
Clinical Assistant Professor, University of Western Ontario, London,

Ontario, Canada; Active Staff, Victoria Hospital, London, Ontario, Canada
Wrist Arthroscopy—Radiocarpal Arthroscopy: Technique and Selected Cases

Alfred B. Swanson, M.D.
Professor of Surgery, Michigan State University, Lansing, Michigan; Director, Orthopaedic and Hand Surgery Training Program of the Grand Rapids Hospital; Director, Hand Fellowship and Orthopaedic Research, Blodgett Memorial Medical Center, Grand Rapids, Michigan
Implant Arthroplasty in the Carpal and Radiocarpal Joints

Genevieve de Groot Swanson, M.D.
Assistant Clinical Professor of Surgery, Michigan State University, Lansing, Michigan; Coordinator, Orthopaedic Research Department, Blodgett Memorial Medical Center, Grand Rapids, Michigan
Implant Arthroplasty in the Carpal and Radiocarpal Joints

H. Kirk Watson, M.D.
Associate Clinical Professor, University of Connecticut Medical School, Farmington, Connecticut; Associate Professor of Orthopaedics and Surgery, University of Massachusetts Medical Center, Worcester, Massachusetts; Assistant Clinical Professor of Plastic Surgery and Orthopaedics, Yale New Haven Medical School, New Haven, Connecticut; Chief, Connecticut Combined Hand Service, Hartford, Connecticut; Chief, Hand Service, Newington Children's Hospital, Newington, Connecticut; Senior Staff, Department of Orthopaedics, Hartford Hospital, Hartford, Connecticut
Degenerative Disorders of the Carpus

Edward R. Weber, M.D.
Associate Clinical Professor, University of Arkansas; Staff, Doctors Hospital, St. Vincent Infirmary, Baptist Medical Center, Veterans Administration, University of Arkansas for Medical Sciences, and Arkansas Children's Hospital, Little Rock, Arkansas
Wrist Mechanics and Its Association with Ligamentous Instability

Craig E. Weil, M.D.
Clinical Instructor in Hand Surgery, Department of Orthopedics, Emory University School of Medicine, Atlanta; Orthopedic and Hand Surgeon, Kennestone–Windy Hill Hospital, Marietta, Georgia
Arthrodesis of the Rheumatoid Wrist: Indications and Surgical Technique

Terry L. Whipple, M.D., F.A.C.S.
Assistant Clinical Professor, Orthopaedic Surgery, The Medical College of Virginia; Consultant, Hand and Sports Medicine Division, Department of Orthopaedics, University of Virginia at Charlottesville; Chief of Orthopaedic Surgery, Humana St. Luke's Hospital, Richmond, Virginia
Clinical Applications of Wrist Arthroscopy

Preface

Prior to 1984, few important textbooks or symposia were devoted to disorders of the wrist. This fact is curious in light of the abundant information available about wrist problems and the acute interest shown by hand surgeons and orthopedic surgeons in this fascinating topic. Perhaps the principal reason for this lack of coordinated reference material is that data accumulated on the wrist have been excessively compartmentalized; for example, articles about scaphoid nonunion were not concerned with the development of carpal instabilities or the subsequent appearance of more extensive degenerative arthritis; discussions of Kienböck's disease frequently omitted carpal kinematics and focused primarily on isolated treatment options for the collapsed lunate; likewise, studies of the distal radioulnar joint overlooked the influence of that structure on carpal kinematics or in the pathogenesis of other carpal derangements.

The absence of an accurate model for wrist kinematics is another significant factor contributing to the lack of cohesiveness of this topic. Traditional concepts of wrist motion and pathomechanics have not been substantiated by direct observations made in the clinical practice of wrist surgery. "Columnar wrist" concepts and "slider-crank" mechanisms may be helpful in visualizing limited aspects of wrist disorders, such as scaphoid fractures and scapholunate instability, but they fail to account for the anatomic derangements seen in perilunate dislocations, midcarpal instabilities, or proximal carpal dissociations. Adherence to concepts that fail to unify the interactions of the entire carpus or to clarify its derangements makes it difficult to visualize separate components of the wrist as having a unified design or purpose.

Fortunately, much has changed in recent years. In 1983, I participated in a panel at the Second Congress of the International Federation of Societies for Surgery of the Hand. The topic for discussion was "The Wrist: Problems and Challenges." Clinical material was easily collected, since most disorders of the wrist are medical challenges, and a good many of them eventually turn into significant problems. Topics discussed were scaphoid nonunion—prognosis and appropriate treatment; Kienböck's disease; the role of silicone replacement arthroplasty; carpal instability—the meaning and mechanics of palpable clunks and clicks; the distal radioulnar joint and its relation to other carpal disorders. The symposium acknowledged the absence of real answers to many of these problems but also assured the audience that much significant research is currently being done.

This textbook exists because of the success of these investigations in recent years. Among current developments is the firm evidence of the interrelationship between structural and kinematic alterations and the pathogenesis of carpal disorders. Variations in ulnar length have been shown to affect the stresses applied to the scapholunate and triquetrolunate joints. Postfracture collapse of a scaphoid fragment or rotation of the entire bone has been shown to have significant prognostic implications for the entire radiocarpal articulation. Limited fusions at either side of the carpus create abnormal stresses and, possibly, secondary planes of motion at other, unaffected, sites in the wrist. Stated simply, the wrist can truly be thought of as a functional entity or *system*. In current practice, there is a greater appreciation of these subtle interrelationships as the body of information constantly expands. And so, a textbook about the wrist and its disorders, drawing upon the work of as many of the original investigators in this field as possible, seemed to be a logical undertaking. My purpose has been to orchestrate a systematic and comprehensive look at the wrist, while preserving the originality and style of each contributing author.

As a functional unit, the wrist includes the proximal metacarpal bones, the carpals, the distal radius, and the ulna, as well as the intervening joint and connective tissue structures. All of these areas are covered here, organized into separate sections with unavoidably overlapping borders.

Section I, on basic science, includes a history of wrist surgery by Sir Geoffrey Fisk, as well as discussions of anatomy, kinematics, and pathomechanics. Although these chapters cover basic science of the wrist as a whole, reference to basic science is again made in later chapters on specific wrist disorders.

Section II is devoted to evaluative techniques, including proper history-taking, physical examination, and an algorithmic approach to the x-ray diagnosis of wrist disorders. A section on arthroscopy is included here because the current state of the art of this technique emphasizes diagnostic applications, although the authors do discuss the treatment potentials of this modality in some detail as well.

Section III, on trauma-related conditions, reviews fractures and dislocations of the carpal bones, the distal radius, and the carpometacarpal joints. A discussion of degenerative disorders of the carpometacarpal joints is included here for continuity. The section also explores carpal instabilities, nerve injuries related to wrist trauma, and injuries of the distal radioulnar joint.

Section IV, on developmental and degenerative conditions, includes discussions of Kienböck's disease, inflammatory and rheumatoid conditions, and tumors of soft tissue and bone. A review of scaphoid nonunion and chronic scapholunate dissociation is included in this section because I believe that the significant problems associated with these conditions involve the treatment of associated degenerative arthritis and are best included in the larger section dealing with arthritic conditions. The chapter on pediatric wrist disorders is unique in that it has not been covered in a single chapter before, yet I believe that a textbook on wrist disorders would not be complete without considering those problems peculiar to the developing wrist joint.

The final section on surgical options is appropriate because many wrist disorders respond satisfactorily to a limited number of procedures, such as total or limited wrist arthrodesis, proximal row carpectomy, and wrist arthroplasty. This point underscores the concept of the wrist as a unified *system*, for when one component of the system fails, secondary changes follow that ultimately lead to generalized problems and require generic solutions.

The Wrist and Its Disorders has been most satisfying to assemble. The participating authors have generously given their time to this project, while continuing to make valuable contributions to the literature on the wrist. Obviously the subject is very dynamic, and eventually much of the material will need to be revised. For now, this material serves as a solid basis for understanding the complexities of wrist disorders and the way in which many individuals have contributed to the synthesis of this topic.

Contents

PART I

Basic Science

CHAPTER 1

The Development of Wrist Surgery: An Historical Review

GEOFFREY R. FISK, M.B., B.S., F.R.C.S. Eng., F.R.C.S. Edin.

Surgery of the wrist and hand is no doubt as old as civilization itself, since the arm is the part of the body most exposed to injury, whether from falls, hunting accidents, or in battle. The endeavors by the Egyptians, Greeks, and Romans to heal and minimize the baleful effects of the crippled hand have continued unabated by their successors to the present day. Amputation of part or the whole of the hand for ceremonial or penal purposes was practiced by early humans and illustrated on the walls of the caves in La Tene and Lascaux at least 30,000 years ago.[1]

A visit to the museum at Epidaurus in Greece, where the first asclepion was established in the fifth century B.C., reveals surgical instruments that are instantly recognizable. Hippocrates (460–356 B.C.) wrote 28 books that contained all contemporary medical knowledge and included one section entitled "Fractures and Reduction of Dislocations." It would seem, however, that at the time amputation of the hand was the only life-saving measure available, and the provision of an artificial hand has an ancient lineage. On July 19th, 1965, an account was written in the London *Times* of an operation to remove an artificial hand from an Egyptian mummy. Pliny the Elder (23–79 A.D.) described a similar case with an artificial hand.[2] Indeed, Johannes Scultatus wrote a learned treatise on the techniques of amputation of the upper extremity entitled *Armamentarium Chirurgicum Bipartum*, that was published in Frankfurt in 1666. Ambroise Paré, the founder of French surgery, also described an artificial hand in a work entitled *Of the Means and Manner to Repair or Supply the Natural or Accidental Defects or Wants in Man's Bodie* (*Oeuvres*, 1664). He was also an early pioneer in the excision and resection of joints.

Paul of Aegina (256–290 A.D.) first described a "ganglion" as a swelling formed around joints, particularly the wrist, but he described this as a "round tumour of tendon." He did not recommend any treatment for such a swelling, but there is little doubt that hitting or squashing it would have occurred to those early surgeons.

Jean Louis Petit (1674–1750) described congenital anomalies and dislocations of the hand and wrist. Jules Desault (1738–1795)[3] also wrote on dislocations of the carpus, and Pierre Brasdor described disarticulation of the hand at the level of the wrist. By the latter part of the eighteenth century, attempts were made to deal with the ravages of infection, particularly tuberculosis, and in 1805 Moreau (father and son) published in Paris *Resection of Articulations Affected by Caries*.

1

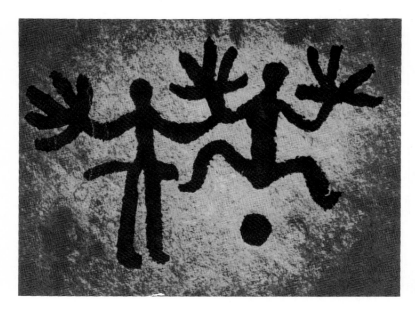

Figure 1–1. Rock carving of Bohus-län, about 3000 years old.

Vesalius (1543) first described and illustrated the wrist joint in his fundamental anatomy textbook, *De humani corporis fabrica*,[107] and these illustrations were copied by Spigelius.[108] The ligamentous structures binding these bones together have also been fully described, but until relatively recently the physiology of the wrist has been neglected. In 1833 Sir Charles Bell regarded the wrist joint as a composite ball and socket articulation.[109] Bryce, through his work in 1896, has been credited with the notion that all carpal movements take place through a single axis that passes through the neck of the capitate bone.[110] In 1925, Destot referred to the bell-like movement of the scaphoid in normal carpal movements,[111] and in 1919 Wood-Jones drew attention to the different ranges of movement that occur at two levels of the carpus.[112] MacConaill also referred to the anatomy of the carpus in his general study of joint movement.[113]

FRACTURES OF THE FOREARM, WRIST, AND HAND

In the nineteenth century, long before the advent of x-rays, surgeons were describing fractures and their treatment. Much of this is anecdotal, with fulsome descriptions of physical signs, techniques of reduction, and the results in single cases. Nevertheless, remarkable clinical acumen was displayed, considering the limited resources available to the diagnostician. Indeed, an anatomist, G.W. Hind, wrote an illustrated manual in

1836 entitled *Fractures of the Extremities* showing from anatomic dissection of the forearm and hand how fractures might occur.[4] He was able to describe the expected deformity from the muscle attachments and their actions. Astley Cooper of Guy's Hos-

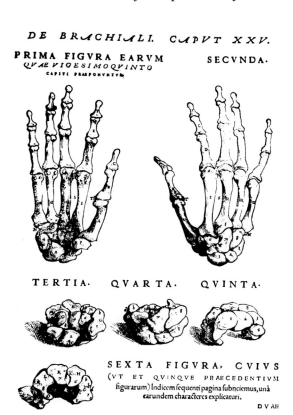

Figure 1–2. Vesalius. De humani corporis fabrica. Liber 1, 115. 1543.

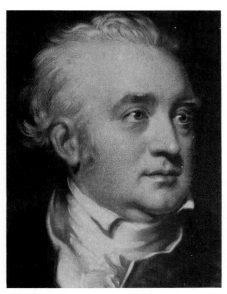

Figure 1–3. Astley Paston Cooper, 1768–1841. (From the Royal College of Surgeons of England.)

pital in London gave a course of lectures and later wrote *A Treatise on Dislocations and Fractures of the Joints* in 1822,[119] and he did in fact describe contracture of the palmar fascia before Dupuytren.[5]

Fractures of the lower radius were described in some detail in writings of this period. Colles' fracture recalls Abraham Colles (1773–1843). He qualified in Dublin, worked at Dr. Steeven's Hospital, obtained his M.D. degree at Edinburgh, and was Professor of Anatomy and Surgery at the Royal College of Surgeons of Ireland. In 1814 he described fracture of the wrist.[6] He prefaced his description by the note that it had not been "described by any other author," and it is doubtful, therefore, that he knew of the work of Petit (1723) and Pouteau (1783). He did, however, differentiate the fracture from a dislocation, and he observed the abnormal mobility of the ulna, but it was not until 1932 that this associated condition was described in some detail by Lippman.[7] In France at this time there were four surgeons quoted by Buxton[8]—Goyrand (1832), Diday (1837), Nelaton (1844), and Malgaigne (1850),[9] who were all treating forearm and wrist injuries. Another Irish surgeon, Robert William Smith (1807–1873), in 1847 described the separation of the lower radial epiphysis and the less common forward displacement.[10]

Barton (1794–1871), an American surgeon working in Pennsylvania, described anteroposterior fracture-dislocations of the wrist, particularly those in which the carpus was displaced forward upon fragments broken from the anterior articular surface of the lower end of the radius.[11] Thomas, in 1957,[12] classified this fracture into three types: (1) an oblique fracture in which the carpus is displaced forward and proximally upon a triangular fragment of the radius, (2) a comminuted fracture of the radial articular surface that carries the carpus anteriorly, and (3) forward angulation of the lower part of the radius with or without comminution. Barton's fracture has proved difficult to hold in a reduced position; in 1965 Ellis described his buttress plate,[13] and there have been many other methods of fixation suggested.

In 1875 Alexander Gordon wrote a book on fractures of the radius, and in 1878, Lewis Pilcher, practicing in Brooklyn, taught the methods of reducing fractures of the wrist. In 1879, Alonzo Ferdinand Carr (1817–1887), who worked in Goff's Town, New Hampshire, described a wooden splint in which the forearm rested on a gutter with a dowel attaching to the distal end and then passing obliquely across the palm. It is remarkable how this universal splint has been the standard fixation procedure for wrist fractures for nearly a century and within living memory of many surgeons alive today; indeed, in many parts of the world this splint may still continue to be used.

Crushing of the lower radial epiphysis, like other injuries in growing bones, may result in premature fusion, which inevitably causes disproportion of the radius and ulna at the wrist joint. Compère drew attention to this in 1935,[14] as did Aitken (1935), writ-

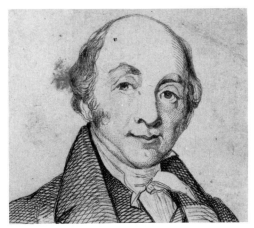

Figure 1–4. Abraham Colles, 1773–1843. (From the Royal College of Surgeons of England.)

ing on fractures of the distal radial epiphysis.[15] The inevitable cessation of growth in the radius leads to severe disproportion and an ugly deformity of the lower forearm, with loss of radioulnar movement. Correction is only possible by shortening the ulna. Excision of the ulnar head was described by William Darrach (1876–1948). Darrach was born in Germantown, Pennsylvania, and graduated from Yale University. His surgical life was spent at the Presbyterian Hospital in Philadelphia, and he described his operation in 1912,[16, 17] although it had first been suggested by Moore in 1880,[18] Tillmanns in 1911,[19] and van Lennep in 1897.[20] However, the operation has the disadvantage of altering the appearance of the wrist joint and disturbing the ulnar aspect of the carpus, particularly its support on the medial side, with later resorption of the ulnar shaft or regrowth of bone fragments if the ulnar head is removed subperiosteally. If an excessive amount of the ulna is removed, the remaining proximal portion becomes hypermobile, and pain and instability result.

However, an account of an operation that preserves the appearance of the wrist, appropriately shortens the ulna, and depends on the development of a pseudarthrosis at the neck of the ulna was published by Baldwin in 1921.[21] Baldwin described his procedure shortly after the 1914–1918 war, while he was still a colonel in the U.S. Army. He practiced in San Francisco and was Bunnell's predecessor.[22] The operation has not enjoyed the popularity it deserves.

A variation of Baldwin's operation has been attributed to Lauenstein.[115] This procedure involves excision of the neck of the ulna, with fusion of the ulnar head to the lower end of the radius by a transversely placed transfixion screw. The transfixion screw will undergo fatigue fracture if persistent movement is allowed. More recently, attempts have been made to realign the inferior radioulnar joint by careful recession of the ulna and internal fixation (Linscheid);[23] but this presupposes normal articular surfaces.

Madelung (1845–1926) practiced in Bonn and drew attention to the dislocation of the inferior radioulnar joint either from congenital or traumatic causes,[24] but this had been previously described by Dupuytren[5] and R.W. Smith.[10] In 1791 Desault also wrote on the dislocation of the inferior radioulnar joint and rightly pointed to the fact that it is the radius that dislocates on the ulna.[3] Dam-

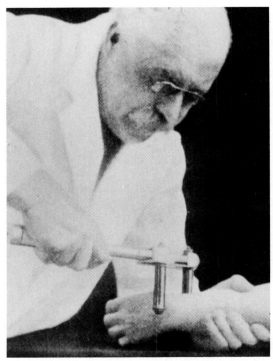

Figure 1–5. Sir Robert Jones (1858–1933) reducing a Colles' fracture using a wrench.

eron classified the types and treatment of traumatic dislocation of the distal radioulnar joint.[25]

Milan, Italy, has the distinction of being the home of two surgeons, Monteggia and Galeazzi, who described fracture-dislocations of the forearm. In 1814, Monteggia (1762–1815) wrote about the fracture of the upper third of the ulna associated with dislocation of the radial head at the elbow joint,[26] and Galeazzi (1866–1962) concentrated on fracture of the lower third of the radius with disruption of the inferior radioulnar joint.[27] Essex-Lopresti also described an injury affecting forearm function—fracture of the head of the radius associated with subluxation of the inferior radioulnar joint.[28]

Many innovations were introduced by Sir Robert Jones and R.W. Lovat in the textbook on *Orthopaedic Surgery*, published in 1929.[29]

In 1966 Buxton[8] reviewed the history of fractures of the lower radius in the *Annals of the Royal College of Surgeons*.

CARPAL TUNNEL SYNDROME

Sir James Paget (1814–1899) of St. Bartholomew's Hospital, London, one of the great surgeons of the later nineteenth century, in

1853 described a case of median nerve compression following a fracture of the lower end of the radius complicated by "ulceration of the thumb, fore and middle fingers" which he was able to alleviate by bandaging the hand in flexion.[30] In 1883 Ormerod accurately described the symptoms of tingling and numbness in the thumb, index, and middle fingers brought on in women at night and exacerbated by "ordinary work of housewives." He made no attempt to postulate the cause, and he attempted treatment by medication only. In 1913, Marie and Foix demonstrated at autopsy bilateral thenar atrophy where the median nerve passed through the carpal tunnel.[31] Indeed, medical students continued to be instructed in the occasional postmortem appearance of "median nerve neuroma" as an anatomic variant, even after its pathology had been appreciated.

Woltman is credited with the first reported case of carpal tunnel syndrome treated surgically in 1941,[32] but sporadic cases of relief of symptoms in the hand by incision around the front of the wrist were reported in the first half of the twentieth century. Learmonth of Edinburgh had reported surgical relief of such symptoms in 1933.[33] Brain, Wright, and Wilkinson, writing in *The Lancet* in 1947, accurately described compression of the median nerve in the carpal tunnel and reported six cases treated surgically.[34] As soon as the condition had been described, it rapidly became universally diagnosed and its repair has become one of the commonest operations in hand surgery. Indeed, in 1966 Phalen was able to report the diagnosis and

treatment of 654 hands with the syndrome.[35] Carroll and Green (1972) drew attention to the risk of damage to the palmar cutaneous branch of the median nerve at the wrist with unwisely placed incisions of the carpal tunnel.[36]

EXCISION, PSEUDARTHROSIS, AND ARTHROPLASTY OF THE WRIST

With the advent of listerian antisepsis, followed by asepsis, surgeons in the latter half of the nineteenth century embarked on wide excision of part or the whole of the carpus in an attempt to eradicate the ravages of infection and to overcome deformity and the complications of fractures and dislocations. This particularly applied to the treatment of tuberculosis of the joints, and pioneer work was performed by Ollier in 1885 in Paris.[37] Many such attempts to retain a mobile useful joint with cure of the disease resulted either unhappily in a flail joint and a useless hand or more happily in spontaneous ankylosis of the remaining bony elements. Steindler stated that the capitate was the commonest bone to be affected by infection in the wrist.[38] In fact, tuberculosis of the wrist was very rare, and Hodgson, writing from Hong Kong, reported an incidence of only 0.7 percent.[39]

Synovectomy was used in preantibiotic days in early cases and was often successful in the rarer forms of tuberculosis in which the onset of bone infection was late. Hodgson (1972) believed that synovectomy was very effective, but in those cases in which suppression of the disease could not be safely achieved by drug therapy, panarthrodesis of the wrist extending from the radius to the third metacarpal gave the best results. He advocated Brittain's arthrodesis.[40]

However, until the advent of antibiotics, surgery of the hand remained limited and was almost totally devoted to overcoming and minimizing the dreadful effects of acute suppurative infections of the wrist and hand. Kanavel (1874–1938) of Chicago was a pioneer in this respect, and his book on infections of the hand became a classic.[41] Indeed, in his publication, coverage of surgery for nonsuppurative conditions is relegated to a few pages.

PARTIAL EXCISION OF THE CARPUS

Partial excision of the carpus or its unreduced elements has long been practiced and

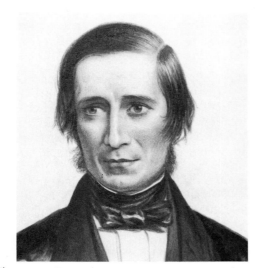

Figure 1–6. Sir James Paget, 1814–1899. (From the Royal College of Surgeons of England.)

in fact can produce improved function. Certainly, excision of the lunate after persistent dislocation or Kienböck's disease is often acceptable. Excision of part or all of the scaphoid for nonunion of a fracture, avascular necrosis, persistent dislocation, or Preiser's disease[42] had its advocates, although there is no unanimity about the wisdom or end results of such practice. In 1964 Crabbe was able to report a series of excisions of the proximal row of the carpus in 24 patients who were followed up over a long period.[43] He advocated this procedure, and although it resulted in the retention of a comfortable and useful wrist inevitably some residual loss of power and movement occurred. In 1949 Dornan reviewed the results of excision of the lunate in Kienböck's disease, and he recorded two thirds of patients as having a good or excellent result and being able to return to full-time work.[44] This has been the general impression among previous generations of orthopedic surgeons, but the advent of prosthetic or soft tissue replacement has superseded simple excision, and Swanson has popularized the use of silicon rubber for this and many other conditions in the wrist and hand.[45] In the same way, excision of the trapezium for painful degenerative arthritis was reported by Gervis[46] and Murley.[47] Lasting, satisfactory results were reported for both series. Here again, the insertion of foreign materials of varying design has required stabilization by tendon or fascial grafts, which is the present fashion.

ARTHRODESIS

In contrast to natural ankylosis, surgical stiffening of the wrist has certainly been practiced for the last hundred years. Albert of Vienna recommended this operation in 1878. At the turn of the century, Tubby advocated arthrodesis of the wrist for paralysis of the hand.[48] Colonna reviewed the methods of fusion of the wrist in 1944.[49] In 1946, Steindler discussed the advantages of fusion.[50] These authors all recommended fusion of the wrist from the base of the second or third metacarpals to the radius without involvement of the inferior radioulnar joint, and most authors have suggested that a small degree of dorsiflexion assisted function of the hand, but it has been agreed more recently that fusion is better performed with a little ulnar flexion and with the wrist in a neutral position. This is particularly impor-

tant in cases with bilateral disease in which attendance to personal hygiene is facilitated. Brittain described his operation of fusing the carpus from the dorsum using a "bail" graft taken from the tibia or iliac crest, i.e., a graft chamfered at either end and slotted into the radius proximally and the third metacarpal distally.[40] Other methods have been recommended by Seddon[51] in which an exposure from the radial aspect protects the dorsal tendons from adherence to the operation site; in 1940 Smith-Petersen advocated the ulnar approach to the wrist using the lower end of the ulna as a free graft.[52] Abbott, Saunders, and Bost advocated panarthrodesis of the wrist using multiple iliac crest grafts.[53]

In 1919 Steindler recommended partial arthrodesis (in reality radiocarpal fusion) by scooping out part of the radius and the scaphoid to produce limited movement in preparation for tendon transfers in cases of paralytic or spastic dropped wrist.[54]

Wedge resection of the carpus from the dorsum in order to overcome fixed flexion deformity has been practiced since the turn of the century, and attempts have been made to correct the deformity of malunited fractures around the wrist; these were reviewed by Durman.[55] Steindler advocated this corrective osteotomy in 1918.[56]

In 1943 White and Stubbins recommended total carpectomy for intractable flexion deformities of the wrist; this induced a pseudarthrosis between the bases of the metacarpals and the radius, although the procedure appears to have been confined to adolescents.[57] They particularly advocated this in congenital contractures and after Volkmann's ischemia.

Partial Arthrodesis

In 1953 O'Rahilly did a comprehensive review of carpal and tarsal anomalies from an anatomic point of view, and he described the incidence and variety of congenital fusion of carpal bones.[58] Clinical observation has indicated a high degree of carpal function in the presence of such anomalies, and this encouraged surgeons in the past to carry out limited fusions in the wrist joint, where degenerative changes, infection, hypermobility, or ununited fractures appeared to have benefited from limited arthrodesis. However, it has not been sufficiently appreciated that congenital anomalies in the carpus can lead to premature degenerative changes in the remaining joints. It is postu-lated that partial arthrodesis may achieve only temporary amelioration, and that in the long term further arthrodeses may become necessary.

Not infrequently infections and injuries have brought about spontaneous radiocarpal or midcarpal ankylosis. These have resulted in the patient's retaining a useful range of movement, usually about half that of normal, and a variable loss of ulnar or radial flexion. Indeed, it has been suggested in the past that the function of the hand is improved if panarthrodesis of the wrist has not been fully achieved!

Localized fusion of the wrist joint was reviewed by Schwartz in 1967. He described localized radioscaphoid fusion of the wrist for old scaphoid fractures, osteoarthritis, and rheumatoid arthritis, especially with ulnar translocation,[59] but this is admittedly diffi-cult to achieve and has no advantage over inclusion of the lunate.

Scapholunate fusion has been advocated in cases of carpal instability or nonunion of the proximal pole of the scaphoid when this fragment has already been excised. In 1960 Maguire advocated this operation for all forms of carpal instability and avascular ne-crosis of the proximal pole of the scaphoid,[60] but unfortunately the scapholunate joint is essential to normal carpal movement.

Scaphotrapezial-trapezoid arthrodesis has likewise been advocated for scaphoid trans-location within the carpus, and Watson, Goodman, and Johnson have described its indications.[61]

Instability of the ulnar column of the car-pus has been similarly treated by triquetro-hamate fusion.[62]

THE FRACTURED CARPAL SCAPHOID

Recognition of this fracture and its subse-quent treatment have gyrated wildly from studied neglect through prolonged immobi-lization to internal fixation with or without bone grafting. The fracture was certainly recognized before the advent of Roentgen's discovery of x-rays. Callender[63] described the fracture in 1866, and Codman and Chase discussed the diagnosis and treatment of the fracture of the carpal scaphoid in 1905.[64] Destot[65] also described the treatment of this fracture in 1921. It had been appreciated quite early that fracture of the carpal sca-phoid could be found incidentally without any definite history of injury and the patient would often be symptom-free. On the other hand, in other patients, symptoms arose and persisted while the fracture remained un-united, and the condition might well have been followed by a periscaphoid degenera-tive arthritis. It was also agreed that this fracture would not normally unite unless it were immobilized, and during the first half of the present century many papers appeared describing the method of fixation, the posi-tion, and the extent of the splintage and its duration, most notably by Adams and Leonard[66] and Berlin.[67]

In 1961 London reviewed the many at-tempts to immobilize the wrist effectively in many different positions.[68] Snodgrass used the flat palmar splint,[69] Speed[116] slight flex-ion, and Hosford hyperextension.[70] Others, including Berlin, advocated extension and radial deviation,[67] while Watson-Jones[74] and Bunnell[22] advocated slight extension and ul-nar flexion. Some authorities, such as Soto-Hall, advocated fixation of the thumb in extension,[72] while others advised a more physiologic position. Others, including Lon-don himself, following Bohler's example, left the thumb free. Still others, such as Verdan,[9] advocated immobilizing the elbow or at least preventing rotation of the forearm. In 1959 Squire advocated immobilization of the forearm fully supinated and in ulnar flexion.[73]

London asserted that, using the criterion of clinical symptoms rather than radiologic appearance, immobilization was not neces-sary for more than six to eight weeks and that some 90 percent or more of these frac-tures united at that stage. Those that were

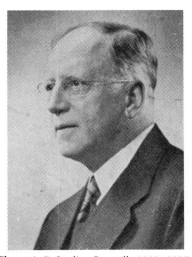

Figure 1–7. Sterling Bunnell, 1882–1957.

ununited on radiologic examination showed only an increased vulnerability to symptoms after heavy use or further injury to the wrist. The present author's experience, gained over some 20 years of wedge grafting ununited fractures of the scaphoid, shows three striking features. First, all the patients seen were male; second, the original injury occurred early in the third decade of life; and third, the fractures had not been treated previously either because the patient had not attended hospital, the wrist had not been x-rayed, or these young men would not tolerate prolonged immobilization (Fisk).[117]

Largely under the influence of Watson-Jones,[74] it became fashionable to immobilize the wrist until union had been achieved as seen on radiographs, even if this meant plaster fixation for many months. This teaching was maintained during World War II, when fracture of the scaphoid was a relatively common injury and a considerable number of servicemen were withdrawn from active service during treatment while the wrist was immobilized in plaster. In the 1930s, several methods were advocated to obtain union of the fracture by longitudinal peg grafts, and Murray published a report of his first series in 1934[75] and then later a report of a series of 100 cases.[76]

In 1939 Matti[118] described inserting a cancellous graft into the anterior aspect of the scaphoid. This operation was developed by Russe in 1960 and remains the most popular method of treatment.[77] However, these authors did not appreciate that in many cases of nonunion the anterolateral aspect of the fracture surfaces had resorbed, leaving a py-

ramidal defect with primary or secondary instability of the carpus. The present author has described a wedge graft that not only restores stability to the wrist but also results in union of the fracture without humpback deformity.[78]

In 1954, McLaughlin introduced the Vitallium lag screw, which was inserted at open operation.[79] This was refined by Maudsley and Chen in 1972, when they cannulated the screw so that it could be fitted over a Kirschner wire inserted under fluoroscopy through a small puncture wound.[80] More recently still, in 1984 Herbert and Fisher introduced a new principle in internal fixation by means of a screw with a recessed head and a screw thread of different pitch at either end.[81]

Removal of the radial styloid in the presence of painful localized scaphostyloid arthritis was studied by Barnard and Stubbins in 1947.[114] These authors particularly recommended the operation of removing the styloid in the presence of nonunion of the scaphoid, but they did not distinguish between fractures that occurred in stable versus those that occurred in unstable wrist joints. They recommended peg grafting of the scaphoid using the bone from the excised radial styloid. Styloidectomy is not approved of by many European authors, who claim that it destroys the ligamentous support on the radial aspect of the carpus, but Barnard and Stubbins reported that there was no appreciable instability of the wrist joint in their cases, and the present author can confirm that this complication is theoretical only and is never seen purely as a result of removing the styloid. The operation is contraindicated, however, when there is an unstable pseudarthrosis of the scaphoid with an unstable carpus.

Other fractures of carpal bones with or without dislocation have been described at least since the days of Astley Cooper,[119] and there has been increasing emphasis not only on early diagnosis and reduction but on internal fixation of the scaphoid by screw or wire if it were involved, and stabilization of the rest of the carpus by impaled Kirschner wires. Destot, one of the pioneers in the investigation of carpal movement, recommended manipulative reduction.[88] Other authors include Conwell in 1925,[89] Schnek in 1930,[90] Watson-Jones in 1928,[91] and Johannson in 1926, who discussed dislocation of the hamate bone.[92]

Watson-Jones classified carpal dislocation

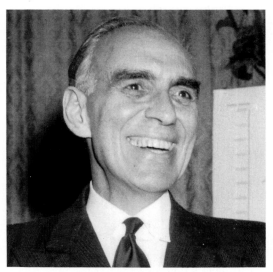

Figure 1–8. Sir Reginald Watson-Jones, 1902–1972.

and fracture dislocations in his textbook.[93] He recommended manipulative reduction and, if necessary, excision of the displaced carpal bone, and he advocated prolonged immobilization of the wrist when a fractured scaphoid was involved. However, he did not differentiate between the first stage of dislocation of the carpus, leaving one or more bones in position, and the second stage, in which the carpus and hand spring back into position, dislocating those bones that origi-

nally were undisplaced. In 1949, Russell reviewed wrist injuries treated in the Royal Air Force during World War II.[94]

CARPAL INSTABILITY

In 1943, Lambrinudi first expounded the principle of zig-zag buckling, which he saw as taking place in the human body where there occurs a chain of three elements in which the central link could become unsta-

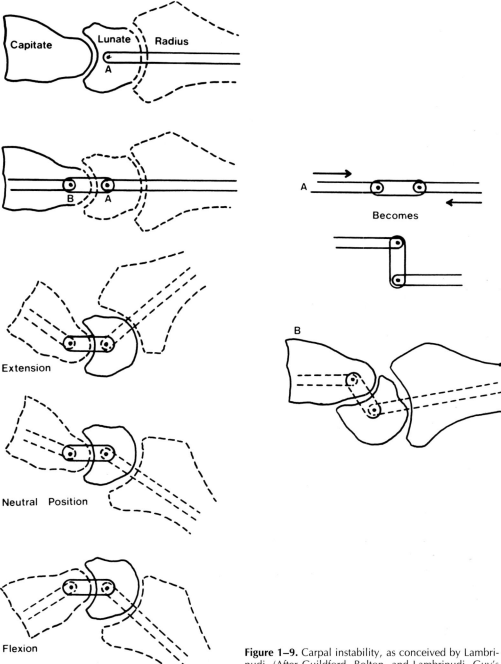

Figure 1–9. Carpal instability, as conceived by Lambrinudi. (After Guildford, Bolton, and Lambrinudi. Guy's Hospital Reports, 92:52, 1943.)

ble.[82] Such an arrangement is seen not only in the fingers and toes but in the carpus. Guildford, Bolton and Lambrinudi, in a fundamental paper, illustrated this in *Guy's Hospital Reports* in 1943.[83] In 1961 Landsmeer further developed this concept.[84] In 1968, the author set out to show that unpredictability of the fractured scaphoid depended upon the associated ligamentous injury, and that if this were recognized early, the treatment of the fractured carpal scaphoid could be logically planned.[85] In 1972, Linscheid and his colleagues further classified traumatic instability of the wrist in a fundamental paper in the *Journal of Bone and Joint Surgery*.[86] Rotational subluxation of the scaphoid within the carpus has long been recognized (Armstrong, 1968),[87] but the exact pathologic process is not yet fully understood and its treatment is insufficiently elaborated. Writers in the past have referred to "sprained wrist" with little attempt to analyze or specifically treat the effects of the injury. Attempts to stabilize the carpus by soft tissue repair are a recent innovation.

TRIANGULAR FIBROCARTILAGE

It has long been thought that triangular fibrocartilage lying between the radius and ulna and contributing to the smooth proximal carpal joint is subject to injury and responsible for pain, clicking, and locking of the wrist. Indeed, many surgeons have regarded this structure as analogous to the meniscus of the knee and have advised its excision. In 1960, Coleman reported a series of 14 cases in which excision of the articular disk was performed,[105] but it is likely that some patients with symptoms suggesting this injury in fact have instability of the medial column of the carpus. In addition, it is now realized that this structure is subject to degenerative change with age, and about half of patients in their middle years show perforation of the fibrocartilage with damage to or erosion of the lunate or the distal ulnar articular surface. In 1981 Palmer and Werner estimated that in the neutral position of the forearm and wrist, some 40 percent of the load crosses the joint and is carried through the disk to the lower end of the ulna.[106]

ARTHROPLASTY OF THE WRIST

Attempts to produce controlled movement of the carpus by the insertion of foreign material are of recent origin and still in the early stages. Various types of pseudarthroses with limited but useful movement have been successfully employed over the last century, and the interposition of autogenous material has been employed with varied success, using fascia lata, skin, and abdominal fat. Bourgeois discussed wrist arthroplasty in 1925[95] and Albee in more general terms in 1931.[96] Foreign material, such as cellophane, has also been used, but the use of flexible material such as silicon rubber has allowed not only the replacement of individual carpal bones or parts of them but also the design of Swanson's prosthesis, giving rise to a "controlled pseudarthrosis."[97] More recently, attempts have been made to design a universal joint for the wrist in metal. They include Meuli in 1973,[98] Volz in 1976 and 1978,[99, 100] and GUEPAR,[101] metal on polyethylene, 1983.

Implant arthroplasty of carpal bones has also been advocated, including the scaphoid, the lunate, and the trapezium, but its durability remains unknown. However, replacement arthroplasty is no doubt the treatment of the future, although for the heavy manual laborer arthrodesis is so satisfactory that replacement will require a very high standard of material and design to supersede it.

CONCLUSION

Although the development of wrist surgery stretches back into the mists of time, it is only over the last 100 years that it has become safe and effective. The postwar period has seen the greatest strides and advances, and the positive deluge of publications makes it impossible to provide a balanced assessment. No author can claim that he has presented an exhaustive review of this exciting development, and the reader's indulgence is sought for any important omissions in this history.

I have relied heavily on Joseph Boyes' notable contribution *On the Shoulders of Giants*,[102] Mercer Rang's *Anthology of Orthopaedics*,[103] and the survey of European hand surgery by Verdan.[104]

References

1. Janssens PA: Medical views on prehistoric representations of human hands. Med Hist 1:318, 1957.
2. Lorthoir J: Essai sur l'histoire de la chirurgie de la main. Acta Orthop Belg Supplement 1, 24:15–27, 1958.
3. Desault J: . . . Sur la luxation de l'extrémité inférieure du radius. J Chir 1:78, 1791.

4. Hind GW: Fractures of the Extremities. 2nd ed, London, Taylor & Walton, 1836.

5. Dupuytren G: Leçons Orales de Clinique Chirurgicale. Paris, Ballière, 1832.

6. Colles A: On the fracture of the carpal extremity of the radius. Edin Med Surg J 182, 1814.

7. Lippman RK: Laxity of the radio-ulnar joint following Colles' fracture. Arch Surg 35:772, 1932.

8. Buxton StJ D: Fractures of the forearm and wrist. Ann R Coll Surg 38:253, 1966.

9. Verdan C: Fractures of the scaphoid. Surg Clin North Am 40:461, 1960.

10. Smith RW: Treatise on Fracture in the Vicinity of Joints. Dublin, Hodges & Smith, 1847.

11. Barton JR: Views and treatment of an important injury of the wrist. Med Exam 1:365, 1838.

12. Thomas FB: Reduction of Smith's fracture. J Bone Joint Surg 39B:463, 1957.

13. Ellis J: Smith's and Barton's fractures. J Bone Joint Surg 47B:724, 1965.

14. Compère EL: Growth arrest in the long bones. JAMA 105:2140, 1935.

15. Aitken AP: End results of fracture dislocation of the radial epiphyses. J Bone Joint Surg 17:302, 1935.

16. Darrach W: Anterior dislocation of the head of the ulna. Ann Surg 56:802, 1912.

17. Dingman PVC: Resection of the distal end of the ulna in the Darrach operation. J Bone Joint Surg 34A:893, 1952.

18. Moore EM: Three cases illustrating luxation of the ulna in connection with Colles' fracture. Med Rec 17:305, 1880.

19. Tillmanns H: Lehrbuch der Algemeinen und Speziellen Chirurgie. Bund 2. S749. Leipzig, Veit, 1911.

20. van Lennep GA: Dislocation forward of the head of the ulna at the wrist joint and fracture of the styloid process of the ulna. Hahnemannian Monthly 32:350, 1897.

21. Baldwin WI: Surgery of the Hand and Wrist. In Jones Sir Robert (ed): Orthopaedic Surgery of Injuries. London, 1921, pp 241–282.

22. Bunnell S: Surgery of the Hand. 3rd ed, Philadelphia and London, JB Lippincott Co, 1956.

23. Linscheid RL: Symposium on distal ulnar injuries. Contemp Orthop 7:81, 1983.

24. Madelung OW: Die spontane subluxation der hand nach vorne. Langenbecks Arch Klin Chir 23:395, 1879.

25. Dameron TB: Traumatic dislocation of the distal radio-ulnar joint. Clin Orthop 83:55, March–April, 1972.

26. Monteggia GB: Instituzioni Chirurgiche. Milan, Maspero, 5:130, 1814.

27. Galeazzi R: Uber ein besonderes syndrom bei verletsungen im bereich der unterarm knocken. Arch Orthop Unfallchir 35:557, 1935.

28. Essex-Lopresti B: Fractures of the head of the radius with distal ulnar dislocation. J Bone Joint Surg 33B:244, 1951.

29. Jones, Sir Robert, Lovat RW: Orthopaedic Surgery. Baltimore, William Wood, 1929.

30. Paget Sir James: Lectures on Surgical Pathology. 50, 3rd ed, Philadelphia, Lindsay & Blakiston, 1865.

31. Marie, Pierre, and Foix: Atrophie isolée de l'éminence thénar d'origine névritique. Rôle du ligament annulaire du carpe dans la pathologie de la lésion. Rev Neurol 26:647, 1913.

32. Woltman. Quoted by Phalen ES. Carpal tunnel syndrome. Clin Orthop 83:29, 1972.

33. Learmonth Sir James: The principle of decompression in the treatment of certain diseases of peripheral nerves. Surg Clin North Am 13:905, 1933.

34. Brain WR, Wright AD, Wilkinson M: Spontaneous compression of both median nerves in the carpal tunnel: Six cases treated surgically. Lancet 1:277–282, 1947.

35. Phalen ES: The carpal tunnel syndrome: Seventeen years' experience in diagnosis and treatment of 654 hands. J Bone Joint Surg 48A:211, 1966.

36. Carroll RE, Green DP: The significance of the palmar cutaneous nerve at the wrist. Clin Orthop 83:24–28, 1972.

37. Ollier L: Traité des résections et des opérations conservatifs quand pratiqués sur le système osseux. Rev Chir 3, Paris, 1885.

38. Steindler A: Postgraduate Lectures on Orthopaedic Diagnosis and Indications. Vol 3, Springfield, Charles C Thomas, 1952.

39. Hodgson AR, Smith TK: Tuberculosis of the wrist. Clin Orthop 73:83, 1972.

40. Brittain HA: Architectural Principles in Arthrodesis. 2nd ed, Edinburgh and London, E. & S. Livingstone, 1952.

41. Kanavel AB: Infections of the Hand. Philadelphia, Lea & Febiger, 1912.

42. Preiser GKF: Zur frage der typischen traumatischen ernahrung storungen der kurzen hand und fuss wurzelknochen. Forschritte A. D. Gebiete der Rontgenstrahlen 17:360–362, 1911.

43. Crabbe WA: Excision of the proximal row of the carpus. J Bone Joint Surg 46B:708, 1964.

44. Dornan A: The results of treatment in Kienböck's disease. J Bone Joint Surg 42B:522, 1960.

45. Swanson AB: Flexible implant resection arthroplasty in the hand and extremities. St. Louis, CV Mosby, 1973.

46. Gervis WH: Excision of the trapezium for osteoarthritis of the trapezio-metacarpal joint. J Bone Joint Surg 31B:537, 1949.

47. Murley AHG: Excision of the trapezium in osteoarthritis of the 1st carpo-metacarpal joint. J Bone Joint Surg 42B:502, 1960.

48. Tubby A: Surgical Treatment of Paralysis by Arthrodesis. London, 1901.

49. Colonna TC: Methods for fusion of the wrist. South Med J 37:195, 1944.

50. Steindler A: Traumatic deformities and disabilities of the upper extremity. Springfield, Ill, Charles C Thomas, 1946.

51. Seddon HJ: Reconstruction surgery of the upper extremity in poliomyelitis. Papers and discussions presented at the 2nd International Poliomyelitis Conference. Philadelphia, London, Montreal, JB Lippincott, 1952, p. 226.

52. Smith-Petersen MN: A new approach to the wrist joint. J Bone Joint Surg 22:122, 1940.

53. Abbott LC, Saunders JB, Bost FC: Arthrodesis of the wrist. J Bone Joint Surg 24:883, 1942.

54. Steindler A: Operative treatment of paralytic conditions of the upper extremity. J Orthop Surg 1:608, 1919.

55. Durman DC: An operation for correction of deformities of the wrist following fracture. J Bone Joint Surg 17:1014, 1935.

56. Steindler A: Problems with reconstruction of the hand. Surg Gynaecol Obstet 27:317, 1918.

57. White, JW, Stubbins SG: Flexion deformities of the wrist. J Bone Joint Surg 26:131, 1944.

58. O'Rahilly R: A survey of carpal and tarsal anomalies. J Bone Joint Surg 35A:626, 1953.

59. Schwartz S: Localised fusion at the wrist joint. J Bone Joint Surg 49A:1591, 1967.

60. Maguire WB: Carpal instability and its surgical management by scapho-lunate fusion. J Bone Joint Surg 62B:266, 1980.

61. Watson HK, Goodman ML, Johnson TR: Limited wrist arthrodesis. No 2. Intercarpal and radiocarpal combination. J Hand Surg 6:223, 1981.

62. Lichtman DM, Schneider JR, Swafford AR: Ulnar midcarpal instability. Clinical and laboratory analysis. J Hand Surg 6:515–523, 1981

63. Callender GW: Fracture of the carpal end of the radius and of the scaphoid. Trans Pathol Soc 17:221, 1866.

64. Codman EA, Chase HM: The diagnosis and treatment of fractures of the carpal scaphoid with dislocation of the semilunar bone. Ann Surg 41:321, 1905.

65. Destot E: Fractures du scaphoïde. Lyon Chir 18:741, 1921.

66. Adams JD, Leonard RD: Fracture of the carpal scaphoid. N Engl J Med 198:401, 1928.

67. Berlin D: Position in the treatment of fractures of the carpal scaphoid. N Engl J Med 201:574, 1929.

68. London PS: The broken scaphoid bone. The case against pessimism. J Bone Joint Surg 43B:237, 1961.

69. Snodgrass LE: End results of carpal scaphoid fractures. Ann Surg 97:209, 1933.

70. Hosford JP: Prognosis in fractures of the carpal scaphoid. Proc R Soc Med 24:982, 1931.

71. Watson-Jones R: Carpal semilunar dislocations and other wrist dislocations with associated nerve lesions. Proc R Soc Med 22:1071, 1929.

72. Soto-Hall R, Haldeman KO: The conservative and operative treatment of fractures of the carpal scaphoid. J Bone Joint Surg 23:841, 1941.

73. Squire M: Carpal mechanics and trauma. J Bone Joint Surg 41B:210, 1959.

74. Watson-Jones R: Fractures and Joint Injuries. 4th ed, 610, Edinburgh and London, E & S Livingstone, 1955.

75. Murray G: Bone graft for non-union of the carpal scaphoid. Br J Surg 22:63, 1934.

76. Murray G: End results of bone grafting for non-union of the carpal navicular. J Bone Joint Surg 28:749, 1946.

77. Russe O: Fracture of the carpal navicular, diagnosis and operative treatment. J Bone Joint Surg 42A:759, 1960.

78. Fisk GR: Wedge grafting of the ununited scaphoid. In Rob C and Smith R (eds): Operative Surgery (Orthopaedics, Part 2). 540, London, Butterworths, 1979.

79. McLaughlin HL: Fracture of the carpal navicular (scaphoid). J Bone Joint Surg 36A:765, 1954.

80. Maudsley RH, Chen SC: Screw fixation in the management of fractured carpal scaphoid. J Bone Joint Surg 54B:432, 1972.

81. Herbert TJ, Fisher WE: Management of the fractured scaphoid using a new bone screw. J Bone Joint Surg 66B:114, 1984.

82. Lambrinudi C: Paper read at British Orthopaedic Association, 1943.

83. Guildford WW, Bolton RH, Lambrinudi C: Mechanism of the wrist joint with special reference to fractures of the scaphoid. Guy's Hospital Reports 92:52, 1943.

84. Landsmeer JMF: Studies in the anatomy of articulation. Acta Morphol Neerl Scand 3:304, 1961.

85. Fisk GR: Carpal instability and the fractured scaphoid (Hunterian Lecture 1968). Ann R Coll Surg London 46:63, 1970.

86. Linscheid RL, Dobyns JH, Beabout JW, Bryans RS: Traumatic instability of the wrist. Diagnosis classification and pathomechanics. J Bone Joint Surg 54A:1612, 1972.

87. Armstrong GWD: Rotational subluxation of the scaphoid. Can J Surg 11:306, 1968.

88. Destot E: Le Poignet et les Accidents du Travail. London, Ernest Benn, 1925.

89. Conwell HE: Closed reduction of dislocation of the semi-lunar. Ann Surg 82:289, 1925.

90. Schnek F: Carpal dislocations. Ergeben D Chir u Orthop 23:1, 1930.

91. Watson-Jones R: Dislocation of the scaphoid. Proc R Soc Med 22:1084, 1928.

92. Johannson S: Dislocation of the os hamatum. Acta Radiol 7:9, 1926.

93. Watson-Jones R: Fractures and Other Bone and Joint Injuries. 2nd ed, 424, Edinburgh, E & S Livingstone, 1941.

94. Russell TB: Intercarpal dislocations and fracture-dislocations. A review of 59 cases. J Bone Joint Surg 31B:524, 1949.

95. Bourgeois P: Contribution à l'Etude de l'Arthroplastie du Poignet. Algiers, These, 1925.

96. Albee FH: Principles of arthroplasty. JAMA 96:245, 1931.

97. Swanson AB: Flexible implant resection arthroplasty in the hand and extremities. St. Louis, C V Mosby, 1973.

98. Meuli HCh: Arthroplastie du poignet. Ann Chir 27:527, 1973.

99. Volz RG: Clinical experience with the new total wrist prosthesis. Arch Orthop Umfallchir 85:205, 1976.

100. Volz RG: Total wrist arthroplasty. Clin Orthop 128:180, 1978.

101. Alnot J-Y: Les arthroplasties du poignet. In Razemon J-P and Fisk GR (eds): Le Poignet. Paris, Expansion Scientifique Française, 1983, p 252.

102. Boyes JH: On the Shoulders of Giants: Notable Names in Hand Surgery. Philadelphia, Toronto, JB Lippincott Co, 1976.

103. Rang M: Anthology of Orthopaedics. Edinburgh and London, E & S Livingstone, 1966.

104. Verdan C: L'histoire de la chirurgie de la main. Ann Chir 34:647, 1980.

105. Coleman HN: Injuries of the articular disc at the wrist. J Bone Joint Surg 42B:522, 1960.

106. Palmer AK, Werner FW: The triangular fibrocartilage complex of the wrist and function. J Hand Surg 6:153, 1981.

107. Vesalius A: De Humani Corporis Fabrica. Libre 7, Basle, Switzerland, 115, 1543.

108. Spigelius: Opera: Omnia Quae Extant. Amsterdam, 1645.

109. Bell Sir Charles: The Hand, Its Mechanism and Vital Endowments as Evincing Design. London, William Pickering, 1833.

110. Bryce TH: On certain points in the anatomy and mechanism of the wrist joints. J Physiol, 1896.

111. Destot E: Traumatismes du Poignet. Paris, Editions Masson, 1923.

112. Wood-Jones F: The Principles of Anatomy As Seen in the Hand. 195, London, Ballière, Tindal & Cox, 1919.

113. MacConaill MA: The mechanical anatomy of the carpus and its bearing on some surgical problems. J Anat 166:75, 1941.

114. Barnard L, Stubbins SG: Styloidectomy of the radius in the surgical treatment of non-union of the carpal navicular. J Bone Joint Surg 30A:98, 1947.

115. Lauenstein C von, Zur Behandlung der nach Karpalen Vorderarmfractur zurückbleibender Störung der Pro- und Supinations Bewegung. Zentralbl Chir 23:433, 1887.

116. Speed K: Traumatic injuries of the carpus. New York, D Appelton and Co, 1925.

117. Fisk GR: Traitement des pseudarthroses au scaphoïde carpien par greffe cunéiforme. In Razemon J-P and Fisk GR (eds): Le Poignet. Expansion Scientifique Française, 1983.

118. Matti H: Über die Behandlung der Navicularefraktur und der Refraktura Patellae durch Plombierung mit Spongiosa. Zentralbl Chir 64:23–53, 1937.

119. Sir Astley Cooper, Bart: Treatise on Dislocations and on Fractures of the Joints. London, Longman, Hurst, Rees, Orme, and Brown, 1822.

CHAPTER 2

Anatomy of the Wrist

GEORGE P. BOGUMILL, Ph.D., M.D.

The wrist is the region that connects the distal forearm to the hand. Its boundaries are somewhat imprecise, depending on the purposes of the description. It consists of the distal radius and ulna, the proximal ends of the five metacarpals, and the intercalated carpal bones. The osseous elements are connected by a complex array of ligaments that are difficult to define, show a fair amount of variability from wrist to wrist, and are given a variety of names by different authors. The mobility of the wrist is determined by the shapes of the bones making up this complex as well as by the attachments and lengths of the various ligaments. This complex osteoligamentous array allows a wide range of motion limited at the extremes by a combination of bone shape and ligamentous attachment. The fibrous capsule, lined by synovium, divides the complex into a series of joints that are separate from each other in the normal wrist but may communicate as the individual ages (e.g., the distal radioulnar joint may communicate with the radiocarpal joint).

THE OSSEOUS ELEMENTS OF THE WRIST

The bony elements that make up the wrist joint consist of the distal end of the radius and ulna with their connecting ligaments and the distal radioulnar joint. Beyond this, there are the eight carpal bones, which are classically described as being in two rows: the scaphoid, lunate, triquetrum, and pisiform in the proximal row; the trapezium, trapezoid, capitate, and hamate in the distal row. Still more distal are the bases of the five metacarpals.

Distal Radius and Ulna

The distal radius is expanded from the cylindrical shape of the diaphysis to the tri-angular shape of the articular surface. The palmar face is flat and smooth. The dorsal face has Lister's tubercle and other less prominent ridges for attachment of the dorsal retinaculum and extensor compartments (Fig. 2–1). The radial surface ends in the prominent radial styloid. The ulnar face has a concavity, the sigmoid notch, which is covered with hyaline cartilage for articulation with the ulna. The distal articular surface is triangular in shape with the apex at the radial styloid process and the base at the rounded notch for articulation with the distal ulna; it is concave in both anteroposterior (AP) and lateral directions and has two recognizable facets separated by an anteroposterior ridge for articulation with the scaphoid and lunate.

The distal ulna ends in an expansion that is covered with hyaline cartilage on its dorsal, lateral, and palmar surfaces as well as on its distal end. The ulnar styloid projects from the posterior aspect of the distal ulna; there is a groove for attachment of the apex of the triangular fibrocartilage where it joins the head of the ulna. In this groove is a small recess containing synovium, which is the source of the erosions seen so commonly in rheumatoid arthritis.

The Carpal Bones

The carpal bones are eight small, irregularly shaped ossicles conveniently described as being in two rows (Fig. 2–2). With the exception of the pisiform, they have some common characteristics. Each is described in terms of its six surfaces: proximal, distal, anterior (palmar), posterior (dorsal), medial, and lateral. Usually, the proximal and distal surfaces are articular; the medial and lateral may also be covered with articular cartilage to a variable extent; the anterior and posterior are usually roughened and irregular for attachments of the capsule and ligaments.

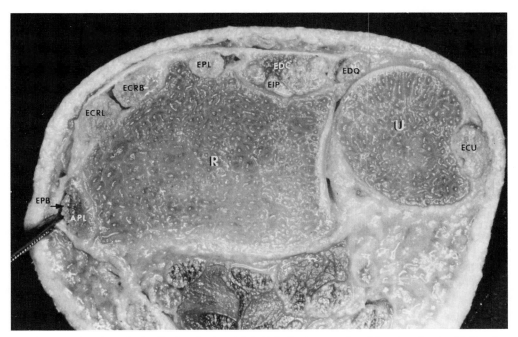

Figure 2–1. Cross section through the distal radioulnar joint. Note the incongruity of the ulnar head with the ulnar notch and also the loose capsule of the joint itself. APL= abductor pollicis longus; ECRB = extensor carpi radialis brevis; ECRL = extensor carpi radialis longus; ECU = extensor carpi ulnaris; EDC = extensor digitorum communis; EDQ = extensor digiti quinti; EIP = extensor indicis proprius; EPB = extensor pollicis brevis; EPL = extensor pollicis longus; R = radius; U = ulna.

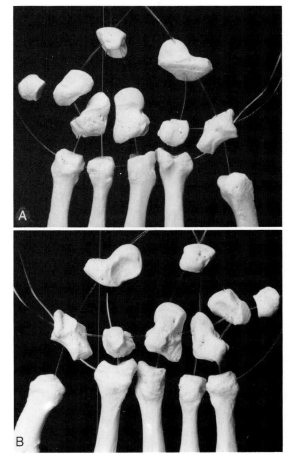

Figure 2–2. A, Dorsal view of carpal and metacarpal bones. B, Palmar view of carpal and metacarpal bones. Despite the irregularities of size, shape, and contour, they can each be assigned six surfaces for purposes of description.

Scaphoid (Navicular)

The scaphoid is the most radially situated bone in the proximal row and is also the largest in that row. Its proximal surface is biconvex for articulation with the scaphoid facet on the distal radius. The distal surface is smooth and convex for articulation with the trapezium and trapezoid. The dorsal surface is rough and irregular and represents a site of attachment of the dorsal radiocarpal ligament and radial collateral ligaments to the waist of the scaphoid. There are numerous perforations in this surface for small blood vessels to pass into the interior of the bone. The palmar surface has an irregular area for the attachment of volar ligaments as well as a rounded projection called the tubercle of the scaphoid to which the transversely placed flexor retinaculum is attached. The medial surface has a small, elongated semilunar articular surface for articulation with the lunate and a large concavity that occupies much of the medial surface of the bone for articulation with the head of the capitate.

The scaphoid articulates with five bones: the radius proximally, the trapezium and the trapezoid distally, and the capitate and lunate medially.

Lunate

This bone is located between the scaphoid radially and the triquetrum medially. It is deeply concave on its distal surface for articulation with the capitate; it is convex proximally for articulation with the lunate facet of the distal radius. Medially it has a large, flattened facet for articulation with the triquetrum, and laterally it has a similar flattened facet for articulation with the proximal end of the scaphoid. There are small areas on dorsal and palmar surfaces for ligamentous attachment, through which the blood supply to the lunate passes. These small areas provide a rather tenuous attachment of ligaments in addition to providing for blood supply. The lunate articulates with five bones: radius proximally, capitate and hamate distally, scaphoid laterally, and triquetrum medially.

Triquetrum

The triquetrum, located on the ulnar side of the proximal row, is pyramid-shaped with its apex medial and distal and its base late-ral. The convex proximal surface has a smooth portion that articulates with the triangular fibrocartilage of the wrist and has a roughened surface for attachment of the ulnar collateral ligament. The distal surface is concave for articulation with the hamate and has a spiral configuration that exerts an important influence on relative motion between the two rows. The palmar surface has an oval facet for articulation with a similar facet on the pisiform; the remainder of this palmar surface as well as the entire dorsal surface is rough, permitting attachment of capsular ligaments. The smooth, flattened lateral surface is covered with hyaline cartilage, which allows for articulation with the lunate. The medial surface, which is the apex of the pyramid, is rough, permitting attachment of the ulnar collateral ligament.

The triquietrum articulates with three bones: the lunate laterally, the pisiform anteriorly, and the hamate distally. It also articulates with the triangular fibrocartilage and occasionally with the distal radius, depending on the position of the wrist.

Pisiform

The pisiform bone is small and rounded on most surfaces; it has a single articular facet by which it articulates with the anterior surface of the triquetrum. The remainder of the bone is rough, allowing for attachment of the flexor carpi ulnaris tendon and its continuations, the pisohamate and pisometacarpal ligaments. It also provides attachment for part of the abductor digiti minimi as well as medial attachment for the flexor retinaculum.

Trapezium (Greater Multangular)

The trapezium is the most radially situated bone in the distal carpal row. On its palmar surface there is a deep groove that is converted by a ligament into a tunnel for the flexor carpi radialis tendon. The proximal surface is smooth and somewhat flattened, where it articulates with the distal end of the scaphoid. The distal surface is saddle-shaped for articulation with the base of the first metacarpal. The dorsal and palmar surfaces are rough and irregular, allowing for ligamentous and capsular attachments. The palmar surface, however, is somewhat smooth where it transmits the flexor carpi radialis tendon. On the lateral aspect of this deep palmar groove is a bony prominence or tuberosity that gives lateral attachment to the flexor retinaculum. The medial surface has two articular facets, the first for articulation with the trapezoid, and the second for articulation with the base of the second metacarpal; this latter facet is quite small but quite distinct.

Trapezoid

The trapezoid is the smallest bone in the distal row. It is wedge-shaped, with the apex on the palmar surface and the base located dorsally. The proximal surface is flattened and smooth, allowing for articulation with the scaphoid. The distal surface is also smooth but has a longitudinal ridge that divides it into two facets, both of which articulate with the proximal end of the second metacarpal. The dorsal and palmar surfaces are rough, permitting attachment of ligaments; the lateral surface is smooth for articulation with the trapezium; the medial surface is convex and smooth for articulation with the capitate. There is usually a fairly strong interosseous ligament between the capitate and the trapezoid in the center of this medial surface.

The trapezoid articulates with four bones: the scaphoid proximally, second metacarpal distally, trapezium laterally, and capitate medially.

Capitate

The capitate is the largest of the carpal bones. It is situated in the center of the wrist and is the center of wrist motion in all planes. Proximally, the surface is convex, smooth, and separated from the remainder of the bone by a relatively constricted area or neck; this proximal head articulates with the scaphoid and lunate bones. The distal surface is divided by two ridges into three facets for articulation with the second, third, and fourth metacarpals. The dorsal surface is broad and rough, permitting attachment of ligaments and capsules and for penetration of blood vessels. The palmar surface is, likewise, rough, allowing for attachment of the very strong thick anterior ligaments and a portion of the adductor pollicis muscle. The lateral surface articulates with the trapezoid distally and the scaphoid proximally; there is a rough area in between that allows for attachment of ligaments. The medial surface articulates with the hamate by an elongated smooth facet that is somewhat irregular in shape but generally flattened (Fig. 2–3).

The capitate, therefore, articulates with seven bones: the scaphoid and lunate proximally, the second, third, and fourth metacarpals distally, the trapezoid radially, and the hamate on the ulnar side.

Hamate

The hamate, the most medial bone in the distal row, is easily identified by the pronounced hook (hamulus) projecting from its palmar surface. The proximal surface is narrow, convex, and smooth for articulation with the lunate. The distal surface articulates with the fourth and fifth metacarpals by two facets that are separated by an anteroposterior ridge. The dorsal surface is triangular in shape, roughened, and provides

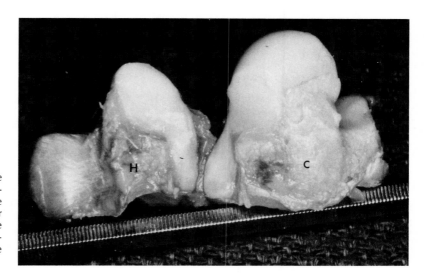

Figure 2–3. Hamate and capitate bones illustrate the long oval sliding joint between them and the heavy capsular ligaments on their anterior surfaces. Note the large hook on the hamate, which is almost as extensive as the hamate itself. C = capitate; H = hamate.

for ligamentous attachment. The palmar surface has the pronounced hook that is curved towards the lateral surface and gives attachment at its apex to the flexor retinaculum as well as to the origin of the flexor digiti minimi and opponens digiti minimi; it also provides insertion to the flexor carpi ulnaris through the pisohamate ligament. The lateral surface has a deep concavity formed by the body and the hamulus; this provides a pulley mechanism for the flexor tendons passing from the forearm to the fingers (see Fig. 2–8C). The ulnar surface articulates with the triquetrum by means of an oval, elongated facet, and the radial surface articulates with the capitate through a similarly elongated and flattened facet (Fig. 2–3). As previously noted, the spiral orientation of the triquetrohamate joint exerts an important influence on the relative motion between the two carpal rows.

The hook of the hamate makes up one of the four prominences on the palmar aspect of the carpus for attachment of the flexor retinaculum. The other three prominences are the pisiform, the tuberosity of the scaphoid, and the oblique ridge of the trapezium. The hamate articulates with five bones: the lunate proximally, the fourth and fifth metacarpals distally, the triquetrum medially, and the capitate laterally.

Metacarpals

The metacarpals participate in the wrist at their proximal ends. They are, in general, elongated bones that are flared both proximally and distally.

The *first metacarpal* has a concavo-convex proximal articular surface for articulation with the similar concavo-convex surface (saddle joint) of the trapezium. It will be described in more detail elsewhere in this volume (Chapter 12).

The *second metacarpal* is the longest of these bones. Its base is elongated medially by a projection that brings it into contact with the capitate. It has four articular surfaces—one medially for articulation with the third metacarpal and three on its proximal surface. The most medial of these is at the apex of the ridgelike projection of bone at the base of the metacarpal; this articulates with the base of the capitate. A concave surface of the center of the proximal end articulates with the trapezoid, and there is a small radial facet for articulation with the trapezium. The extensor carpi radialis lon-

gus inserts into the dorsal surface, and there may be a bony projection in this area at the tendinous attachment.

The *third metacarpal* is almost as large as the second. A dorsal projection on its base extends proximally to the distal surface of the capitate. It is just proximal to the insertion of the extensor carpi radialis brevis, and this metacarpal boss may be enlarged enough to cause concern about its being a tumor or to be confused with a ganglion. The proximal end of the third metacarpal articulates with the capitate through a flattened articular surface, and on the medial and lateral sides of the base there are articulations for the fourth and second metacarpals, respectively. The configuration of the second and third metacarpal bones together and the strong ligamentous attachment binding them to each other and to the trapezoid and capitate renders this the so-called fixed point of the hand with movements of the remainder of the hand described around these two bones as the axis.

The *fourth metacarpal* is smaller than the third but larger than the fifth; however, it usually has the narrowest medullary cavity of any of the metacarpal bones. The base is small and almost square; the medial and lateral surfaces are flattened and smooth allowing for articulation with the fifth and third metacarpals, respectively; the proximal surface is smooth for articulation with the lateral portion of the base of the hamate, and the dorsal and palmar surfaces are rough, permitting attachment of ligaments.

The *fifth metacarpal* has an articular facet at its proximal end for the hamate and a flattened surface on its lateral side for articulation with the fourth metacarpal. The remainder of the base of the fifth metacarpal is rough, allowing for attachment of ligaments as well as for insertion of the flexor and extensor carpi ulnaris tendons.

WRIST JOINTS

Distal Radioulnar Joint

The distal radioulnar joint is a pivot joint formed between the head of the ulnar and the ulnar (sigmoid) notch of the distal radius (Fig. 2–1). The capsule of this joint is quite loose, in order to allow rotation of the radius about the ulna. Although anterior and posterior transverse fibers reinforce the capsule, they do not add stability to the joint. The bones are held together primarily by the

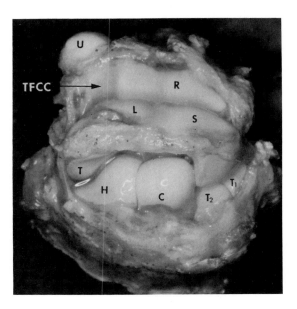

Figure 2–4. Dorsal view of opened radiocarpal and midcarpal joints illustrates their separation. Well illustrated is the smooth contour provided by the interosseous ligaments between lunate and scaphoid as well as between the radial articular surface and the triangular fibrocartilage. The distal radioulnar joint is separated from the radiocarpal joint by the triangular fibrocartilage. In the same way, the radiocarpal joint is separated from the midcarpal joint by the dorsal and volar capsule connecting the proximal carpal row and by the interosseous ligaments between scaphoid and lunate, and lunate and triquetrum. C = capitate; H = hamate; L = lunate; R = radius; S = scaphoid; T = triquetrum; T_1 = trapezium; T_2 = trapezoid; TFCC = triangular fibrocartilage complex; U = ulna.

interosseous membrane, which is present to the level of the joint, and by the triangular fibrocartilage complex (TFCC) or articular disk (Figs. 2–4, 2–5, and 2–6). This latter structure is the chief uniting element of the joint. It is thicker peripherally than centrally but is usually not perforated in younger individuals. It is attached by its base to the medial margin of the distal radius and by its apex to the lateral side of the base of the styloid process of the ulna. It is biconcave and articulates with the distal ulna proximally and with the proximal carpal row, primarily the triquetrum, on its distal surface. The triangular fibrocartilage is reinforced anteriorly and posteriorly by fibrous

bands that extend into the anterior and posterior radioulnar capsule. The capsule is only minimally reinforced and does not provide any support to the joint nor does it limit joint movement. The triangular fibrocartilage is at maximum tension in approximately midposition between pronation and supination, and lax in full pronation and supination; at these latter positions, the interosseous membrane is under tension.

A synovial cavity extends between the distal radius and ulna and then across the distal ulna; it is, therefore, L-shaped in longitudinal section. The synovial membrane of the joint is usually completely separated from that of the radiocarpal joint. Occasion-

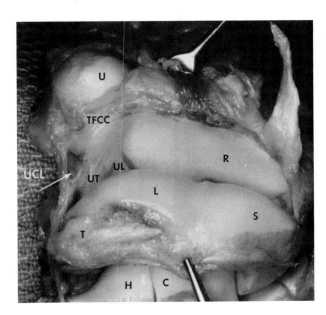

Figure 2–5. Dorsal view of the opened radiocarpal joint illustrating the triangular fibrocartilage complex and the anterior ligaments arising from it. The *arrow* indicates the prestyloid recess. C = capitate; H = hamate; L = lunate; R = radius; S = scaphoid; TFCC = triangular fibrocartilage complex; U = ulna; UCL = ulnar collateral ligament; UL = ulnolunate ligament; UT = ulnotriquetral ligament; T = triquetrum.

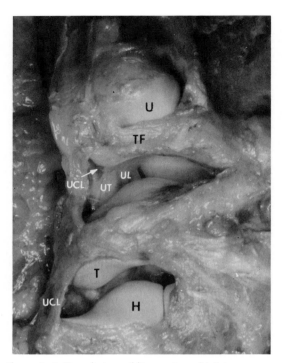

Figure 2–6. Dorsal view of ligaments and joint spaces on the ulnar aspect of the wrist. The ulnar collateral ligament is clearly shown as a separate, distinct entity from the triangular fibrocartilage complex. It extends from the outer aspect of the ulnar styloid to the triquetrum and continues to the hamate and the fifth metacarpal. The ulnolunate and ulnotriquetral ligaments originate from the anterior aspect of the triangular fibrocartilage and extend distally to attach to the lunate and triquetrum, respectively, on their anterior surfaces. H = hamate; T = triquetrum; TF = triangular fibrocartilage; U = ulna; UCL = ulnar collateral ligament; UL = ulnolunate ligament; UT = ulnotriquetral ligaments.

present. The articular capsule encloses the joint and is strengthened by dorsal and palmar radiocarpal ligaments and ulnocarpal ligaments. The radiocarpal ligaments are composed of fibers that run downward and toward the ulna from both the dorsal and palmar surfaces of the radius to the three carpal bones of the proximal row. This determines that the hand will follow the radius passively in movements of pronation and supination of the radius. The lax synovial membrane lines the deep surface of the capsule and presents numerous folds that may extend into the pisiform-triquetral joint as shown by arthrography in approximately one third of normal wrists. The dorsal and palmar surfaces of the proximal carpal row are sites of attachment of the dorsal and palmar capsule, respectively, thus sealing the radiocarpal joint into a single unit that does not communicate with other joints (Fig. 2–8).

ally, the center of the articular fibrocartilage is perforated; this usually occurs in older individuals and is so common that it may be due to normal wear and tear.[2]

Radiocarpal Joint

This joint is formed by the distal surface of the expanded end of the radius and the triangular fibrocartilage proximally, and the scaphoid, lunate, and triquetrum distally (Figs. 2–4 and 2–5). The proximal row of carpal bones is joined by the interosseous ligaments at their proximal edges (Figs. 2–4 and 2–7), forming a smooth biconvex surface that fits into the biconcave articular surface of the radius and articular disk. The loosely congruent surfaces allow free movement in flexion/extension, in abduction/adduction, and in circumduction. True rotation is not

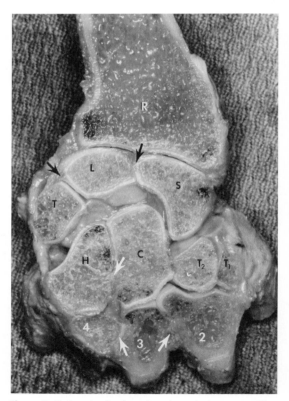

Figure 2–7. Longitudinal section through the carpus illustrating the separation of the radiocarpal joint from the midcarpal joint and the continuity of the midcarpal joint with the carpometacarpal joint. *Arrows* indicate interosseous ligaments between the various carpal and metacarpal bones. C = capitate; H = hamate; L = lunate; R = radius; S = scaphoid; T = triquetrum; T_1 = trapezium; T_2 = trapezoid; 2,3,4 = second, third, and fourth metacarpals.

Midcarpal Joint

The midcarpal joint is formed by the scaphoid, lunate, and triquetrum in the proximal row and the trapezium, trapezoid, capitate, and hamate in the distal row (Figs. 2–7 and 2–8). The distal pole of the scaphoid articulates with the two trapezial bones as a gliding type of joint; the proximal end of the scaphoid combined with the lunate and triquetrum form a deep concavity that articulates with the convexity of the combined capitate and hamate in a form of diarthrodial, almost condyloid joint.* The cavity of the midcarpal joint is very extensive and irregular (Figs. 2–7 and 2–8A). The major portion of the joint cavity is located between the distal surfaces of scaphoid, lunate, and triquetrum and the proximal surfaces of the four bones of the second row. Proximal prolongations of the cavity occur between the scaphoid and lunate and between the lunate and triquetrum (Figs. 2–7 and 2–8). These extensions reach almost to the proximal surface of the bones in the proximal row and are separated from the cavity of the radiocarpal joint by the thin interosseous ligaments (Fig. 2–7). There are three distal prolongations of the midcarpal joint cavity between the four bones of the distal row (Fig. 2–8C). The joint space between trapezium and trapezoid or that between trapezoid and capitate may communicate with the cavities of the carpometacarpal joints,

---

*The importance of the triquetrohamate and the scaphotrapezial articulations in guiding intercarpal motion in both physiologic and pathologic conditions is discussed in Chapter 18.

most frequently the second and third. The cavity between the first metacarpal and carpus is always separate from the midcarpal joint; the joint cavity between the hamate and fourth and fifth metacarpals is a separate cavity more often than not but may communicate normally with the midcarpal joint.

Carpometacarpal Joints

The first carpometacarpal joint is quite complex and is described in Chapter 12; the second and third joints are also complex and extend between the bases of the metacarpals. The second and third may frequently communicate with the midcarpal joint or with the hamate-metacarpal joint.

Pisotriquetral Joint

The pisiform articulates with the palmar surface of the triquetrum in a flat, planar type of joint. It may occasionally communicate with the radiocarpal joint as is shown in approximately one third of normal wrist arthrograms.

LIGAMENTOUS APPARATUS OF THE WRIST

Interosseous Ligaments

The bones of the proximal carpal row are joined by interosseous ligaments that are located at the proximal articular surfaces of the lunate, with its adjoining scaphoid and triquetral bones. The ligaments connect the bones from palmar to dorsal surfaces; they

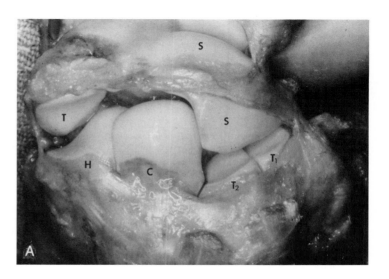

Figure 2–8. *A,* Dorsal view of the midcarpal joint, illustrating condyloid nature of the combined hamate-capitate and the gliding articulation between the distal scaphoid and the trapezium-trapezoid.

Illustration continued on following page

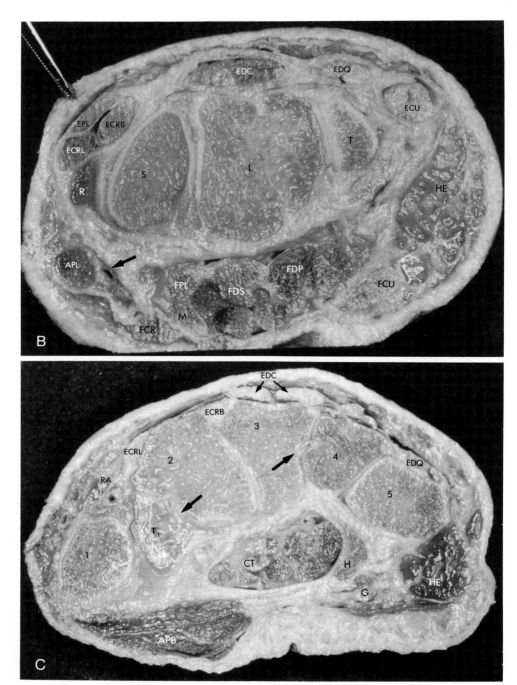

Figure 2–8 *Continued B,* Cross section through the proximal carpal row, demonstrating the extensions of the midcarpal joint between the bones making up the proximal row. It also illustrates clearly the location of the various tendons as they cross the wrist. The *arrow* indicates the position of the radial artery. *C,* Cross section through the bases of the metacarpals to illustrate extensions of the midcarpal and carpometacarpal joints between the metacarpal bases. The *large arrows* indicate interosseous ligaments. The *small arrows* indicate divisions of the extensor digitorum communis tendon. 1, 2, 3, 4, and 5 indicate the respective metacarpal bones. Note that the wedge shape of the metacarpal bases provides for the dorsal carpal arch. APB = abductor pollicis brevis; APL = abductor pollicis longus; C = capitate; CT = carpal tunnel; ECRB = extensor carpi radialis brevis; ECRL = extensor carpi radialis longus; ECU = extensor carpi ulnaris; EDC = extensor digitorum communis; EDQ = extensor digiti quinti; EPL = extensor pollicis longus; FCR = flexor carpi radialis; FCU = flexor carpi ulnaris; FDP = flexor digitorum profundus; FDS = flexor digitorum superficialis; FPL = flexor pollicis longus; G = Guyon's canal; H = hamate; HE = hypothenar eminence; L = lunate; M = median nerve; R = radial styloid; S = scaphoid; T = triquetrum; T_1 = trapezium; T_2 = trapezoid; RA = radial artery.

are approximately 1 to 2 mm thick and are quite short. They are actually covered by a thin layer of hyaline cartilate that conceals on gross inspection the line between the contiguous bones (Fig. 2–5).

The distal carpal row has three interosseous ligaments that unite the trapezium with the trapezoid, the trapezoid with the capitate, and the capitate with the hamate. These do not usually extend from volar to dorsal capsules; consequently, continuations of the midcarpal joint space can connect with the carpometacarpal joint spaces. The interosseous ligament between the capitate and hamate is the strongest in the distal row and is situated near the anterior distal portion of the two bones (Fig. 2–7).

Radial Collateral Ligament

The radial collateral ligament of the wrist joint extends from the tip of the styloid process of the radius to attach at the waist of the scaphoid on its radial aspect. The fibers then extend to the trapezium, where they blend with the transverse carpal ligament and the dorsal capsular ligament. The radial collateral ligament is crossed by the radial artery as it courses around the lateral aspect of the wrist from palmar to dorsal aspect. The ligament is fairly lax in the neutral position of the wrist joint and becomes tight only at the extreme of ulnar deviation.

Ulnar Collateral Ligament

The ulnar collateral ligament is attached to the base and body of the styloid process of the ulna. Usually, the tip of the styloid process is free of ligamentous attachments and projects into the prestyloid recess (Fig. 2–5), a space between the ulnar collateral ligament and the triangular fibrocartilage complex. The proximal attachment of the ligament also extends into the anterior and posterior borders of the triangular fibrocartilage. As it passes distally, it narrows and attaches to the pisiform and transverse carpal ligament as well as to the triquetrum. It then extends more distally and inserts into the ulnar border of the hamate and into the base of the fifth metacarpal.

Dorsal Radiocarpal Ligament

This is an obliquely placed thickening in the dorsal capsule, which extends toward the ulna and distally from the dorsal lip of the articular surface of the radius toward the dorsal surface of lunate and triquetrum (Fig. 2–9). When the forearm pronates, this ligament draws the attached carpus and hand passively along into pronation.

Palmar Radiocarpal Ligaments

These are described in standard anatomy texts as a broad triangular band of fibers extending from the palmar edge and the

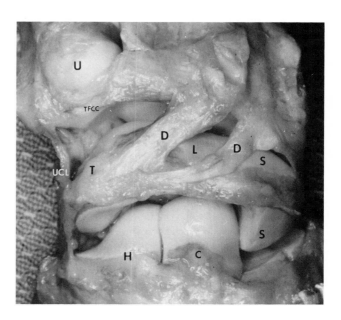

Figure 2–9. Dorsal view of the wrist showing clearly the dorsal radiocarpal ligament extending from the dorsal lip of the radius near Lister's tubercle to the dorsal aspect of the triquetrum. The dorsal capsule had been removed, leaving the reinforced fibers intact. C = capitate; D = dorsal radiocarpal ligament; H = hamate; L = lunate; S = scaphoid; T = triquetrum; TFCC = triangular fibrocartilage complex; U = ulna; UCL = ulnar collateral ligament.

styloid process of the distal radius to the palmar surfaces of the scaphoid, lunate, and triquetrum in the proximal row and in prolongation from there to the capitate and hamate of the distal row (Fig. 2–10). More recently, these ligaments have been assigned subdivisions by a number of authors after careful dissection of fresh specimens. These subdivisions have been shown to have functional value in terms of kinematics of the wrist and appropriate treatment of injuries and are best visualized from inside the joint (Fig. 2–11).

The *palmar radiocapite ligament* is a strong intracapsular ligament that arises from the volar and radial aspects of the radial styloid process and extends distally and ulnarly. It traverses a groove in the waist of the scaphoid and may have an attachment

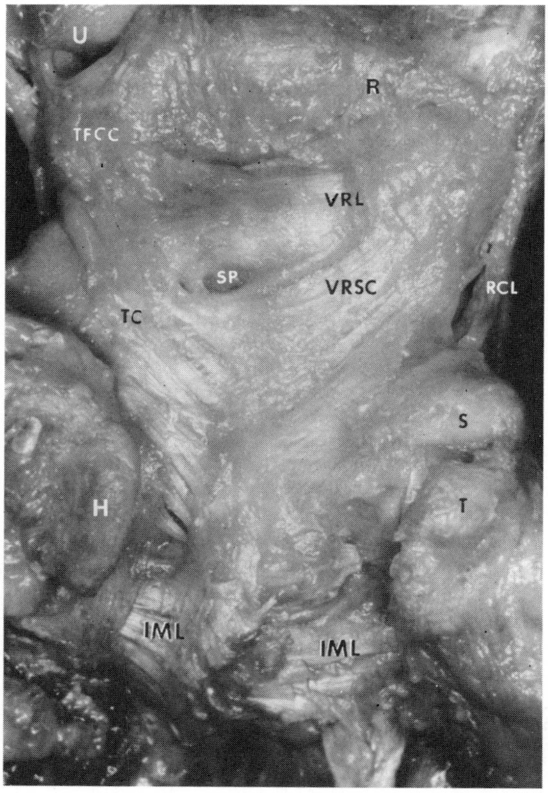

Figure 2–10. Volar aspect of wrist joint illustrating the heavy interlacing fibers of the volar ligaments. The carpal tunnel is open and its contents have been removed. The synovial lining has also been removed. H = hamate; IML = intermetacarpal ligament; R = radius; RCL = radial collateral ligament; S = tuberosity of the scaphoid; SP = space of Poirier; T = oblique ridge of trapezium; TC = triquetral capitate ligament; TFCC = triangular fibrocartilage complex; U = ulna; VRL = volar radiolunate ligament; VRSC = volar radioscaphoid capitate ligament.

to the waist of the scaphoid in some individuals. It then continues to its end in the center of the volar aspect of the capitate; thus, it may be termed a radioscaphocapitate ligament.

The *radiotriquetral ligament* (radiolunatetriquetral) is medial to the palmar radiocapite. It is also an intracapsular ligament arising from the volar lip and styloid process of the radius; it is directed toward the ulna across the volar aspect of the lunate, to which it has a variable attachment, and it ends in the palmar surface of the triquetrum. This ligament acts as a volar sling for the lunate. There may be a space between this ligament and the preceding one (the space of Poirier), through which dislocations of the lunate occur.

The *volar radioscapholunate ligament* is the third component. It is placed more medially and slightly deeper than the preceding one and inserts into the proximal volar surface of the scapholunate joint. This is a large ligament that is consistently present and must be divided before complete scapholunate dissociation can occur.

Triangular Fibrocartilage Complex

The palmar ulnocarpal ligament is formed by fibers that extend from the anterior edge of the triangular fibrocartilage and base of the ulnar styloid process downward and laterally to the carpal bones (Figs. 2–5, 2–6, and 2–9). Again, recent studies have demonstrated that this is more complex than has previously been acknowledged or recognized. The triangular fibrocartilage and adjacent ulnocarpal meniscus share a common origin from the attachment to the dorsal ulnar corner of the ulnar notch of the radius. The meniscus swings around the ulnar border of the wrist to insert into the triquetrum. There is a small triangular prestyloid recess filled with synovium surrounding the tip of the ulnar styloid and found between the meniscus and the triangular fibrocartilage. Extending from the anterior border of the triangular fibrocartilage is the ulnolunate ligament, which inserts into the lunate. Medial to this is another diagonal band that attaches to the triquetrum, and then extends onto the palmar aspect of the capitate and hamate. This extension may represent the ulnar arm of the arcuate ligament from the capitate to the triquetrum described by Alexander and Lichtman in Chapter 20. It adds stability to

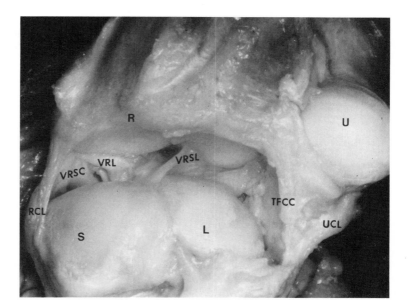

Figure 2–11. Open view of the radiocarpal joint illustrates the intracapsular portions of the volar radiocarpal ligaments. L = lunate; R = radius; RCL = radial collateral ligament; S = scaphoid; TFCC = triangular fibrocartilage complex; U = ulna; UCL = ulnar collateral ligament; VRL = volar radiolunate ligament; VRSC = volar radioscaphoid ligament; VRSL = volar radioscapholunate ligament.

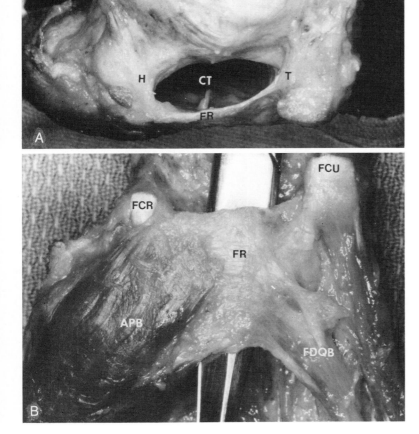

Figure 2–12. *A,* End-on view of carpal tunnel. *B,* Anterior view of flexor retinaculum, illustrating its attachment to the carpal bones and showing its extent. APB = abductor pollicis brevis; CT = carpal tunnel; FCR = flexor carpi radialis; FCU = flexor carpi ulnaris; FDQB = flexor digiti quinti brevis; FR = flexor retinaculum; H = hook of hamate; T = trapezium.

the ulnar aspect of the midcarpal joint. Since the triangular fibrocartilage is strongly attached to the radius, the ligaments arising from it attach the palmar aspect of the ulnar carpus to the radius and not to the ulna. The wrist is thus suspended primarily from the radius by both palmar and dorsal ligaments.

Flexor Retinaculum

This is a strong, broad ligament attached to the pisiform and hook of the hamate medially and to tuberosities of the scaphoid and trapezium laterally (Fig. 2–12). Its primary function is to hold the flexor tendons of the digits in place during wrist flexion to prevent the loss of power that would occur with bowstringing. The amount of support it provides the carpus is unknown, but it is under constant tension and is probably a factor in the maintenance of the contour of the carpal arch.

SUMMARY

The wrist is a pliable osteoligamentous complex situated between the forearm and the palm of the hand. Its movements are permitted and restrained by the complex shape and ligamentous attachments of the various bones. Large portions of the surface of the involved bones are covered with articular cartilage. The ligamentous attachments are the sites for vascular access for the nourishment of the individual carpal bones. When these ligaments are disrupted, the vessels are also frequently disrupted, with variable effects on the individual bones.

The mobility of the wrist results from its complex structure. The stability of the wrist is also a result of the complex shapes of the bones and the array of ligaments.

References

1. Linscheid RL, Dobyns JN, Beabout JW, and Bryan RS: Traumatic instability of the wrist: diagnosis, classification and pathomechanics. J Bone Joint Surg 54A:1612–1632, 1972.
2. Palmer AK, and Werner FW: The triangular fibrocartilage complex of the wrist—anatomy and fuction. J Hand Surg 6:153–162, 1981.
3. Taleisnik J: Wrist: anatomy, function and injury. AAOS Inst Course Lect 27:61–87, 1978.
4. Taleisnik J: The ligaments of the wrist. J Hand Surg 1:110–118, 1976.
5. Mayfield JK: Wrist ligamentous anatomy and pathogenesis of carpal instability. Orthop Clin North Am 15:209–216, 1984.
6. Mayfield JK, Johnson RP, and Kilcoyne RF: The ligaments of the human wrist and their functional significance. Anat Rec 186:417–428, 1976.
7. Mayfield JK, Johnson RP, and Kilcoyne RF: Carpal dislocations: pathomechanics and progressive perilunar instability. J Hand Surg 5:226–241, 1980.

CHAPTER 3

Vascularity of the Carpus

RICHARD H. GELBERMAN, M.D.
and MICHAEL J. BOTTE, M.D.

Relatively few studies investigating the vascular patterns of the carpus have been performed. Technical difficulties in identifying small vessels in three dimensions and in determining their location within thick capsules and ligaments about the wrist have led to conflicting anatomic reports.[1, 5, 8, 19] Cadaver studies utilizing improved techniques with arterial injection, chemical débridement, and decalcification have allowed the arterial anatomy of the carpus to be more accurately delineated.[4-7, 16] This chapter discusses these arterial patterns, with attention to both the extraosseous and intraosseous vascularity.

EXTRAOSSEOUS VASCULAR PATTERNS

The extraosseous vascularity of the carpus consists of a series of dorsal and palmar transverse arches connected by anastomoses formed by the radial, ulnar, and anterior interosseous arteries.[6]

Dorsal Carpal Vascularity

The vascularity to the dorsum of the carpus consists of 3 dorsal transverse arches: the radiocarpal,[6, 8] the intercarpal,[2, 3, 6, 8, 13, 20] and the basal metacarpal transverse arches (Figs. 3–1 and 3–2).[6] These arches are approximately 1 mm in diameter; their branches are less than 1 mm. The presence of each arch is variable.

The dorsal radiocarpal arch, present in 80 percent of cadaver specimens studied,[6] is the most proximal. Located at the level of the radiocarpal joint, it lies deep to the extensor tendons. The radiocarpal arch provides the main nutrient vessels to the lunate and the triquetrum. It is usually supplied by branches of the radial and ulnar arteries and the dorsal branch of the anterior interosseous artery. Occasionally, the dorsal radiocarpal arch is supplied by the radial and

ulnar arteries alone or by the radial and anterior interosseous arteries.[6]

The dorsal intercarpal arch is the largest of the dorsal transverse arches and is consistently present.[6] It runs transversely across the dorsal carpus between the proximal and the distal carpal rows, supplying the distal carpal row and anastomosing with the radiocarpal arch to supply the lunate and the triquetrum. Like the radiocarpal arch, it receives variable contributions. It is supplied by the radial, ulnar, and anterior interosseous arteries in 53 percent of cadavers studied, by the radial and ulnar arteries alone in 20 percent, by the radial and anterior interosseous in 20 percent, and by the ulnar and anterior interosseous arteries in 7 percent.[6]

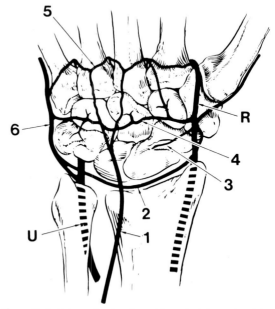

Figure 3–1. Schematic drawing of the arterial supply of the dorsum of the wrist. R = radial artery, U = ulnar artery; 1 = dorsal branch, anterior interosseous artery; 2 = dorsal radiocarpal arch; 3 = branch to the dorsal ridge of the scaphoid; 4 = dorsal intercarpal arch, 5 = basal metacarpal arch; 6 = medial branch of the ulnar artery. (From Gelberman RH, Panagis JS, Taleisnik J, et al. J Hand Surg 8:367–375, 1983.)

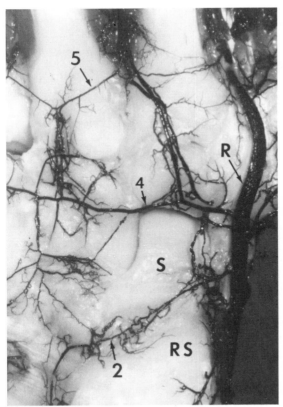

Figure 3–2. View of the three dorsal transverse arches. RS = radial styloid; S = scaphoid; R = radial artery; 2 = dorsal radiocarpal arch; 4 = dorsal intercarpal arch; 5 = basal metacarpal arch. (From Gelberman RH, Panagis JS, Taleisnik J, et al: J Hand Surg 8:367–375, 1983.)

The basal metacarpal arch is the most distal of the dorsal transverse arches and is located at the base of the metacarpals just distal to the carpometacarpal joints. It is the smallest of the dorsal arches and is actually a series of vascular retia; its presence is the most variable among these arches. It is complete in 27 percent of specimens, absent in 27 percent, and present in its radial aspect alone in 46 percent.[6] The basal metacarpal arch is supplied by perforating arteries from the second, third, and fourth intraosseous spaces.[6] It contributes to the vascularity of the distal carpal row through anastomoses with the intercarpal arch.

The dorsal arches are connected longitudinally at their medial and lateral aspects by the ulnar and radial arteries. They are connected centrally by the dorsal branch of the anterior interosseous artery.

Palmar Carpal Vascularity

Similar to the dorsal vascularity, the palmar vascularity is composed of 3 transverse arches: the palmar radiocarpal, the palmar intercarpal, and the deep palmar arch (Fig. 3–3).

The palmar radiocarpal arch is the most proximal, extending transversely 5 to 8 mm proximal to the radiocarpal joint at the level of the distal metaphysis of the radius and the ulna. It lies within the wrist capsule. It is consistently present and is formed by branches of the radial, anterior interosseous, and ulnar arteries in 87 percent of specimens, and by radial and ulnar arteries alone in 13 percent. This arch supplies the palmar surface of the lunate and the triquetrum.

The intercarpal arch, located between the proximal and distal carpal rows, is the most variable in occurrence. Present in 53 percent of specimens, it is formed by branches of the radial, ulnar, and anterior interosseous arteries in 75 percent and by the radial and ulnar arteries alone in 25 percent. This arch is small and is not a major contributor of nutrient vessels to the carpus.

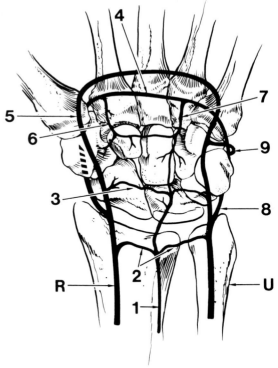

Figure 3–3. Schematic drawing of the arterial supply of the palmar aspect of the wrist. R = radial artery; U = ulnar artery; 1 = palmar branch, anterior interosseous artery; 2 = palmar radiocarpal arch; 3 = palmar intercarpal arch; 4 = deep palmar arch; 5 = superficial palmar arch; 6 = radial recurrent artery; 7 = ulnar recurrent artery; 8 = medial branch, ulnar artery; 9 = branch off ulnar artery contributing to the dorsal intercarpal arch. (From Gelberman RH, Panagis JS, Taleisnik J, et al: J Hand Surg 8:367–375, 1983.)

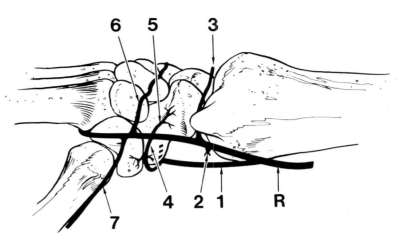

Figure 3–4. Schematic drawing of the arterial supply of the lateral aspect of the wrist. R = radial artery; 1 = superficial palmar artery; 2 = palmar radiocarpal arch; 3 = dorsal radiocarpal arch; 4 = branch to the scaphoid tubercle and trapezium; 5 = artery to the dorsal ridge of the scaphoid; 6 = dorsal intercarpal arch; 7 = branch to the lateral trapezium and thumb metacarpal. (From Gelberman RH, Panagis JS, Taleisnik J, et al: J. Hand Surg 8:367–375, 1983.)

The deep palmar arch, the most distal of the palmar transverse arches, is located at the level of the metacarpal bases, 5 to 10 mm distal to the palmar carpometacarpal joints. It is consistently present and contributes to the radial and ulnar recurrent arteries and sends perforating branches to the dorsal basal metacarpal arch and to the palmar metacarpal arteries.

The 3 palmar arches are connected longitudinally by the radial, ulnar, anterior interosseous, and deep palmar recurrent arteries.

Specific Vessels

The 5 major arteries that supply the carpus are the radial artery, ulnar artery, anterior interosseous artery, deep palmar arch, and accessory ulnar recurrent arteries.

Radial Artery

Of the major arteries supplying the carpus, the radial artery is the most consistent. It has 7 major carpal branches: 3 dorsal, 3 palmar, and a final branch that continues distally (Figs. 3–4 and 3–5). The most proximal branch of the radial artery is the superficial palmar artery. It leaves the radial artery 5 to 8 mm proximal to the tip of the radial styloid, passes between the flexor carpi radialis and brachioradialis, and continues distally to contribute to the superficial palmar arch (Fig. 3–4). The second branch contributes to the palmar radiocarpal arch. This branch leaves the radial artery approximately 5 mm distal to the superficial palmar artery and runs toward the ulna. A third branch originates at the level of the radiocarpal joint and runs dorsally and ulnarly, penetrating the radiocarpal ligament deep to the extensor tendons. This branch supplies the dorsal radiocarpal arch. The fourth branch arises palmarly at the level of the scaphotrapezial joint. It supplies the tubercle of the scaphoid and the radiopalmar

Figure 3–5. Vascularity of the lateral aspect of the wrist. RS = radial styloid; S = scaphoid; T = trapezium; R = radial artery; 1 = superficial palmar branch of the radial artery; 3 = dorsal radiocarpal arch; 4 = branch to the tubercle of the scaphoid and trapezium; 5 = artery to dorsal ridge of scaphoid; 6 = dorsal intercarpal arch; 7 = branch to the lateral trapezium and thumb metacarpal; 8 = medial branch of radial artery (seen in 22 percent of the specimens) penetrating the base of the index–long finger web space. (Note: In this view, 2, the palmar radiocarpal arch, cannot be seen.) (From Gelberman RH, Panagis JS, Taleisnik J, et al: J Hand Surg 8:367–375, 1983.)

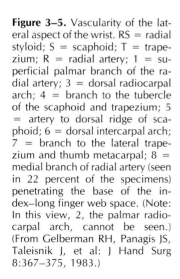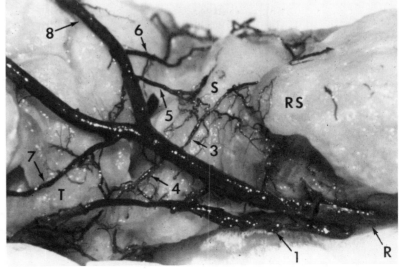

surface of the trapezium. It then anastomoses with the superficial palmar artery. This vessel is absent in 25 percent of specimens; in 25 percent, it anastomoses with a branch of the superficial palmar artery prior to entering the scaphoid tubercle.[6] The fifth branch of the radial artery, the artery to the dorsal ridge of the scaphoid, originates directly from the radial artery in 75 percent of specimens and from the radiocarpal or intercarpal arch in 25 percent (Fig. 3–4). It takes an ulnar retrograde course to supply the scaphoid. The sixth branch leaves the radial artery 5 mm distal to the branch to the scaphoid and contributes to the dorsal intercarpal arch. This arch courses ulnarly across the trapezoid and the distal half of the capitate prior to branching and anastomosing with both the dorsal branch of the anterior interosseous artery and the dorsal branches of the ulnar artery. The last branch of the radial artery originates at the level of the trapezium and courses radially and distally to supply the trapezium and the lateral aspect of the thumb metacarpal.[6]

ULNAR ARTERY

At the level of the carpus, the ulnar artery gives off a latticework of fine vessels that span the dorsal and palmar aspects of the medial carpus (Figs. 3–1 and 3–3). Proximal to the end of the ulna, there are 3 branches: a branch to the dorsal radiocarpal arch, one to the palmar radiocarpal arch, and one to the proximal pole of the pisiform and to the palmar aspect of the triquetrium. Several small branches supply the lateral aspect of the pisiform, and a single branch joins the palmar intercarpal arch. Distally, a branch supplies the distal pisiform and the medial hamate and continues dorsally between the pisohamate and the pisometacarpal ligaments to contribute to the dorsal intercarpal arch. At the midcarpal joint level, the medial branch of the ulnar artery contributes to the intercarpal arch (Fig. 3–1). Distally, at the level of the metacarpal bases, the basal metacarpal arch receives its contribution from the medial branch of the ulnar artery. The medial branch of the ulnar artery then continues distally toward the base of the metacarpal of the little finger. A distal branch of the ulnar artery arises proximal to the origin of the superficial palmar arch and continues dorsally to supply the basal metacarpal arch. A deep palmar branch is given off distally that contributes to the deep palmar arch.

The ulnar artery continues distally and radially to contribute to the superficial palmar arch.

ANTERIOR INTEROSSEOUS ARTERY

At the proximal border of the pronator quadratus muscle, the anterior interosseous artery bifurcates into dorsal and palmar branches. The dorsal branch continues distally on the interosseous membrane to the carpus, where it supplies the dorsal radiocarpal arch (89 percent of specimens).[6] Small branches extend radially to supply the lunate and to anastomose with several small radial artery branches supplying the dorsal ridge of the scaphoid. The dorsal branch of the anterior interosseous artery bifurcates at the intercarpal level, each branch contributing to the intercarpal arch (83 percent of specimens).[6] The dorsal branch of the anterior interosseous artery terminates by anastomosing with recurrent vessels from the basal metacarpal arch at the third and fourth interosseous spaces (70 percent of specimens) (Fig. 3–1).[6]

The palmar branch of the anterior interosseous artery continues deep to the pronator quadratus and bifurcates 5 to 8 mm proximal to the radiocarpal arch. It usually contributes at least one branch to the palmar radiocarpal arch to supply the ulnar lunate and triquetrum and then terminates by anastomosing with recurrent vessels from the deep palmar arch.

DEEP PALMAR ARCH

The deep palmar arch provides the primary arterial supply to the distal carpal row by way of 2 branches—the radial and ulnar recurrent arteries (Fig. 3–3). These branches run in a distal-to-proximal direction and are consistently present.[6] The radial recurrent artery is slightly smaller, originates from the arch just lateral to the base of the index metacarpal, and runs proximally to bifurcate on the palmar aspect of the trapezoid. It anastomoses with the ulnar recurrent artery in 45 percent of specimens.

The ulnar recurrent artery originates from the deep arch between the bases of the long and ring metacarpals. It courses proximally within the ligamentous groove between the capitate and the hamate, supplying both bones. It anastomoses with the terminal portion of the anterior interosseous artery in 80 percent of specimens.

ACCESSORY ULNAR RECURRENT ARTERY

In 27 percent of specimens, an accessory ulnar recurrent artery is present. It originates from the deep arch 5 to 10 mm medial to the ulnar recurrent artery and supplies the medial aspect of the hook of the hamate. When this vessel is not present, the medial aspect of the hamate is supplied by direct branches from the ulnar artery.[6]

POSTERIOR INTEROSSEOUS ARTERY

The posterior interosseous artery does not reach the carpus and does not directly contribute to its dorsal vascularity.[6, 20]

The contributions of the major arteries and arches to the carpus are summarized in Figures 3–6 and 3–7.

VASCULAR ANATOMY OF SPECIFIC CARPAL BONES

The specific vascular supply, including the intraosseous vascularity of each bone, is described below.[16] Nutrient arteries usually en-

Dorsal

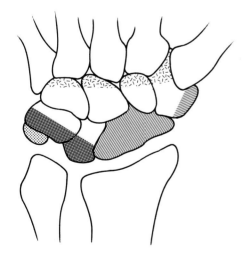

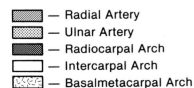

  — Radial Artery
  — Ulnar Artery
  — Radiocarpal Arch
  — Intercarpal Arch
  — Basalmetacarpal Arch

Figure 3–6. Schematic drawing of the dorsum of the wrist, showing the major artery and arch contributions to the carpal bones. (From Gelberman RH, Panagis JS, Taleisnik J, et al: J Hand Surg 8:367–375, 1983.)

Volar

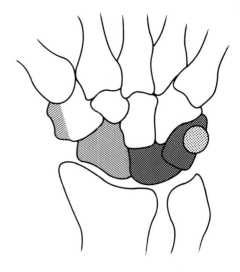

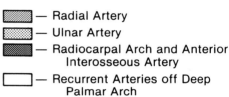

  — Radial Artery
  — Ulnar Artery
  — Radiocarpal Arch and Anterior Interosseous Artery
  — Recurrent Arteries off Deep Palmar Arch

Figure 3–7. Schematic drawing of the palmar aspect of the wrist, showing the major artery and arch contributions to carpal bones. (From Gelberman RH, Panagis JS, Taleisnik J, et al: J Hand Surg 8:367–375, 1983.)

ter the bone through the noncartilaginous areas of ligament attachment and then branch to form an intraosseous vascular network within each bone.[4, 7, 8, 16, 20]

Scaphoid

The scaphoid receives its blood supply primarily from the radial artery (Fig. 3–8). Vessels enter palmarly and dorsally through nonarticular areas of ligamentous attachment.[1, 5, 8, 19]

The palmar vascular supply accounts for 20 percent to 30 percent of the internal vascularity, all in the region of the distal pole.[5] At the level of the radioscaphoid joint, the radial artery gives off the superficial palmar branch. Just distal to the origin of the superficial palmar branch, several smaller branches course obliquely and distally over the palmar aspect of the bone to enter the scaphoid through the region of the tubercle.[5, 8] These branches, the palmar scaphoid branches, divide into several smaller

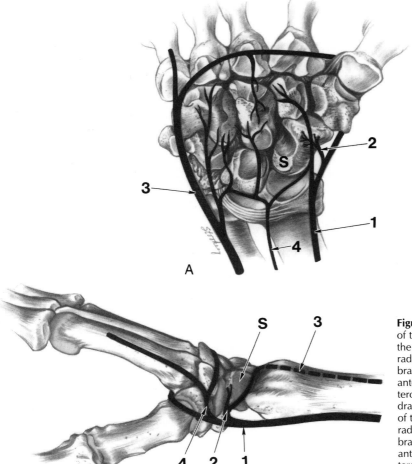

Figure 3–8. *A*, Schematic drawing of the volar external blood supply of the scaphoid. S = scaphoid; 1 = radial artery; 2 = volar scaphoid branches; 3 = ulnar artery; 4 = anterior division of the anterior interosseous artery. *B*, Schematic drawing of the dorsal blood supply of the scaphoid. S = scaphoid; 1 = radial artery; 2 = dorsal scaphoid branch; 3 = dorsal division of the anterior interosseous artery; 4 = intercarpal artery. (From Gelberman RH, and Menon J: J Hand Surg 5:508–513, 1980.)

branches just prior to penetrating the bone. In 75 percent of specimens, these arteries arise directly from the radial artery.[5] In the remainder, they arise from the superficial palmar branch of the radial artery. Consistent anastomoses exist between the palmar division of the anterior interosseous artery and the palmar scaphoid branch of the radial artery, when the latter arises from the superficial palmar branch of the radial artery. There are no apparent communicating branches between the ulnar artery and the palmar branches of the radial artery that supply the scaphoid. Vessels in the palmar scapholunate ligament do not penetrate the scaphoid. The palmar vessels enter the tubercle and divide into several smaller branches to supply the distal 20 percent to 30 percent of the scaphoid. There are no apparent anastomoses between the palmar and dorsal vessels (Fig. 3–9).[5]

The dorsal vascular supply to the scaphoid accounts for 70 percent to 80 percent of the internal vascularity of the bone, all in the proximal region (Fig. 3–10).[5] On the dorsum of the scaphoid, there is an oblique ridge that lies between the articular surfaces of the radius and of the trapezium and trapezoid. The major dorsal vessels to the scaphoid enter the bone through small foramina located on this dorsal ridge (Fig. 3–9).[1, 5] At the level of the intercarpal joint, the radial artery gives off the intercarpal artery, which immediately divides into two branches: a transverse branch to the dorsum of the wrist and a branch that runs vertically and distally over the index metacarpal. Approximately 0.5 cm proximal to the origin of the intercarpal vessel at the level of the styloid process of the radius, another vessel is given off that runs over the radiocarpal ligament to enter the scaphoid through its waist along

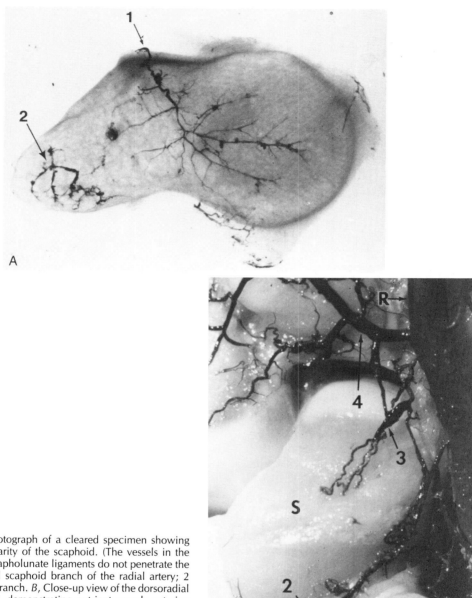

Figure 3–9. *A,* Photograph of a cleared specimen showing the internal vascularity of the scaphoid. (The vessels in the dorsal and volar scapholunate ligaments do not penetrate the bone.) 1 = Dorsal scaphoid branch of the radial artery; 2 = volar scaphoid branch. *B,* Close-up view of the dorsoradial aspect of the wrist, demonstrating nutrient vessels entering the dorsal ridge of the scaphoid. RS = radial styloid; S = scaphoid; R = radial artery; 2 = dorsal radiocarpal arch; 3 = branch to the dorsal ridge of the scaphoid; 4 = dorsal intercarpal arch. (From Panagis JS, Gelberman RH, Taleisnik J, et al: J Hand Surg 8:367–375, 1983.)

the dorsal ridge. In 70 percent of specimens, the dorsal vessel arises directly from the radial artery. In 23 percent, the dorsal branch has its origin from the common stem of the intercarpal artery. In 7 percent, the scaphoid receives its dorsal blood supply directly from the branches of both the intercarpal artery and the radial artery. There are consistent major anastomoses between the dorsal scaphoid branch of the radial artery and the dorsal branch of the anterior interos-

seous artery in each specimen (Fig. 2–8). There are no vessels that enter the proximal-dorsal region of the bone through the dorsal scapholunate ligament and no vessels that enter through dorsal cartilaginous areas.

The dorsal vessels usually enter the scaphoid through foramina located on the dorsal ridge at the level of the scaphoid waist; however, in a few of the specimens studied, they entered just proximal or distal to the waist. The dorsal vessels usually divide into

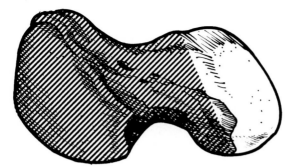

Figure 3–10. The proximal 70 to 80 percent of the bone is supplied by dorsal vessels (shaded area). The distal 20 to 30 percent is supplied by volar branches of the radial artery (white area). (From Gelberman RH, and Menon J: J Hand Surg 5:508–513, 1980.)

2 to 3 branches soon after entering the scaphoid. These branches run palmarly and proximally, dividing into smaller branches to supply the proximal pole as far as the subchondral region (Fig. 3–9).

Trapezium

The trapezium receives vessels from distal branches of the radial artery (Figs. 3–1, 3–3, and 3–4).

Nutrient vessels enter the trapezium through its 3 nonarticular surfaces (Fig. 3–11). These surfaces include the dorsal and lateral aspects, which are rough and serve as sites for ligament attachment, and the prominent palmar tubercle from which the thenar muscles arise. Dorsally, 1 to 3 vessels

enter and divide in the subchondral bone to supply the entire dorsal aspect of the bone. Palmarly, 1 to 3 vessels enter the midportion and divide and anstomose with the vessels entering through the dorsal surface. Laterally, 3 to 6 very fine vessels penetrate the lateral surface and anastomose freely with the dorsal and palmar vessels. The dorsal vascular supply predominates. There are frequent anastomoses among all three systems.[16]

Trapezoid

The trapezoid is supplied by branches from the dorsal, the intercarpal, and the basal metacarpal arches and the radial recurrent artery (Figs. 3–1, 3–2, and 3–3).

The nutrient vessels enter the trapezoid through its 2 nonarticular surfaces (Fig. 3–12). These surfaces include the dorsal surface, which is broad and round, and the palmar surface, which is narrow and flat. Both surfaces are rough and serve as sites for ligament attachment. Dorsally, 3 to 4 small vessels enter the central aspect of the rough, nonarticular surface. After penetrating the subchondral bone, the vessels branch to supply the dorsal 70 percent of the bone. Primarily, the dorsal vessels provide the vascularity of the trapezoid.[16]

Palmarly, one to two small vessels penetrate the central palmar area and branch several times to supply the palmar 30 percent of the bone. The palmar vessels do not anastomose with the dorsal vessels.[16]

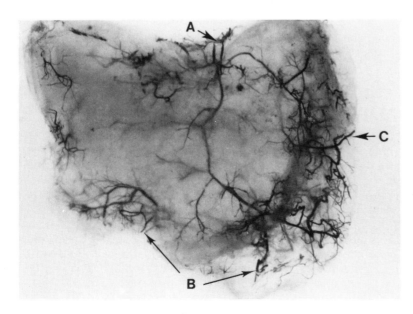

Figure 3–11. Trapezium: Distal view from articular surface at thumb trapeziometacarpal joint, showing dorsal (A), palmar (B), and lateral (C) nutrient vessels, with anastomoses of the three. (From Panagis JS, Gelberman RH, Taleisnik J, et al: J Hand Surg 8:375–382, 1983.)

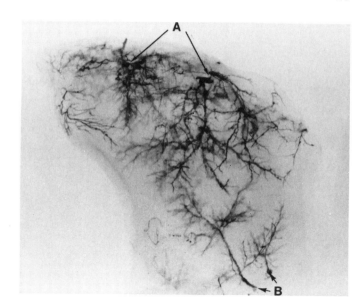

Figure 3–12. Trapezoid: Lateral view, showing dorsal nutrient vessels (A) supplying dorsal 70% of the bone and palmar vessels (B) supplying palmar 30%. There were no intraosseous anastomoses. (From Panagis JS, Gelberman RH, Taleisnik J, et al: J Hand Surg 8:375–382, 1983.)

Capitate

The capitate receives vessels from the dorsal intercarpal and the dorsal basal metacarpal arches and also from anastomoses between the ulnar recurrent and the palmar intercarpal arches.

The vessels enter through the two nonarticular surfaces on the dorsal and palmar aspects of the capitate. The dorsal surface is broad, deeply concave, and rough, serving for ligamentous attachment. Two to 4 vessels enter the distal two thirds of the concavity (Fig. 3–13). Smaller vessels occasionally enter more proximally near the neck. The dorsal vessels course palmarly, proximally, and ulnarly in a retrograde fashion to supply the body and head of the capitate. This dorsal

supply predominates on the convex, rough palmar surface (Fig. 3–14).[16]

On the palmar surface, 1 to 3 vessels enter the distal half of the capitate and course proximally in a retrograde fashion. In 33 percent of the specimens, vascularity to the capitate head originates entirely from the palmar surface. There are significant anastomoses between the dorsal and the palmar blood supplies in 30 percent of specimens.[16]

Hamate

The hamate receives vessels from the dorsal intercarpal arch, the ulnar recurrent artery, and the ulnar artery (Figs. 3–1 and 3–3).

Vessels enter through the 3 nonarticular surfaces of the hamate: the dorsal, the pal-

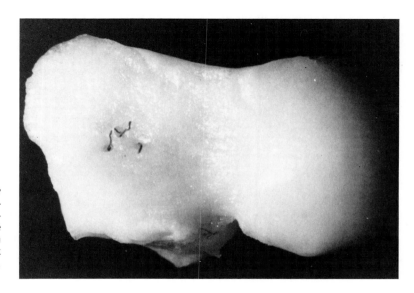

Figure 3–13. Capitate: Dorsal view prior to clearance with the Spalteholz technique, showing three arteries entering nutrient foramina in the distal one third of the bone. (From Panagis JS, Gelberman RH, Taleisnik J, et al: J Hand Surg 8:375–382, 1983.)

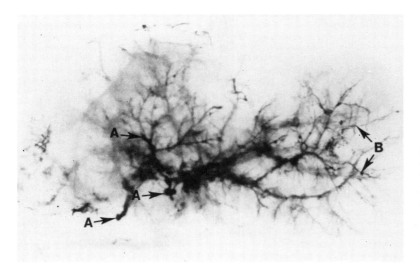

Figure 3–14. Capitate: Dorsal view, following clearing by Spalteholz technique. Nutrient vessels (A) enter distal third with retrograde course toward the proximal articular surface. Terminal vessels (B) in the head of the capitate. (From Panagis JS, Gelberman RH, Taleisnik J, et al: J Hand Surg 8:375–382, 1983.)

mar, and the medial surface through the hamate hook (Fig. 3–15). The dorsal surface is triangular in shape and receives 3 to 5 vessels. These branch in multiple directions to supply the dorsal 30 percent to 40 percent of the bone.[16]

The palmar surface is triangular in shape and receives 1 large vessel that enters through the radial base of the hook. It then branches and anastomoses with the dorsal vessels in 50 percent of specimens studied.[16]

The hook of the hamate receives 1 to 2 small vessels that enter through the medial base and tip of the hook. These vessels anastomose with each other but usually not with the vessels to the body of the hamate.

Triquetrum

The triquetrum is supplied by branches from the ulnar artery, the dorsal intercarpal arch, and the palmar intercarpal arch. Nutrient vessels enter through its 2 nonarticular surfaces, the dorsal and the palmar.

The dorsal surface is rough and contains a ridge that runs from the medial to the lateral aspect. Two to 4 vessels enter this dorsal ridge and radiate in multiple directions to supply the dorsal 60 percent of the bone (Fig. 3–16). This network is the prodominant blood supply to the triquetrum in 60 percent of specimens.[16]

The palmar surface contains an oval facet that articulates with the pisiform. One to 2 vessels enter proximal and distal to the facet. The vessels have multiple anastomoses with each other and supply the palmar 40 percent of the bone. This palmar vascular network

is predominant in 20 percent of specimens studied (Fig. 3–17).[16]

The dorsal and the palmar vascular networks have significant anastomoses in 86 percent.[16]

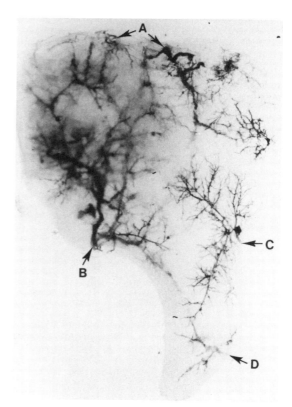

Figure 3–15. Hamate: End view from the distal surface, demonstrating dorsal (A) and palmar (B) supplies. Vessels to the hook enter at the medial base (C) and at the tip of the hook (D). (From Panagis JS, Gelberman RH, Taleisnik J, et al: J Hand Surg 8:375–382, 1983.)

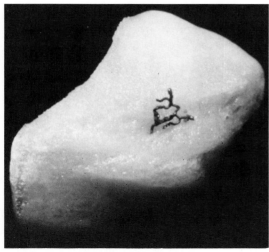

Figure 3–16. Triquetrum: Dorsal view prior to clearance with Spalteholz technique, showing a branching nutrient vessel entering the center of the obliquely running dorsal ridge. (From Panagis JS, Gelberman RH, Taleisnik J, et al: J Hand Surg 8:375–382, 1983.)

Pisiform

The pisiform is a sesamoid bone within the tendon of the flexor carpi ulnaris. Dorsally, it articulates with the triquetrum. The remainder of the bone is rough and serves for ligament and muscle attachment. It receives its blood supply through the proximal and distal poles from branches of the ulnar artery. Proximally, 1 to 3 vessels enter inferior to the triquetral facet and divide into multiple branches. Two superior branches run parallel beneath the articular surface of the facet. One to 2 inferior branches run along the palmar cortex and anastomose with the superior branches.[16]

Distally, 1 to 3 vessels enter inferior to the facets, divide into superior and inferior branches, run parallel to the palmar cortex, and anastomose with the proximal vessels. The superior vessels run beneath the facet and anastomose with the proximal superior vessels, forming an arterial ring beneath the facet. There are multiple anastomoses between the proximal and the distal vascular networks (Fig. 3–18).[16]

Lunate

The lunate receives its nutrient vessels from both palmar and dorsal surfaces in 80 percent of specimens, and palmarly alone in 20 percent.[16] The remainder of the surface of the lunate is covered by articular cartilage. Dorsally, these nutrient vessels receive their supply from the dorsal radiocarpal arch, from the dorsal intercarpal arch, and occasionally from smaller branches of the dorsal branch of the anterior interosseous artery.[4, 6, 16] Palmarly, the lunate nutrient vessels are supplied by the palmar intercarpal arch, the palmar radiocarpal arch, and anastomosing vessels from the anterior interosseous artery and the ulnar recurrent artery (Fig. 3–3).

The nutrient vessels that enter dorsally are slightly smaller than the palmar vessels. Major vessels branch proximally and distally after entering the bone and terminate in the subchondral bone. The dorsal and palmar vessels anastomose intraosseously just distal to the midportion of the lunate. The proximal pole is relatively avascular. There are 3 major intraosseous patterns forming "Y", "I", or "X" patterns (Figs. 3–19, 3–20, and

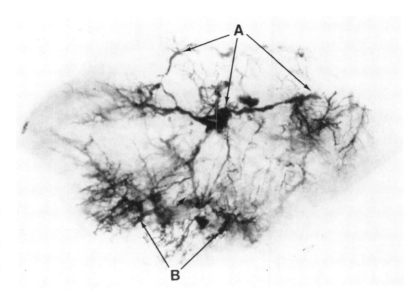

Figure 3–17. Triquetrum: Lateral view, showing three dorsal (A) and two palmar (B) nutrient vessels with intraosseous anastomoses in the middle one third of the bone. This pattern is seen in 80 percent of the specimens. (From Panagis JS, Gelberman RH, Taleisnik J, et al: J Hand Surg 8:375–382, 1983.)

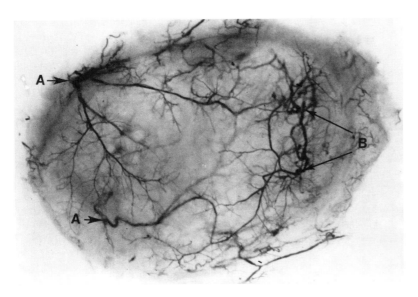

Figure 3–18. Pisiform: Dorsal view looking onto the facet for the triquetrum, with the proximal superior (*A*) and distal superior (*B*) vessels forming an arterial ring beneath the facet. (From Panagis JS, Gelberman RH, Taleisnik J, et al: J Hand Surg 8:375–382, 1983.)

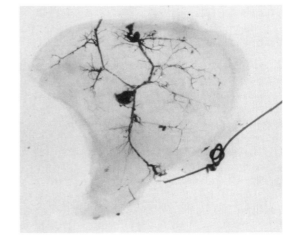

Figure 3–19. Lunate: The most common intraosseous vascular pattern—the "Y" pattern. (From Gelberman RH, Bauman RD, and Menon J: J Hand Surg 5:272–278, 1980.)

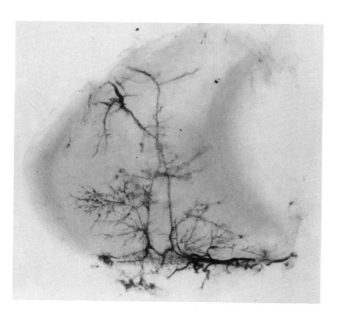

Figure 3–20. The "X" intraosseous vascular pattern formed by two dorsal and two volar vessels anastomosing in the midportion of the lunate. (From Gelberman RH, Bauman RD, and Menon J: J Hand Surg 5:272–278, 1980.)

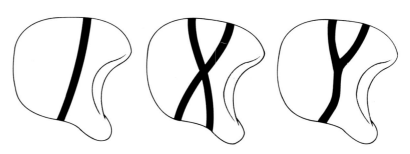

Figure 3–21. Schematic representation of "I", "X", and "Y" intraosseous vascular patterns. (From Gelberman RH, Bauman RD, and Menon J: J Hand Surg 5:272–278, 1980.)

3–21).[4] The "Y" pattern is the most common (59 percent), the stem of the Y occurring dorsally or palmarly with equal frequency. The "I" pattern, occurring in approximately 30 percent, consists of a single dorsal and a single palmar vessel that anastomose in a straight line. The "X" pattern, occurring in 10 percent, consists of 2 dorsal and 2 palmar vessels that anastomose in the center of the lunate.[4, 16]

In 20 percent of specimens studied, a single palmar supply was shown to be present. This consists of a single large vessel that enters on the palmar surface and branches within the bone to provide the sole blood supply (Fig. 3–22).

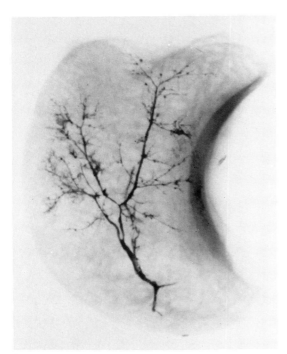

Figure 3–22. Lunate: Lateral view, showing single large vessel entering palmar surface and branching within the bone to provide the sole blood supply. This pattern is seen in 20 percent of the specimens. (From Panagis JS, Gelberman RH, Taleisnik J, et al: J Hand Surg 8:375–382, 1983.)

SUMMARY

The extraosseous arterial pattern is formed by an anastomotic network of 3 dorsal and 3 palmar arches connected longitudinally at their medial and lateral borders by the ulnar and radial arteries. Additional longitudinal anastomoses are provided by the dorsal and palmar branches of the anterior interosseous artery. The most distal of the palmar arches is the deep palmar arch, formed by the anastomosis of the radial artery and the deep palmar branch of the ulnar artery. Two consistent recurrent arteries, 1 radial and 1 ulnar, arise from the concavity of this arch and traverse proximally to frequently anastomose with the terminal branches of the anterior division of the anterior interosseous artery. This anastomosis provides the major collateral circulation about the wrist.

The bones of the carpus can be placed into 3 general groups based on the size and location of nutrient vessels, on the presence or absence of intraosseous anastomoses, and on the dependence of large areas of bone on a single intraosseous vessel.[16] Group I includes the scaphoid, the capitate, and, in approximately 20 percent of specimens, the lunate. Each has large areas of bone dependent on a single intraosseous vessel and is considered at greater risk to develop avascular necrosis following fracture. Group II includes the trapezoid and the hamate, both of which have 2 areas of vessel entry but lack intraosseous anastomoses. Group III includes the trapezium, the triquetrum, the pisiform, and, in approximately 80 percent of specimens, the lunate. These receive nutrient arteries through 2 nonarticular surfaces, have consistent intraosseous anastomoses, and have no large area of bone dependent upon a single vessel. The clinical incidence of avascular necrosis in Groups II and III is low.

The arterial anatomy of the carpus presents a technically demanding area of study. With recently improved techniques of investigation, the anatomy of this area can be more clearly defined. The results of a number of these recent studies have been summarized in this report.

References

1. Barber H: The intraosseous arterial anatomy of the adult human carpus. Orthopedics 5:1–19, 1972.
2. Coleman SS, and Anson BJ: Arterial patterns in the hand. Surg Gynecol Obstet 113:409–429, 1961.
3. Edwards EA: Organization of the small arteries of the hand and digits. Am J Surg 99:837–846, 1960.
4. Gelberman RH, Bauman RD, and Menon J: The vascularity of the lunate bone and Kienböck's disease. J Hand Surg 5:272–278, 1980.
5. Gelberman RH, and Menon J: The vascularity of the scaphoid bone. J Hand Surg 5:508–513, 1980.
6. Gelberman RH, Panagis JS, Taleisnik J, et al: The arterial anatomy of the human carpus. Part I: The extraosseous vascularity. J Hand Surg 8:367–373, 1983.
7. Gelberman RH, and Gross MS: The vascularity of the wrist—identifying arterial patterns at risk. Clin Orthop 202:40–49, 1986.
8. Grettve S: Arterial anatomy of the carpal bones. Acta Anat 25:331–345, 1955.
9. Hollingshead WH: Anatomy for Surgeons, Vol 3, New York, Harper & Row, Publishers, Inc, 1969.
10. Lawrence HW, and Bachuber AE: The Collateral Circulation After Ligature of Both Radial and Ulnar Arteries at the Wrist, Thesis. University of Wisconsin, Department of Anatomy, 1923.
11. Lawrence HW: The collateral circulation in the hand. Indust Med 6:410–411, 1937.
12. Lee MCH: The intraosseous arterial pattern of the carpal lunate. Acta Orthop Scand 33:43–55, 1963.
13. Mestdagh H, Bailleu JP, Chambou JP, et al: The dorsal arterial network of the wrist with reference to the blood supply of the carpal bones. Acta Morphol Neerl Scand 17:73–80, 1979.
14. Meyers MH, Wells R, and Harvey JP: Naviculocapitate fracture syndrome. J Bone Joint Surg 53:1383–1386, 1971.
15. Minne J, Depreux R, Mestdagh H, et al: Les pédicules artériels du massif carpien. Lille Méd 18:1174–1185, 1973.
16. Panagis JS, Gelberman RH, Taleisnik J, et al: The Arterial Anatomy of the Human Carpus. Part II: The Intraosseous Vascularity. J Hand Surg 8:375–382, 1983.
17. Quiring AP: Collateral Circulation. Philadelphia, Lea & Febiger, 1949.
18. Rockwood CA, and Green DP: Fractures, Vol. 1. Philadelphia, J. B. Lippincott Co, 1975, 421–428.
19. Taleisnik J, and Kelly PJ: Extraosseous and intraosseous blood supply of the scaphoid bone. J Bone Joint Surg 48(6):1125–1137, 1977.
20. Travaglini E: Arterial circulation of the carpal bones. Bull Hosp J Dis Orthop Inst 20:19–36, 1959.
21. Vance RM, Gelberman RH, and Evans EF: Scaphocapitate fracture. J Bone Joint Surg 62:271–276, 1980.

CHAPTER 4

Wrist Mechanics and Its Association with Ligamentous Instability

EDWARD R. WEBER, M.D.

INTRODUCTION

Understanding the mechanics of the wrist is becoming increasingly important. The recent surge in interest in the wrist has resulted in many new operative procedures and many strongly held opinions. Some procedures, such as scaphotrapeziotrapezoidal arthrodesis, have found a valid place in the surgical correction of wrist pathology. Indiscriminate use of this procedure, however, will lead to unnecessary wrist impairment. Other procedures, such as ligamentous repairs, direct suture of damaged structures, and changes in the length relationship of the radius and the ulna, also have their uses and abuses.

The development of diagnostic procedures has been concomitant with the development of new operations. Wrist arthrography, midcarpal wrist arthrography, videotaped motion studies, magnetic resonance imaging (MRI), and, now, wrist arthroscopy have led to the ability to diagnose previously undetected pathology.

The proliferation of these new techniques demands that the surgeon undertaking the care of the wrist-injured patient have an understanding of the basic wrist mechanics. This chapter relates concepts I have developed over the past ten years, many based on inductive reasoning. Happily, those concepts that have been experimentally tested by myself and others have been validated. Minor variations are likely to occur clinically, but I believe that the overall picture of wrist mechanics presented here will withstand the test of time and further investigations.

We owe a great debt to people from the past who have studied and written about the wrist: Wagner, Landsmeyer, Fisk, Destot, and Navaro all contributed greatly to our basic understanding of the subject. Currently, Taleisnik, Linscheid, Dobyns, Lichtman, Palmer, and Watson have offered concepts and documentation related to wrist mechanics and wrist surgery. All of these people have encouraged and stimulated me, either through their writings or directly.

WRIST MECHANICS

The human carpus is the portion of the upper extremity that extends from the distal radius to the metacarpal shafts. The distal radial and ulnar articular surfaces as well as the carpometacarpal joints are properly included in the carpal unit. The motor units affecting the carpus arise from the forearm and insert distal to the wrist. Landsmeer has likened this arrangement to an intercalated segment in a mechanical linkage.[2] In fact, it is the proximal carpal row that acts as the intercalated segment.

Understanding the interactions of the scaphoid, lunate, and triquetrum with their neighboring bones and within the proximal row is the key to comprehending how the wrist maintains its stability while allowing a wide range of motion.

Functionally, the carpal unit transmits forces, generated or applied, through the hand of the forearm. It also acts as part of a kinematic linkage system with the remainder of the body as the final adjuster of the hand in space. The requirements for the carpal unit to perform both of these functions (that is, force transmission and adjustment) without direct motor control present a unique problem in design.

Basically, the carpus is able to accomplish both of its tasks simultaneously by utilizing

41

a dual articular system. The most proximal joint in this system is the radiocarpal articulation, and the more distal joint is the midcarpal articulation. Modest motion in the stable range in one joint is amplified at the second joint without loss of stability. In the carpal system, where motion between the proximal and midcarpal joints is controlled and coordinated without the necessity of a motor unit, stability becomes a matter of mechanical linkage.

Much has been written about the role of the ligaments in controlling the relative motion of the two carpal joints.[1, 3–5, 7–9] One basic truth concerning ligaments is that they are static structures; thus, they have only two possibilities of action: They are either active, limiting the excursion of the joint system involved, or they are lax, not affecting joint motion. There is no partial action imposed by the static constraints. The single exception to this rule occurs when a ligament is oriented axially and at right angles to the plane of motion of a joint, as in the proximal interphalangeal joint of the finger. If we are to fully understand the function of the carpus, we must look to additional factors controlling joint motion.

The other possibility for control of the carpal intercalated segment is through the contact surfaces of the carpal joints. A contact surface type of control system would provide stability throughout the entire range of motion while transmitting loads. A ligamentous control system provides stability only at the extremes of joint motion. The wrist relies on both ligamentous and contact surface constraints during normal function.

As the wrist ranges from radial to ulnar deviation, the proximal carpal row rotates in a dorsal direction. Simultaneously, translocation of the proximal carpal row occurs in the radial direction at the radiocarpal and midcarpal articulations. These combined motions of the carpal rows have been called the rotational shift of the carpus (Fig. 4–1). Regarded as a unit, however, the center of wrist motion remains in the head of the capitate throughout this complex interaction of motions.[9]

To facilitate the understanding of how joint contact acts to control the rotational shift of the intercalated carpal segment, it is useful to think of the wrist in terms of longitudinal columns (Fig. 4–2). These are the force-bearing column, which constitutes the central core of the wrist, the ulnar or

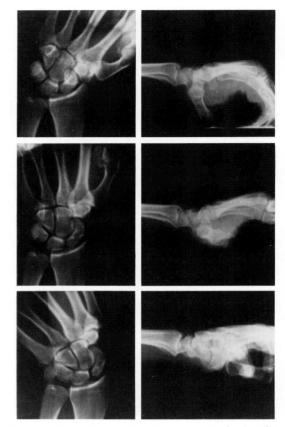

Figure 4–1. Rotational shift of the carpus. Biplanar radiographs of a normal wrist in radial deviation (*top*), neutral deviation (*middle*), and ulnar deviation (*bottom*). Note the attitude of the lunate with reference to the capitate and radius as the wrist goes from radial to ulnar deviation. Also note the relationship of the triquetrum to the hamate during this motion. (From Weber ER: Orthop Clin North Am 15:2, 193–206, 1984.)

control column, and a partial radial column, which acts to support the thumb base.

The Force-Bearing Column

The main function of the force-bearing column is to transmit the forces generated by the hand to the forearm unit. Proximally to distally, it is composed of the distal radial articular surface, the lunate, the proximal two thirds of the scaphoid, the capitate, the trapezoid, and the articulations of the second and third metacarpals.

When viewing the distal articular surface of the radius, one notices two prominent features (Fig. 4–3). The first of these is a distal projection of the dorsal articular surface of the radius. The function of this dorsal projection is to provide a bone constraint to dorsal shear forces, thus eliminating capsu-

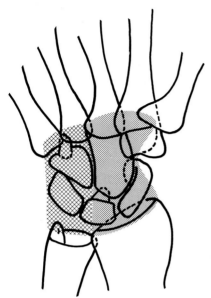

Figure 4–2. Longitudinal carpal columns. The control column occupies the ulnar portion of the wrist (*cross-hatched area*), while the majority of force transmission takes place on the radial side (*stippled area*). (From Weber ER: Orthop Clin North Am 15:2, 193–206, 1984.)

lar feedback. Activities such as pushing, with the wrist in dorsiflexion, are made possible by this feature. The second prominent feature of the distal radial articular surface is a volar projection known as the radial styloid. This bony prominence also acts as a shear constraint to eliminate capsular feedback in power grip. The majority of the force transmitted by the carpus is received on the distal radius.

Force transmission by the ulnar column is limited because the distal ulnar joint is covered by a triangular fibrocartilage disk, that

is, the triangular fibrocartilage (TFC) (Fig. 4–4). This substance has a greater compliance to applied load and therefore yields, allowing the radius to sustain the major portion of the transmitted load.

The articular chain that transmits loads begins at the fixed carpometacarpal joints of the index and long fingers. The load is transmitted through the capitate to an acetabulum-shaped joint forming part of the midcarpal row. The force-receiving acetabulum is formed by the distal articular surface of the lunate and the proximal two thirds of the scaphoid. The scaphoid and lunate transmit the load to the radius through two sulci in the radial articular surface. These sulci are separated by an intersulcal ridge. The most radial receives the convex surface of the lunate (Fig. 4–3). All of these surfaces interact to form the major force-bearing axis of the wrist.

The Control Column

The column on the ulnar side of the wrist has quite a different configuration (Figs. 4–1 to 4–3). Beginning with the distal ulna, a well-formed styloid process is present. Arising near the radial side of the styloid is the apex of the triangular fibrocartilage, which increases in its anteroposterior diameter as it extends radially to attach to the entire ulnar surface of the distal radial articulation. The surface of the triangular fibrocartilage is continuous with that of the distal radius.

The next most distal bone in the ulnar column is the triquetrum. It possesses a broad and relatively nondescript articulation with the triangular fibrocartilage. The distal

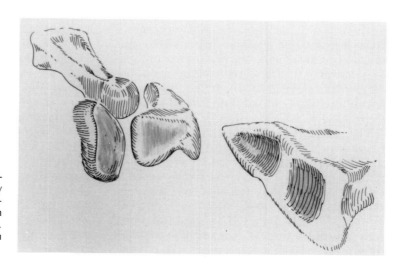

Figure 4–3. Distal radial articular surface. The radial styloid is placed radially and volarly on the radial articular surface. It acts to support the wrist in dorsiflexion and in ulnar deviation. (From Weber ER: Ortho Clin North Am 15:2, 193–206, 1984.)

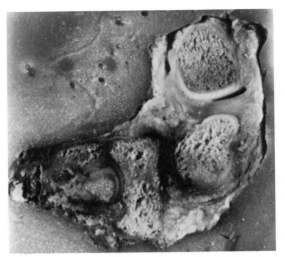

Figure 4–4. Triangular fibrocartilage. This is a sagittal section of a wrist loaded in 100° of dorsiflexion. Included on this section are the distal ulna, triangular fibrocartilage, triquetrum, hamate, and fifth metacarpal base. (From Weber ER: Orthop Clin North Am 15:2, 193–206, 1984.)

articular surface of the triquetrum and the proximal surface of the hamate form a fascinating articulation. The triquetrum has a smallish cartilaginous surface that is mildly saddle-shaped. The proximal surface of the hamate has three separate components. The ulnarmost component is also the most volar, nestled adjacent to the hook of the hamate. This articular surface faces volarly and is of the size necessary to accommodate the triquetral surface. The central portion of the hamate's articular surface faces the same plane as the body of the hamate. It is larger than the reciprocal surface of the triquetrum and offers little restriction of rotation. In addition, the midportion of the hamate is several millimeters dorsal to that of the ulnar surface. The radial surface of the hamate is, again, more dorsal than the midportion and faces dorsally. This surface becomes continuous with the articular crown of the capitate. The surface of the hamate has been described as helicoid or screw-shaped in configuration. This configuration is well suited to provide rotational control.

The joint between the hamate and the capitate presents a planar surface, thus transmitting only normal forces (right angle to joint surface). It is attached to the capitate by an interosseous ligament on both the dorsal and volar surfaces. The ligaments allow for approximately 2° of rotation and 2 mm of translation in the proximal distal direction. This joint acts as a shock absorber to compressive forces placed on the ulnar column of the wrist, transmitting forces to the more stable capitate through the hamatocapitate ligaments.

The next most distal joints in the ulnar column are the carpometacarpal joints of the ring and small fingers. These joints are mobile, with the ring finger allowing approximately 15° in the flexion-extension arc and the small finger allowing an even greater flexion-extension arc—between 25° and 30°. Because these joints are functional, they decrease the lever arm distance of the metacarpals and, therefore, the amount of force delivered through their carpal attachments. Thus, the rotational and compressive forces delivered to the capitohamate articulation are dampened. In addition, the amount of compressive force delivered through the hamate is changed into shear force by the inclination of the proximal surface of the hamate. Therefore, compressive forces transmitted by the hamate are applied on the triquetrum, tending to rotate this bone and to displace it ulnarly. Because of these considerations (the compliance of the triangular fibrocartilage, the slope of the hamate's surface, the shock-absorbing configuration of the hamatocapitate articulation, and the flexion-extension arc allowed at the carpometacarpal joints of the ring and small fingers), the compressive loads carried by the ulnar column are considerably dampened. Thus, the major loads transmitted by the carpus are conveyed by the force-bearing column onto the distal radius.

The Thumb Axis

The thumb axis includes the distal third of the scaphoid, the trapeziotrapezoid joint, and the first carpometacarpal joint. Because only one digit is included in this axis, considerably less force will be transmitted from these articulations to the carpus. The great mobility at the carpometacarpal joint of the thumb tends to dampen most of the bending load generated along the thumb axis. The joints interfacing between the thumb axis and the force-bearing column are again oriented in a planar fashion, transmitting only normal forces. The ligament attachments between the scaphoid pole and the capitate, however, are much looser than those of the hamatocapitate joint, allowing for approximately 30° of flexion-extension of the scaphoid relative to the axis of the capitate.

Measurements of relative motion between the scaphoid and the lunate are also between 20° and 30° in flexion and extension.

THE ROLE OF LIGAMENTOUS STRUCTURES OF THE CARPUS

In general, two types of carpal ligaments can be described: those crossing the carpal rows and those contained within the carpal rows. The function of the ligaments crossing the carpal rows is to guide the excursion of one row (the proximal row) upon the second row (the distal row). These ligaments include the radiolunatotriquetral ligament, the dorsal carpal ligament, the ulnotriquetral ligament, and the radioscapholunate ligament. The second type of ligaments are those contained within the carpal row. These ligaments act to limit the relative motion between the carpals within that row.

The interosseous ligaments of the proximal carpal row (that is, the scapholunate and lunatotriquetral ligaments) are positioned circumferentially around two thirds of the joint surface, with the distal articular surface remaining open. These ligaments provide strong rotational stability in the frontal plane because they are placed away from the axis of rotation and thus possess maximal mechanical advantage as rotational constraints. They bind the proximal row into a unit of rotational stability. Thus, in radial and ulnar deviation, the amount of intercarpal rotation allowed by this system is approximately 4° at the lunatotriquetral joint and 4° at the scapholunate joint. However, in flexion and extension, there can be as much as 30° at the scapholunate joint and 8° at the lunatotriquetral joint.

The interosseous ligament of the distal carpal row (hamatocapitate ligament) binds the surface of the capitate to that of the hamate. This ligament acts as a shock absorber, allowing limited excursion in the proximal-distal direction—approximately 1 to 2 mm. Only a few degrees of rotation are permitted to occur.

The radiocapitate ligament crosses the proximal carpal row to insert into the distal carpal row on the radial volar surface of the capitate. Because this ligament crosses two joint systems, it falls into a category of its own and is therefore considered an exception. The function of this ligament is to loosely bind the distal carpal row to the radius. Because of its location and the fact

that it does cross the proximal carpal row without inserting into the scaphoid, the radiocapitate ligament can also act as a sling, stabilizing the scaphoid waist and proximal pole. The fibers of the volar capsule between the proximal and distal carpal rows are oriented parallel to the intercarpal joint. Thus, these fibers possess little strength in binding the midcarpal and proximal carpal rows together. On the extreme ulnar side of the wrist, there are dorsal and palmar fibers connecting the triquetrum to the hamate. These fibers are oriented at 90° to the plane of motion of the triquetrohamate joint. They are attached radial to the hamate, so that the excursion of the triquetrum on the hamate inscribes the circumference of a circle centered at the ligament's hamate attachment. Therefore, this ligamentous connection provides stabilization in all phases of joint excursion.

KINEMATIC LINKAGE OF THE WRIST

Let us now look at how these different columns and structures interact with one another as the wrist displays its range of motion. It is well known that as the wrist goes from ulnar to radial deviation in neutral flexion, the scaphoid pole flexes, and that as the reverse motion occurs, the scaphoid pole extends. How do these actions take place? Two contact surfaces and the ligamentous attachments acting on the carpal rows are involved. The contact surface between the distal pole of the scaphoid and the trapezio-trapezoid joint forms a passive control surface. The ulnar control surface is contained in the triquetrohamate joint. As the hand moves from neutral position toward ulnar deviation, the triquetrum is translated ulnarly on the hamate's slope (Figs. 4–5A through 4–5E). Because of the relative volar position of the ulnar facet of the hamate, the triquetrum is also forced in a palmar direction (Fig. 4–5E). This palmar displacement of the triquetrum on the hamate brings the lunate axis palmar to the axis of the capitate. Compressive forces transmitted by the capitate also act on the lunate to rotate it into the dorsally facing attitude (Fig. 4–5C). This dorsiflexion of the lunate is transmitted through the scapholunate articulation by the interosseous ligament and results in elevation of the distal pole of the scaphoid. The

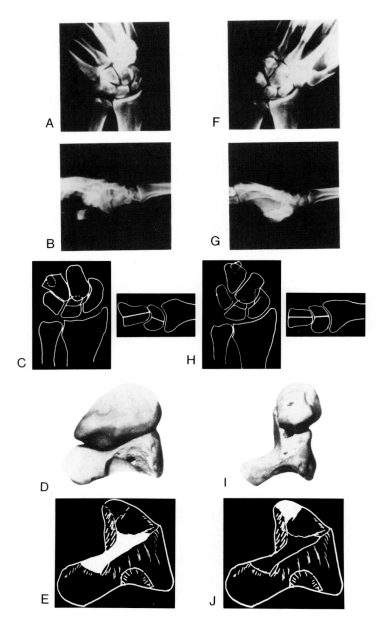

Figure 5. Wrist kinematics: Ulnar deviation. *A,* Anteroposterior radiograph of a wrist in ulnar deviation. Note the position of the triquetrum on the hamate and the extended scaphoid. *B,* Lateral radiograph of a wrist in ulnar deviation. Note dorsiflexion position of the lunate. *C,* Line drawing of the ulnarly deviated wrist, with the axes of the capitate and lunate added. As the axis of the lunate drops below the axis of the capitate, the lunate goes into dorsiflexion. *D,* Position of the triquetrum on the hamate with the wrist in ulnar deviation. View from ulnar side with volar to the left and distal to the bottom of the photograph. *E,* Line drawing of hamate in the same orientations as above. White area is the volar radial facet that is occupied by the triquetrum in ulnar deviation.

Wrist kinematics: Radial deviation. *F,* Anteroposterior radiograph of a wrist in radial deviation. Note the change in the relationship between the triquetrum and the hamate and the flexed position of the scaphoid. *G,* Biplanar lateral radiograph. Note that the lunate is facing slightly palmar. *H,* Line tracing of biplanar radiographs in radial deviation demonstrating above relationships. *I,* The position of the triquetrum on the hamate when the wrist is in full radial deviation. Note that the triquetrum has moved dorsally as well as laterally. *J,* Line drawing of hamate with the radial facet highlighted. (From Weber, ER: Orthop Clin North Am 15:2, 193–206, 1984.)

extension of the scaphoid is accommodated at the distal scaphotrapeziotrapezoid joint.

As the wrist moves from ulnar to radial deviation (Figs. 4–5F through 4–5J), the triquetrum translates radially and dorsally on the slope of the hamate (Fig. 4–5I). As this occurs, the lunate becomes coaxial with the capitate as the triquetrum enters the midzone on the hamate articulation. Simultaneously, the axis of the scaphoid flexes to its neutral position. As radial deviation is continued from the neutral position, the triquetrum continues to slide up the slope of the hamate. As the last 10° of radial deviation are achieved, the triquetrum enters the

radial dorsal facet of the hamate articulation (Fig. 4–5J). As this occurs, the lunate, by virtue of its ligamentous attachments with the triquetrum, is brought dorsal to the axis of the capitate, and compressive forces, transmitted through the capitate, cause the lunate to go into slight palmar flexion (Fig. 4–5H). The circumferential ligamentous articulation between the lunate and the scaphoid transmits this flexion force to the scaphoid, resulting in palmar flexion of the scaphoid. This motion is again accommodated at the scaphotrapeziotrapezoid joint.

Because the thumb base maintains full mobility in both extremes of deviation, strong radial compressive forces initiating the scaphoid and proximal row flexion, although theoretically possible, seem unlikely. Thus, in my view, the major control surface for rotation of the proximal row is contained on the ulnar side of the wrist, that is, the triquetrohamate articulation.

In summary, the wrist employs a Class I lever system (the inclined plane) to control the attitude of the intercalated segment. The slope of the hamate acts as the inclined plane, positioning the lunate relative to the stable capitate. The compressive forces delivered through the capitate provide the power, producing the attitudinal change in the proximal row. Thus, the contrl surface is removed from the axis of maximal force, where less energy is required to achieve effective positioning.

FLEXION-EXTENSION

Next, let us look at the kinematics that take place in the flexion-extension arc of the wrist. As dorsiflexion is initiated at the mid-

carpal articulation, the triquetrum is translated further up the slope of the hamate, and simultaneously, the radiolunatotriquetral ligament becomes taut. The radiocapitate ligament also comes into play. As it tightens, a sling is created across the scaphoid waist, dorsiflexing the scaphoid and the capitate as a unit. The sling effect is translated through the scapholunate joint to cause the lunate to dorsiflex as well. Thus, the capitate and the lunate remain coaxial as dorsiflexion proceeds. The tendency for the lunate to palmar flex as a result of the triquetrum's elevation on the hamate is checked by the sling effect of the radiocapitate ligament. From the lateral view, the effect of the radiocapitate ligament can be seen, as most dorsiflexion appears to be taking place at the proximal carpal articulation (Fig. 4–6A).

As palmar flexion occurs from a neutral position, the dorsal carpal ligament becomes taut, and the palmar capsular ligaments become lax. The taut dorsal carpal ligament translates the triquetrum on the slope of the hamate toward the dorsal radial facet. While

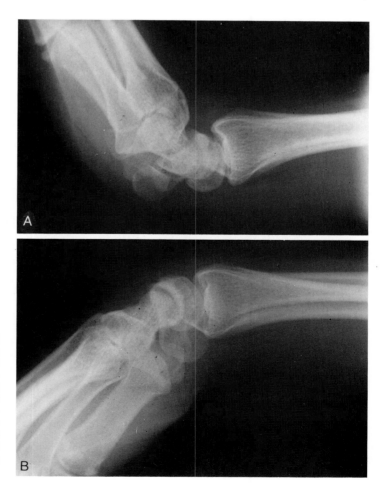

Figure 4–6. Anteroposterior and lateral radiographic views of wrist in dorsiflexion (A) and palmar flexion (B). A, Note that most of the dorsiflexion appears to be occurring at the radiocarpal joint. This is because of the locking of the motion of the proximal and distal rows by the radiocapitate ligament. B, Palmar flexion occurs primarily at the midcarpal joint because the capitate compressive forces tend to extend the lunate. (From Weber ER: Orthop Clin North Am 15:2, 193–206, 1984.)

this is occurring, most of the palmar flexion takes place at the midcarpal articulation (Fig. 4–6B). Some palmar flexion of the lunate also occurs with simultaneous flexion of the scaphoid. As the distal carpal row becomes narrower, the triquetrum is constrained by the dorsal carpal ligament as this structure tightens. The effect of the tightening of the dorsal carpal ligament is to lock the triquetrum to the triangular fibrocartilage and against the slope of the hamate. Flexion of the proximal row is limited by the taut dorsal ligament. In fact, flexion of the proximal row becomes synchronous with radial translocation of the triquetrum, with this movement being allowed by the narrower articular surface of the hamate and capitate on their dorsal and proximal aspects (Fig. 4–7).

The loss of radial and ulnar deviation in the extremes of flexion and extension can also be explained by this model. In dorsiflexion, as the radiocapitate ligament and the radiolunatotriquetral ligaments become fully taut, the ability of the scaphoid to flex is lost. Thus, the scaphoid blocks any chance for radial deviation to occur. Similarly, the tight radiocapitate and radiolunatotriquetral ligaments lock the two carpal rows to the radius, resisting any attempt at ulnar deviation. In palmar flexion, the taut dorsal carpal ligament restricts ulnar translocation of the proximal row. In addition, the scaphoid in the flexed position acts as a buttress to radial deviation, and the relatively flexed positions of the capitate and hamate present a planar surface to the fully constrained triquetrum. Thus, a bony mortise joint is achieved.

NATURAL HISTORY OF THE DORSALLY FACING INTERCALATED SEGMENT COLLAPSE

The natural history of a dorsally facing intercalated segment collapse consists of the development of osteoarthritis in two characteristic locations, the radial styloid and the lunatocapitate joints. The reason osteoarthritis develops in these locations follows directly from the kinematics previously described. The loss of rotational stability of the proximal carpal row between the scaphoid and the lunate allows the scaphoid to assume an abnormally flexed position. This scaphoid flexion causes the wrist to shorten. This shortening results in ulnar displacement of the lunate and triquetrum on the hamate (Fig. 4–8). The ulnar displacement brings the axis of the lunate palmar to the axis of the capitate, so that compressive forces result in a dorsally facing attitude of the lunate.

As a consequence of the aforementioned events, the force transmission in the wrist is altered. In particular, the acetabular joint for the capitate head is disrupted.

The disruption of the force of the acetab-

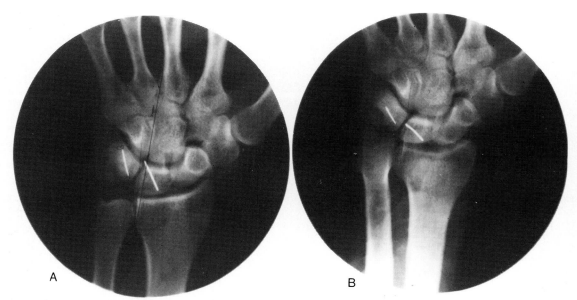

Figure 4–7. Anteroposterior radiographs of the wrist in neutral (*A*) and in full palmar flexion (*B*). Note position of triquetrum relative to the distal radioulnar joint, in its radial migration as the wrist flexes. (From Weber ER: Orthop Clin North Am 15:2, 193–206, 1984.)

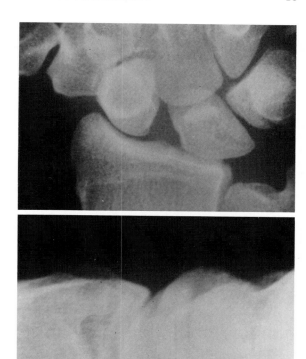

Figure 4–8. Dorsal intercalated segment collapse. Antero-posterior and lateral radiographs of a wrist with a dorsal intercalated segment collapse deformity. Disruption of the rotational stability of the proximal carpal row between the scaphoid and the lunate results in ulnar displacement of the lunate and triquetrum. (From Weber ER: Orthop Clin North Am 15:2, 193–206, 1984.)

ulum results in an abnormal concentration of pressures on the remaining articular surfaces. The lunate and the triquetrum no longer carry their share of the load because compression has displaced them ulnarly. The remaining surface available for load-bearing is the proximal pole of the scaphoid. The concentration of force crossing this articulation exceeds the capacity of the reduced surface area's ability to cope with it, and osteoarthritis results. This leads to the well-described picture of radial styloid osteoarthritis that is associated with this injury.

A secondary area of arthritis develops along the ulnar border of the capitate, which is now articulating with the lunate. This results from abnormal shearing forces on this articulation as the lunate tries to slide medially under the influence of compressive loads.

Repair of these injuries must be aimed at increasing the surface area available for force transmission. This can be partially accomplished by extending the scaphoid and fusing it in this position, such as in the tris-caphe fusion described by Watson.[6] An alternative procedure is to realign the carpus and repair the ligaments between the scaphoid and the lunate. Arthrodesis between the scaphoid and the lunate will completely restore the force-bearing surface. More experience must be gained with this procedure before it can be wholeheartedly recommended.

PATHOGENESIS OF ISOLATED TEARS OF THE LUNATOTRIQUETRAL LIGAMENT

As the wrist is palmar flexed from the neutral position, the angular change between the lunate and the triquetrum measures 8° in the clockwise direction. This increase in excursion is allowed as the radiolunatotriquetral ligament becomes lax. Because of the tightening of the dorsal carpal ligament, the triquetrum is translated up the slope of the hamate to contact the dorsal radial facet. The shape of this facet causes the triquetrum to flex. At the same time, the capitate has achieved a high position in the acetabular joint (Fig. 4–6B), driving the lunate into extension. Loads applied to the back of the hand in this position cause the lunatotriquetral fibers to fail. A characteristic of this injury is that the palmar fibers of the lunatotriquetral joint (that is, the radiolunatotriquetral ligament) are spared because they are carrying a relatively small portion of the load and are stronger than the central and dorsal fibers. The maintenance of these fibers, however, is insufficient to restore rotational integrity, since only one side of the lunatotriquetral joint is maintained. The palmar fibers become the rotational axis of the joint and a palmar intercalated segment collapse results (Fig. 4–9). This is the most common injury affecting the ulnar side of the carpus and can be caused by relatively small forces directed to the dorsum of the hand with the wrist in flexion.

Patients with lunatotriquetral tears complain of a clicking sensation and wrist weakness. The click is reproduced when the wrist is loaded and moved from ulnar to radial deviation. The diagnosis is confirmed by midcarpal arthrography. Leakage of contrast material between the midcarpal and proximal carpal rows, with a palmarly facing attitude of the lunate, is diagnostic of disruption between the lunate and the triquetrum. This injury rarely progresses to arthritis because the major force-bearing joints of the wrist remain intact.

Treatment of this condition is the re-establishment of the rotational integrity of the proximal row. This may be achieved by

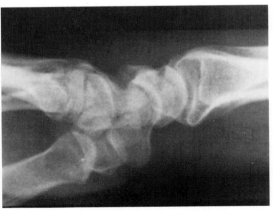

Figure 4–9. Palmar intercalated segment instability. Lateral radiograph of a wrist with a palmar intercalated segment instability deformity. This deformity is produced by disruption of the rotational stability of the proximal carpal row between the lunate and the triquetrum. Shortening of the carpal unit is accompanied by scaphoid flexion. Because interosseous ligaments between the scaphoid and the lunate are intact, scaphoid flexion and lunate flexion occur together and a palmar-facing lunate results. (From Weber ER: Orthop Clin North Am 15:2, 193–206, 1984.)

arthrodesis or capsulodesis of the lunatotriquetral joint. When performing arthrodesis, care must be taken to preserve the spatial relationships of the bones of the carpus. Excising the joint and fixing the bones together will decrease the volume of the concavity of the proximal row, leading to osteoarthritis of the tip of the hamate.

NONDISSOCIATIVE INSTABILITY

This entity is defined as the loss of stability of the proximal row of the carpus without disruption of the ligaments within the proximal carpal row. The proximal row usually assumes the palmar flexed attitude. Occasionally, dorsiflexed posture is seen. If the patient presents with the dorsal-facing lunate, no gap between scaphoid and lunate can be detected.

The angular measurements between the bones of the proximal row remain within normal ranges because no damage to the interosseous ligaments has occurred. The causes of nondissociative collapse are multiple, and I doubt that this or any list is exhaustive. So far identified are fractures of the distal radius with change in inclination of the radial articular surface, ulnar plus variance, midcarpal instability, and loss of integrity of the scaphotrapeziotrapezoidal joint.

Distal radial fracture may result in loss of the normal volar inclination of the distal radial articular surface. If the angle of the distal radius exceeds 10 percent of dorsiflexion, normal bone containment of dorsally directed shear forces is lost. Compressive loading of the carpus will result in dorsal displacement of the lunate to the extent allowed by the palmar capsular constraints. If the amount of displacement is sufficient to allow the axis of the lunate to rise above the axis of the capitate, then palmar flexion of the lunate will result. The same mechanism is present for the proximal pole of the scaphoid. If both the lunate and the scaphoid palmar flex, the wrist reaches a new state of entropy through shortening. If the ligaments are complaint, this state may become permanent. The result is the commonly observed fixed palmar flexion intercalated segmental instability (PISI) associated with distal radial fracture. Rupture or partial damage to the radioscapholunate and ulnolunate ligaments may contribute to this deformity, but I do not believe that they are an essential part of the mechanism.

Dorsal intercalated segment instability (DISI) with distal radial fractures is, I believe, the result of damage to the ligaments stabilizing the midcarpal joint. These ligaments, the radiocapitate and the hamatotriquetral, each keep the capitate from rising dorsally. If they are stretched or divided, the capitate migrates dorsally, causing the lunate and the scaphoid to extend. Again, this posture becomes permanent as a new state of entropy is achieved. I believe that stretching or division of the hamatotriquetral ligament is the key in this injury, since division of the radiocapitate ligament alone allows the capitate to migrate dorsally only in maximal ulnar deviation.

Midcarpal instability results from the attenuation of the ligaments stabilizing the hamatotriquetral joint. There are a dorsal and a volar ligament oriented at 90° to the plane of motion of this joint; hence, they are true collateral ligaments. The palmar ligament appears to be much stronger than the dorsal ligament. These ligaments are reinforced by the ulnar wrist tendons. These tendons are sufficient to compensate for the absence of the hamatocapitate complex in most circumstances. If concomitant synovitis of the midcarpal joint prevents the normal functioning of these tendons, a collapse of the proximal row into palmar flexion may occur when the wrist is in neutral deviation. As the wrist is ulnarly deviated, a "clunking" reduction results from the normal tendency of the triquetrum to assume its low dorsiflexed position as it rides ulnarly on the hamate. Strong, active ulnar wrist flexor and extensor tendons usually correct any functional loss resulting from this condition.

The last condition in the nondissociative category is caused by laxity of the ligaments. My experimental studies checking the flexion of the distal pole of the scaphoid indicate that this joint is normally passive insofar as scaphoid flexion and extension are concerned. It does function to limit the amount of flexion that the scaphoid undergoes. If these restraints are weakened, the scaphoid will assume a more flexed attitude, allowing the capitate to assume a more palmar position relative to the lunate and the proximal pole. Patients with this condition present with wrist synovitis. The diagnosis is made on lateral x-rays with the wrist in radial and ulnar deviation. On these views, it can be seen that, in ulnar deviation, the lunate is in a neutral to slightly dorsiflexed attitude instead of its normal, noticeably dorsiflexed

position. In radial deviation, the lunate is in a marked palmar flexed attitude instead of the normal neutral to slight palmar flexion. Hence, the rotation of the proximal row is intact but now displays its range of motion at a new state of entropy allowed by the abnormal flexion of the scaphoid. The flexor carpi radialis (FCR) tendon seems to play a key role in this entity and, like midcarpal instability, this condition can often be improved by strengthening the FCR muscle tendon unit.

PARTIAL TEARS

The final entity is that of partial tears of the interosseous ligaments. These include partial tears of the lunotriquetral and the scapholunate ligaments as well as tears of the triangular fibrocartilage. Partial tears of the lunotriquetral and scapholunate ligaments cause an abnormal amount of flexion about a vertical axis drawn through the joint involved. This instability is expressed in synovitis with use of the wrist and in the feeling of wrist insecurity. Patients often comment that the wrist "just doesn't feel right." There is no instability pattern displayed on x-ray films. The diagnosis is established by midcarpal arthrography with videotape storage of the passage of the dye between the midcarpal and proximal carpal rows. Suturing of these partial tears shortly after injury results in resolution of the symptoms.

The most common tear of the triangular fibrocartilage is one that is located near or at the radial attachment. The tear is oriented in a dorsal to volar direction and does not include either the dorsal or the volar ligamentous portions of the triangular fibrocartilage complex. This tear also results in wrist synovitis that is occasionally associated with chondromalacia of the lunate, triquetrum, or head of the ulna. In my experience, the symptom of diffuse wrist pain is present and is only resolved after surgical correction.

Ulnar recession appears to be the key surgical procedure in correcting this entity. I also repair the tear in the TFC by direct suture; aggressive excision is not recommended and will often worsen the patient's symptoms by creating ulnocarpal instability.

Wrist synovitis is a symptom of all partial tears. These injuries do not appear to progress to frank osteoarthritis, but they are disabling to the patient whose work or lifestyle requires heavy use of the wrists.

SUMMARY

A kinematic model of the wrist has been presented. The basis for this model is the control of the proximal carpal row provided by the hamatotriquetral articulation. Many of the heretofore confusing patterns of wrist sprains may now be seen to follow logically, when viewed with an understanding of kinematic linkage. It is my hope that this knowledge will lead to new therapies for the treatment of these troublesome injuries.

References

1. Dobyns J, Linscheid R, Chao E, et al: Traumatic instability of the wrist. Instructional Course Lectures 24:182–199, 1975.
2. Gilford WW, Bolton RH, and Lambrinudi G: The mechanism of the wrist joint with special reference to fractures of the scaphoid. Guy's Hospital Report 92:529, 1943.
3. Mayfield JK: Mechanism of carpal injuries. Clin Orthop 149:45–54, 1980.
4. Taleisnik J: Post-traumatic carpal instability. Clin Orthop 149:73–82, 1980.
5. Taleisnik J: The ligaments of the wrist. J Hand Surg 1:110–118, 1976.
6. Watson HK: Limited wrist arthrodesis. Clin Orthop 149:126–137, 1980.
7. Weber ER, and Chao EY: An experimental approach to the mechanism of scaphoid waist fracture. J Hand Surg 3:142, 1978.
8. Weber ER: Biomechanical implications of scaphoid waist fractures. Clin Orthop 149:83–90, 1980.
9. Youm Y, and Flatt A: Kinematics of the wrist. Clin Orthop 149:21–32, 1980.

CHAPTER 5

Pathogenesis of Wrist Ligament Instability

JACK K. MAYFIELD, M.D., M.S., F.A.C.S.

Carpal instability represents persistent carpal bone malalignment, primarily as a result of ligamentous injury. A spectrum of ligamentous damage is now recognized, and various patterns of carpal instability have been elucidated.

In 1943, Gilford and associates were the first to recognize carpal instabiltity. They described the carpus as a link mechanism, with the scaphoid serving as the link between the proximal and the distal carpal rows. A disturbance of this connecting rod (the scaphoid) led to longitudinal carpal collapse. They noted that this phenomenon occurred primarily as a result of scaphoid fractures. Fisk[12] later described this same phenomenon of intercarpal instability as a "concertina deformity." He also recognized this instability pattern in other conditions, such as Kienböck's disease. This longitudinal collapse of the carpus is well recognized on a lateral roentgenogram, and the associated scaphoid instability has been well described by various authors, using terms such as scaphoid subluxation, rotational subluxation, and so forth.*

Linscheid and associates[27] later described a frequently observed post-traumatic intercarpal instability collapse deformity. Their classification was based primarily on the capitolunate angle seen on lateral roentgenograms. They described two basic patterns: dorsal intercalary segment instability, or DISI deformity (Fig. 5–1), and volar intercalary segment instability, or VISI deformity (Fig. 5–2). In their observations and analyses, they found that these collapse defor-

mities of the carpus were due directly to the loss of various ligamentous restraints.

The concept of progressive ligamentous damage with progressive loading was described by Mayfield and associates.[29] Increased degrees of perilunar instability were noted with increased degrees of ligamentous damage. The degrees of associated perilunar instability were described in Stages I to IV. Taleisnik,[44] in addition, described the direct relationship between various patterns of carpal instability and overt wrist ligament tears or attenuation or relaxation of these ligaments.

Until recently, attention in the literature has been focused principally on describing patterns of radiocarpal instability (perilunar and scapholunate instabilities). Lichtman and coworkers[1, 25, 26] described the phenomenon of midcarpal instability and the implications of ulnar carpal instability patterns.

The mechanism of carpal injuries has been a subject of considerable controversy. Although some authors have suggested that hyperflexion is an important mechanism,[12, 15] many authors consider hyperextension to be the major mechanical factor leading to these injuries.* Many authors have been impressed with the wide spectrum of injuries that seem to occur about the carpus (perilunate and lunate dislocations; scaphoid fractures; trans-scaphoid perilunate fracture-dislocations; radial styloid, triquetral, and, occasionally, capitate fractures). Logically, it would seem unlikely that a single mechanism such as hyperextension could account for such a variety of fractures

---

*References 2, 3, 7–10, 18, 19, 22, 43, 44.

*References 12, 20, 27, 40, 43, 46–48, 50.

53

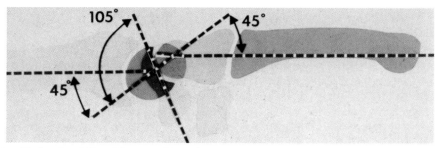

Figure 5–1. Dorsiflexion instability. Diagram of lateral roentgenogram of the wrist showing dorsiflexion of the lunate relative to the radius, a scapholunate angle of 105°, and palmar flexion of the capitate relative to the lunate of 45°. (From Linscheid RL, et al: J Bone Joint Surg 54A:1615, 1972.)

and dislocations. For this reason, investigators have looked for additional mechanisms.

Tanz[43] suggested that a rotational component might be important in perilunar dislocations. He considered lunate dislocations a result of compression, dorsiflexion, ulnar deviation, and pronation. He thought that perilunate dislocations were a result of the same mechanics, with the exception that supination, rather than pronation, of the hand was involved.

Explanations of the mechanism of scaphoid fractures have also been controversial. Fisk suggested that extension and ulnar deviation were the principal mechanical components.[12] Squire[42] was convinced that forced radial deviation would fracture the scaphoid over the tip of the radial styloid. Verdan and Narakis showed that pronation and supination cause shearing forces at the scaphoid waist,[47] implying that a rotational load would create shear stress in the scaphoid, leading to fracture, as suggested by Gilford and associates.[15] Recent experimental investigations[21, 50] have shown that the scaphoid can be fractured in cadaver specimens by hyperextension and ulnar deviation. Until recently, knowledge of the mechanism of trans-scaphoid perilunate fracture-dislocations has been only speculative, although Fisk was convinced that supination caused dorsal dislocation of the capitate.[12]

In 1974, Johnson and associates were able to create these complex injuries in fresh cadaver specimens with extension, ulnar deviation, and a rotational component, i.e., supination.[21]

In addition to scaphoid fractures and perilunate dislocations, other associated injuries are frequent. Many authors have noted the association of radial and ulnar styloid fractures with carpal injuries.[5, 7, 9, 49] The association of triquetral fractures with scaphoid fractures has been reported by Bartone and Grieco,[4] and Borgeskov and colleagues.[6]

It is well known clinically that various carpal instability patterns are a result of previous carpal dislocations.[7–9, 12, 26–31, 34, 46] However, the pathomechanics of scaphoid subluxation and instability are largely unknown.

Since it has been difficult to identify a single planar mechanism as the cause of the many types of carpal injuries, recent investigations have focused on a three-dimensional mechanical concept to explain the pathogenesis of these enigmatic injuries.[21, 29, 30]

As our knowledge of carpal instability increases, we see that the role of the wrist ligaments in the development of this condition is exceedingly important. In order to understand the multitude of instability patterns that can develop with various combi-

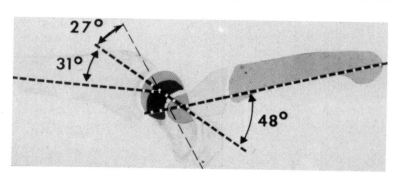

Figure 5–2. Palmar flexion instability. Diagram of lateral roentgenogram showing palmar flexion of the lunate, relative to the radius, of 31°, a scapholunate angle of 27° (somewhat less than normal), and dorsiflexion of the capitate, relative to the lunate, of 48°. (From Linscheid RL, et al: J Bone Joint Surg 54A:1615, 1972.)

nations and degrees of ligamentous damage, a fundamental knowledge of wrist anatomy and wrist ligament biomechanics is essential.

WRIST LIGAMENT ANATOMY[30]

Descriptive Anatomy

The intimate relationship between the carpal bones and the distal radius and ulna is maintained in all planes of motion by a complex arrangement of ligaments. Three types of ligaments are present across the wrist joint: intercarpal, capsular, and intracapsular.[30, 45]

The dorsal radiocarpal ligament is a thickening of the dorsal wrist capsule.[14, 16, 17, 41] It originates from the dorsal lip of the radial styloid process, passes obliquely across the dorsal surface of the lunate, to which it is also attached, and terminates in the dorsal aspect of the triquetrum. It also has connections to the hamate, but the major portion of this ligament is directed into the dorsal triquetrum (Fig. 5–3).

The proximal and distal rows of carpal bones are united by dorsal and volar intercarpal ligaments and by interosseous intercarpal ligaments.[17, 41]

The main functional ligaments of the wrist joint are volar and intracapsular.* In a func-

*References 24, 29, 30, 32–34, 45, 46.

tional sense, the complex intercarpal motion in radial and ulnar deviation and in dorsiflexion and volar flexion is dependent upon the specific arrangement and integrity of these volar intracapsular ligaments.

The volar or palmar radiocarpal ligament (lig. radiocarpeum palmare) is a large, thick intracapsular ligament seen only after the capsule is meticulously dissected from the volar aspect of the wrist or after the wrist joint is opened dorsally and the wrist is volar flexed (Figs. 5–4 and 5–5). This ligament is divided into three separate discrete ligaments, the first connecting the radius with the capitate (distal carpal row), the second connecting the radius with the triquetrum (proximal carpal row), and the third connecting the distal radius to the proximal scaphoid. The radiocapitate ligament (pars radiocapitate), the smaller and weaker of the first two, originates from the volar aspect of the radial styloid process, traverses a groove in the waist of the scaphoid, and terminates in the center of the volar aspect of the capitate body (Fig. 5–4). The second ligamentous band is thick and tendinous in appearance and is the strongest of the volar intracapsular ligaments. This volar radiotriquetral ligament (pars radiotriquetral) originates from the volar aspect of the radial styloid process next to the radiocapitate ligament and, acting as a sling, passes under the lunate (to which it is also attached) and

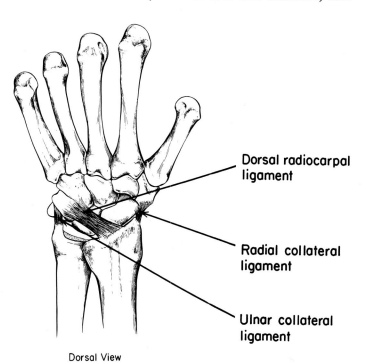

Figure 5–3. Dorsal view of the wrist joint. DRC = Dorsal radiocarpal ligament. (From Mayfield JK, et al: Anat Rec 186:417–428, 1976.)

Dorsal radiocarpal ligament

Radial collateral ligament

Ulnar collateral ligament

Dorsal View

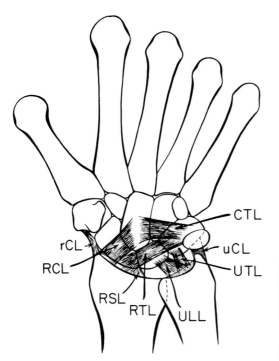

Figure 5–4. Volar view of the wrist joint: Intracapsular ligaments. Lig. radiocarpeum palmare: RCL = pars radiocapitate; RTL = pars radiotriquetral; RSL = pars radioscaphoid. Lig. ulnocarpeum palmare: ULL = pars ulnolunate; UTL = pars ulnotriquetral. Lig. intercarpea palmaria; CTL = pars capitotriquetral.

Volar view of the wrist joint: Capsular collateral ligaments. rCL = lig. collaterale carpi radiale; uCL = lig. collateral carpi ulnare. (From Mayfield JK, et al: J Hand Surg 5:226–241, 1980.)

terminates in the volar surface of the triquetrum (Figs. 5–4 and 5–5).

The separation of the radiocapitate ligament from the volar radiotriquetral ligament (the space of Poirier) over the volar aspect of the capitolunate joint was evident in many of the specimens[30, 38] (Figs. 5–6A and 5–6B). The significance of this interligamentous space became evident when carpal motion was later evaluated and after experimentally injured wrists were studied. A volar intracapsular ligament that was di-

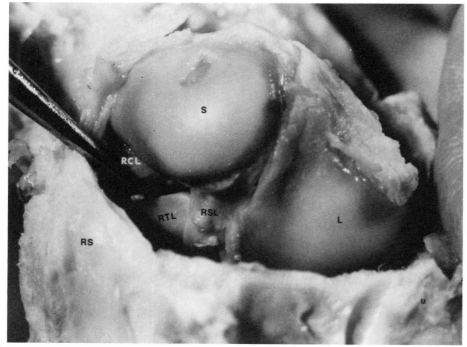

Figure 5–5. Intra-articular view of the radiocarpal joint. S = scaphoid; L = lunate; RS = radial styloid; u = ulna; RCL = radiocapitate ligament; RTL = radiotriquetral ligament; RSL = radioscaphoid ligament.

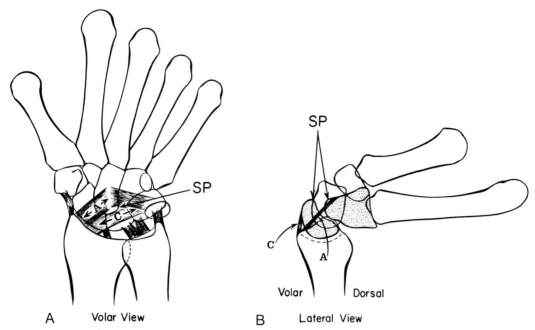

A   Volar View   B   Lateral View

Figure 5–6. *A,* Space of Poirier, volar view. A = radiocapitate ligament; C = radiotriquetral ligament; SP = space of Poirier. *B,* Space of Poirier, lateral view. A = radiocapitate ligament; C = radiotriquetral ligament; SP = space of Poirier. (From Mayfield JK, et al: Anat Rec 186:417–428, 1976.)

rected into the proximal pole of the scaphoid was consistently found. This ligament (the radioscaphoid ligament) actually originates from the volar surface of the radial styloid process ulnar to the radiotriquetral ligament and is directed vertically to terminate in the proximal volar pole of the scaphoid (Figs. 5–4 and 5–5). It also has some small attachments to the volar aspect of the lunate, hence it is also known as the radioscapholunate ligament. It is classified as the third portion of the palmar radiocarpal ligament. The major portion (pars radioscaphoid) is separate from the interosseous intercarpal ligament connecting the scaphoid to the lunate.

Sectioning of the scapholunate interosseous intercarpal ligament did not allow the scaphoid to separate from the lunate; only after additional sectioning of the stabilizing radioscaphoid ligament from the scaphoid did it separate from the lunate on volar flexion and ulnar deviation. The size of the radioscaphoid ligament varied (it was frequently very large and massive), but it was consistently present.

A significant palmar intercarpal ligament, the capitotriquetral ligament (pars capitotriquetral) is only evident after the overlying capsule is dissected away. It is directed from the volar surface of the center of the capitate body across the volar surface of the hamate, to terminate in the volar surface of the tri-

quetrum (Fig. 5–4). This ligament is also known as the ulnar arm of the arcuate or deltoid ligament.

Ligamentous stabilization on the ulnar side of the wrist, in addition to the ulnar collateral ligament, is formed by the intracapsular ulnocarpal ligament. This is a thick, discrete ligament that originates from the volar aspect of the intra-articular triangular wrist meniscus and actually divides and continues in two separate directions, one to the lunate (pars ulnolunate) and the other to the triquetrum (pars ulnotriquetral) (Fig. 5–4).

This descriptive analysis of the wrist ligaments forms a model that is useful in the functional analysis of the wrist joint. These ligaments resemble parts of a puzzle, each having little significance alone, but when combined to form a unit, they become the basis of carpal motion.

The Ligamentous Anatomy of the Scapholunate Joint

Since fractures of the scaphoid are a common source of wrist instabilities, the scaphoid's ligamentous connections to the lunate and to the proximal carpal row have great significance.

In dissections of 34 cadaver wrists, Nash and Mayfield[36] were able to differentiate the

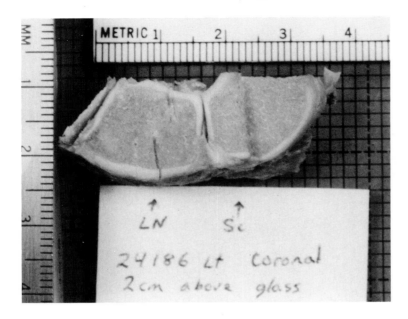

Figure 5–7. Cross section of scapholunate joint. Note triangular shape and peripheral position of the scapholunate interosseous ligament. LN = lunate; SC = scaphoid.

intricate ligamentous attachments of this joint. In their dissections, they found that the scapholunate interosseous ligament is triangular in cross section, occupying nearly one third of the articular surface of this joint (Fig. 5–7), and is peripherally attached at the joint (Fig. 5–8). A portion of the innermost aspect of the ligament is not attached to the bone but is free in the joint (Fig. 5–8). The fibers of the scapholunate interosseous ligament run in several directions. The fibers at the dorsum of the joint run transversely or perpendicular to the joint and form a thick bundle that is tendinous in appearance. The fibers of the peripheral portion of the ligament run peripherally and obliquely along the arc of the joint from the scaphoid downward to the lunate. The volar portion of the ligament runs obliquely between the volar aspects of the lunate and the scaphoid (Fig. 5–9). The orientation of these fibers is such that they allow mobility of the volar aspect of the joint about a fixed dorsal axis.[23, 36] In addition to the three portions of the scapholunate interosseous ligament, the volar aspect of the proximal pole of the scaphoid and, to a lesser extent, the lunate are stabilized to the distal radius by the radioscaphoid ligament (Figs. 5–5 and 5–9).[30, 45] In some specimens, the volar radiotriquetral ligament (VRT) also had some fibrous attachments to the proximal inferior pole of the scaphoid (Fig. 5–9).

This unique arrangement of the directions of the fibers occurs in the three portions of the scapholunate interosseous ligament and,

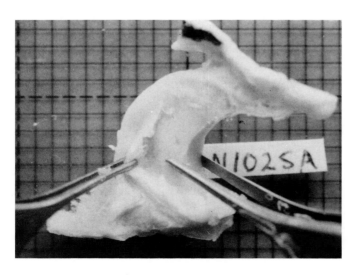

Figure 5–8. Intra-articular view of scapholunate joint, lunate side. Note peripheral aspect of interosseous ligament and dorsal thickening of the interosseous ligament. Tweezers are holding back loose portion of the ligament.

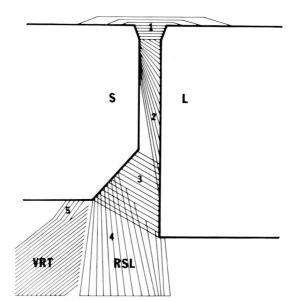

Figure 5–9. Drawing showing the direction of the fibers of the ligaments that stabilize the scapholunate joint. (Scapholunate interosseous ligament consists of portions 1,2, and 3.) S = scaphoid; L = lunate; RSL = radioscaphoid ligament; VRT = volar radiotriquetral ligament.

in conjunction with the radioscaphoid ligament, allows for certain movements at this joint. The joint is basically hinged at the dorsum by the transverse portion of the interosseous ligament, allowing volar opening of the joint[23, 36] (Figs. 5–10 and 5–11). In addition, the scaphoid can rotate on the lunate about a dorsal transverse axis. This fact has significance, since many carpal injuries are initiated by a hyperextension movement causing the scaphoid to rotate dorsally through a dorsal scapholunate axis. Since there is volar mobility at this joint, some of the load can be dissipated. However, if forced extension occurs, then failure of the scapholunate interosseous ligaments begins in the volar region first.[31]

WRIST LIGAMENT BIOMECHANICS

In order to understand the different patterns of injury that can occur in the different wrist ligaments, it is helpful to understand the biomechanics of the wrist ligaments themselves.

Recent investigations[32] using 11 fresh or fresh frozen human wrists have helped elucidate the biomechanical properties of these ligaments. In this study, bone-ligament-bone complexes for each ligament of the wrist were dissected free. The length of all ligaments was measured using an area micrometer with a standardized blade pressure.[51] The ends were mounted in aluminum cups, fixed to an 810 MTS materials testing sys-

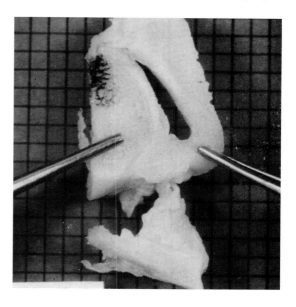

Figure 5–10. Transverse section through the base of the scapholunate joint (the blackened area marks the dorsum of the scaphoid.) Note the mobility of the volar part of this joint.

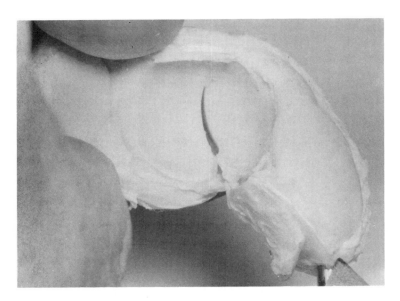

Figure 5–11. Distal view of the intact scapholunate complex with all ligaments attached. The triangle on the right at the bottom of the picture indicates the direction of force being applied to the distal scaphoid pole. Note the volar opening of the scapholunate joint.

tem, and tested in tension to failure with simultaneous graphic recording. Cinematography provided correlative data during ligament elongation and failure. A strain rate of 1 cm/sec was utilized, since a strain rate of 50 to 100 percent of ligament length per second most closely approximates the strain rate of a physiologic injury. The strain rate used for the scapholunate interosseous ligament (SCLN) was 1 mm/sec because of its short length. Histologic analysis with light microscopy was performed on selected ligaments using both hematoxylin and eosin and elastin stains. The results of this study are particularly pertinent.

Failure Location and Mode

The *radiocapitate ligament* failed proximally between the radial styloid and the scaphoid waist in 80 percent of fresh specimens. There were no avulsions.

The *radiotriquetral ligament* failed distally more frequently than proximally, with 56 percent failing between the lunate and the triquetrum. Of the distal failures, four were ligament failures and one was a triquetral avulsion.

When testing the *radiotriquetral attachment to the lunate*, it was found that less than one half of specimens had strong ligamentous insertion, and most of the specimens (55 percent) experienced insertional failure (i.e., the ligament "pulled off" the lunate) with very low forces, averaging 64 newtons. This weak attachment to the lunate

may explain the phenomenon of dorsiflexion instability after hyperextension injuries.

The *radioscaphoid ligament* (RS) failed in its substance in all specimens, the failures being equally divided between proximal and distal ends.

The *dorsal radiocarpal ligament* (DRC) failed at its distal end in 90 percent of the specimens, eight in the ligament and one by triquetral avulsion.

The *scapholunate interosseous ligament* (SCLN) rarely failed in its substance, owing to its remarkable stiffness and strength. In 56 percent of specimens, ligament failure occurred at 359 newtons, and in 44 percent of specimens, bone avulsion or cement failure occurred at 410 newtons.

Tensile Properties

The radiocapitate and radiotriquetral ligaments were found to be approximately the same *length* (30 mm). The radioscaphoid was the shortest of all ligaments, except for the scapholunate interosseous (not shown), which averaged 5.7 mm in length. The dorsal radiocarpal ligament, which is the dorsal proximal row stabilizer, was shorter than its volar mirror image, the radiotriquetral ligament. The ulnar collateral ligament was over twice the length of the radial collateral ligament (Fig. 5–12).

No significant difference was found between the *cross-sectional areas* of the radiocapitate and the radiotriquetral ligaments. The radioscaphoid was the smallest, the dor-

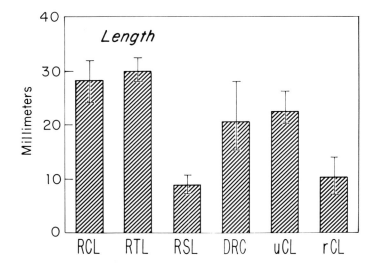

Figure 5–12. The length of the wrist liga-ments. (For abbreviations, see Fig. 5–4.) DRC = dorsal radiocarpal ligament.

sal radiocarpal was smaller than the radio-triquetral, and the ulnar collateral was larger than the radial collateral ligament (Fig. 5–13).

The *maximum force* required for failure of the radiotriquetral ligament was the great-est required for any of the volar intracapsular ligaments, significant at the 0.05 level. On the dorsal aspect of the wrist, the maximum force of 240 newtons for the dorsal radiocar-pal ligament was not significantly different from that for the radiotriquetral ligament. The average radiocapitate ligament failed at 170 newtons, while the distal segment of this ligament required 190 newtons, sup-porting the clinical evidence that in carpal injuries the scaphoid follows the capitate. The radioscaphoid ligament was the weakest of all volar ligaments, failing at 54 newtons.

Of the two collateral ligaments, the radial collateral required the least force (70 new-tons) to reach failure. The scapholunate in-terosseous ligament was the strongest of all ligaments tested in the wrist, with ligament failure occurring at a maximum force of 359 newtons (Fig. 5–14).

Of equal significance is the fact that the scapholunate interosseous ligament was found to be the *stiffest* of all wrist ligaments tested. The radiotriquetral was significantly stiffer than the radiocapitate at the 0.01 sig-nificance level (Fig. 5–15).

The *elastic modulus* of the radioscaphoid ligament was the lowest and that of the dorsal radiocarpal ligament was the highest, suggesting that the dorsal radiocarpal is the least elastic and the radioscaphoid is the most elastic of the carpal ligaments. The

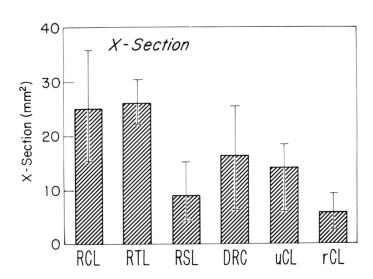

Figure 5–13. The cross-sectional area of the wrist ligaments. (For abbreviations, see Figs. 5–4 and 5–12.)

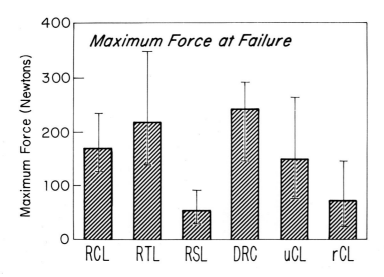

Figure 5–14. The maximum force at failure of the wrist ligament. (For abbreviations, see Fig. 5–4.)

radial collateral ligament was more elastic than the ulnar collateral ligament (Fig. 5–16).

Maximum stress, or tensile strength, is the maximum force per unit cross-sectional area. Of interest, the DRC, or dorsal radiocarpal ligament, had the highest tensile strength, which may explain why lunate dislocations are less frequent than perilunate injuries when this ligament is ruptured (Fig. 5–17).

Maximum strain is the percent elongation at total failure. The two ligaments that elongated the most at failure were the radioscaphoid ligament and the scapholunate interosseous ligament. The scapholunate ligament doubled its length prior to total failure, with a maximum strain of 225 percent. The radioscaphoid ligament lost its continuity at 140 percent strain. The radiocapitate ligament, the distal carpal row stabilizer, had a maximum strain that was significantly

greater than the radiotriquetral ligament at the 0.05 significance level (Fig. 5–18).

Partial Failure

Partial or sequential failure occurred in all ligaments to various degrees. In every ligament filmed, there was evidence of partial failure (ligament elongation), even though the ligaments appeared intact. The RC ligament in particular, was grossly intact at 50 percent, 70 percent, and 80 percent strain, and only at approximately 100 percent strain was total failure evident. The gross continuity of a ligament, therefore, does not always reflect its biomechanical integrity.

Histology

Twenty-two ligaments from 10 fresh wrists were studied by light microscopy using he-

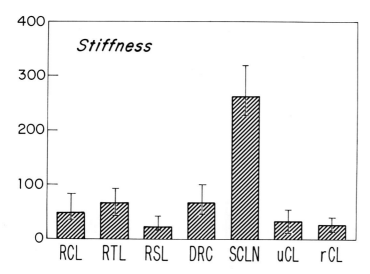

Figure 5–15. The stiffness of the wrist ligaments. (For abbreviations, see Fig. 5–4.) SCLN = scapholunate interosseous ligament.

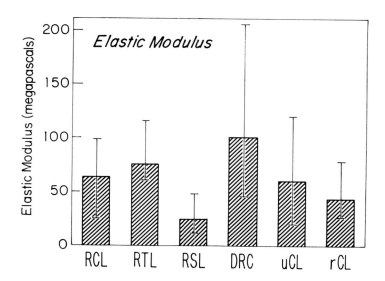

Figure 5–16. The elastic modulus of the wrist ligaments. (For abbreviations, see Fig. 5–4.)

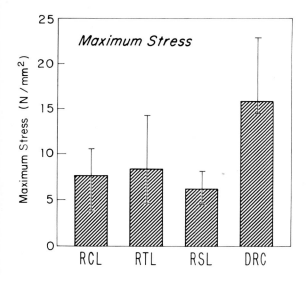

Figure 5–17. The maximum stress of the wrist ligaments. (For abbreviations, see Figure 5–4.)

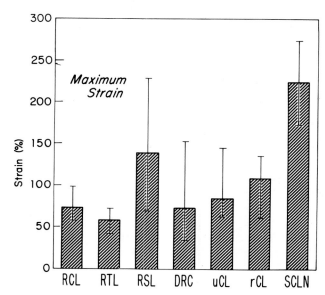

Figure 5–18. The maximum strain of the wrist ligaments. (For abbreviations, see Fig. 5–4.) (From Mayfield J: Orthop Clin North Am 15:2, 209–216, 1984.)

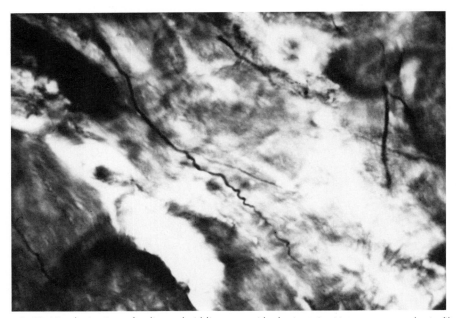

Figure 5–19. Histologic view of radioscaphoid ligament with elastin stain. Note numerous elastin fibers.

matoxylin and eosin and elastin stains.[36] A relative abundance of elastic fibers was noted in the radioscaphoid ligament and less frequently in the scapholunate interosseous ligament. This fact lends itself to speculation concerning the mechanics of the scapholunate articulation, since these two ligaments stabilize this joint, both have high strains at failure, and the radioscaphoid ligament is biomechanically elastic with a very low elastic modulus (Fig. 5–19).

WRIST JOINT KINEMATICS AND CARPAL INJURY

In several studies using sonic digitalization[53] and stereophotography,[11, 37] the apex of carpal rotation in the anteroposterior (AP) plane has been shown to be in the center of the capitate or at the junction of the radiocapitate and the capitotriquetral ligaments.[30]

When the wrist moves from neutral position to maximum extension, the palmar ligaments become progressively more taut and achieve their maximum tautness in complete extension. Movement of the wrist in radial deviation relaxes the radiocapitate ligament. Movement of the wrist in ulnar deviation tightens the radiocapitate ligament (RCL) and relaxes the radiotriquetral ligament (RTL) (Fig. 5–20). When the wrist is progressively extended, an interligamentous space develops palmarly because of the separation of the radiocapitate ligament (RCL)

and the radiotriquetral ligament (RTL). This space overlies the capitolunate joint palmarly and is called the space of Poirier.[29, 30]

It is interesting to note that recent anatomic[36] and kinematic[39] studies have shown that the scapholunate joint has a dorsal axis of rotation (Fig. 5–21). This is particularly pertinent, since most carpal injuries are initiated by hyperextension and intercarpal supination.[33] During impact loading over the thenar eminence, the scaphoid rotates dorsally on the lunate through a dorsal axis of the scapholunate joint. The anatomic arrangement of the fibers of the scapholunate interosseous and radioscaphoid ligaments in turn allows mobility of the volar inferior pole of the scaphoid,[23, 36] which allows the inferior and proximal poles of the scaphoid to rotate about this dorsal axis. The ligamentous fiber orientation of this joint also allows separation of the scaphoid and the lunate at the inferior portion of this joint (Figs. 5–9, 5–10, and 5–11). Mechanically, the scapholunate joint has a specialized design that enhances stability but also allows load-dampening during excessive loads applied to the wrist in hyperextension and intercarpal supination.

The following facts are useful in developing a mechanical concept of carpal injuries: (1) the weakest ligaments of the wrist are on the radial side; (2) the radiocapitate ligament (RCL) is maximally taut in maximum extension and in ulnar deviation; (3)

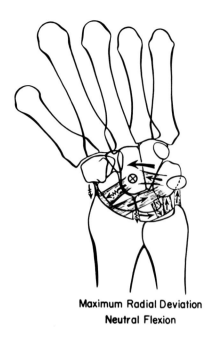
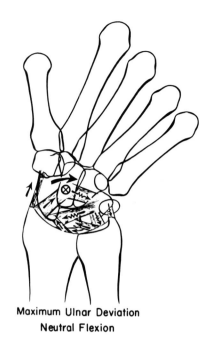

Maximum Radial Deviation
Neutral Flexion

Maximum Ulnar Deviation
Neutral Flexion

⊗ = *axis of AP rotation*

Figure 5–20. Wrist kinematics. → = taut ligament, ⇝ loose ligament. (From Mayfield JK, et al: Anat Rec 186:417–428, 1976.)

the proximal carpal row is stabilized to the distal forearm by five ligaments, whereas the distal carpal row is stabilized to the forearm by only one—the radiocapitate ligament (RCL); (4) the weakest link between the distal carpal row and the distal forearm is the radiocapitate ligament.

MECHANISM OF CARPAL INSTABILITY

Carpal Dislocations

The actual mechanism of injury is difficult, if not impossible, to document in the clinical setting. Not infrequently, however, there is clinical evidence supporting a certain mechanism of injury.

Case 1. A 31-year-old male accountant suffered a hyperextension injury to his *right* wrist when he fell from a diving board. He sustained a dorsal perilunate dislocation and a radial styloid fracture. A large abrasion was noted over the thenar side of his palm in the area of the scaphoid tuberosity.

Case 2. A 25-year-old man sustained a hyperextension injury to his *left* wrist and also a dorsal perilunate dislocation in a motorcycle accident. A large impact abra-

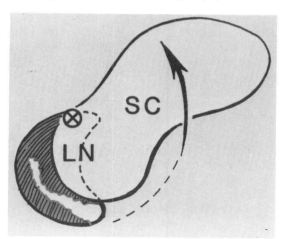

Figure 5–21. Dorsal axis of rotation of the scapholunate joint, side view. Note the volar, interosseous ligament tear. LN = lunate, SC = scaphoid; ⊗ = axis. (From Mayfield JK: Clin Orthop 187:36–42, 1984.)

sion was noted over the thenar aspect of his palm.

These two cases and other similar ones would suggest that hyperextension was an important cause in these dislocations. Forced ulnar deviation and intercarpal supination could also be implicated, since the injuries were on the radial side of the palm. Experimental loading studies have helped to clarify these impressions.

Experimental Loading[29]

MATERIALS AND METHODS

Thirty-two fresh and embalmed cadaver wrists were loaded to failure using two loading machines, one fast loading and gravity-dependent, the other hydraulic and slow loading. The average age of the specimens was 53 years (range 5 to 89 years). All specimens were stripped of soft tissue to within 2 cm of the wrist joint, leaving the interosseous membrane, radius, and ulna intact. They were then cemented in 2-in steel pipes and secured in the loading machines with the wrist extended for various roentgenographic and loading studies. Specimens subjected to fast loading were loaded with an average of 19 kg from an average height of 68 cm. The force plate was placed across the metacarpal heads with the fingers free, and the angles of loading were varied with combinations of extension, extension with ulnar deviation or extension, and ulnar deviation and intercarpal supination (equivalent to pronation of the forearm on the carpus, as observed in actual clinical injuries). Specimens subjected to hydraulic slow loading were positioned in such a way that a 1 cm by 2 cm pressure plate engaged the scaphoid tuberosity in maximum extension. All loading studies included preload radiographs, loading lateral cineradiographs at 60 and 120 frames/sec, and postloading radiographs. All specimens were dissected after loading to assess bony and ligamentous damage and carpal instability.

RESULTS

Thirteen dorsal perilunate dislocations were produced. The mechanism of injury was extension, ulnar deviation, and intercarpal supination in 12 and extension alone in one. Intercarpal supination was a major mechanical component, since all loading was on the radial side of the wrist. All specimens had rupture of the radioscaphoid and scapholu-

nate interosseous ligaments. Scaphoid rotation was noted in six specimens. Two patterns of palmar ligamentous damage were noted.

One pattern was represented by radiocapitate and radial collateral ligament failure and scapholunate ligamentous failure (scapholunate interosseous and radioscaphoid ligaments) with capitate and scaphoid dislocation and opening of the space of Poirier (Fig. 5–22). The other pattern with more severe ligamentous damage had similar findings, except that radiotriquetral ligament failure between lunate and triquetrum was evident with triquetral dislocation (Fig. 5–23).

Two lunate dislocations were also produced, and the pathomechanics were the same as those of most of the perilunate dislocations (extension, ulnar deviation, and intercarpal supination). Scaphoid rotation and scapholunate diastasis were noted in both specimens (Fig. 5–24). The palmar ligamentous damage in the lunate dislocations was the same as that of the severe perilunate dislocation, but, in addition, dorsal radiocarpal ligament failure allowed palmer lunate rotation.

Scaphoid rotation was a direct result of progressive failure of the scapholunate ligamentous complex. Ligamentous failure began in the palmar aspect of the scapholunate joint and progressed dorsally, owing to the intercarpal supination component of the loading mechanics (Fig. 5–25).

Seven radial styloid fractures were produced by avulsion.

Triquetral fractures were associated with perilunate and lunate dislocations in five specimens; their mechanism was by avulsion of either the radiotriquetral (RTL) or the ulnotriquetral ligament (UTL) (Fig. 5–24).

All dislocations had varying degrees of perilunar instability. As the loading forces of extension, intercarpal supination, and ulnar deviation progressed, the scaphoid, capitate, and then the triquetrum were progressively dislocated from the lunate, creating progressive carpal instability. The degree of perilunar instability (PLI) has been divided into four stages, according to the degree of carpal dislocation and ligamentous damage that starts at the scapholunate joint and progresses around the lunate: Stage I PLI— scaphoid dislocation or instability with scapholunate interosseous and radioscaphoid ligament injury; Stage II PLI—capitate

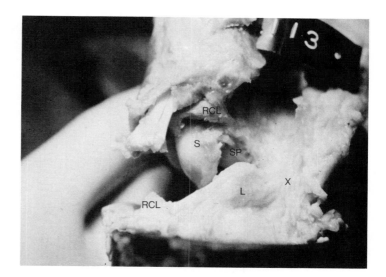

Figure 5–22. Carpal tunnel view of Stage II PLI (perilunar instability) in an experimentally loaded wrist. Notice the scaphoid and capitate dislocations, radiocapitate ligament (RCL) failure, and opening of the space of Poirier (SP). S = scaphoid; L = lunate; X = axis of intercarpal supination. (From Mayfield JK: Clin Orthop 149:49, 1980.)

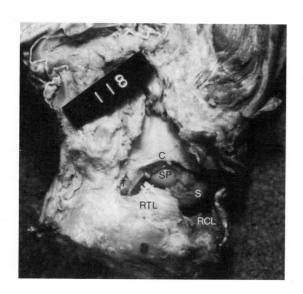

Figure 5–23. Volar view of Stage III PLI in an experimentally loaded wrist. Notice the scaphoid (S), capitate (C), and triquetral (T) dislocations. The space of Poirier (SP) is open wide. The torn ligaments are the radiocapitate (RCL) and the radiotriquetral (RTL) between the lunate and triquetrum. (From Mayfield JK: Clin Orthop 143:45–54, 1980.)

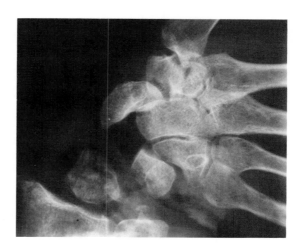

Figure 5–24. Experimentally loaded wrist with Stage IV PLI. The lunate has been reduced. Notice the scaphoid rotation and the triquetral avulsion fracture. (From Mayfield JK: Clin Orthop 149:45–54, 1980.)

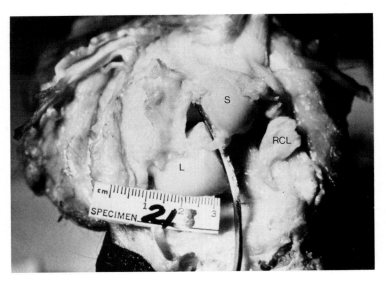

Figure 5–25. Experimentally loaded wrist showing the effects of intercarpal supination (dorsal view). Notice the dorsal rotational dislocation of the scaphoid. Probe is under the remaining portion of the scapholunate interosseous ligament. Notice also the failed radiocapitate ligament (RCL) avulsed from the capitate. S = scaphoid; L = lunate. (From Mayfield JK: Clin Orthop 149:45–54, 1980.)

dislocation and opening of the space of Poirier; Stage III PLI—triquetral dislocation and radiotriquetral ligament failure; Stage IV PLI—RCL, RTL, and dorsal radiocarpal ligament failure with lunate dislocation (Fig. 5–26).

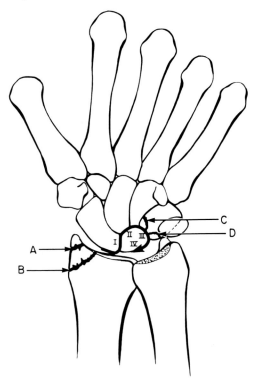

Figure 5–26. Progressive perilunar instability (PLI) Stage I—scapholunate failure; Stage II—capitolunate failure; Stage III—triquetrolunate failure; Stage IV—dorsal radiocarpal ligament failure, allowing lunate rotation volarly. A = radial styloid tip fracture, B = radial styloid body fracture, C = radiotriquetral ligament avulsion, D = ulnotriquetral ligament avulsion. (From Mayfield JK et al: J Hand Surg 5:226–241, 1980.)

Scaphoid Fracture and Fracture-Dislocation

It has been stated for a long time that the scaphoid acts like a connecting rod between the proximal and the distal carpal rows. It is a recognized fact that in most carpal dislocations or fracture-dislocations the scaphoid must either fracture or dislocate from the lunate. Fracture of the waist of the scaphoid is the most common injury to the carpal bones. In reviewing carpal fractures, Borgeskov and coworkers noted that of all carpal fractures, the scaphoid was the bone most frequently fractured (71.2 percent), but, interestingly, the triquetrum was the next most frequently fractured bone (20.4 percent).[6] This association of scaphoid fractures with triquetral fractures has been a clinical curiosity, but the explanations for this association have been speculative. Seventy to 80 percent of scaphoid fractures occur at the waist, with the remainder occurring equally often at the proximal pole and at the tubercle.[12, 28]

Displaced unstable fractures of the scaphoid associated with other carpal fractures and dislocations usually have a poor prognosis. This relationship between scaphoid fractures and perilunar dislocations is well known clinically.* The degree of instability of the scaphoid fracture seems to be directly related to the degree of ligamentous damage and associated perilunar instability, but this has never been documented. Recent experimental work by Johnson and colleagues[21] and Weber and Chao[50] have aided our un-

*References 12, 13, 20, 21, 27, 35, 40, 49.

derstanding of the pathomechanics of these fractures and fracture-dislocations.

Experimental Loading[21]

MATERIALS AND METHODS

Twenty-nine fresh cadaver specimens, including hand, wrist, and forearm, were stripped of soft tissue to within 2 cm of the distal articular surface of the radius and were cemented in steel pipes. Each prepared specimen was placed in a hydraulic machine and secured. A 1 cm by 2 cm pressure plate was positioned over the distal portion of the scaphoid with the wrist in maximum extension. Each wrist was subjected to progressive hydraulic loading. The loading sequence created extension, ulnar deviation, and intercarpal supination. All specimens were obtained fresh and were loaded within 72 hours post mortem. All specimens had preloading radiographs (anteroposterior supination and lateral views, and oblique and lateral views in flexion and extension). The loading sequence was recorded with the use of lateral cineradiography at 120 frames/sec. All wrists were loaded to either bone or ligament failure and then were dissected to assess the bony and ligamentous damage.

RESULTS

Of the twenty-nine wrists loaded, five scaphoid waist fractures, two proximal pole fractures, and six tuberosity fractures were produced. Five scaphoid fractures were associated with Stage I perilunar instability (PLI) and three scaphoid fractures were associated with Stage III PLI. In addition, seven fractures of the distal radius, three of the trapezium, and two of the triquetrum were produced as well as two scaphotrapezial dislocations.

Nonphysiologic hyperextension and ulnar deviation were the primary mechanisms of the scaphoid waist fractures, with the dorsal aspect of the scaphoid engaging the dorsal rim of the radius, thereby creating an anvil effect leading to fracture.

Scaphoid waist fractures were described according to their stability. Type I was stable, not associated with significant ligamentous damage, and could not be displaced with extension, intercarpal supination, ulnar deviation, or distraction. Types II and III were unstable and were associated with moderate to severe degrees of ligamentous damage and perilunar instability (Fig. 5–27).

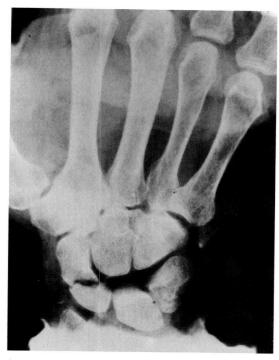

Figure 5–27. Displaced Type III scaphoid waist fracture with Stage III PLI (perilunar fracture-dislocation). Notice the triquetral fracture (avulsion of the UTL ligament). (Courtesy of Roger P. Johnson, M.D.)

They could be displaced with any of the preceding maneuvers and could be reduced by reversing the loading mechanism (i.e., radial deviation, flexion, or intercarpal pronation with compression).

The mechanism of fracture was hyperextension, with the scaphoid fracture beginning on the palmar side and progressing dorsally. In Type I fractures, the dorsal soft-tissue hinge remained intact, and palmar flexion produced fracture stability. Types II and III scaphoid fractures had more severe ligamentous damage and associated carpal instability, and in these, the soft-tissue hinge was lost.

Eight of the 12 scaphoid fractures were associated with varying degrees of perilunar instability as a result of associated ligamentous failure (trans-scaphoid perilunar fracture-dislocations) (Fig. 5–27). Associated ligamentous damage and resultant perilunar instability were a direct result of the rotational component of intercarpal supination. This rotation of the scaphoid, distal carpal row, and triquetrum as a unit about the fixed lunate was also responsible for avulsion fracture of the triquetrum (avulsion of the radiotriquetral and ulnotriquetral ligaments) (Fig. 5–27).

Fractures of the proximal pole of the scaphoid were caused by subluxation of the scaphoid dorsally, before it was fractured over the dorsal rim of the radius. Scaphoid tuberosity fractures were caused by compression forces.

Cineradiography documented failure occurring first on the radial side of the wrist. This failure was either a scaphoid fracture or a scapholunate joint disruption (Stage I PLI) or both. Any further degrees of perilunar instability (Stage III PLI) were a result of intercarpal supination. Virtually all of the scaphoid fractures had some degree of scapholunate interosseous ligament failure. The spectrum stretched from a small tear palmarly to a complete disruption of the ligament.

A SPECTRUM OF WRIST LIGAMENT INJURY

Carpal injuries present a spectrum of bone and ligament damage. The name given to the various injuries (for example, lunate dislocation, perilunate dislocation, scaphoid fracture, trans-scaphoid perilunate fracture-dislocation) only describe the resultant damage apparent on radiographs. Each injury is not a separate entity, but part of a continuum. The character of the final injury is determined by (1) the type of three-dimensional loading, (2) the magnitude and duration of the forces involved, (3) the position of the hand at the time of impact, and (4) the biomechanical properties of the bones and ligaments.

Progressive Perilunar Instability

Impact on the thenar side of the wrist levers the wrist progressively into hyperextension, ulnar deviation, and intercarpal supination.[15, 32] The intercarpal injuries begin at the scapholunate joint and proceed around the lunate, progressively creating ligamentous injury as well as scapholunate, capitolunate, and triquetrolunate instability. In Stage I perilunar instability (PLI), the primary instability is limited to the scapholunate joint. In Stage II PLI, there is also ligamentous damage at the capitolunate articulation, and in Stage III PLI, ligamentous damage at the triquetrolunate joint is added to the preceding damage (Fig. 5–26).[15]

In Stage IV PLI, dorsal disruption of the dorsal radiocarpal ligament (as a result of intercarpal supination) allows the lunate to rotate volarly on its volar radiotriquetral and ulnolunate ligamentous hinge. In Stages I and II PLI, spontaneous reduction of the capitolunate and triquetrolunate joints frequently occurs as the wrist recoils from injury. In this situation, persistent scapholunate diastasis may be the only manifestation of these more severe injuries. In Stage IV PLI (lunate dislocation), the roentgenographic manifestations are more obvious. Experimental and clinical investigations[29, 33] have also shown that the spectrum of carpal instability previously described can also be expected and can be associated with scaphoid and capitate fractures as well as avulsion fractures of the radial and ulnar styloid processes and of the triquetrum.

Scapholunate Instability

Patients frequently complain of persistent pain over the radial aspect of the wrist joint after various hyperextension injuries of this joint. If scapholunate diastasis is present with or without stress roentgenograms, then the diagnosis is clear. However, in many cases no appreciable scapholunate diastasis can be clinically documented. This can be explained by two distinct types of incomplete ligamentous injury that occur at this joint.

In the first type, limited volar interosseous and radioscaphoid ligament failure occurs. Studies by Kauer[23] and Nash and Mayfield[36] have substantiated that the axis of motion of the scapholunate joint is in the dorsal part of the joint. Some wrist injuries can be associated with an intact dorsal interosseous ligament, along with volar interosseous ligament disruptions, since the scaphoid rotates on the lunate through the dorsal axis of this joint. I have verified this surgically in patients who had chronic wrist pain after a hyperextension injury.[31] Scapholunate diastasis was not present on stress roentgenograms[31] (Fig. 5–21) (Case 1).

In the second type of limited scapholunate ligamentous injury, elongation of the scapholunate interosseous and the radioscaphoid ligaments occurs without complete ligament failure. Experimental studies[32] have documented sequential elongation of these ligaments prior to failure (Fig. 5–18). This phenomenon has been substantiated in my clinical practice; such ligament elongation leads to varying degrees of persistent scapholunate instability (Fig. 5–28).

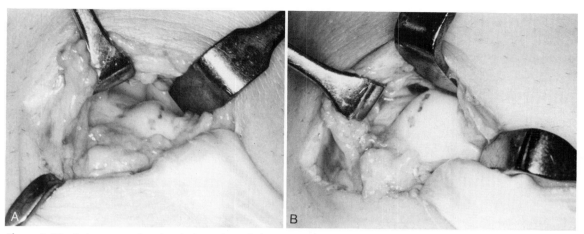

Figure 5–28. A, Intra-operative dorsal view of scapholunate joint. Note the step-off at this point. B, Surgeon is pushing longitudinally on the thumb, causing marked increase in the degree of step-off at the scapholunate joint. (From Mayfield JK: Orthop Clin North Am 15:215, 1984.)

The syndrome of chronic wrist pain located about the scapholunate joint associated with various degrees of scapholunate instability remains a common and vexing problem.

Anatomic studies by Kauer[23] and unpublished data of Nash[35] have demonstrated the relative hypermobility of the volar aspect of the scapholunate joint. Biomechanical studies[32] have verified the relative weakness and elasticity of the radioscaphoid ligament. This information suggests that the weakest ligamentous attachments at this joint are volar. Since the axis of rotation of this joint is dorsal, wrist hyperextension is accommodated to some degree by this volar scapholunate mobility. Conversely, in extremes of extension and intercarpal supination, this area will be the first to tear. This subtle finding has been verified clinically in the following case.

Case 1. A 22-year-old student was evaluated for chronic wrist pain after sustaining an extension injury a year earlier. Clinically, his pain was localized to the scapholunate joint area. Stress roentgenograms in ulnar deviation and extension under fluoroscopic control revealed only a minimal incongruity of the midcarpal scapholunate joint surfaces, which suggested mild instability. Surgical exploration verified a complete tear of the volar aspect of the scapholunate interosseous ligament. The dorsal aspect of the ligament was intact (Fig. 5–21).[32]

The preceding case suggests that a spectrum of ligament injury may be present at the scapholunate joint in Stage I perilunar instability. The earliest injury begins with a partial volar scapholunate interosseous ligament tear that proceeds to complete failure, or it could begin by ligament elongation that proceeds to complete failure.

It is the impression of this author that many patients plagued by chronic wrist pain similar to this type have partial interosseous ligament failure with volar tears or ligament elongation associated with minor degrees of scapholunate instability.

SUMMARY

The mechanism responsible for carpal injuries is elusive. Direct results of the inability to identify the mechanism clinically include a confusing system of classification and the lack of a rational plan of treatment for the many fractures and fracture-dislocations that occur about the carpus. The mechanism of injury determined experimentally was three-dimensional, including extension, ulnar deviation, and intercarpal supination. The resultant spatial vector, in conjunction with the magnitude and duration of loading, determined the combination of injuries produced. Carpal dislocations resulted from a force vector that emphasized ulnar deviation and intercarpal supination. Scaphoid fractures were produced by a vector that emphasized extension, and these bones were fractured by the dorsal rim of the radius. The degrees of carpal instability produced experimentally were divided into four stages, depending upon the amount of ligamentous damage and joint instability present. Stage I (scapholunate instability) was the most stable, and Stage IV (lunate dislocation) was the least stable. Scaphoid fractures started on the palmar surface and progressed dorsally. Type I fractures had an intact dorsal soft-tissue hinge, and fracture stability could be created by flexion. Types II and III scaphoid fractures were associated with significant perilunar instability (PLI) and were classified as fracture-dislocations.

References

1. Alexander CE, and Lichtman DM: Ulnar carpal instabilities. Orthop Clin North Am 15:307–320, 1984.
2. Andrews FT: A dislocation of the carpal bones—the scaphoid and the semilunar: report of a case. Mich Med 31:269–271, 1932.
3. Armstrong BWD: Rotational subluxation of the scaphoid. Can J Surg 11:306–314, 1968.
4. Bartone NF, and Grieco RV: Fractures of the triquetrum. J Bone Joint Surg 38A:353, 1956.
5. Bonnin JG, and Greening WP: Fractures of the triquetrum. Br J Surg 31:278, 1943.
6. Borgeskov S, Christiansen B, Kjaer A, et al: Fractures of the carpal bones. Acta Orthop Scand 37:276, 1966.
7. Campbell RD Jr, Lance EM, and Yeoh CB: Lunate and perilunar dislocations. J Bone Joint Surg 46B:55–72, 1964.
8. Campbell RD Jr, Thompson TC, Lance EM, et al: Indications for open reduction of lunate and perilunate dislocations of the carpal bones. J Bone Joint Surg 47A:915–937, 1965.
9. Destot E: Injuries of the Wrist, A Radiographic Study. New York, Paul B Koeker Co, 1926.
10. England JPS: Subluxation of the carpal scaphoid. Proc R Soc Lond, 63:581–582, 1970.
11. Erdman AG, Mayfield JK, Dorman F, et al: Kinematic and kinetic analysis of the human wrist by stereoscopic instrumentation. 1978 Advances in Bioengineering, American Society of Mechanical Engineers, 1978, pp 79–82.
12. Fisk G: Carpal instability and the fractured scaphoid. Ann R Coll Surg Engl 46:63–76, 1970.
13. Friedenberg ZB: Anatomic considerations in the treatment of carpal navicular fractures. Am J Surg 78:379, 1949.
14. Gardner EE, Gray J, and O'Rahilly R: Anatomy. 3rd ed. WB Saunders Co, Philadelphia, 1969, pp 160–163.
15. Gilford W, Bolton R, and Lambrinudi C: The mechanism of the wrist joint. Guy's Hospital Report 92:52–59, 1943.
16. Grant JCB: An Atlas of Anatomy. 5th ed. Williams & Wilkins, Baltimore, 1962, plates 90–94.
17. Goss CM: Gray's Anatomy of the Human Body. 29th ed. Lea & Febiger, Philadelphia, 1973, pp 333–336.
18. Green DP, and O'Brian ET: Classification and management of carpal dislocations. Clin Orthop 149:55–72, 1980.
19. Howard FM, Fahey T, and Wojcik E: Rotatory subluxation of the navicular. Clin Orthop 104:134, 1974.
20. Hill NA: Fractures and dislocations of the carpus. Orthop Clin North Am 1:275, 1970.
21. Johnson RP, Mayfield JK, and Kilcoyne RF: Scaphoid fractures and fracture-dislocations—pathomechanics and perilunar instability. (Unpublished study, 1974.)

22. Johnson RP: The acutely injured wrist and its residuals. Clin Orthop 149:33–44, 1980.
23. Kauer JMG: The interdependence of carpal articulation chains. Acta Anat 88:481, 1974.
24. Lewis OJ, Hamshere RJ, and Bucknill TM: The anatomy of the wrist joint. J Anat 106:539–552, 1970.
25. Lichtman DM, et al: Dynamic triquetrolunate instability: case report. J Hand Surg 9:186, 1984.
26. Lichtman DM, Schneider JR, Swofford AR, et al: Ulnar midcarpal instability—clinical and laboratory analysis. J Hand Surg 6:515–523, 1981.
27. Linscheid RL, Dobyns JH, Beabout JW, et al: Traumatic instability of the wrist. Diagnosis, classification, and pathomechanics. J Bone Joint Surg 54A:1612–1632, 1972.
28. London PS: The broken scaphoid bone. J Bone Joint Surg 43B:237, 1961.
29. Mayfield JK, Johnson RP, and Kilcoyne RK: Carpal dislocations: pathomechanics and progressive perilunar instability. J Hand Surg 5:226–241, 1980.
30. Mayfield JK, Johnson RP, and Kilcoyne RF: The ligaments of the human wrist and their functional significance. Anat Rec 186:417–428, 1976.
31. Mayfield JK: Patterns of injury to carpal ligaments. A spectrum. Clin Orthop 187:36–42, 1984.
32. Mayfield JK, Williams WJ, Erdman AG, et al: Biomechanical Properties of Human Carpal Ligaments. Orthop Trans 3:143, 1979.
33. Mayfield JK: Mechanism of carpal injuries. Clin Orthop 149:45–54, 1980.
34. Mayfield JK: Wrist ligamentous anatomy and pathogenesis of carpal instability. Orthop Clin North Am 15:209–216, 1984.
35. Mazet R, and Hoal M: Fractures of the carpal navicular. J Bone Joint Surg 45A:82, 1963.
36. Nash D, and Mayfield JK: The ligamentous anatomy of the scapholunate joint. Unpublished study, 1979.
37. Peterson JW, Robbin ML, Erdman AG, et al: Screw axis measurement of the human wrist. 1982 Advances in Bioengineering, American Society of Mechanical Engineers, 1982.
38. Poirier P, and Charpy A: Traité de l'Anatomie Humaine. Tome I. Masson et Cie, Paris, 1911, pp 226–231.
39. Robbin ML, Erdman AG, Mayfield JK, et al: Kinematic measurement of relative motion in the human wrist. 1981 Advances in Bioengineering, American Society of Mechanical Engineers, 1981.
40. Russell TB: Intercarpal dislocations and fracture-dislocations. J Bone Joint Surg 31B:524, 1949.
41. Schaeffer JP: Morris' Human Anatomy. 11th ed. McGraw-Hill, Inc, New York, pp 339–347, 1965.
42. Squire M: Carpal mechanics and trauma. J Bone Joint Surg 41B:210, 1959.
43. Tanz SS: Rotational effect in lunar and perilunar dislocations. Clin Orthop 57:147–152, 1968.
44. Taleisnik J: Post-traumatic carpal instability. Clin Orthop 149:73–82, 1980.
45. Taleisnik J: The ligaments of the wrist. J Hand Surg 1:110–118, 1976.
46. Taleisnik J: Wrist anatomy, function and injury. American Academy of Orthopaedic Surgeons, Instructional Course Lectures, Vol XXVII, St Louis, CV Mosby Co, 1978, p 61.
47. Verdan C, and Narakas A: Fractures and pseudarthrosis of the scaphoid. Surg Clin North Am 48:1083, 1968.
48. Wagner CJ: Perilunar dislocations. J Bone Joint Surg 38A:1198, 1956.

49. Wagner CJ: Fracture-dislocations of the wrist. Clin Orthop 15:181, 1959.

50. Weber ER, and Chao EY: An experimental approach to the mechanism of scaphoid waist fractures. J Hand Surg 3:142, 1978.

51. Williams WJ, Erdman AG, and Mayfield JK: Design and analysis of a ligament cross-sectional area micrometer. 1980 Advances in Bioengineering, American Society of Mechanical Engineers, 1980, pp 50–52.

52. Wright RD: A detailed study of movement of the wrist joint. J Anat 70:137, 1935.

53. Youm Y, McMurtry RY, Flatt AE, et al: Kinematics of the wrist I: an experimental study of radial-ulnar deviation and flexion-extension. J Bone Joint Surg 60A:423, 1978.

PART II

Evaluation

CHAPTER 6

Physical Examination
of the Wrist

DAVID E. BROWN, M.D.
and DAVID M. LICHTMAN, M.D.

INTRODUCTION

Successful examination of the wrist requires a thorough knowledge of topical anatomy and underlying structures. The ability to correlate the mechanism of injury with localized physical findings, such as tenderness, abnormal motion, or "clicks," enables the examiner to formulate a differential diagnosis (Table 6–1) and to plan further investigative studies or treatments.

CLINICAL HISTORY

A careful history of the mechanism of injury is essential. Attention should be paid to the specific position of the wrist during initial loading and to the subsequent direction and degree of stress to which the wrist was subjected. Dorsiflexion and supination forces usually produce perilunate injuries, whereas palmar flexion and pronation forces are more likely to affect the ulnar side of the wrist. The location, intensity, and duration of pain that occurred after the acute injury should be noted. Careful questioning of the patient will often enable the examiner to more accurately localize the pain.

When wrist pain has become chronic, it is necessary to determine the frequency with which it occurs and any particular movements or activities that aggravate or relieve the discomfort. The extent to which occupational or avocational activities aggravate

the symptoms should be ascertained and considered later, when the physician is deciding upon a course of treatment. Many patients can live with their symptoms if advised to eliminate or modify certain nonessential activities.

Information should be obtained about the presence of swelling, abnormal clicks (some may be better described as clunks, snaps, or crackles), limitation of motion, burning, or tingling. The effects of previous immobilization, medications, injections, or surgery are defined. The efficacy of prior treatment is an important factor in choosing treatment alternatives for many chronic wrist disorders.

After the history of injury is completed, a thorough medical history should be obtained, including information about other orthopedic or rheumatologic disorders, concurrent acute or chronic medical disease (such as diabetes or thyroid dysfunction), and a complete family history of orthopedic conditions.

PHYSICAL EXAMINATION OF THE WRIST

It is important to obtain complete relaxation of the patient's forearm, wrist, and hand while performing an examination of the wrist. Following acute injury, this is performed with the involved extremity in a

Table 6–1. DIFFERENTIAL DIAGNOSIS OF WRIST PAIN*

I. Traumatic/Degenerative
  A. Fractures
  B. Fracture nonunions
  C. Carpal instability
    1. Perilunate
      a. Scapholunate
      b. Triquetrolunate[6]
    2. Midcarpal
      a. Intrinsic[3]
      b. Extrinsic[8]
    3. Radiocarpal
      a. Ulnar translocation
      b. Dorsal subluxation
      c. Volar subluxation
  D. Postinstability arthrosis (SLAC wrist)[9]
  E. Distal radioulnar joint disruption
    1. Dislocation/subluxation
    2. Triangular fibrocartilage complex tears[5]
    3. Ulnar abutment syndrome[4]
II. Developmental
  A. Synovial inflammatory diseases
  B. Osteoarthritis
  C. Simple bone cysts
III. Infectious
  A. Bacterial
  B. Granulomatous
IV. Neoplastic
  A. Enchondroma
  B. Osteoid osteoma
  C. Metastasis
  D. Miscellaneous
V. Miscellaneous
  A. Peripheral nerve entrapment
    1. Carpal tunnel syndrome
    2. Ulnar tunnel (Guyon's canal) syndrome
  B. Kienböck's disease
  C. Tendonitis
  D. Neuromata
  E. Ganglia
    1. Intraosseus
    2. Extraosseus
  F. Subluxating extensor carpi ulnaris tendon[2]

*Modified from Brown DE, and Lichtman DM: Orthop Clin North Am 15:184, 1984.

splinted position or lying flat on a soft examination table. For chronic wrist pain, the patient rests the ipsilateral elbow on his or her thigh (or a low table), while the physician gently holds the patient's distal forearm and hand to support the wrist (Fig. 6–1). This allows the examiner to carefully position the wrist as desired, while permitting free and easy motion of the wrist and forearm.

A thorough and methodical examination is performed. It begins with inspection of the surface features and evaluation of the range of motion of the extremity and is followed by careful palpation of the topographic anatomy. More specific tests can be performed as indicated by the history and physical examination.

Inspection

Inspection should begin with a search for localized swelling, nodules, or masses. Any erythema, abrasions, lacerations, or incisions are identified and their presence is recorded. Any deformities of soft tissues or bony landmarks are noted.

The wrist should be tested for active and passive motion in dorsiflexion, palmar flexion, radial deviation, and ulnar deviation. Forearm pronation and supination are measured. Testing the range of motion may be indicated for the elbow, shoulder, and neck. All values are compared with those of the opposite extremity. Particular attention is given to any abnormal noises or pain that occurs during motion testing, since they can help to localize the site of many lesions.

Palpation and Topographic Anatomy

The osseus and soft tissue topographic anatomy should be systemically palpated to define areas of tenderness (the key feature in localizing pathology). Palpation should be done to localize fine crepitus and the gross clicks and clunks of instabilities. Any abnormal gaps or dissociations between anatomic elements should be appreciated.

A systemic approach to the topographic anatomic examination is achieved by dividing the wrist into five zones: three dorsal and two palmar. With an organized approach to osseous and soft tissue palpation, the physician can perform a comprehensive examination of the diffusely painful wrist or a precise regional examination when the symptoms are well localized.

Prominent bony landmarks are utilized as reference points to begin the examination. The landmarks on the dorsal side are the radial styloid, Lister's tubercle, and the ulnar styloid process (Fig. 6–2). The landmarks on the palmar surface are the radial styloid, the pisiform, and the tubercle of the trapezium (see Fig. 6–7). These prominences should be palpable in most individuals.

RADIAL DORSAL ZONE

The bony features palpable in the radial dorsal zone include the radial styloid, the scaphoid and scaphotrapezial joint, the trapezium, the base of the first metacarpal, and the first carpometacarpal (CMC) joint. Soft tissue structures include the tendons of the first dorsal compartment (abductor pollicis

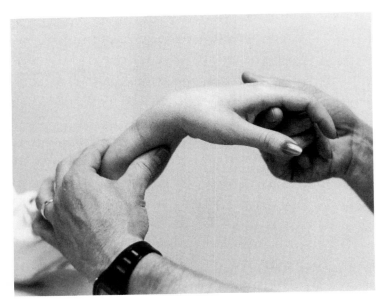

Figure 6–1. Examination of the wrist. The elbow, forearm, and hand must be supported to obtain relaxation of the arm muscles. Gently grasping the distal forearm and hand of the injured extremity also allows the physician to position the wrist as desired.

longus and extensor pollicis brevis) and the extensor pollicis longus (Fig. 6–3).

The scaphoid is present just distal to the radial styloid on both sides of the tendons of the first dorsal compartment (Fig. 6–3). The scaphoid tuberosity is just palmar and ulnar to the first compartment tendons and is more prominent in dorsiflexion and radial deviation. The classic "anatomic snuffbox" lies between the tendons of the first compartment and the extensor pollicis longus.

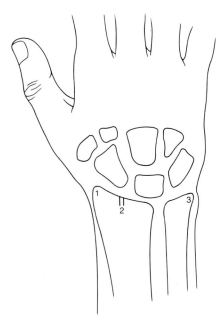

Figure 6–2. Landmarks of the dorsal side of the wrist. Identification of the radial styloid (1), Lister's tubercle (2), and the ulnar styloid (3) provides an important starting point for the examination of the dorsal surface of the wrist.

The scaphoid waist is palpable deep in the snuffbox. Tenderness in the snuffbox may be caused by an occult scaphoid fracture or by a scaphoid nonunion.

Distal to the scaphoid are the scaphotrapezial joint and the trapezium. Gentle rotation of the thumb will help the examiner to differentiate the trapezium from the first metacarpal.

The first CMC joint is easily identified in thin individuals. If the examiner's finger is slowly moved in a proximal direction along the dorsomedial aspect of the first metacarpal, a small depression can be felt and represents the CMC joint. The grind test is performed by effecting axial compression on the thumb, while palpating the first CMC joint. Pain that is reproduced by this test is frequently caused by CMC arthrosis. Tenderness over the palmar aspect of the CMC joint is confirmatory. This should be differentiated from pain that originates one joint more proximal, at the scaphotrapezial joint. Roentgenograms will further aid in this differential diagnosis.

Examination of the radial dorsal zone is completed by palpation of the extensor pollicis brevis, abductor pollicis longus, and extensor pollicis longus tendons for tenderness, crepitation, or localized nodules. De Quervain's tenosynovitis (inflammation of the first dorsal compartment tendons) is a common cause of pain in this region. Pain and tenderness occur over the radial aspect of the wrist, accentuated by active thumb extension and abduction. Pain may be reproduced by passive flexion of the metacarpo-

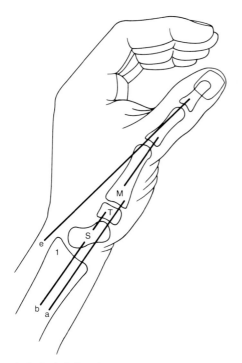

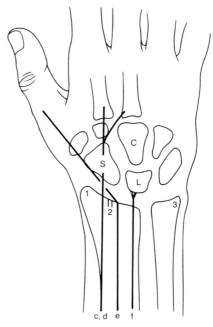

Figure 6–3. Radial dorsal zone. On the radial side of the wrist lie the radial styloid (1), the scaphoid (S), the trapezium (T), and the first metacarpal (M). The important tendons in the zone are the extensor pollicis brevis (a), the abductor pollicis longus (b), and the distal segment of the extensor pollicis longus (e).

Figure 6–4. Central dorsal zone. In this zone are the scaphoid (S), the lunate (L), the capitate (C), and Lister's tubercle (2). The respective joints should also be evaluated, since pathology is frequent here. The superficial tendons are the extensor carpi radialis brevis and longus (c, d), the proximal portion of the extensor pollicis longus (e), and the common finger extensors (f).

phalangeal joint, adduction of the thumb, and ulnar deviation of the wrist (Finklestein's test). Some normal individuals may be very sensitive to this test, so results must be compared with the opposite wrist.

CENTRAL DORSAL ZONE

The central dorsal zone includes Lister's tubercle, the scapholunate joint, the lunate, the capitate, and the base of the second and third metacarpals and their CMC joints. The soft tissue structures in this zone are the distal aspects of the extensor carpi radialis brevis and longus and the extensor digitorum communis tendons (Fig. 6–4).

The lunate is present distal and ulnar to Lister's tubercle. It is much more prominent with the wrist held in palmar flexion (Fig. 6–5). Lunate tenderness should raise the suspicion of Kienböck's disease (idiopathic osteonecrosis). There is often associated local swelling or synovitis.

The wrist should be moved into radial and ulnar deviation, while an examining finger is placed over the scapholunate interval and an assessment made of the integrity of the joint. Tenderness, clicking, or an increase in the size of the scapholunate depression may

indicate dissociation. Tenderness alone may be caused by "occult" ganglia, a frequent cause of chronic wrist pain. These occult ganglia are often palpable as pea-sized tender nodules in the distal aspect of the scapholunate joint. Palmar flexion may make them more prominent.

The capitate is present just distal to the lunate and is located beneath a mild depres-

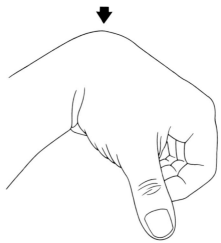

Figure 6–5. The lunate. Palmar flexion of the wrist makes the lunate (*solid arrow*) more prominent.

sion between the lunate and the base of the third metacarpal.

The extensor carpi radialis longus and brevis are located immediately radial to Lister's tubercle at the wrist. Ulnar to Lister's tubercle is the extensor pollicis longus, whereupon it courses toward the radius to the thumb. It becomes quite prominent when the thumb interphalangeal joint is hyperextended. Ulnar to the extensor pollicis longus is the extensor digitorum communis. Tenderness over any of these tendons may be due to localized inflammation or to impingement beneath the extensor retinaculum.

Ulnar Dorsal Zone

The ulnar dorsal zone includes the ulnar styloid, the distal radioulnar joint (DRUJ), the triquetrum and hamate, and the base of the fourth and fifth metacarpals. The principal soft tissue structures located in this zone are the triangular fibrocartilage complex (TFCC) and the extensor carpi ulnaris tendon (Fig. 6–6).

The distal radioulnar joint is located just radial to the prominent ulnar head. When an examining finger is placed over the DRUJ, the patient's forearm should be rotated into maximum pronation and supination, and

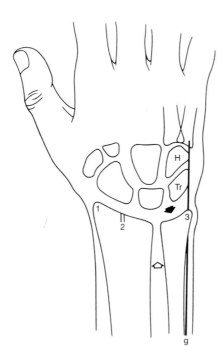

Figure 6–6. Ulnar dorsal zone. The ulnar dorsal zone includes the ulnar styloid (3), the triquetrum (Tr) and the hamate (H), the distal radioulnar joint (*open arrow*), the triangular fibrocartilage complex (*solid arrow*), and the extensor carpi ulnaris (g).

any changes in the relationship between the distal ulna and radius should be noted. The ulna is normally more prominent in full pronation. Pain that occurs with forearm rotation may indicate DRUJ disease.

Immediately distal to the DRUJ lies the TFCC. Exquisite tenderness is noted with tears of the TFCC or when ulnocarpal abutment causes triquetral chondromalacia. Either of these disorders may be associated with clicking in the wrist. Unlike the DRUJ disorders, forearm rotation is generally pain-free.

The hamate is palpable proximal to the base of the fifth metacarpal. With the wrist in radial deviation, the triquetrum can be found in an apparent sulcus between the hamate and the ulnar styloid. In the patient with midcarpal instability, localized pain, swelling, and tenderness will be most noticeable in this area. In addition, the wrist will seem to sag on the ulnar side. As the wrist is moved from neutral to ulnar deviation, a pronounced "clunk" will signal the reduction of the midcarpal subluxation.

The triquetrolunate joint should be identified and will be tender in the presence of sprains or dissociations. There may be an associated wrist click. The findings of the triquetrolunate ballottement test[6] are positive in the unstable joint. To perform this test, the examiner stabilizes the lunate with the thumb and index finger of one examining hand, while attempting to displace the triquetrum dorsally. In a positive test, there is excessive laxity, pain, and crepitus.

The extensor carpi ulnaris tendon is located ulnar to the ulnar styloid, becoming quite prominent in supination and in active ulnar deviation. Occasionally, recurrent subluxation of the tendon can be detected by a sudden palpable snap when the wrist is moved into this position.

Radial Volar Zone

In the radial volar zone, the examiner should locate the scaphoid tuberosity and the tubercle of the trapezium, the flexor carpi radialis, the palmaris longus (if present), the long finger flexors, and the median nerve (Fig. 6–7).

The scaphoid tuberosity can be detected just distal to the radial styloid. It is most prominent when the wrist is radially deviated. Distal to the scaphoid is the trapezial ridge, which is tender when fractured. Special radiographic views are usually necessary to demonstrate this fracture.

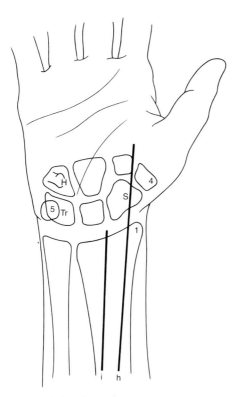

Figure 6–7. Radial volar zone. Examination of the radial volar zone is begun by identifying the radial styloid (1) and the tubercle of the trapezium (4). The scaphoid (S) and its tuberosity lie between these two structures. The flexor carpi radialis (h) and palmaris longus (i) tendons are very superficial.

The volar aspect of the first CMC joint lies next to the trapezial ridge. When CMC joint inflammation is present, this area will be exquisitely sensitive. Crepitation and pain can be elicited by applying axial compression to the joint, while moving it through a range of motion.

Ulnar to the scaphoid tuberosity is the prominent flexor carpi radialis tendon, which disappears into its synovial tunnel alongside the trapezium. Tenderness and fullness are found over this tunnel when tenosynovitis occurs. The palmaris longus tendon lies ulnar to the flexor carpi radialis and is present in 87 percent of limbs.[7] If present, it can be identified best when active wrist flexion is accompanied by opposition of the thumb and small finger. The long finger flexors (flexor digitorum superficialis and profundus) lie beneath the palmaris and are difficult to identify individually.

The median nerve is present immediately deep and ulnar to the palmaris longus. A tight transverse carpal ligament causing irritation of the median nerve can be detected by tapping directly over the nerve at the proximal wrist flexion crease. This can elicit or reproduce dysesthesias along the distribution of the median nerve (Tinel's sign). Numbness or tingling can also be induced by holding the wrist in full passive volar flexion for 15 to 60 seconds (Phalen's test).

ULNAR VOLAR ZONE

In this zone are located the pisiform and the hook of the hamate, the ulnar nerve and artery, and the tendon of the flexor carpi ulnaris (Fig. 6–8).

The pisiform is the bony prominence located at the base of the hypothenar eminence. When the wrist is relaxed, the pisiform is mobile and can be balloted against the triquetrum. This causes pain and possibly crepitation in cases of pisotriquetral arthrosis.

If the examiner palpates in a slightly radial and distal direction, the hook of the hamate is easily located. It can fracture when the loaded wrist is suddenly dorsiflexed, such as when a golfer strikes a tree or firm ground with a golf club. As in the case of the

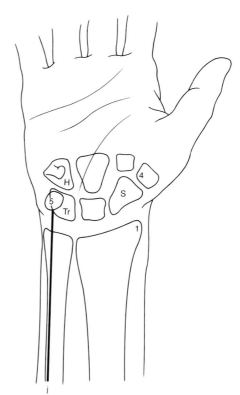

Figure 6–8. Ulnar volar zone. Structures that are easily identified in the ulnar volar zone are the pisiform (5), the hook of the hamate (H) and the flexor carpi ulnaris (j). The triquetrum (Tr) lies beneath the pisiform. Guyon's canal is between the pisiform and the hook of the hamate.

trapezial ridge fracture, special radiographic projections are required to demonstrate this fracture. The presence of isolated tenderness will alert the astute clinician to order these views.

Between the pisiform and the hook of the hamate (anatomically termed Guyon's canal) lie the ulnar nerve and artery. Usually the ulnar nerve can be detected under the palpating finger with a gentle rolling motion over this canal. In this area, small ganglia or pulsatile masses should be sought, especially when vascular or neurologic symptoms are present in the distal ulnar nerve distribution.

The flexor carpi ulnaris tendon is located by having the patient flex and ulnar deviate the clenched fist. This tendon inserts into and around the pisiform.

Discussion

When palpating each of these bony or soft tissue structures, attention should be focused on any pain that is produced by the palpation or by gentle movement of the involved area. If possible, the patient should repeat the motions and positions that reproduce the wrist discomfort, while the examiner is again palpating over the area of pain.

The examiner should detect and localize any clicks or clunks, as they may indicate occult carpal instability. These are most significant if pain and a spontaneous noise are reproduced by the patient who is actively moving the wrist into the position that causes discomfort. The noise should be anatomically localized by the previously discussed examination techniques. If the patient cannot reproduce the click, it may often be brought out passively by the examiner. However, these passive clicks are significant only if they reproduce the clinical symptoms, as many loose-jointed individuals have painless clicks that can be reproduced unwittingly and misinterpreted by the inexperienced examiner.

The most common clicks are those seen in patients with scapholunate dissociation or midcarpal instability. Clicks from scapholunate dissociation occur as the wrist is moved from radial deviation toward the neutral position. This occurs when the scaphoid rotates from its palmar flexed position and "catches up" with the lunate, which is already excessively dorsiflexed. Occurrence of the click can be facilitated by placing the examining index finger and thumb dorsal and palmar to the scaphoid, with the patient's hand in radial deviation. As the wrist is moved toward the neutral position, pressure is gently applied from palmar to dorsal aspects. The click is felt as the scaphoid jumps back into its normal relationship with the lunate.

The midcarpal instability clunk occurs at the triquetrohamate joint. With the wrist held in a relaxed neutral position, a slight sag is noted over the ulnar border of the wrist. When the patient actively pronates and ulnarly deviates the wrist, a painful clunk occurs, and the sag disappears. Passive manipulation may duplicate this clunk, and its occurrence is facilitated by gentle axial compression.

Neurovascular Examination

A complete neurovascular evaluation, when indicated, includes examination of motor strength, sensation, arterial patency, and capillary filling.

Allen's test verifies the ulnar and radial arterial patency by exsanguinating the hand after applying direct (occlusive) pressure over each of the arteries. When pressure is released over one artery, the return of normal color to the hand indicates adequate arterial function. The test is then repeated and the other artery is evaluated.

Sensation is tested using the static two-point discrimination method. Other suitable sensory tests include the Semmes-Weinstein and the moving two-point[1] methods. Gross motor strength is recorded using the grip and pinch measurements. Specific tests for intrinsic muscle function should be performed when lesions of the carpal tunnel or Guyon's canal are present.

Differential Injections

Differential injection of specific structures with short-acting local anesthetic agents can be performed to confirm the location and source of a patient's pain. It is also useful in the patient with pain in several distinct anatomic areas of the wrist. In these patients, injection of one specific region will often determine the proportion of the symptoms that arise from that location. A good example is the injecting of anesthetic into the DRUJ to distinguish DRUJ from radiocarpal symptoms (when the TFCC is intact). Aspiration of cystic masses and specific joints is useful when the presence of infection or a ganglion is suspected. The return of thick, clear material confirms that there is a ganglion. Any other fluid obtained may be sent for routine laboratory and microbiologic analysis.

SUMMARY

Wrist pain has often been called the low back pain of hand surgery. Both of these areas provide the clinician with significant diagnostic and therapeutic challenges. As in the evaluation of the lower back, a careful history and physical examination are important for arriving at an accurate diagnosis of wrist pathology. Emphasis during the history-taking is placed on the mechanism of any injuries, a careful localization of the apparent source of pain, and a detailed description of any prior treatment. The patient's occupational and avocational requirements should be considered. Physical examination will then localize the anatomic site of bone or soft tissue disorder. This will allow the physician to narrow the differential diagnosis and will enable him or her

to order more appropriate radiographic and laboratory tests in order to arrive at the correct diagnosis.

References

1. Dellon AL, and Kallman CH: Evaluation of functional sensation in the hand. J Hand Surg 8:865, 1983.
2. Eckardt WA, and Palmer AK: Recurrent dislocation of the extensor carpi ulnaris tendon. J Hand Surg 6:629, 1981.
3. Lichtman DM et al: Ulnar midcarpal instability—clinical and laboratory analysis. J Hand Surg 7:515, 1982.
4. Palmer AK, Glisson RR, and Werner FW: Ulnar variance determination. J Hand Surg 7:376, 1982.
5. Palmer AK, and Werner FW: The triangular fibrocartilage complex of the wrist—anatomy and function. J Hand Surg 6:153, 1981.
6. Reagin DS, Linscheid RL, and Dobyns JH: Lunotriquetral sprains. J Hand Surg 9:502, 1984.
7. Reimann RF et al: The palmaris longus muscle and tendon: a study of 1600 extremities. Anat Rec 89:495, 1944.
8. Taleisnik J, and Watson HK: Midcarpal instability caused by malunited distal radius fractures. J Hand Surg 9:350, 1984.
9. Watson HK, and Ballet FL: The SLAC wrist: scapholunate advanced collapse pattern of degenerative arthritis. J Hand Surg 9:358, 1984.

CHAPTER 7

Roentgenographic Diagnosis of Wrist Pain and Instability

JUDY M. DESTOUET, M.D., LOUIS A. GILULA, M.D.
and WILLIAM R. REINUS, M.D.

INTRODUCTION

Injuries to the wrist often result in subtle clinical and roentgenographic findings that necessitate a careful, organized evaluation of the carpal bones, ligaments, and joint capsule for an appropriate diagnosis to be reached. An algorithm for the imaging approach to the painful wrist is presented. When combined with a thorough history and clinical examination, this approach allows early diagnosis and appropriate definitive treatment of an underlying wrist disorder.

One of the greatest diagnostic challenges that faces both the orthopedic surgeon and the radiologist is the patient with a subacute or chronic wrist injury who has no obvious clinical or radiographic abnormality to explain the pain. Most of these problems are post-traumatic, and many of the injuries are work-related. In some cases, a pre-existing, normal variant, such as a negative ulnar variance, places a patient at greater risk for injury, and only with additional radiologic views, such as an instability series, specialized views, or tomography, does the underlying disorder become evident.[31]

Roentgenographic evaluation of the wrist should not proceed until a careful history describing the mechanism of injury is obtained and a complete physical examination has been performed. Guidelines for such a detailed physical examination of the wrist have been published.[1, 25] An important step in the physical examination is to relate the site of maximum tenderness to an underlying anatomic structure, such as a particular carpal bone or ligament. If a diagnosis is not

made following the physical examination, the radiographic work-up may proceed according to an algorithm (Fig. 7–1). Asymmetric progression through the algorithm should result in a definitive roentgenographic diagnosis, if one is possible. The following sections will enlarge on this algorithm.

IMAGING TECHNIQUES FOR EVALUATION

The tools available to the radiologist include the following: (1) routine four-view wrist survey, (2) detailed carpal bone views, (3) fluoroscopic spot films, (4) instability series, (5) videotape or cine evaluation, (6) bone scan (scintigraphy), (7) tomography, (8) wrist arthrography, (9) computed tomography (CT), and (10) magnetic resonance imaging (MRI). A description of each procedure with a proposed sequence in which to use these studies follows.

Routine Wrist Survey. Four standard views centered on the wrist, not the hand, should be performed and should include the posteroanterior (PA), scaphoid (proximally angled beam or ulnar-deviated PA), oblique, and lateral views. On each view, the soft tissues should be surveyed first in order to identify any area of swelling that may indicate an underlying bone abnormality.[11, 13] Soft tissue swelling is most easily identifiable on the lateral projection, especially along the dorsal surface of the wrist. Normally, the dorsal soft tissues of the wrist are concave, and any straightening or convexity in this region is indicative of swelling. The pronator

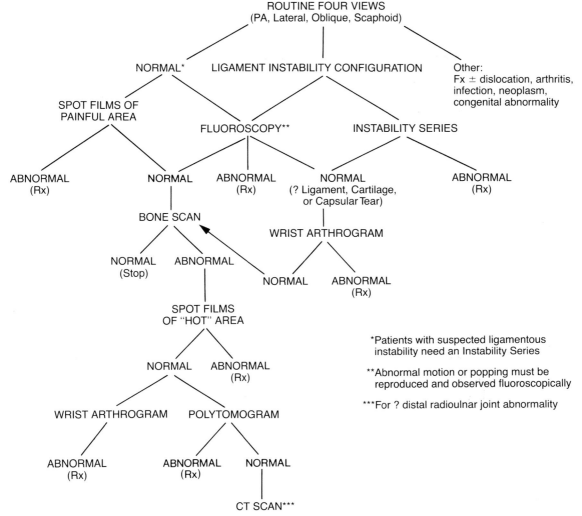

Figure 7–1. Roentgenographic approach to the painful wrist.

fat line along the ventral aspect of the wrist should be straight. Bulging or convexity of this line also implies soft tissue swelling.

The navicular fat stripe is a thin, radiolucent line that parallels the lateral surface of the scaphoid.[29] Obliteration or bowing of this fat stripe indicates localized hemorrhage or edema around the scaphoid, a finding that may occasionally be the only sign of an acute scaphoid fracture (Fig. 7–2).

Once the soft tissues have been carefully examined, the bones should be scrutinized for evidence of malalignment, fracture, or other abnormality. The PA view should be obtained with the palm of the hand flat on the table or the film cassette, with the elbow resting on the table and the shoulder level with the elbow. Such standardization will enable better evaluation of ulnar variance at the distal end of the ulna.[24] Normally, the radiocarpal and intercarpal joints form three smooth arcs on the PA view (Fig. 7–3). Disruption of these arcs or overlapping of adjacent bones indicates carpal malalignment, i.e., subluxation or dislocation (Fig. 7–4).[13] The normal scapholunate joint space width is the same as that between the other carpal bones. This space usually measures 1 or 2 mm in maximum width and remains constant with different degrees of medial or lateral deviation of the wrist. Abnormal widening to more than 3 to 4 mm (Fig. 7–5) suggests a scapholunate ligament tear or laxity. When in question, this abnormality may be confirmed with arthrography. In the scaphoid view, which is performed with ulnar deviation of the hand or with angulation of the x-ray tube toward the elbow, dorsiflexion of the scaphoid and elongation of the scaphoid waist allow a better profile of the

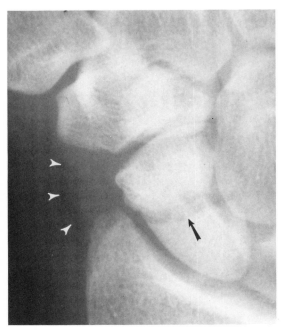

Figure 7–2. An acute, nondisplaced scaphoid waist fracture (*arrow*) causes bowing of the scaphoid fat stripe (*arrowheads*).

scaphoid waist (Fig. 7–6).[10] Subtle scaphoid fractures may be evident on only one of these views, because the scaphoid bone is frequently foreshortened on the PA view (Fig. 7–6).

The semipronated oblique view profiles the scaphotrapeziotrapezoidal joints and is the best view to profile the trapeziotrape-

zoidal joint. In addition, the scaphocapitate and lunocapitate joints may be profiled in this view. Osteoarthritis involving the base of the thumb and processes involving the trapeziotrapezoidal joints are frequently best visualized on this view.

At times, the overlap of the carpal bones on the lateral view makes it difficult to identify all the carpal bones and their relationships. However, this view is essential to detect certain significant carpal injuries and ligament instabilities.[1]

Radiography of the wrist in the lateral position may be standardized by having the laterally placed hand and wrist in a straight plane with the shoulder and elbow (the shoulder is the same height above the floor as the wrist) and with the elbow flexed 90°. Mere pronation of the supinated hand from the PA to the lateral position does not provide a true lateral view of the ulna. A well-positioned lateral view of the wrist can be recognized by identifying the position of radial- and ulnar-sided bones of the carpus. The distal pole or distal third of the scaphoid should be ventral to the ventral surface of the pisiform (Fig. 7–7). If the pisiform is visible ventral to or overlaps the distal scaphoid pole, the wrist is off-lateral or semisupinated. The ulna may be more ventral in this position. Also, in this position, the lunate may falsely appear abnormally tilted. With semipronation, the pisiform is not readily, if at all, apparent, and more than

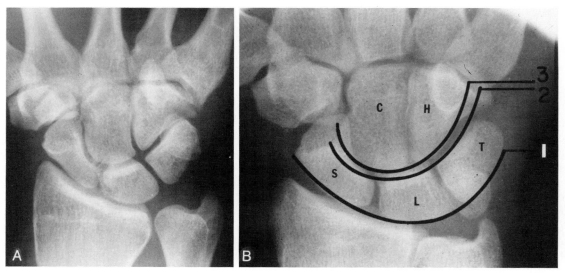

Figure 7–3. *A*, PA view of a normal wrist. *B*, Same view with the three arcs drawn. Arc 1 connects the proximal articular surfaces of the scaphoid (S), lunate (L), and triquetrum (T). Arc 2 joins the distal concave surfaces of these same carpal bones. Arc 3 outlines the proximal convexities of the capitate (C) and hamate (H).

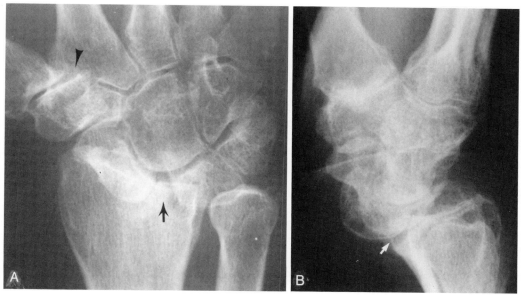

Figure 7–4. Chronic right wrist pain is present three years after injury. *A,* PA view shows ulnar translocation of the entire carpus with respect to the distal radius. The scapholunate joint is abnormally wide (*arrow*) from disruption of the scapholunate ligament. Overlap of the scaphoid and lunate bones and the distal articular surface of the radius indicates dislocation at the radiocarpal joint. Degenerative spurring of the trapezial first metacarpal joint (*arrowhead*) is evident. *B,* The lateral projection shows ventral dislocation of the carpus with pseudojoints (*arrow*) suggested at the radiolunate and radioscaphoid junctions. (From Bellinghausen HW, Gilula LA, and Young LV: J Bone Joint Surg 65A:998–1006, 1983.)

the distal one third to one half of the scaphoid projects free of the other carpal bones, as in the standard semipronated oblique view. As suspected, the ulna will be more dorsal in this view. Although much emphasis has been placed on the position of the dorsal surface of the ulna lying over the

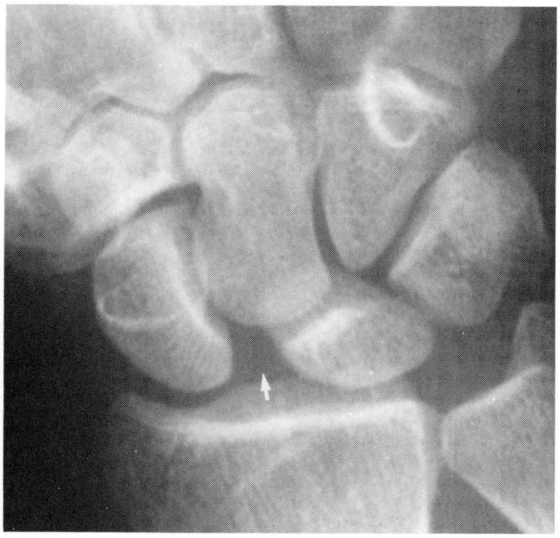

Figure 7–5. Abnormal widening of the scapholunate joint (*arrow*) and signet ring appearance (foreshortening) of the scaphoid bone indicate scapholunate ligament disruption with resultant rotary subluxation of the scaphoid.

dorsal surface of the radius to indicate a good lateral wrist view, variations in the shape and position of the distal ulna make the above method of checking the relative position of various carpal bones more reliable for recognizing true laterality of the wrist on a roentgenogram.

The lateral view affords evaluation of the articulation between the radius, carpus, and metacarpals as well as alignment of the scaphoid, lunate, and capitate (Fig. 7–7). Although it can be readily suspected on the PA view, final diagnosis of lunate, perilunate, or radiocarpal dislocation is generally best verified on the lateral projection (Fig. 7–4).[1, 11, 13] When evaluating the position of the carpal rows on the lateral view, the lunate may be used to identify the proximal carpal row, whereas the capitate can represent the distal carpal row. When an intercarpal dislocation occurs, usually either the lunate or the capitate remains centered over the radius. Therefore, with a lunate dislocation, the capitate head remains centered over the radius. Conversely, with a perilunate dislocation, the capitate is dorsal or ventral to the lunate and the distal radius, but the lunate normally remains aligned with the radius.[13, 20, 22] In both of these conditions, typically the triquetrum, hamate, trapezium,

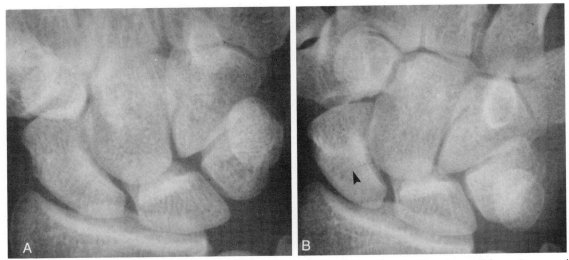

Figure 7–6. A, PA view of the wrist appears normal in this young patient with pain over the snuff box. On second inspection, after examination of Figure 7–6B, a subtle lucency is evident at the junction of the proximal and middle thirds of the scaphoid. B, A scaphoid view of the hand in ulnar deviation profiles the scaphoid waist and reveals a subtle, nondisplaced fracture (*arrowhead*). (The ulnar edges of the lunate and radius are in line, the distal end of the triquetrum is closer to the distal end of the hamate, and the proximal pole of the hamate has moved radially toward the central portion of the lunate.)

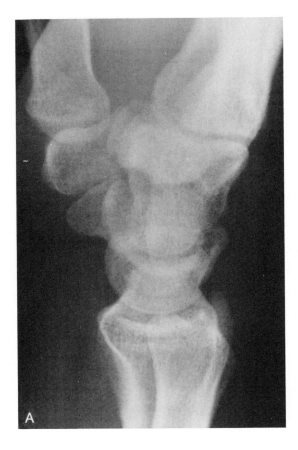

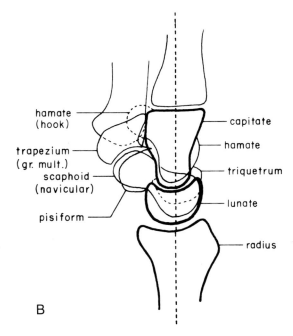

Figure 7–7. A and B, Normal lateral view with the carpal bones labeled. (Fig. 7–7B from LA Gilula: Carpal injuries: Analytic approach and case exercises. AJR, 133:503–517, © by The Endocrine Society, 1979.)

trapezoid, and distal portion of the scaphoid (if there is a scaphoid fracture present) will move as a unit with the capitate, away from the lunate. The presence or absence of parallel articulating surfaces (seen best on the PA view) will allow the physician to detect dissociation or probable normal articulation between adjacent carpal bones.[13]

On the lateral view, the scaphoid can be identified with its proximal convexity overlapping the mid-portion of the lunate and its distal pole projecting proximal to the trapezium. The scaphoid axis can be drawn by passing a line tangent to the distal and proximal convexities of the scaphoid.[16] This line will serve as a reproducible axis of the scaphoid and is helpful in evaluating rotary subluxation of the scaphoid (Fig. 7–5).[10, 16]

Specific Carpal Bone Views. In order to evaluate cortical margins of the carpal bones that are not routinely visualized on the wrist survey, detailed views, such as the carpal tunnel view (Fig. 7–8), the carpal boss view,[8] and semisupination (off-lateral) and reverse oblique views, may be obtained. The carpal tunnel view may be obtained with the wrist dorsiflexed and either the ventral aspect of the wrist or the palm placed on the x-ray cassette. The x-ray beam is angled to profile the carpal tunnel. The hamate hook, trapezium, pisiform, and ventral surface of the capitate or lunate are profiled.

A slightly semisupinated off-lateral view to tangent a dorsal carpal boss will enable distinction among (1) a separate os styloideum, (2) a bony prominence attached to the second or third metacarpal base or apposing surface of the trapezoid or capitate

bones, and (3) degenerative osteophytes in this same area. Ventrally, the semisupination oblique view demonstrates the pisotriquetral joint, pisiform, triquetrum, and hook of the hamate.

With the PA reversed oblique view (thenar eminence on the table and hypothenar eminence elevated off the table or film cassette), avulsion fractures of the dorsum of the scaphoid waist and ulnar aspect of the hamate and triquetrum can be detected. If a specific point of tenderness is detected and the previous views are unrevealing, multiple views at 5° to 10° of obliquity can be obtained, locating the point of tenderness or focal hot spot noted on bone scan. Angulation of the x-ray beam with respect to the carpal bones may also provide information not seen previously, i.e., it may profile a fracture line not shown on routine views.

Fluoroscopic Spot Films. When detailed carpal views fail to demonstrate an abnormality in a clinically suspicious area, the wrist may be studied with fluoroscopy, and special attention can be paid to particular areas of tenderness, and to popping or grinding. Specifically, precisely profiled spots of cortical surfaces and joints can easily be accomplished with good fluoroscopic spot filming techniques. In patients with midcarpal pain, manipulation under fluoroscopy may reveal capitolunate or other intercarpal instability, when routine films are normal.[32]

Ligament Instability Series. (See the section in this chapter entitled Carpal Instability.) If there is any clinical or plain film radiographic indication of carpal ligament damage, i.e., widening of the scapholunate space

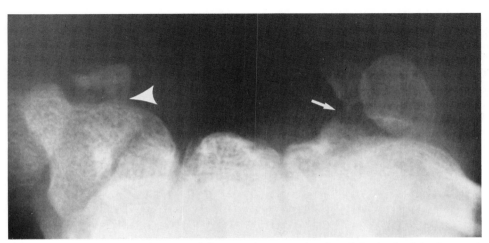

Figure 7–8. On a carpal tunnel view, fractures of the trapezium (arrowhead) and the hook of the hamate (arrow) are evident.

or dorsiflexion or palmar flexion ligamentous instability patterns,[16, 20] an instability series should be performed to detect abnormal carpal motion.[14, 16, 20] A routine series includes AP clenched fist and PA views in neutral, radial, and ulnar deviation; a semipronated oblique view (30° from PA); lateral views in neutral, full flexion, and extension; and semisupinated off-lateral (30° from lateral) oblique views. Comparison views of the opposite side are helpful for detecting motion abnormalities and normal variations.

Videotape or Cine Evaluation. Active and assisted carpal motions may also be studied using fluoroscopy, videotape, or cinematography as the patient or the examiner or both performs flexion-extension, medial and lateral deviation, and twisting maneuvers. This method of examination is of particular use in detecting dynamic ligament instabilities and for patients with a history of clicking or popping even though the wrist appears normal on plain films. The movement that causes the sound should be reproduced as closely as possible.[14] Use of a recording medium such as videotape will enable repeated

review of all motions, and some machines will allow slowing of the film, which may provide ease of motion analysis.

Scintigraphy. Technetium-[99m] bone scans are useful in evaluating subtle wrist injury when the preceding roentgenographic workup is normal. The procedure is especially valuable for excluding osteochondral or osseous abnormalities. Technical aspects of this exam should be closely monitored, especially the type of collimator used, so as to facilitate identification of areas of abnormality or the identification of individual abnormal carpal bones. The bone scan must be detailed enough to examine both wrists in dorsal and ventral views with additional lateral or oblique views to enable localization of any "hot spots" to a specific carpal bone or to a particular site in the wrist (Fig. 7–9A). Detection of such an abnormal area can direct more detailed spot films or tomography.

Radioisotope uptake occurs in specific sites of increased bone turnover secondary to an osseous or chondral fracture or to one of the various causes of local hyperemia, i.e.,

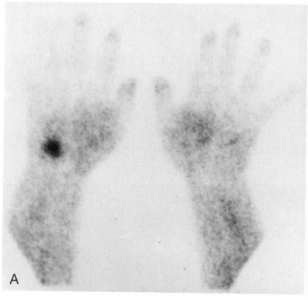

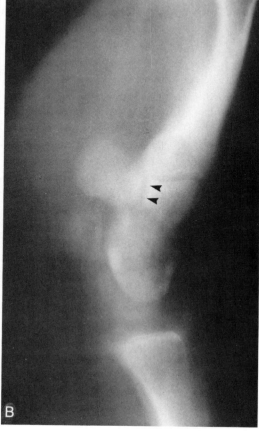

Figure 7–9. *A,* A ventral (AP) view of a technitium-99m bone scan (end of vascular phase) in an early static image shows increased uptake in the hamate bone. *B,* Polytomography of the wrist in a lateral projection shows a healing fracture of the hamate hook (*arrowheads*).

infection or synovitis. Broader areas of increased uptake are seen in synovitis as well as other inflammatory processes involving the soft tissues. It is uncertain whether purely ligamentous injuries without bone involvement can produce hot spots.

Tomography. If any questionable bone abnormality is seen following routine and detailed spot views and especially if there is a focally abnormal bone scan, polytomography should be performed. Sections are taken at 2 or 3 mm intervals in two positions at 90° to each other. Occasionally, 1 mm sections may be necessary to show an abnormality such as the small bone component of an osteochondral fracture suspected because of clinical symptoms and a focally hot bone scan. The best position for polytomography is determined by the specific bone in question, and the wrist should be placed in the position that most optimally profiles this

bone (Fig. 7–9B). The proper position can be determined fluoroscopically, just prior to tomographic positioning.

Wrist Arthrography. When a patient's history, plain films, and instability series suggest an intercarpal ligamentous problem, arthrography may be used to confirm the diagnosis. Contrast medium may be injected into any of the three normally noncommunicating spaces in the carpus. These include the distal radioulnar joint, the radiocarpal joint, and the midcarpal joint space between the proximal and the distal carpal rows.

The technique for wrist arthrography has been described in the literature.[15, 18, 26, 30] Ordinarily, we inject the radiocarpal joint at either the radioscaphoid or radiolunate joints away from the site of point tenderness, using a dilute, water-soluble contrast material such as Conray 43 (iothalamate meglumine) (Fig. 7–10A). Filling of the distal ra-

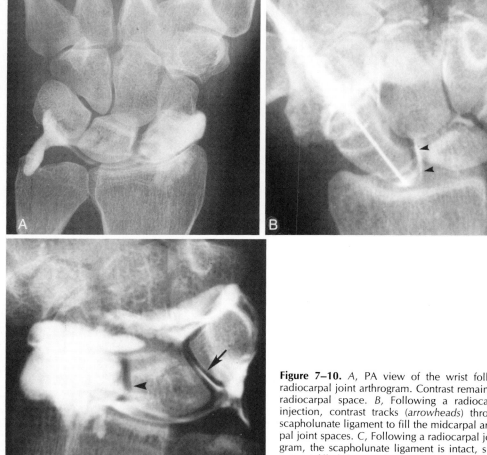

Figure 7–10. *A,* PA view of the wrist following a normal radiocarpal joint arthrogram. Contrast remains confined to the radiocarpal space. *B,* Following a radiocarpal joint space injection, contrast tracks (*arrowheads*) through a disrupted scapholunate ligament to fill the midcarpal and carpometacarpal joint spaces. *C,* Following a radiocarpal joint space arthrogram, the scapholunate ligament is intact, since contrast has not yet filled the scapholunate space (*arrowhead*); however, contrast tracks through the lunotriquetral joint space (*arrow*) as a result of lunotriquetral ligament disruption.

dioulnar joint after injection of the radiocarpal joint indicates a tear in the triangular fibrocartilage complex. When contrast material injected into the radiocarpal joint enters the midcarpal joint, the site of communication indicates a tear of that structure, i.e., the scapholunate ligament, the lunotriquetral ligament, or the radial or ulnar capsule (Fig. 7–10B). Fluoroscopic spot films should be obtained during injection in order to determine which ligament is torn, since on the complete filling phase the anatomy may be obscured by overlying contrast material.[15] Alternatively the injection may be recorded with videotape, cine, or digital subtraction arthrography.[26]

Since the scapholunate ligament is frequently torn, the wrist is maintained in a position with the scapholunate joint profiled during the filling phase (Fig. 7–10C). If no tears have been detected after injection of contrast material, stress views may be obtained to facilitate visualization of small tears that may not fill during routine injection. Radial- and ulnar-deviated views with the wrist in both PA and AP positions are diagnostically valuable maneuvers to create moderate stress in a wrist distended with contrast material.

If no abnormalities are detected to explain the patient's problem and the patient has ulnar-sided wrist pain, a distal radioulnar joint injection may be performed to diagnose partial proximal surface tears of the triangular fibrocartilage complex. A scapholunate or lunotriquetral ligament can falsely appear normal when one of these torn ligaments has been bridged with scar tissue. Additional information as to the origin of pain may be gained by mixing a small amount of anesthetic with the contrast agent and, after injection of one or more of these wrist compartments, noting whether the patient's presenting symptoms have been relieved.[19]

Computed Tomography. This procedure is valuable to confirm a clinical diagnosis of distal radioulnar joint subluxation, when pain or cast immobilization prevents optimum positioning of the wrist for plain radiographs; it is also valuable in situations in which, even with adequate radiographs, the diagnosis is still uncertain.[5, 7, 23] Both wrists should be symmetrically positioned with the palms flat on the table top inside the CT scanner. Ideally, the wrist should be scanned a second time in the position that produces symptoms in the patient. This second position may produce the distal ulnar subluxation that may be missed when the wrist is in a comfortable position.

With this same hand position, hamate hook fractures can be easily demonstrated with CT.[12] However, CT is usually not necessary to demonstrate a hamate hook fracture, since the carpal tunnel view, detailed tangential views, or routine polytomography can usually demonstrate this fracture at much less expense to the patient. Except for clinically evident ganglia, CT is also useful in evaluating the character of some soft tissue masses about the wrist. The extent of soft tissue and bone processes is often easily determined with CT. The degree of lunate fragmentation in Kienböck's disease can readily be visualized by CT scan.

As a general rule, CT of the wrist, except when used for distal radioulnar, lunate, and hamate hook problems, can be performed to show the margins of the carpal bones for more optimal osseous detail. This is done with the wrist elevated off the CT table and dorsiflexed and the gantry tilted toward the elbow of the patient. The resultant CT sections display the carpus in the coronal plane, which provides sections looking like PA tomograms of the wrist. These sections allow much easier interpretation of subtle and gross wrist abnormalities.[3, 4]

Magnetic Resonance Imaging. Magnetic resonance imaging (MRI), although a new modality, promises to be valuable in assessing not only the wrist in particular but also the musculoskeletal system in general. MRI, unlike other imaging modalities, does not rely on ionizing radiation. Instead, using a magnetic field, it generates a proton map of the patient's anatomy. This mapping may have different appearances, depending on the manner in which the scan is performed. Scans may be performed to take advantage of different tissue characteristics, e.g., relative fat and water concentrations in the tissue examined.

Patients with wrist pain, normal plain films, and an abnormal bone scan are especially suited for MRI. In a recent study of patients with unexplained wrist pain, MRI aided in the diagnosis of avascular necrosis with a high degree of specificity and its use suggested a more specific diagnosis than did bone scan in a significant proportion of the cases.[9] This technique promises to be particularly useful in patients suspected of having Stage I Kienböck's disease[17] and for patients

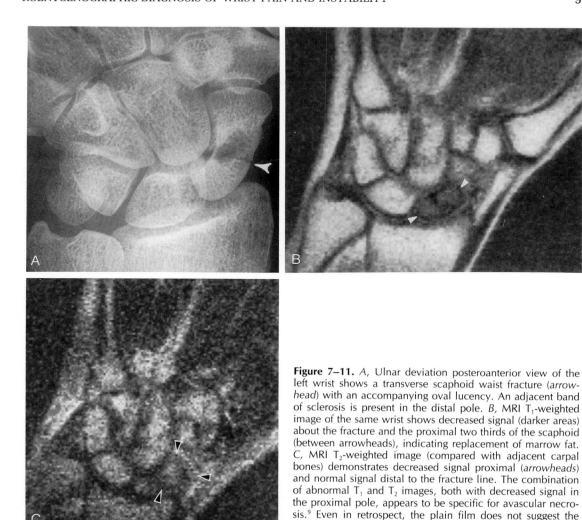

Figure 7–11. *A,* Ulnar deviation posteroanterior view of the left wrist shows a transverse scaphoid waist fracture (*arrowhead*) with an accompanying oval lucency. An adjacent band of sclerosis is present in the distal pole. *B,* MRI T$_1$-weighted image of the same wrist shows decreased signal (darker areas) about the fracture and the proximal two thirds of the scaphoid (between arrowheads), indicating replacement of marrow fat. *C,* MRI T$_2$-weighted image (compared with adjacent carpal bones) demonstrates decreased signal proximal (*arrowheads*) and normal signal distal to the fracture line. The combination of abnormal T$_1$ and T$_2$ images, both with decreased signal in the proximal pole, appears to be specific for avascular necrosis.[9] Even in retrospect, the plain film does not suggest the diagnosis of avascular necrosis.

with scaphoid fracture in whom a diagnosis of proximal pole avascular necrosis is entertained[27] (Fig. 7–11).

Carpal Instability

Carpal instabilities are conditions in which carpal bones have lost some of their normal alignment and intercarpal motion because of interruption of some of the intercarpal or radiocarpal ligaments or both, resulting in hand dysfunction.[2, 16, 21, 28] Recognition of these conditions is necessary for proper patient treatment. At times, patients can have instability patterns without symptoms; however, in many cases this instability progresses to further disruption between carpal bones. The end result of many of these problems is advanced degenerative joint disease, with the patient suffering severe weakness and inability to perform routine tasks. Indeed, carpal ligament instability may be the single reason a patient receives major compensation for loss of hand and wrist function. Carpal ligamentous instabilities may be static, i.e., due to intercarpal malalignment, which is recognizable on routine radiographs, or dynamic, i.e., due to abnormal motion between carpal bones, which is recognizable only during motion observed fluoroscopically.

At least five static carpal instability patterns have been described.[16, 20] These include dorsiflexion instability (DISI—dorsal intercalated segmental instability), palmar flexion instability (VISI—ventral intercalated segmental instability), ulnar translocation, dorsal carpal subluxation, and palmar carpal subluxation[2] (Table 7–1) (Fig. 7–12). A complete classification of carpal instabilities can

Table 7–1. **LIGAMENTOUS INSTABILITY OF THE WRIST***

Ligamentous Instability	Scapholunate Angle	Capitolunate Angle	Comments
NORMAL (Fig. 7–12A and B)	30°–60°	0°–30°	—
DORSIFLEXION (DISI) (lateral view) Lunate tilts dorsally and scaphoid tilts palmarly (Fig. 7–12C and D)	60°–80° = ? abnormal > 80° = abnormal	Normal or increased	Present when either the scapholunate and/or the capitolunate angle is abnormal and abnormal intercarpal motion exists
PALMAR FLEXION (VISI) (lateral view) Both lunate and scaphoid tilt palmarly (Fig. 7–12E and F)	< 30°	< 30° or normal	Present when abnormal intercarpal motion exists
ULNAR TRANSLOCATION (PA view) Carpal bones are ulnar in position (Fig. 7–3A)	Normal	Normal	Space increases between scaphoid and radial styloid; over 50 percent of lunate is medial to radius on neutral PA hand position
DORSAL SUBLUXATION (Lateral view) Carpal bones are dorsal to mid-plane of the radius (Fig. 7–12G)	Normal	Normal	Usually this has an associated dorsally impacted distal radius fracture
PALMAR SUBLUXATION[2] (lateral view) Carpal bones are palmar to mid-plane of the radius (Fig. 7–12H and 7–3B)	Normal	Normal	In reported cases, there is associated ulnar translocation[2]

*Modified from Gilula LA, Totty WG, Weeks PM, et al: Clin Orthop 187:56, 1984, Table I.

be found in Chapter 18. The key to recognizing each of these instability patterns is to identify the lunate on PA and lateral roentgenograms and to determine if the lunate is tilting ventrally or dorsally or if it is displaced ulnarly, dorsally, or ventrally, as compared with the opposite wrist.

The lateral roentgenogram is a more reliable indicator of most of the carpal instability patterns (other than ulnar translocation) than is the PA or AP view. On the lateral view, which is made with the wrist in neutral position, the dorsum of the metacarpals and radius are in a straight line. The scapholunate angle ranges from 30° to 60° and is borderline abnormal up to 80° (Fig. 7–12A), and the capitolunate angle is less than 30° (Fig. 7–12B) (Table 7–1).

Dorsiflexion ligament instability may be suspected on the PA view by the presence of scaphoid foreshortening, lunate tilting, and an increased overlap of the proximal and distal carpal rows, particularly of the lunate over the capitate.[16] On the lateral view, this instability pattern is recognized by dorsal tilting of the lunate; that is, the

Figure 7–12. Ligament instability patterns of the wrist (see Table 7–1). *A*, The scapholunate angle is normal between 30 and 60° and is sometimes normal up to 80°. Although here the scaphoid axis (S) is drawn through the center of the scaphoid, it is easier and is also adequate to draw a scaphoid axis line tangent to the proximal and distal ventral convexities of the scaphoid.[11] (See axis "S" in Figure 7–12E.) C = capitate axis; L = lunate axis. *B*, The capitolunate angle is normally less than 30°. C = capitate axis; L = lunate axis. *C*, Dorsiflexion instability (DISI) is suspected when there is dorsal tilting of the lunate and ventral tilting of the scaphoid with resultant increased scapholunate angle, with or without an increased capitolunate angle. *D*, Dorsiflexion instability. As the lunate tilts dorsally and the scaphoid tilts ventrally, the lunate tends to move ventrally and the capitate dorsally. *E*, Palmar flexion instability (VISI) is suspected with a scapholunate angle decreased to less than 30° and/or a capitolunate angle of 30° or more. C = capitate; S = scaphoid; L = lunate axes. *F*, In palmar flexion instability, the scaphoid and lunate both tilt ventrally. The lunate tends to move or slide dorsally; in the capitate, although the distal pole tends to tilt dorsally, the head (or proximal end) tends to move ventrally. *G*, With dorsal carpal subluxation, the center of the carpus is dorsal to the center of the mid axis of the radius. *H*, Palmar carpal subluxation is recognized when the central axis of the carpus and lunate is ventral to the mid axis of the radius. (From Gilula LA, and Weeks, PM: Post-traumatic ligamentous instabilities of the wrist. Radiology, 129:641–651, 1978.)

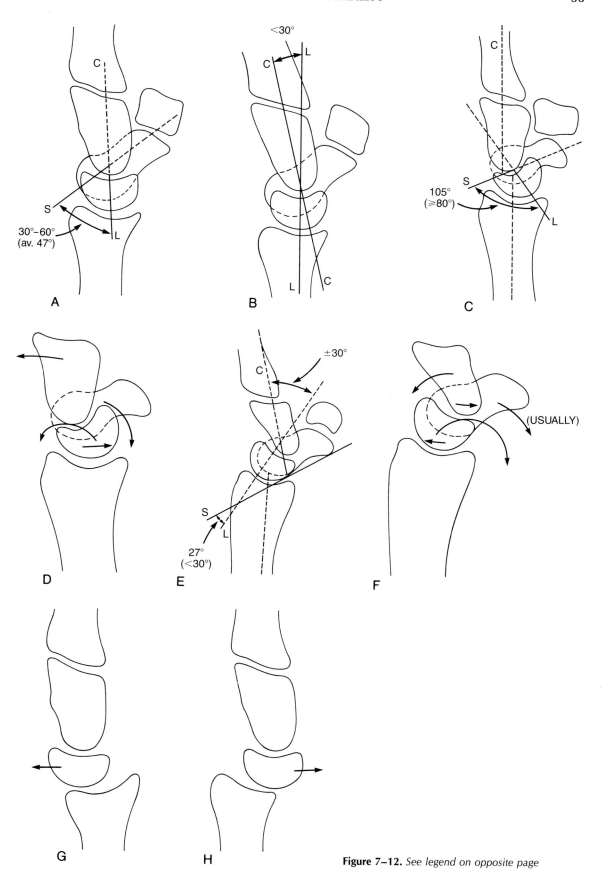

Figure 7–12. *See legend on opposite page*

lunate tilts so that its distal articular surface faces more dorsally than normal (Table 7–1) (Figs. 7–12C and D). Also, there is dissociated movement between the lunate and scaphoid; that is, while the lunate is tilted dorsally, the scaphoid is rotated volarly.

Palmar flexion instability is a condition also known as VISI (Table 7–1). The diagnosis may be suspected on the PA view when there is both foreshortening of the scaphoid and tilting of the lunate and adjacent surfaces of the scaphoid and lunate are parallel. On the lateral view, there is volar flexion of both the lunate and the scaphoid, so that there is decreased scapholunate or increased capitolunate angles or both (Figs. 7–12E and F). The distal carpal row, as identified by the capitate, may also be displaced volarly so that the lunate overlaps the capitate, and on the PA view, this overlap appears to be greater than that on the opposite, normal side.

When either DISI or VISI is suspected, the scapholunate and capitolunate angles should be measured, and, at minimum, the three lateral views (neutral, full flexion, and extension) mentioned in the discussion of the ligament instability series should be performed. The lateral neutral view should be obtained with the dorsum of the metacarpals and the radius in a straight line. With flexion and extension, there should be normal carpal motion; that is, the carpal bones should *flex on flexion* and *extend on extension*. The lunate can be used to identify the proximal, the capitate, and the distal carpal rows.[16, 20]

Ulnar Translocation

In this condition, the carpus has subluxated ulnarly, so that on the PA view, more than one half of the proximal articular surface of the lunate lies ulnar to the radius, and there may be increased space (more than the width of other intercarpal spaces) between the radial styloid process and scaphoid (Fig. 7–4A). Ulnar translocation is common in synovium-based processes, such as rheumatoid arthritis.

Dorsal Carpal Subluxation

This condition is recognized by the presence of dorsal displacement of the carpus onto the distal articular surface of the radius (Fig. 7–12G, Table 7–1). It is usually associated with an old, dorsally impacted fracture of the distal radius.

Palmar Carpal Subluxation

Palmar subluxation of the carpus (Fig. 7–12H) is very uncommon[2] and often has an associated ulnar carpal subluxation. This condition is recognized on the lateral radiograph when the central axis of the lunate and carpus is ventral to the mid-axis of the shaft of the radius.

Delayed recognition or unsuccessful conservative treatment of carpal ligament instabilities can lead to irreversible scar formation in and about the carpus, with atypical alignment and abnormal function of the carpal bones. Malaligned carpal bones may be associated with early degenerative arthritis and the formation of pseudojoints (Fig. 7–4).

DISCUSSION

A thorough clinical history and physical examination form the most solid basis for reaching a definitive diagnosis of wrist pain. When a definite clinical diagnosis can be made, a radiographic examination may not be necessary. However, such diagnoses as ganglion, tenosynovitis, or de Quervain's disease may be associated with underlying, unsuspected disease. A routine wrist survey is recommended in all patients, in order to exclude anatomic variants,[31] osteophytes, ischemic necrosis, degenerative joint disease, or even old, ununited fractures that are not clinically suspected. This survey may change the surgical approach to the patient's problem and may alter expectations for full recovery.

Following the initial clinical investigation, if no definitive diagnosis is made, routine plain films of the wrist should be obtained. When the plain films are normal, the work-up should proceed as described in the algorithm (Fig. 7–1), depending upon whether bone or soft tissue abnormality is suspected.

If a bone abnormality is suspected, detailed spot views or fluoroscopic spot films of a tender site may be helpful. If these do not reveal the cause of the patient's problem, a bone scan is the next step used to localize and verify subtle bone abnormalities, such as hairline fractures, avulsion injuries, or chondral-osteochondral abnormalities. Once the bone scan has detected an abnormal region, plain films, fluoroscopic detailed views, or tomography (plain or CT) may be useful for further definition of the abnormality.

If a ligamentous injury is suspected, an instability series may demonstrate static ligamentous instabilities and abnormal intercarpal motion. Dynamic motion studies or stress views may detect dynamic ligamentous instabilities, or they may define the cause of popping or clicking. Wrist arthrography may then be used to further define the nature of the ligamentous or capsular abnormality, particularly when the patient has point tenderness localized over the dorsum of the wrist. Again, if these radiographic measures fail to demonstrate an anatomic abnormality, a bone scan may reveal an area of abnormal uptake of radioisotope. In the face of a persistent focal bone scan abnormality, as much work-up as is possible and practical should be done to try to explain the abnormality, since such findings are rarely, if ever, meaningless.

CONCLUSION

An organized approach to wrist pathology will, in most cases, lead to a diagnosis. When clinical information is combined with appropriate roentgenographic tests, an early diagnosis can be made and can lead to prompt definitive treatment of the underlying disorder.

References

1. Beckenbaugh RD: Accurate evaluation and management of the painful wrist following injury: an approach to carpal instability. Orthop Clin North Am 15:289–306, 1984.
2. Bellinghausen HW, Gilula LA, and Young LV: Posttraumatic palmar carpal subluxation. J Bone Joint Surg 65A:998–1006, 1983.
3. Biondetti PR, Vannier MW, Gilula LA et al: CT of the wrist. Coronal versus transaxial approach. Radiology. (In press.)
4. Biondetti PR, Vannier MD, Gilula LA, et al: CT of the wrist. Enhancing the three-dimensional reconstruction. Comput Radiol. (In press.)
5. Bowers WH: Problems of the distal radioulnar joint. Adv Orthop Surg 7:289–303, 1984.
6. Chernin MM, and Pitt MJ: Radiographic disease patterns at the carpus. Clin Orthop 187:72–80, 1984.
7. Cone RO, Szabo R, Resnick D, et al: Computed tomography of the normal radioulnar joints. Invest Radiol 18:541–545, 1983.
8. Conway WF, Destouet JM, Gilula LA, et al: The carpal boss: an overview of radiographic evaluation. Radiology 156:29–31, 1985.
9. Reinus WR, Conway WF, Totty WG, et al: Carpal avascular necrosis: MR imaging. Radiology 160:689–693, 1986.
10. Cope JR: Rotatory subluxation of the scaphoid. Clin Radiol 35:495–501, 1984.
11. Curtis DJ: Injuries of the wrist: an approach to diagnosis. Radiol Clin North Am 19:625–644, 1981.
12. Egawa M, and Asai T: Fracture of the hook of the hamate: report of six cases and the suitability of computerized tomography. J Hand Surg 8:393–398, 1983.
13. Gilula LA: Carpal injuries: analytic approach and case exercises. AJR 133:503–517, 1979.
14. Gilula LA, Destouet JM, Weeks PM, et al: Roentgenographic diagnosis of the painful wrist. Clin Orthop 187:52–64, 1984.
15. Gilula LA, Totty WG, and Weeks PM: Wrist arthrography: the value of fluoroscopic spot viewing. Radiology 146:555–556, 1983.
16. Gilula LA, and Weeks PM: Post-traumatic ligamentous instabilities of the wrist. Radiology 129:641–651, 1978.
17. Kuzma GR: Kienböck's Disease. Adv Orthop Surg 8:250–263, 1985.
18. Levinsohn EM, and Palmer AK: Arthrography of the traumatized wrist. Radiology 146:647–651, 1983.
19. Linscheid RL: Personal communication, 1986.
20. Linscheid RL, Dobyns JH, Beabout JW, et al: Traumatic instability of the wrist. J Bone Joint Surg 54A:1612–1632, 1972.
21. Linscheid RL, and Dobyns JH: Athletic injuries of the wrist. Clin Orthop 198:141–151, 1985.
22. Mayfield JK: Patterns of injury to carpal ligaments. A spectrum. Clin Orthop 187:36–42, 1984.
23. Mino DE, Palmer AK, and Levinsohn EM: Radiography and computerized tomography in the diagnosis of incongruity of the distal radioulnar joint. J Bone Joint Surg 67A:247–252, 1985.
24. Palmer A: Personal communication, 1986.
25. Polley HF, and Hunder GG: The wrist and carpal joints. In Polley HG and Hunder GG (eds): Rheumatologic Interviewing and Physical Examination of the Joints. 2nd ed. Philadelphia, WB Saunders Co, 1978, pp 90–111.
26. Resnick D, Andre M, Kerr R, et al: Digital arthrography of the wrist: a radiographic-pathologic investigation. AJR 142:1187–1190, 1984.
27. Ruby LK, Stinson, J, and Belsky MR: The natural history of scaphoid nonunion. A review of fifty-five cases. J Bone Joint Surg 67A:428–432, 1985.
28. Sebald JR, Dobyns JH, and Linscheid, RL: The natural history of collapse deformities of the wrist. Clin Orthop 104:140–148, 1974.
29. Terry DW, and Ramin JE: The navicular fat stripe: a useful roentgen feature for evaluating wrist trauma. AJR 124:25–28, 1975.
30. Tirman RM, Weber ER, Snyder LL, et al: Midcarpal wrist arthrography for detection of tears of the scapholunate and lunotriquetral ligaments. AJR 144:107–108, 1985.
31. Voorhees DR, Daffner RH, Nunley JA, et al: Carpal ligamentous disruptions and negative ulnar variance. Skeletal Radiol 13:257–262, 1985.
32. White SJ, Louis DS, Braunstein EM, et al: Capitatelunate instability: recognition by manipulation under fluoroscopy. AJR 143:361–364, 1984.

CHAPTER 8

Soft Tissue Radiography of the Wrist

EDWARD F. DOWNEY, JR., D.O.
and DAVID J. CURTIS, M.D., F.A.C.R.

The soft tissues of the hand and wrist, even though integrally involved in trauma, have received relatively little radiographic attention. Most descriptions of trauma deal strictly with bone abnormalities. When soft tissue findings are given, they usually refer to the deep structures of the hand or wrist.[1, 2] However, a new approach that systematically details the soft tissue abnormalities of the hand and wrist has been useful in avoiding misdiagnosis.[3, 4] This approach evaluates the soft tissue abnormalities as well as bone and joint abnormalities, correlates the two findings, and resolves any discrepancies between soft tissue and bone abnormalities. Additional views are sometimes necessary to resolve a particular discrepancy. Supplemental findings observed in accordance with this method may lead to a more complete description and understanding of the injury sustained.

In evaluating a film for soft tissue abnormalities, the radiographically visible fat planes that have been disturbed by trauma must be adequately demonstrated.[5] Good film quality is necessary to see the fat planes without diminishing bone detail. New extremity cassettes seem to provide one solution to the need for high quality film. Soft tissue swelling with subsequent disturbance of the fat planes is most usefully observed in posteroanterior (PA) and lateral radiographs of the hand and wrist. The relevance of these soft tissue abnormalities can be confirmed by correlating other anatomic findings with the observed distribution of the swelling.[6]

A systematic approach to soft tissue swelling patterns in the diagnosis of subtle fractures will be discussed. The use of radio-graphs during traction to demonstrate ligamentous injuries may help explain soft tissue swelling seen in the absence of a fracture.[7]

RADIOGRAPHIC ANATOMY

The Deep Fat Planes

Two deep fat planes useful in the evaluation of trauma radiographs of the wrist are the *pronator quadratus fat pad* and the *scaphoid fat pad*. The pronator quadratus fat pad lies between the pronator quadratus muscle and the volar tendon sheaths. This fat plane is seen on the lateral radiograph of the wrist as a lucent crescent closely applied to the volar aspect of the normal distal radius (Fig. 8–1). It is obliterated in trauma to the distal radius or ulna (Fig. 8–2A). The scaphoid fat plane lies between the radial collateral ligament and the abductor pollicis brevis tendon. This fat plane is seen on the posteroanterior radiograph as a lucent stripe extending from the radial styloid to the trapezium, almost paralleling the radial aspect of the scaphoid (Fig. 8–2B).

The Superficial Fat Planes

Seven superficial fat planes, which include the continuous skin-subcutaneous fat zone, are useful in localizing the site of bone abnormality.[3] Four sites should be scrutinized on the PA view (Fig. 8–3A). These are the *thenar*, overlying the proximal aspect of the first metacarpal; the *hypothenar*, at the level of the proximal fifth metacarpal and hamate; the *paraulnar*, superficial to the distal aspect of the ulna; and the *pararadial*, superficial to the distal aspect of the radius.

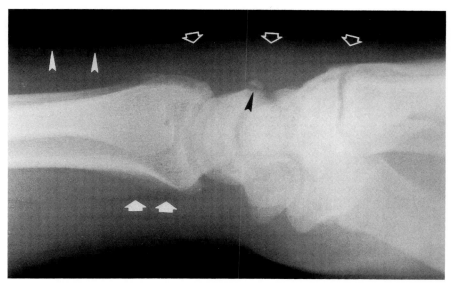

Figure 8–1. Triquetral fracture, lateral wrist. A normal dorsal forearm (*white arrowheads*), dorsal hand, and pronator fat pad (*white arrows*) are seen. Dorsal wrist swelling only is seen (*open arrows*). An avulsion of the triquetrum explains this swelling (*black arrowhead*).

The remaining three fat planes involve the dorsal aspect of the wrist seen on the lateral radiograph (Fig. 8–1 and 8–3B). The normal *dorsal superficial skin subcutaneous fat zones* appear to be continuous; however, fresh cadaver dissections demonstrate that a superficial compartmentalization of the soft tissues deep to the skin-subcutaneus fat zone exists.[6] Three distinct anatomic areas are created by fascial planes that connect the dorsal retinaculum to the skin. This anatomic configuration makes the localization of swelling useful in determining the site of bone injury.

Analysis of Soft Tissue Changes

Swelling that conforms to the observed fractures or dislocations is always present within the acute period of the injury. A fracture or dislocation must be excluded with particular care in the presence of soft tissue swelling of two or more complementary fat planes (Fig. 8–4A and B). Similarly,

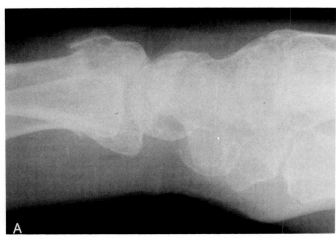

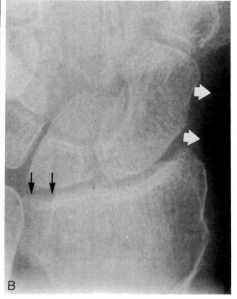

Figure 8–2. Lateral and PA views of wrist with intra-articular distal radius fracture. *A,* Lateral view of the wrist. The pronator fat pad is obliterated and dorsal forearm swelling is seen. Dorsal and volar cortical radial fractures are noted, explaining these soft tissue abnormalities. *B,* PA view. A normal scaphoid fat plane is seen (*white arrows*). A comminuted fracture of the distal radius is seen with a depressed medial articulating surface (*black arrows*).

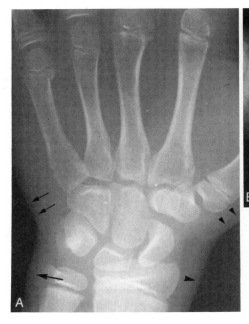

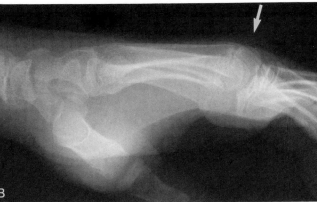

Figure 8–3. PA and lateral views of hand and wrist with fifth metacarpal head fracture. *A,* PA view of the hand. Radial deviation makes the scaphoid fat plane difficult to interpret. Normal pararadial (*large arrowhead*) and paraulnar (*large arrow*) skin-subcutaneous fat interfaces are seen. The hypothenar region also appears normal (*small arrows*). The thenar region is also normal (*small arrowheads*). Salter-Harris II fracture of the fifth metacarpal is seen. *B,* Lateral view of the hand. Localized soft tissue swelling is seen over the head of the metacarpals (*arrows*).

the presence of unequivocal soft tissue swelling in one location should be considered strongly suggestive of a fracture, even though the routine views of the bones are "normal." The absence of soft tissue swelling virtually excludes the presence of a fracture, but the converse is not necessarily true. Additional views should be considered to better demonstrate the area beneath soft tissue swelling, especially if the morbidity is high for a given injury without therapy. Re-examination with radiographs after immo-

bilization should be undertaken when swelling exists without a detectable fracture. This is especially true in scaphoid fractures (Fig. 8–5). A statistical analysis of soft tissue swelling in wrist trauma revealed practical associations between the soft tissue changes and bone abnormalities (Table 8–1).[7]

Initial evaluation of fat planes in the lateral view narrows the radiologic search for injury to only the hand, wrist, or forearm, in the presence of swelling involving the dorsal hand, dorsal wrist, dorsal forearm, or

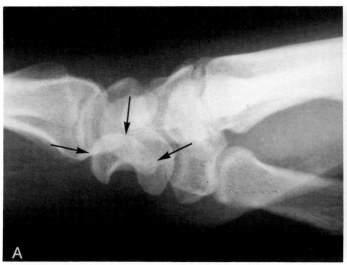

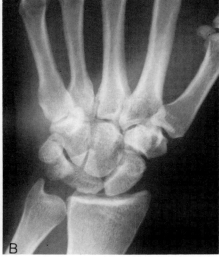

Figure 8–4. Lunate dislocation. *A,* Lateral view of the wrist. The pronator fat is obliterated. Mild obliquity makes it difficult to confirm dorsal forearm and dorsal wrist swelling. The lunate is dislocated volarly (*arrows*). *B,* PA view of the wrist. Minimal scaphoid swelling is noted. There is loss of normal scapholunate, radiolunate, and proximal carpal row joint spaces, and the lunate appears to have a triangular shape.

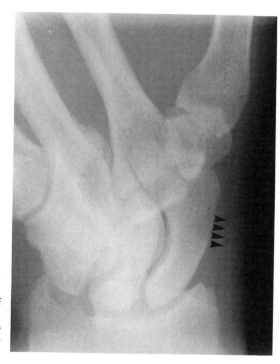

Figure 8–5. Wrist sprain. Scaphoid view shows partial loss of distinct scaphoid fat pad (*arrowheads*). No fracture is noted. Mild scapholunate joint diastasis is seen (the space appears triangular rather than parallel). Immobilization and re-examination may be helpful in this type of case.

Table 8–1. **POSSIBLE ASSOCIATIONS BETWEEN SOFT TISSUE SWELLING AND BONE FRACTURES AND DISLOCATIONS**

	Soft Tissue (Fat Plane) Swelling								
	Dorsal Hand	Dorsal Wrist	Dorsal Forearm	M. Pronator Quadratus	Thenar	Hypothenar	Scaphoid	Pararadial	Paraulnar
Fractured Bone									
Thumb (First Metacarpal)					§		†		
Second to Fifth Metacarpal	§	‡				*			
Scaphoid		§					§		
Greater Multangular (Trapezium)		*			*		*		
Lunate		§							
Capitate		*							
Triquetrum		§							*
Hamate		*				*			
Pisiform									*
Radius			§	§			†	§	*
Ulna			*	*					§
Dislocated Bone									
Radiocarpal		*	*	*			*	*	*
Second to Fifth Metacarpal	§	*			*	*			
Thumb					§				

*Occasionally
†Radial styloid only
‡Associated with dislocated metacarpal base only
§Usually

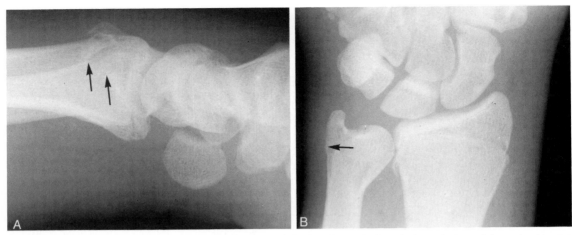

Figure 8–6. Minimally displaced extra-articular fractures of distal radius and ulna. *A*, Lateral view of the wrist. Normal dorsal hand soft tissue is seen. The dorsal wrist and forearm fat planes are obliterated. No pronator is seen. A dorsal cortical fracture of the radius is noted. Less distinctly seen is a volarly displaced ulnar fracture (*arrows*). *B*, PA view. Normal thenar and hypothenar fat planes are seen. Pararadial, paraulnar, and scaphoid fat planes are obliterated. Cortical fractures are noted medially and laterally on the radius. What appears to be a cortical fracture is also seen medially on the ulna (*arrow*). Dorsal wrist and scaphoid swelling are not well explained by the radioulnar fracture.

pronator fat planes, respectively (Fig. 8–6A). Careful inspection of the PA view will direct attention to the radial side (thenar, scaphoid, and pararadial) or ulnar aspect (hypothenar and paraulnar), if further swelling is detected (Fig. 8–6B). A routine oblique view helps evaluate the radial side of the wrist, as does the scaphoid view, The reverse oblique (ball catcher's oblique) view assists in the evaluation of ulnar aspect injuries. Stress views, such as clenched fist and distraction views, assist in the evaluation of midcarpal wrist injuries (Figs. 8–7A, B, and C).[8]

SPECIFIC SWELLING ASSOCIATED WITH SPECIFIC INJURIES

The most important and certainly one of the most common post-traumatic soft tissue abnormalities in the wrist is *swelling of the scaphoid fat pad*. One third of all carpal fractures have swelling of this fat pad associated with them. Most of these are scaphoid fractures (Fig. 8–8). The best position for observing the swelling of the scaphoid fat pad is an ulnar-deviated (PA) view. This position accentuates the fat pad and allows its contour to be visualized in its entirety, from the radial styloid to the trapezium. The ulnar-deviated PA view also allows the diagnosis of subtle changes in the scaphoid fat pad that are caused by edema deep to the fat pad. Displacement of the fat pad without its obliteration may be seen in subtle scaphoid fractures that otherwise might not be

apparent. Since scaphoid fractures are often extremely subtle, and since nondiagnosis with its resultant lack of immobilization can have a high morbidity, we believe the PA radiograph with ulnar deviation of the wrist should be a part of the wrist trauma series.

While other carpal fractures may have associated swelling of the scaphoid fat pad, there is usually other compartmental swelling as well. This most often occurs in the dorsal wrist region. In fact, most scaphoid fractures also have swelling in this area (Fig. 8–9).[10] One rare carpal fracture, that of the trapezium, may also have swelling of the scaphoid fat pad associated with it. A radial styloid or other radial fracture with an intra-articular component may cause swelling of the scaphoid fat pad without a carpal fracture (Fig. 8–10A). The most important fact about swelling of the scaphoid fat pad following trauma is that it is almost always associated with a bone abnormality and, therefore, can be used as a predictor of scaphoid fractures not readily seen on the initial radiographs. The major exception to this statement is scapholunate dissociation, which may cause swelling, but scapholunate dissociation is not usually associated with scaphoid fracture.

Swelling of the pronator quadratus fat pad, the other deep fat plane, is also a good indicator of bone abnormality, since swelling is not usually present at this site unless there is a fracture of the distal forearm. The fracture is usually of the radius and less

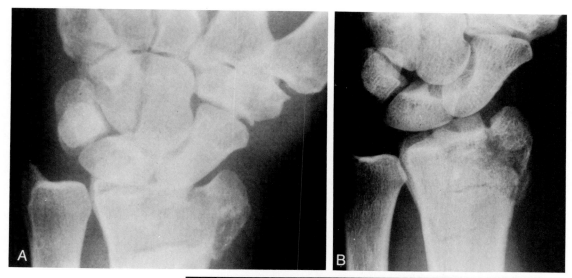

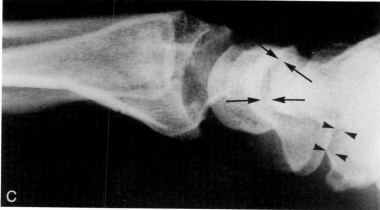

Figure 8–7. Comminuted radial styloid fracture with capitate fracture and carpal ligamentous injuries. *A*, Nondistracted PA view of the wrist shows radial styloid comminuted fracture with some scapholunate widening, a nonparallel midintercarpal row, and a triangular scapholunate joint space, which suggest disrupted intercarpal ligaments. The capitate appears irregular, and there is intercarpal joint widening. A distraction view should help illustrate the carpal injuries. *B*, PA view of the wrist with distraction. The severely comminuted radial styloid and radius articulating surface fragments are more anatomically aligned. There is widening of the radiocarpal joint, midintercarpal row, and ulnar scaphotrapezial joints. The scapholunate joint is not parallel (the proximal scaphoid surface is seen; no lunate articulating surface is seen). *C*, Lateral distraction view shows radiocarpal, volarly asymmetric capitolunate joint (*arrows*), and symmetric scaphotrapezial joint widening (*arrowheads*). These ligamentous disruptions better explain the distribution of subsequent post-traumatic osteoarthritis than do the fractures themselves.[9]

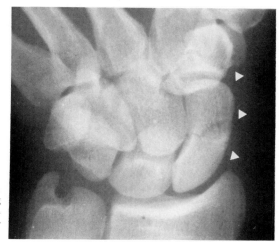

Figure 8–8. Fracture of the scaphoid. Ulnar deviation, PA view, shows an acute fracture of the scaphoid associated with swelling pushing the scaphoid fat pad laterally (*arrowheads*). The proximal pole of the scaphoid is relatively dense, suggesting a prior loss of blood supply.

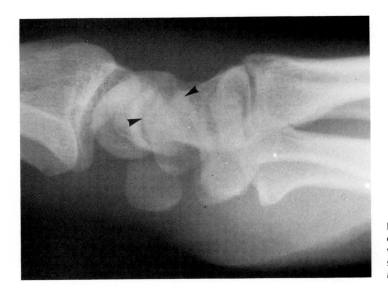

Figure 8–9. Fracture of the scaphoid. Mildly obliqued lateral view. Significant dorsal wrist swelling is seen. An angulated scaphoid waist fracture is seen (*arrowheads*).

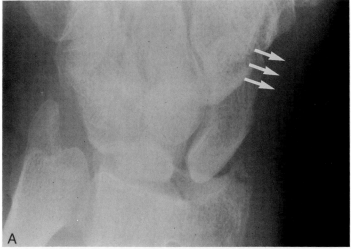

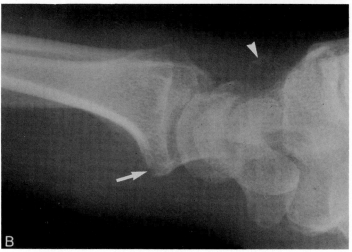

Figure 8–10. Radial styloid fracture, triquetral fracture, and scapholunate ligamentous injury. *A*, Angled scaphoid view shows radial styloid fracture and scapholunate diastasis. Pararadial swelling is prominent. The proximal scaphoid fat plane is obliterated. Only the distal portion of the scaphoid fat pad is normal (*arrows*). *B*, Lateral view. Wrist swelling is present. An avulsion of the dorsal triquetrum is seen (*arrowhead*). The pronator fat pad is bowed and almost obliterated. Dorsal forearm swelling is present. A volar radial cortical break is barely visible (*arrow*). Dorsal hand swelling is not seen.

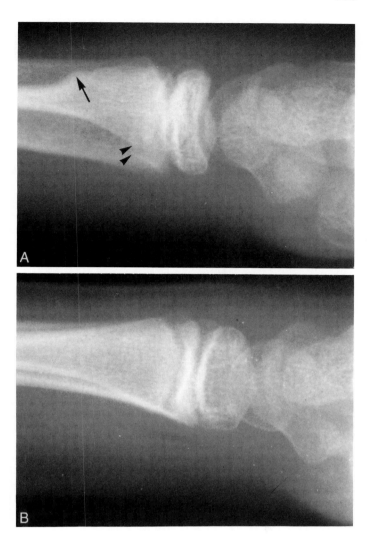

Figure 8–11. Comparison views of minimally displaced wrist fracture in a child. *A,* Lateral view of the wrist. No pronator fat pad is seen. There is dorsal forearm and dorsal wrist swelling as well. A minor dorsal radius cortical fracture is seen (*arrow*). A volar ulnar fracture is also present, suggesting a Salter-Harris II fracture component (*arrowheads*). *B,* Lateral view of the opposite wrist shows a normal pronator fat pad. Minimal wrist swelling is seen. No fracture or definite diastasis is seen.

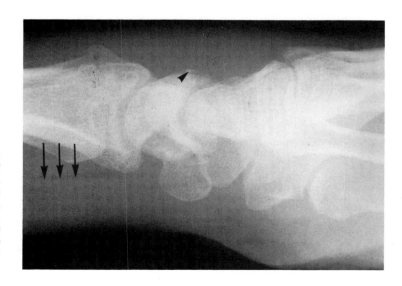

Figure 8–12. Cortical fracture of radius with triquetral avulsion. Lateral view of the wrist. Dorsal wrist and dorsal forearm swelling are seen. The pronator is minimally bowed volarly (*arrows*). A dorsal radius cortical fracture is seen, with loss of the normal articulating angle of the distal radius. An avulsion of the dorsum of the triquetrum is also seen (*arrowhead*).

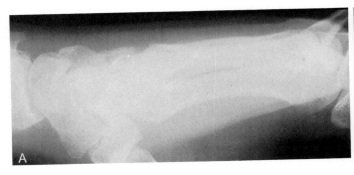

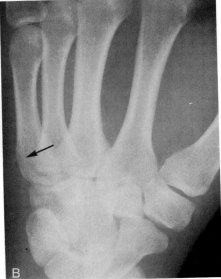

Figure 8–13. Fracture of the base of the fifth metacarpal. *A,* Lateral view of the hand and wrist shows swelling of the dorsum of the hand. *B,* Oblique view of the hand. A nondisplaced fifth metacarpal fracture is seen (*arrow*).

frequently of the ulna (Figs. 8–2A, 8–4A, 8–6A, and 8–10B). Swelling of the pronator fat pad in the absence of an obvious fracture is presumptive evidence of the presence of a fracture. This is especially true in children, since the fat pad disruption may be the only

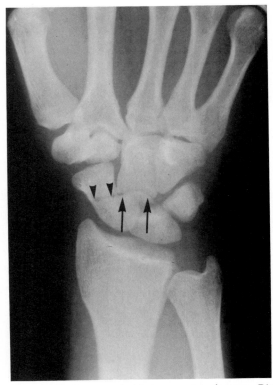

Figure 8–14. Trans-scaphoid, transcapitate fracture. Distraction PA view shows radiocarpal and midcarpal distraction. The scaphoid waist fracture (*arrowheads*) was not seen prior to distraction. An associated capitate fracture with inversion of the fragment is present (*arrows*).

radiographic abnormality in a Salter I or II fracture of the distal radius (Fig. 8–11A and B). Immobilization and re-examination are probably warranted in this situation. A poor lateral radiograph may create a false-positive impression about the abnormality of this fat plane. A repeat image with better positioning is indicated in questionable cases. Palmar bulging is also suggestive of fracture (Fig. 8–12) but less so than radiographic obliteration of the pronator fat pad.

The remaining fat planes are all superficial skin-subcutaneous fat interface zones. The most important regions for evaluation are the three planes visualized on the lateral radiographs. *Dorsal hand swelling* is strongly associated with a fracture of the second through fifth metacarpals (Fig. 8–13A and B). If swelling is localized over the metacarpal heads, close attention to the distal metacarpal will often reveal the fracture (Fig. 8–3B). However, swelling of the dorsal hand or any of the superficial fat planes can be present from direct soft tissue trauma without fracture; therefore, a fracture must be diligently sought, with the diagnosis of soft tissue trauma only made when a fracture has been excluded.

Dorsal wrist swelling is strongly associated with carpal fractures or dislocations (Figs. 8–1, 8–2A, 8–6A, 8–9, 8–10B, 8–11A, and 8–12). However, soft tissue swelling may be observed without a fracture being found. In one study, dorsal wrist swelling was the most commonly observed swelling when no fracture was seen.[4] A recent article has confirmed the usefulness of this fat plane

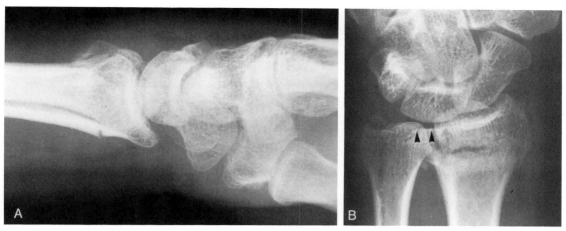

Figure 8–15. Intra-articular distal radius and ulna fracture. *A,* Lateral view of the wrist shows bowing and near-obliteration of the pronator fat pad. Dorsal forearm and dorsal wrist swelling are seen. There is a reversal of the normal distal radius angle because of an impacted fracture. *B,* PA view of the wrist. Pararadial and paraulnar swelling is noted. A comminuted radial fracture is seen with a depressed medial fragment (*arrowheads*). An ulnar styloid fracture is seen.

swelling, when coupled with swelling of the scaphoid fat plane, in diagnosing scaphoid fractures.[8] However, other fractures must be excluded, and if the swelling is remarkable, a distraction view may be useful (Fig. 8–14).

When both dorsal hand and dorsal wrist swelling are present, the cause is (1) a carpometacarpal dislocation, (2) an intra-articular fracture of one or more of the second through fifth metacarpal bases, or (3) both a metacarpal and a carpal fracture. Longitudinally oriented radial fractures that involve the radiocarpal articulating surface accounted for all wrist swelling seen in isolated forearm fractures (Figs. 8–2 and 8–15A). However, if a nonarticular fracture

of the radius is seen and dorsal wrist swelling is present, a carpal fracture, diastasis, or wrist dislocation should also be sought.

Dorsal forearm swelling is a common finding. Two thirds of all forearm fractures have dorsal forearm swelling. Radial or ulnar fractures accounted for all cases with dorsal forearm swelling when only one bone was fractured.[4] When both dorsal wrist and dorsal forearm swelling are present, the cause is (1) a radial fracture involving the radiocarpal articulating surface, (2) a dislocation (Figs. 8–4 and 8–16), or (3) a carpal fracture associated with a forearm fracture (Figs. 8–9 and 8–12). Dorsal forearm swelling may be the only radiographic finding in nondis-

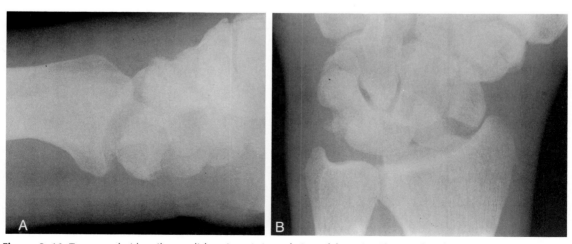

Figures 8–16. Trans-scaphoid perilunate dislocation. *A,* Lateral view of the wrist. There is dorsal wrist, dorsal forearm, and pronator fat pad swelling. A perilunate dislocation is seen. *B,* PA view of a "clenched fist" wrist. There is mild widening of the capitohamate and hamatotriquetral joints. Radiolunate widening is seen. Scaphoid, pararadial, and paraulnar fat plane swelling is prominent. A nonaligned midscaphoid fracture is seen. No joint is seen between the lunate and capitate. Bone fragments in the ulnar aspect of the wrist were avulsed from the triquetrum.

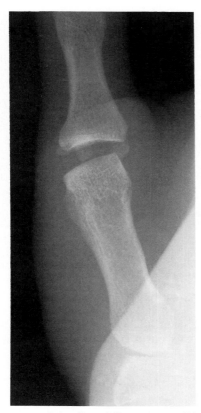

Figure 8–17. Radial collateral ligament tear. PA view of thumb shows loss of skin-subcutaneous fat interface. A widened first metacarpal phalangeal joint is seen with medial deviation of the phalanx.

placed Salter-Harris I or II fractures, as has been seen with swelling of the pronator quadratus.

The remaining superficial fat planes are all seen on the anteroposterior radiograph.

Thenar swelling usually indicates a first metacarpal fracture. Occasionally, this fat plane may be disrupted by a more distal injury to the first metacarpophalangeal joint or proximal first phalanx (Fig. 8–17). Rarely is it associated with a trapezial fracture.

Hypothenar swelling is seen in the majority of cases of second through fifth metacarpal fractures (Fig. 8–18) However, it may be subtle or not present in these fractures. Swelling in the hypothenar region may indicate a hamate fracture, especially when dorsal wrist swelling is present and dorsal hand swelling is absent. Hamate fractures are often difficult to diagnose, and the presence of this soft tissue disruption can help to indicate whether further views are necessary.

Pararadial swelling is strongly indicative of a radial fracture (Figs. 8–6, 8–10A, 8–15B, and 8–19). However, carpal dislocations may also show swelling adjacent to the radial styloid without a fracture of the radius (Fig. 8–16B). In children, pararadial swelling with either pronator quadratus or dorsal forearm swelling is presumptive evidence of a Salter I or II fracture in the appropriate clinical setting, even in the absence of definite bone abnormality. In adults, an ulnar fracture as well as a radial fracture should be looked for, since less than 20 percent of radial fractures occur alone. Similarly, when an ulnar styloid fracture is present, another fracture should be sought, since only 6 percent of ulnar styloid fractures occur alone.[4]

Last, *paraulnar swelling*, like pararadial swelling, is strongly indicative of a forearm

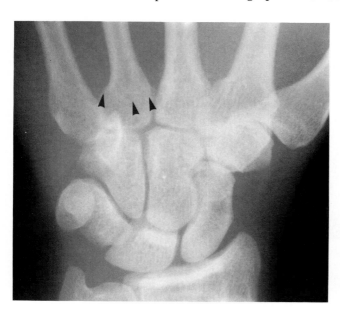

Figure 8–18. Fracture of the fourth metacarpal base. PA view of the wrist. Hypothenar swelling is seen. A careful look shows the metacarpal fracture (*arrowheads*). A reverse (ball catcher's) oblique view would further elucidate this and help to determine if the fifth metacarpal base is subluxed or fractured.

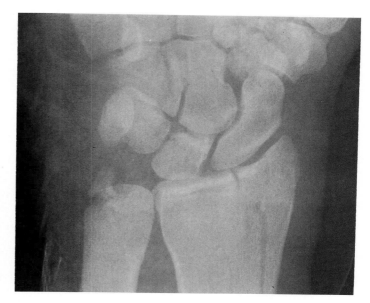

Figure 8–19. Severely comminuted intra-articular radius fracture with lunate and capitate waist fracture. PA view of the wrist. There is pararadial, paraulnar, and scaphoid swelling. A comminuted, longitudinally oriented radius fracture is noted, disrupting the articulating surface of the radius. The ulnar styloid has been fractured. The distal articulating surface of the lunate is fragmented. The waist of the capitate shows a nondisplaced fracture.

injury (Figs. 8–6, 8–15B, 8–16B, 8–19). It is rarely present without swelling in some other soft tissue compartment. When no other soft tissue swelling is seen, it suggests a pisiform fracture (the result of a direct blow to the volar surface of the wrist).

The authors wish to thank Barbara A. Hamer and Pearl Mulraine for manuscript preparation, and George Holborow and Douglas Worman for anatomic laboratory assistance.

References

1. Terry DW Jr, and Ramish JE: The navicular fat stripe; a useful roentgen for evaluating wrist trauma. AJR 124:25–28, 1975.
2. MacEwan DW: Changes due to trauma in the fat plane overlying the quadratus muscle: a radiologic sign. Radiology 82:879–886, 1964.
3. Curtis DJ: Injuries of the wrist: an approach to diagnosis. Radiol Clin North Am 19:625–644, 1981.
4. Curtis DJ, Downey EF Jr, Brower AC, et al: Importance of soft-tissue evaluation in hand and wrist trauma: statistical evaluation. AJR 142:781–788, 1984.
5. Melon GL, Staple TW, and Evans RG: Soft tissue radiographic technique. Semin Roentgenol 8:19–24, 1973.
6. Curtis DJ, Downey EF Jr, and Brahman SL: Letter to the editor. Compartmentalized swelling in hand and wrist trauma. AJR 145:195, 1985.
7. Curtis DJ, Downey EF, Jr, and Brahman SL: Soft tissue support of the hand and wrist: a laboratory study of sprains. (In preparation.)
8. Yousefzadeh DK: The value of traction during roentgenography of the wrist and metacarpophalangeal joints. Skeletal Radiol 4:29–33, 1979.
9. Watson HK, and Ryu, J: Degenerative disorders of the carpus. Orthop Clin North Am 15:337–353, 1984.
10. Carver RA, and Barrington NA: Soft-tissue changes accompanying recent scaphoid injuries. Clin Radiol 36:423–425, 1985.
11. Downey EF Jr, and Curtis DJ: Patient-induced stress test of the first metacarpophalangeal joint. Radiology 158:679–683, 1986.

CHAPTER 9

Wrist Arthroscopy

Radiocarpal Arthroscopy: Technique and Selected Cases

JAMES H. ROTH, M.D., F.R.C.S.(C)

INTRODUCTION

Clinical use of the arthroscope in North America began in the 1970s and revolutionized the management of knee problems. The knee surgeon is now able to accurately diagnose intra-articular pathology. Knee arthroscopy has been shown to be a significant improvement over arthrography[1-5] and to provide more information than arthrotomy, allowing direct visualization of meniscal, anterior cruciate ligament, articular cartilage, and synovial pathology. The experienced knee arthroscopist performs the majority of intra-articular surgical procedures arthroscopically. Patients undergoing arthroscopic knee surgery tend to rehabilitate more quickly and to have less pain postoperatively than patients who have had surgery through an arthrotomy. Infections following arthroscopy of the knee are rare. Arthroscopic procedures are performed on an outpatient surgery basis in most cases. We have had extensive experience with knee arthroscopy at our center and are convinced of its advantages over arthrotomy.

Following the success knee surgeons have had with the arthroscope, orthopedists have become proficient at performing arthroscopy on smaller joints, including the shoulder[6] and the ankle.[7] We have been interested in arthroscopic surgery of the wrist, since the diagnosis of intra-articular pathology can be elusive, and wrist arthrotomy is a procedure with a high morbidity rate, with prolonged rehabilitation and, in some cases, residual stiffness and pain. This is particularly frustrating if the results of the arthrotomy were negative with no pathologic condition dem-

onstrated. For the past four years, we have been developing a technique of radiocarpal arthroscopy in hopes of improving the diagnosis and treatment of internal wrist derangement.

The purpose of this chapter is to present this technique of radiocarpal arthroscopy. Illustrative cases demonstrating intra-articular radiocarpal problems amenable to arthroscopic surgery techniques are also presented.

TECHNIQUE

The technique and instrumentation of radiocarpal arthroscopy continue to evolve. Our present technique is presented. The procedure is performed in the operating room under general or regional anesthesia, with the majority of procedures performed on an outpatient surgery basis.

The surgeon must be comfortable when performing wrist arthroscopy. A chair with arm supports (Fig. 9–1) is recommended. The arm supports are adjusted so that the surgeon can comfortably rest his elbows on them and have his hands in a working position. Without such support, the surgeon will experience neck and shoulder discomfort owing to fatigue after a short period of time, which may affect his ability to persevere with a difficult or prolonged case. The chair is draped with sterile sheets (Fig. 9–2). The surgeon wears a plastic bib or impermeable gown to prevent discomfort from soakage by the irrigation fluid. The patient is positioned supine on the operating room table. The torso on the operated side is

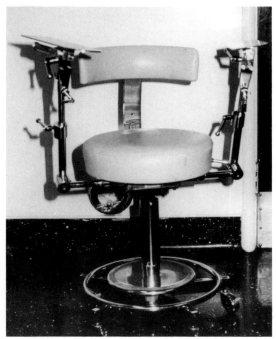

Figure 9–1. A chair with arm supports is recommended.

placed close to the edge of the table so that when the shoulder is abducted, the arm hangs free from the table (Fig. 9–3). An above-elbow tourniquet is elevated to 250 mm Hg. We prefer to perform arthroscopic procedures, both of the knee and the wrist, with a proximal tourniquet, elevated to prevent hemorrhage, which can hinder visualization. Many knee arthroscopists prefer not to use a tourniquet for fear of tourniquet-related nerve paralysis, and it is possible that wrist arthroscopic procedures could also be performed without tourniquet elevation.

A sling is applied over the patient's arm (Fig. 9–3). The hand and forearm are prepared with tincture of iodine. Sterile finger traps are applied to the fingers. We attach the traps to the radial digits when we are primarily interested in the radial aspect of the radiocarpal joint, and to ulnar digits when interested in the ulnar portion of the radiocarpal articulation. Multiple finger traps are attached with wire to a bar, so that

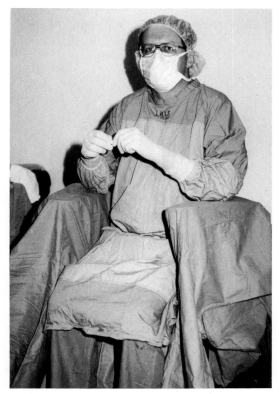

Figure 9–2. The chair is covered with sterile drapes. The arm supports have been adjusted so that the surgeon can comfortably rest his elbows on the supports and have his hands in a working position.

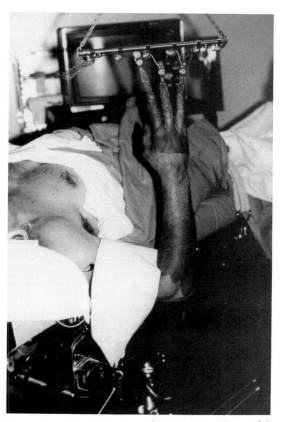

Figure 9–3. The patient is in the supine position and is brought to the edge of the operating table. The fingers are suspended from sterile traps. Seven pounds of weight are applied to a sling over the arm. An above-elbow tourniquet is elevated to 250 mm of mercury.

the entire unit can be autoclaved; sterile finger traps facilitate draping. The hand-holding apparatus is suspended from a "sky-hook" that has been mounted into the ceiling of our operating room. Seven pounds of weight are attached to the sling over the arm (Fig. 9–3). The weight provides some distention of the carpus and helps stabilize the wrist so that it is less mobile during the procedure. A sterile paper U drape with adherent edges is applied.

The surgeon sits comfortably in the arthroscopy chair, with easy access to the dorsum of the wrist (Fig. 9–4). Usually, two arthroscopy portal sites are used. The mid-dorsal portal is located 1 cm distal to Lister's tubercle. Placing a 22-gauge needle into the radiocarpal joint at the planned portal site helps to ensure appropriate placement. The radiocarpal joint is distended with saline (Fig. 9–5). A stab incision with a number 15 blade is made through skin and dorsal capsule (Fig. 9–6). It is important to incise the capsule. Capsular penetration is heralded by a return of saline through the portal site.

The second portal is located dorsoulnarly. The triquetrum is palpated. At the proximal edge of the triquetrum, a stab incision is made. Again, the capsule is incised, with the return of saline indicating when this has

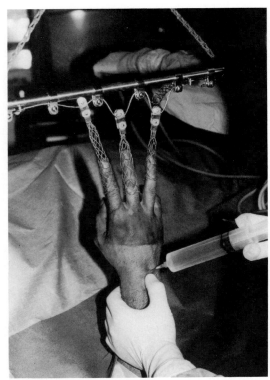

Figure 9–5. The radiocarpal joint is distended with an injection of saline.

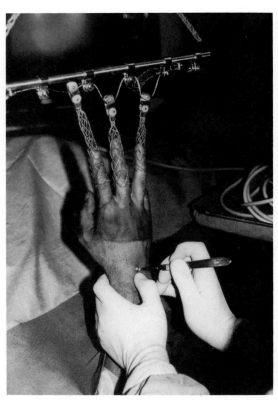

Figure 9–6. The middorsal portal site is located 1 cm distal to Lister's tubercle. A stab incision is made through the skin, subcutaneous tissue, and dorsal capsule.

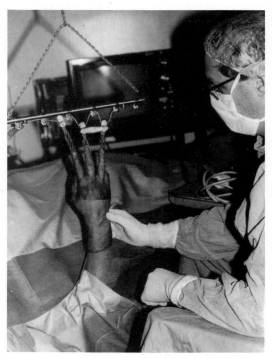

Figure 9–4. The surgeon sits comfortably in the arthroscopy chair, with easy access to the dorsum of the wrist.

been accomplished. A 30° angled arthroscope is inserted through the dorsoulnar portal (Fig. 9–7). A lightweight "chip camera" is applied to the arthroscope (Fig. 9–8). Viewing the arthroscopy on a monitor has the advantages of improved surgeon comfort, improved sterility of the procedure, ability to document the pathologic disorder and the procedure itself, as well as improved ability to help and better morale of assistants.

An irrigation bag is connected by intravenous tubing to the arthroscope. The bag is elevated on a pole to maintain constant joint distention. A small hook probe is inserted through the mid-dorsal portal site. The arthroscope is then inserted in the mid-dorsal portal site. This provides a different orientation and often helps clarify the pathologic condition demonstrated when the arthroscope was in the ulnar portal. The hook probe is important and should be used at all times; it helps to orient the arthroscope so that the surgeon does not "get lost." Palpating structures such as the triangular fibrocartilage and intercarpal articulations may demonstrate disorders not appreciated by visualization alone. The hook probe also aids in determining the size of defects, which is often difficult to do because of the

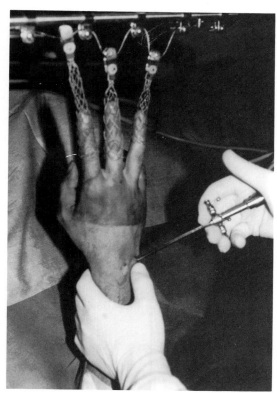

Figure 9–7. The dorsoulnar portal site is located just next to the proximal border of the triquetrum.

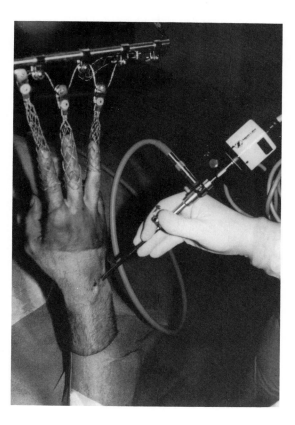

Figure 9–8. A 30° angled arthroscope with "chip camera" is recommended.

magnification of the image by the arthroscope (Figs. 9–9 and 9–10). Numerous other instruments have been developed to aid in arthroscopic surgery. Various punches and small rongeurs can help to remove portions of synovium, bone, or torn triangular fibrocartilage. Motorized cutters with suction can be valuable in many ways (Fig. 9–11).

At the end of the procedure, the radiocarpal joint is injected with 10 ml of 0.5 percent bupivacaine hydrochloride to diminish postoperative discomfort. A bulky below-elbow hand dressing incorporating volar and dorsal plaster splints is applied and the tourniquet released. The patient is examined in 5 to 7 days, the dressing removed, and the appropriate therapy regimen instituted.

SELECTED CASES

Triangular Fibrocartilage Perforations

Chronic ulnar wrist pain can present a diagnostic and therapeutic dilemma. Radiocarpal arthroscopy can be helpful in these cases. The normal triangular fibrocartilage has a smooth surface without a perforation (Figs. 9–12 and 9–13). The distal radius and lunate are normally covered with smooth, glistening articular cartilage (Fig. 9–14).

D.B. is a 36-year-old chambermaid who injured her right (dominant) wrist 18 months prior to arthroscopy, when lifting a garbage bag. She felt something "crack" on the ulnar side of her wrist, and she had immediate pain and swelling. She was seen in the emergency room on the day of the injury. X-rays were taken and demonstrated no gross bone abnormality. The diagnosis of a "wrist sprain" was made by the emergency physician. She was placed in a below-elbow cast for two weeks and then started on a course of physiotherapy. However, disabling ulnar pain and weakness persisted, preventing her from returning to work. A radiocarpal arthrogram was performed (Fig. 9–15) and demonstrated leakage of contrast into the distal radioulnar joint, suggesting a triangular fibrocartilage perforation.

Radiocarpal arthroscopy was performed on an outpatient surgery basis. A Type I[8] perforation (Fig. 9–16) of the triangular fibrocartilage was visualized. Chondromalacia of the lunate and triquetrum was present. The centrum of the triangular fibrocartilage adjacent to the perforation was mobile, and the articular cartilage changes in the lunate and triquetrum appeared to be secondary to

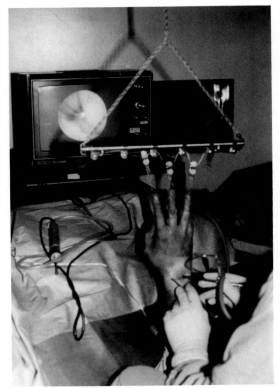

Figure 9–9. The arthroscope is in the dorsoulnar portal site. The hook probe is in the middorsal portal site. This patient had a scaphoid implant performed one year ago and is continuing to have pain.

mechanical trauma from the unstable centrum of the triangular fibrocartilage. A partial triangular fibrocartilage excision was performed using arthroscopic surgery tech-

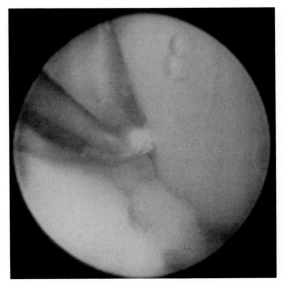

Figure 9–10. The scaphoid implant is visualized. The hook probe is palpating the radial aspect of the implant. Synovitis is seen about the implant.

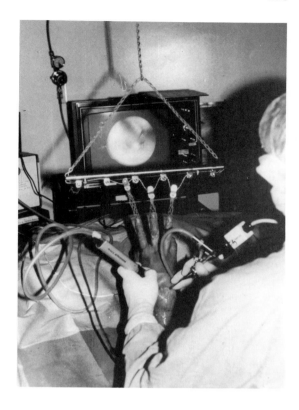

Figure 9–11. Motorized cutters with suction are helpful in joint débridement. Note the fluid extravasation on the dorsum of the wrist. This has not been a problem clinically.

niques, excising only the centrum (Fig. 9–17) and preserving the anterior and posterior distal radioulnar ligaments.

After operation, the wrist was immobilized in a bulky hand dressing for seven days. Physiotherapy was restarted. The patient was able to return to all activities of daily living within six weeks and returned to work as a chambermaid four months fol-

lowing arthroscopy. She has occasional aching wrist discomfort, which is most likely due to the chondromalacia of the lunate and triquetrum, but she is able to tolerate this. She no longer has the episodes of acute pain and swelling that were so disabling.

This case illustrates several important points. The radiocarpal arthrogram demonstrated a leak of contrast into the distal

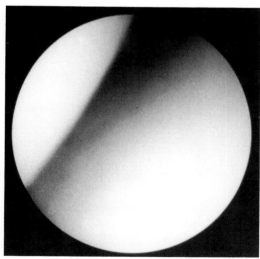

Figure 9–12. This is a normal wrist. We are looking directly at the triangular fibrocartilage complex centrally. The lunate articular cartilage is to the left.

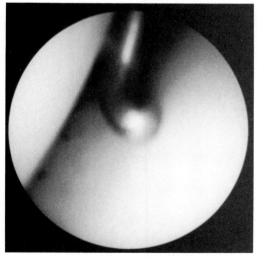

Figure 9–13. The normal triangular fibrocartilage complex is being palpated with the hook probe.

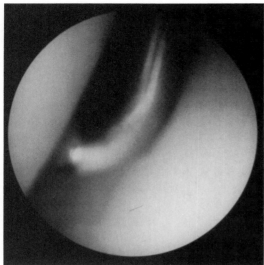

Figure 9–14. The normal articular cartilage of the lunate is being palpated by the hook probe.

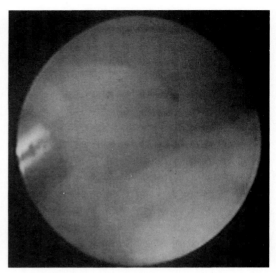

Figure 9–16. Arthroscopy demonstrated a Type I perforation of the triangular fibrocartilage complex and chondromalacia of the triquetrum and lunate.

radioulnar joint, and the disorder was interpreted as a triangular fibrocartilage perforation; however, even with this confirmed, the size and type of tear could not have been predicted. Similarly, the chondromalacia of the lunate and triquetrum could not be diagnosed arthrographically. Arthroscopy, on the other hand, allows exact diagnosis of intra-articular radiocarpal disorder. In a pro-

spective study comparing radiocarpal arthrography and arthroscopy,[9] we found that there were patients with negative arthrograms whose arthroscopic examination showed triangular fibrocartilage tears. Therefore, we feel that the best diagnostic procedure for suspected triangular fibrocartilage disorders is arthroscopy.

Arthroscopic surgery techniques can be

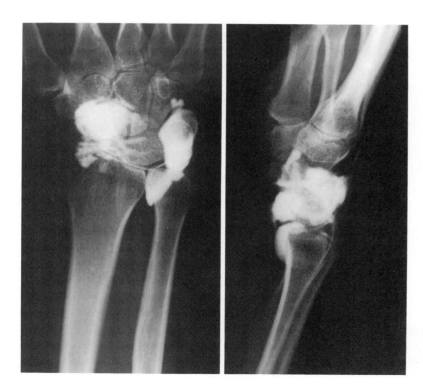

Figure 9–15. D.B.'s radiocarpal arthrogram demonstrated leakage of contrast material into the distal radioulnar joint.

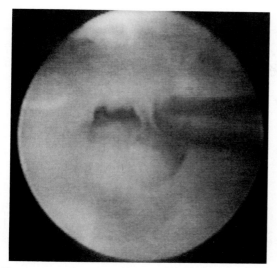

Figure 9–17. The unstable centrum of the triangular fibrocartilage was excised using arthroscopic surgery techniques. The articular surface of the distal ulna is visible through the triangular fibrocartilage complex. The hook probe has been inserted under the anterior aspect of the remaining triangular fibrocartilage complex to ensure that it is stable.

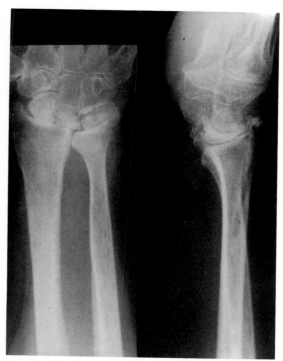

Figure 9–18. D.S.'s x-rays demonstrated severe radiocarpal arthritis with collapse.

used to manage the internal derangements found at arthroscopy. The procedures are not new; they are done using different techniques and instrumentation. Partial triangular fibrocartilage excision for perforation has been described previously.[10] The advantage of arthroscopic partial excision is that an arthrotomy is avoided. This diminishes the postoperative discomfort, shortens rehabilitation time, and prevents formation of a scar. Also, the tear can often be better seen arthroscopically than during open surgery, allowing minimum excision and, perhaps, a cleaner procedure.

Radiocarpal Arthritis

The extent of radiocarpal arthritis and synovitis can be accurately documented arthroscopically. Arthroscopic débridements can be performed as well.

B.S. is a 65-year-old grandmother, who presents with a 10-year history of right (dominant) wrist discomfort. Initially, her pain was intermittent and tolerable, but now the pain is persistent and so severe that she has difficulty sleeping at night. Pain has not been relieved significantly by wrist splinting or anti-inflammatory medications. Radiographs demonstrated severe radiocarpal arthritis (Fig. 9–18). Radiocarpal arthroscopy demonstrated erosion of articular cartilage to

subchondral bone, involving the distal radius and ulna as well as the scaphoid, lunate, and triquetrum.

The proximal poles of the scaphoid, the lunate, and the triquetrum were excised using arthroscopic surgery techniques (Figs. 9–19 and 9–20). B.S. had immediate, decreased wrist pain after arthroscopic proximal row carpectomy. Physiotherapy was started seven days postoperatively. Eight months after surgery, the patient has returned to all activities of daily living and is no longer troubled with night pain.

The extent of the intra-articular pathology caused by degenerative or rheumatoid arthritis can be accurately documented arthroscopically. This provides important information on which to base treatment decisions. As demonstrated in this case, arthroscopic surgery techniques can be used to débride the radiocarpal joint. We have performed synovectomies arthroscopically, as well as excision of the proximal pole of the scaphoid for proximal nonunion, removal of loose bodies, joint irrigation for pseudogout and infection, and partial excision of the distal ulna.

Arthritic derangements are particularly amenable to arthroscopic surgery, since most often excision is the treatment of choice. Such "ectomy" surgery may be better per-

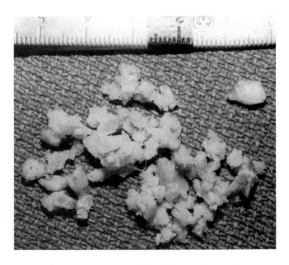

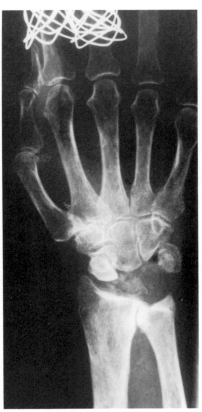

Figure 9–19. Proximal row carpectomy was performed using arthroscopic surgery techniques. A small cervical rongeur was used to remove the carpal bones piecemeal.

formed arthroscopically than through an arthrotomy.

Radiocarpal Trauma

C.B. is a 22-year-old electrician who fell off a ladder onto his outstretched left (nondominant) hand. He sustained a comminuted intra-articular distal radial fracture (Fig.

9–21). Reduction under hematoma block was not satisfactory. Using arthroscopic surgery techniques (Figs. 9–22 and 9–23), the intra-articular fragments were reduced anatomically (Fig. 9–24). An external fixator was applied at the time of arthroscopy. Minimal irrigation was used. The patient was monitored closely for the development of compartment syndrome postoperatively. The external fixator was removed eight weeks later; the fracture had united in excellent position.

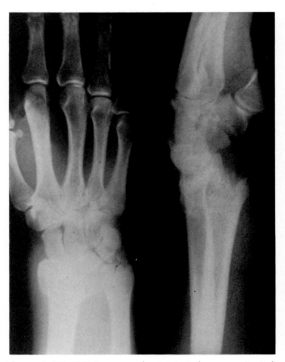

Figure 9–20. An x-ray in the operating room demonstrates that the lunate, triquetrum, and proximal portion of the scaphoid have been excised satisfactorily.

Figure 9–21. C.B.'s x-rays demonstrated a comminuted, intra-articular, distal radius fracture with angulation apex volar.

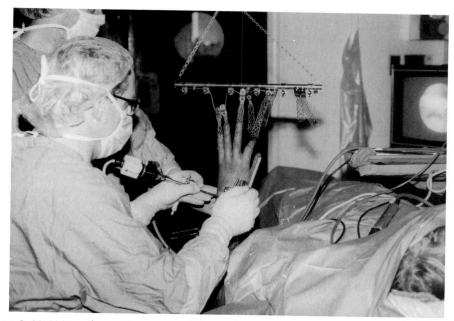

Figure 9–22. Using arthroscopic surgery techniques, the intra-articular fracture fragments were reduced.

Although we have only had limited experience with arthroscopy in acute injuries of the radiocarpal joint, we are enthusiastic about its potential in the treatment of such injuries. We have been able to reduce displaced intra-articular distal radial fractures, as illustrated in the case study presented. In one case, an acute scapholunate dissociation was evident arthroscopically but not on preoperative x-rays. With improved instrumentation and techniques, it is probable that

more acute injuries will be diagnosed and managed arthroscopically.

SUMMARY

A technique of radiocarpal arthroscopy has been presented. Illustrative cases demonstrating intra-articular problems amenable to arthroscopic surgical techniques have also been presented.

We do not have long-term follow-up stud-

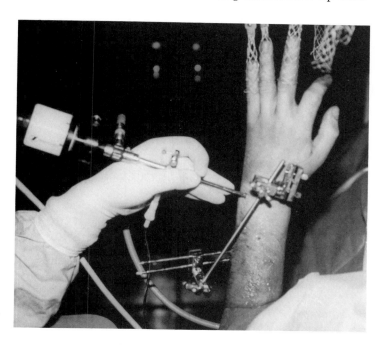

Figure 9–23. Following fracture reduction, an external fixation apparatus was tightened.

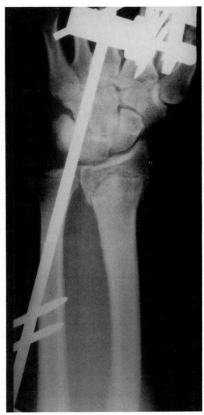

Figure 9–24. Fracture fragment positioning was satisfactory, as demonstrated on this x-ray taken at the time of arthroscopic reduction.

ies of these procedures. The cases presented are illustrative only. The indications, techniques, and instrumentation for arthroscopic wrist surgery are evolving, and careful clinical reviews comparing arthroscopic surgery

technique results with more conventional treatment are required. However, considering its success in the treatment of disorders of other joints, there is reason to believe that results of arthroscopic surgery of the wrist will be equally good, if not better.

References

1. St Pierre RK, Sones PJ, and Fleming LL: Arthroscopy and arthrography of the knee: a comparative study. South Med J 74:1322–1328, 1981.
2. McGinty SB, and Freedmand PA: Arthroscopy of the Knee. Clin Orthop 121:173, 1976.
3. Poehling GL, Bassett FH III, and Goldner JL: Arthroscopy: its role in treating nontraumatic and traumatic lesions of the knee. South Med J 70:465–469, 1977.
4. Dehaven KB, and Collins HR: Diagnosis of internal derangement of the knee: the role of arthroscopy. J Bone Joint Surg 57A:802, 1975.
5. Jackson RW, Abe I: The role of arthroscopy in the management of disorders of the knee: An analysis of 200 consecutive examinations. J Bone Joint Surg 54B:310–322, 1972.
6. Andrews JR, Caron WG, and Ortega K: Arthroscopy of the shoulder: techniques and normal anatomy. Am J Sports Med. 12:107, 1984.
7. Pritsch M, Horoshovski H, and Farine I: Ankle arthroscopy. Clin Orthop 184:137–140, 1984.
8. Blair WF, Berger RA, and El-Khoury GY: Arthrotomography of the wrist. An experimental and preliminary clinical study. J Hand Surg 10A:350–359, 1985.
9. Roth JH, and Haddad RG: Radiocarpal arthroscopy and arthrography in the diagnosis of ulnar wrist pain. Presented at the Annual Meeting of the Arthroscopy Association of North America, San Francisco, California, March 21, 1986.
10. Menon J, Wood VE, Schoene HR, et al: Isolated tears of the triangular fibrocartilage of the wrist: results of partial excision. J Hand Surg 9A:527–530, 1984.

Clinical Applications of Wrist Arthroscopy

TERRY L. WHIPPLE, M.D., F.A.C.S.

Although wrist arthroscopy is a modality of relatively recent development, it is rapidly gaining widespread application. The wrist is a complex joint composed of 15 bones and 27 articular surfaces. It is crossed by 24 tendons, two major arteries, and five primary nerves and branches. This anatomic complexity provides numerous opportunities for the development of joint symptoms that are often difficult to attribute to a specific anatomic structure. The diagnostic aids conven-

tionally used to evaluate wrist pain include radiography, arthrography, cineradiography, and computed tomography. Recently, magnetic resonance imaging has been investigated as a potential modality for wrist evaluation.[11] With the exception of magnetic resonance imaging, however, these ancillary techniques primarily display the skeletal tissues of the wrist and are of limited use in the evaluation of soft tissue disorders. There are numerous subtle instability patterns and intra-articular soft tissue disorders involving the ligaments, the triangular fibrocartilage complex (TFCC), the articular cartilage, and the synovium, which are impossible to diagnose or confirm without the advantage of direct tissue inspection.

Arthroscopy of the wrist provides this advantage.[12] A minimally invasive technique, as discussed in the first part of this chapter, wrist arthroscopy affords a means of direct visualization of intra-articular tissues with magnification and remarkable clarity. These structures may be explored by palpation and manipulation, using various accessory instruments (Fig. 9–25). The procedure may be performed under regional anesthesia and results in virtually no morbidity.

Disruptions of intercarpal ligaments can be demonstrated by wrist arthrography when dye passes from one isolated compartment of the wrist to another. However, it is not possible by use of arthrography to identify the pattern or size of the tear in a specific ligament or in the triangular fibrocartilage complex, nor is arthrography helpful in indicating the mechanical significance of the tear in relation to wrist function or symptoms. These latter considerations have important implications in the formulation of prognoses and appropriate treatment regimens. Central perforations of the triangular fibrocartilage occurring from attrition may be of little long-term significance and require no surgical intervention. An unstable flap tear of the triangular fibrocartilage, however, may cause symptoms of impingement or limitation of motion if the flap is displaced or may even contribute to subtle instabilities of the distal radioulnar joint. While the arthrographic appearance of these two lesions is similar, arthroscopic examination of the TFCC can disclose the size, shape, and precise location of the tear as well as its functional significance in relation to position and stress (Fig. 9–26).

The volar radiocarpal and ulnocarpal ligaments represent specific bulky condensations of fibers in the volar wrist capsule. These concentrated bundles protrude into the joint and can be seen clearly by use of arthroscopy. When these ligaments are torn, palpation of the volar side of the wrist will displace these fiber bundles farther into the joint, and such injuries can be readily confirmed arthroscopically (Fig. 9–27). Chondromalacia and other lesions of articular cartilage without underlying bone sclerosis

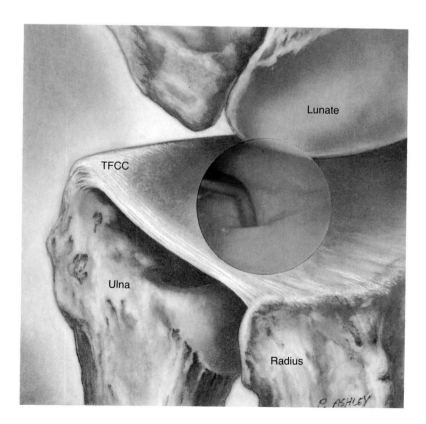

Figure 9–25. Exploration of the soft triangular fibrocartilage complex with a hook probe. Viewed through a 1.9-mm arthroscope from a dorsal approach between the third and fourth extensor compartments.

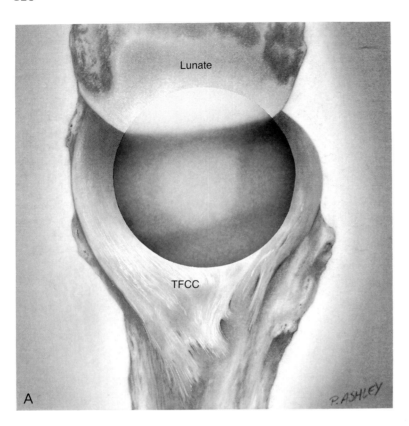

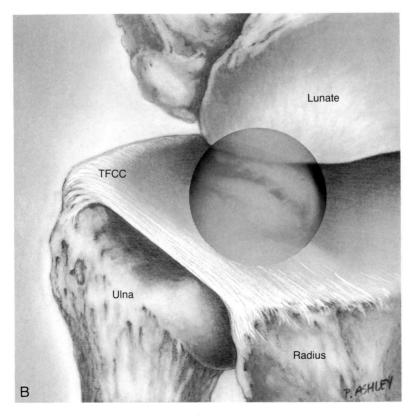

Figure 9–26. *A*, Central perforation of the TFCC viewed from the ulnar side of the wrist. The ulnar head is seen through the perforation. The lesion is smooth and stable, however, and no surgical treatment is indicated. *B*, Unstable flap tear of the TFCC adjacent to its insertion on the ulnar notch of the radius. Turned-up flap of cartilage catches beneath the lunate, causing impingement and pain aggravated by pronation and ulnar deviation. Viewed arthroscopically from dorsal radial approach between first and second extensor compartments.

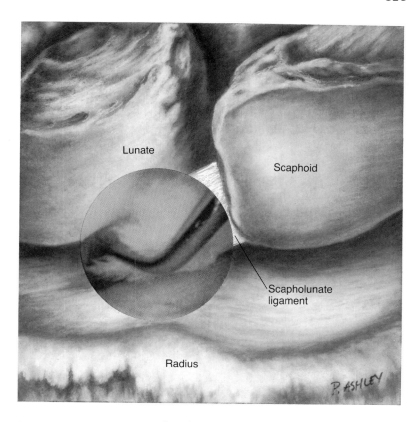

Figure 9–27. A tear of the volar radiolunate triquetral ligament is viewed from a dorsal approach between the third and fourth extensor compartments with a hook probe introduced between the fourth and fifth extensor compartments. Palpation of the volar side of the wrist displaces this ligament into the radiocarpal space.

or osteopenia are best revealed by direct visual inspection of the articular surfaces but do not necessarily require arthrotomy (Fig. 9–28).

While precise indications for wrist arthroscopy are still evolving, early experience has defined certain specific circumstances in which the procedure is extremely useful.[13] Certain surgical procedures may also be performed under arthroscopic control, with the advantage of reduced operative morbidity, as compared with similar procedures performed through arthrotomy. In the evaluation of wrist symptoms, there can be no substitute for a thorough physical examination based on discovery of the mechanism of injury, localization of symptoms, and complete familiarity with wrist anatomy. Conventional diagnostic imaging techniques should then be employed to the greatest possible advantage. However, when these techniques are insufficient to provide the necessary information for a definitive treatment plan, arthroscopy may then be considered.

SPECIFIC INDICATIONS

Through initial clinical experience with wrist arthroscopy, certain specific indica-

tions for this procedure have become apparent. The first group of indications pertains to *lesions of soft tissue.*

If an individual suspected of having an injury to one of the intercarpal ligaments or to the triangular fibrocartilage has a positive arthrogram that demonstrates communication between normally isolated intra-articular spaces, arthroscopy is indicated to assess the size of the defect and to determine whether or not an open procedure is necessary for definitive repair. If, on clinical examination, cineradiography, or stress x-rays, intercarpal instability is proved to be severe enough to warrant surgical stabilization or ligament reconstruction, arthroscopy is indicated for evaluation of articular surfaces; the condition of these surfaces may influence the selection of preferred stabilization procedures. Carpal instability invariably produces abnormal stress on articular surfaces; therefore, certain stabilization procedures that may result in additional stress to already worn articulations would seem to be contraindicated. It is useful as well to know of any associated pathologic conditions of soft tissue that may be present in the wrist when an open procedure is contemplated.

Many patients have a history of *allergic*

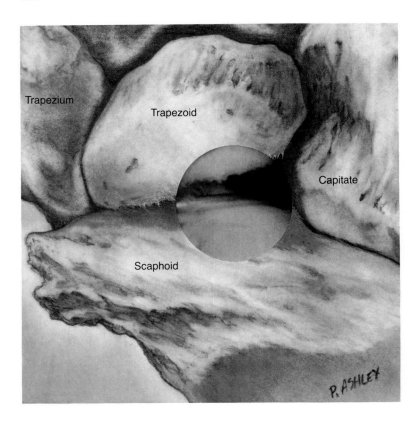

Trapezium

Trapezoid

Capitate

Scaphoid

P. ASHLEY

Figure 9–28. Articular cartilage changes on the distal pole of the scaphoid and the proximal articular surface of trapezoid are explored and palpated with a 23-gauge needle. The triscaphe joint is examined through a 1.9-mm arthroscope introduced in the midcarpal space between the scaphoid and capitate.

reactions to iodine-based radiographic contrast material or to shellfish or other foods with significant iodine content. In these individuals, contrast arthrography is contraindicated. However, if intercarpal ligament tears or injury to the triangular fibrocartilage complex is suspected in such individuals, arthroscopic examination can demonstrate the presence of these disorders.

Finally, in *undiagnosed cases of monarticular synovitis* or when the wrist is the largest joint involved with *synovial hypertrophy*, arthroscopy provides a convenient and straightforward means of synovial biopsy or limited therapeutic synovectomy.

A few case examples will demonstrate these points.

A 32-year-old male fell on his pronated outstretched left hand, causing severe dorsoradial pain and swelling in the wrist. His radiographs demonstrated a minimally displaced fracture of the radial styloid process and widening of the scapholunate interval that was not obviously acute (Fig. 9–29). An arthrogram showed dye passing through the scapholunate interval. Arthroscopy confirmed that the scapholunate ligament was completely ruptured from dorsal to volar aspects and that the injury was indeed acute.

Under arthroscopic control, the scapholunate joint was reduced and pinned with two Kirschner wires, and the radial styloid fracture was managed in a short arm cast. No arthrotomy was performed. Two years postoperatively, the scapholunate joint remains stable and asymptomatic.

A 45-year-old female had scapholunate dissociation that caused pain on flexion and radial deviation. Symptoms were chronic and progressive. A triscaphe arthrodesis was considered,[14] but arthroscopy showed moderately advanced chondromalacic changes on the proximal pole of the scaphoid and early degenerative changes on the radial styloid cartilage. Reconstruction of the dorsal radioscapholunate ligament was performed with a tendon graft, which, although not as durable, does not transfer axial load excessively to the scaphoid.

A 27-year-old professional football player injured his dominant wrist early in the playing season, and an arthrogram showed leakage of dye across the triangular fibrocartilage complex into the distal radioulnar joint. His wrist had slight, positive ulnar variance, pain with pronation against resistance, and tenderness over the triangular fibrocartilage complex. The presence of positive ulnar var-

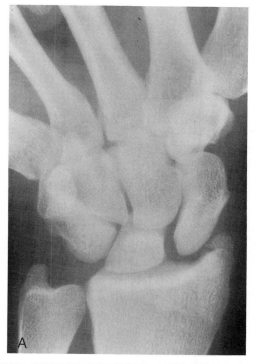

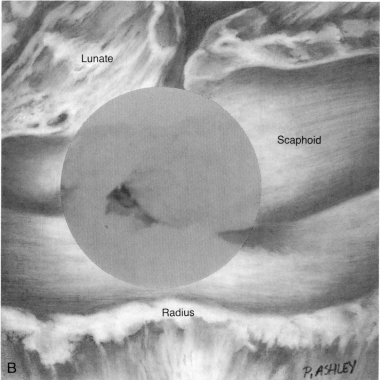

Figure 9–29. *A*, Radiograph shows separation between the scaphoid and lunate association, with transverse fracture of the radial styloid. *B*, Arthroscopic view of proximal edge of the scapholunate interval. Freshly torn tissue confirms acute nature of injury. The defect is viewed arthroscopically through a dorsal approach between the third and fourth extensor compartments.

Illustration continued on following page

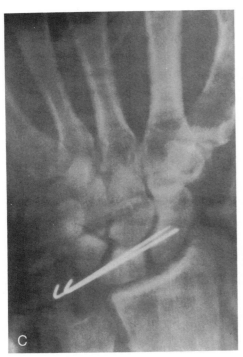

Figure 9–29 *Continued C*, Radiograph of two K wires used to reduce, under arthroscopic control, and stabilize the scapholunate interval.

iance raised the question of the significance and acuteness of the TFCC defect demonstrated on the arthrogram. However, if arthrotomy had been performed to explore and possibly resect the fibrocartilage, it would have eliminated the patient from playing for the remainder of the season and would have caused him significant loss of income. Arthroscopy was done instead and revealed a flap tear of the TFCC near its attachment to the radius. The unstable portion of the TFCC was resected under arthroscopic control, and the patient returned to play within four weeks (see Fig. 9–26B).

Other indications for wrist arthroscopy involve certain cases of *intra-articular fractures*, such as *displaced die-punch fractures* and *comminuted intra-articular fractures of the radius*. Arthroscopy provides the means of thoroughly evacuating hemarthrosis and fibrin precipitate. It also permits reduction of individual fracture fragments to restore a more normal contour to the articular surfaces. In addition, small osteochondral loose bodies may be removed with minimal surgical morbidity, using arthroscopic techniques.

Again, case examples will help illustrate the advantages of arthroscopy in such circumstances.

A 34-year-old male had suffered a nondisplaced distal radial fracture 16 years previously. He complained of pain in the midcarpal space on wrist extension and on radial deviation, aggravated particularly by lifting or power grip. He had a full range of motion, but his wrist was tender to palpation in the midcarpal space. Radiographs showed a small osseous loose body between the distal pole of the scaphoid and the radial side of the capitate (Fig. 9–30A). Under arthroscopic control, the loose body was identified (Fig. 9–30B) and extracted from the midcarpal space with complete relief of the patient's discomfort and full restoration of pain-free function. The wrist required only splint protection for five days postoperatively.

A 21-year-old male roofer fell from a ladder, injuring both wrists. He had a displaced Colles' fracture on the nondominant side and a three-part intra-articular fracture of the distal radius on the dominant side, with a transverse fracture of the ulnar styloid. With conventional management, these fractures would have required bilateral long arm casts, and the likelihood of achieving nonoperative reduction of the radial articular surface on the dominant side would have been extremely small. At arthroscopy, the dominant wrist was cleansed of hemarthrosis and small cartilaginous loose bodies. An occult fracture of the waist of the scaphoid was identified. With transcutaneous Kirschner wires, the articular fragments of the radius were reduced anatomically to restore a near-perfect relationship of the articular surface, and the unstable fragments were pinned with a transcutaneous Kirschner wire. A short arm, thumb spica cast on the dominant side permitted bending at the elbow postoperatively, which allowed the patient to attend to independent feeding and personal hygiene (Fig. 9–31).

Shortly before the state championship game, a 17-year-old high school football lineman fractured his dominant scaphoid. Under arthroscopic control, a Herbert screw was placed across the fracture, compressing the fragments. The patient was comfortable enough with a ¼-in skin incision and stabilization of the fracture to play in a latex thumb spica cast (Fig. 9–32).

A 58-year-old amateur golfer with a chronic nonunion of an old scaphoid fracture had developed increased wrist pain but had an opportunity to play in a "pro-am" tournament as a representative of his prestigious

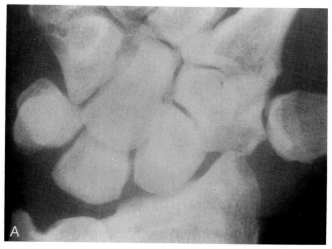

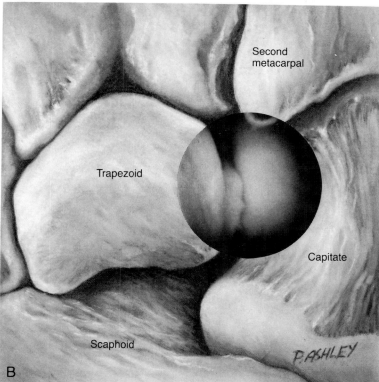

Figure 9–30. *A*, Radial deviation radiograph shows small osseous loose body in the interval between capitate, scaphoid, and trapezoid. *B*, Arthroscopic view of loose body between capitate and trapezoid, seen through a 1.9-mm arthroscope introduced dorsally between capitate and scaphoid.

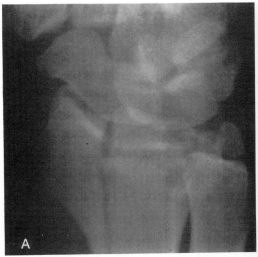

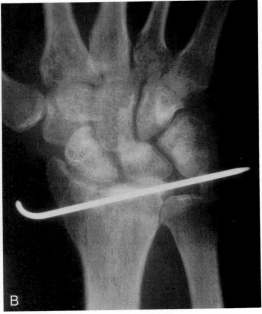

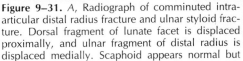

Figure 9–31. *A,* Radiograph of comminuted intra-articular distal radius fracture and ulnar styloid fracture. Dorsal fragment of lunate facet is displaced proximally, and ulnar fragment of distal radius is displaced medially. Scaphoid appears normal but has an occult transverse fracture confirmed on arthroscopic examination. *B,* Radiograph following arthroscopic reduction and K-wire fixation. Articular surface of distal radius has been restored by transcutaneous manipulation of individual fragments.

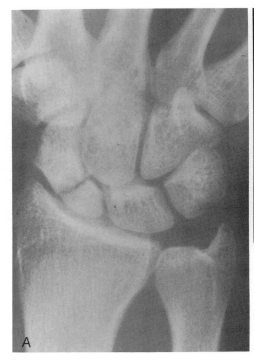

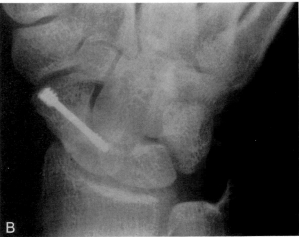

Figure 9–32. *A,* Nondisplaced fracture of right scaphoid. *B,* Appearance of scaphoid compression and internal fixation following arthroscopic placement of a Herbert screw. Procedure was performed with 1.9-mm arthroscope introduced dorsally between the third and fourth extensor compartments, the Herbert screw guide introduced radially between the first and second extensor compartments, and the screw inserted through a small incision over the scaphoid tubercle.

corporation. He was able to play with greatly reduced pain following resection of the proximal pole fragment and resection of the tip of the radial styloid, performed under arthroscopic control (Fig. 9–33).

Although these illustrative case histories may seem to involve extenuating circumstances, they are not atypical in a busy hand surgery practice.

Arthroscopic examination of the wrist has been found to be useful in symptomatic individuals who have an unconfirmed diag-nosis despite thorough conventional work-up. Patients with persistent symptoms with no reliable objective evidence for diagnosis should undergo arthroscopy for direct visual examination of intra-articular tissues. Patients with equivocal conventional work-up results are candidates for arthroscopy when objective findings are inconsistent with the stated symptoms and history. Patients who have been diagnosed by use of conventional techniques may become candidates for wrist arthroscopy when the definitive treatment

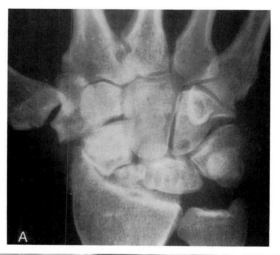

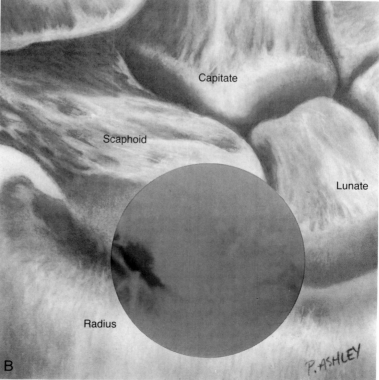

Figure 9–33. A, X-ray appearance of arthritic radiocarpal interval resulting from chronic nonunion of scaphoid fracture. The radial styloid is enlarged and impinges upon the distal scaphoid fragment. B, Arthroscopic appearance of the loose proximal scaphoid fragment. Articular surface of radius is eburnated and devoid of cartilage. Viewed arthroscopically through a dorsal approach between the third and fourth extensor compartments.

has a high morbidity or complication rate and the necessity or urgency of surgical intervention is in question. Such cases typically involve a need to evaluate the status of the articular cartilage or the size and mechanical significance of lesions of the triangular fibrocartilage complex, as previously noted.

In such circumstances, arthroscopy of the wrist provides a safe, simple, and convenient means of direct inspection of the joint as an adjunctive diagnostic technique with virtually no surgical morbidity. If it is practiced beforehand in a surgical skills laboratory and performed with appropriate instrumentation, this minimally invasive technique may well continue to open new vistas in the surgical treatment of certain wrist disorders.

References

11. Koman LA: Magnetic resonance imaging of the wrist. Orthopedic Research of Virginia: The carpal connection—diagnostic and therapeutic approaches to the painful wrist. Orlando, Florida, May 22, 1986.
12. Whipple TL, Powell JH III, Hutton PMJ, et al: Techniques of wrist arthroscopy. Arthroscopy 2(4):244, 1986.
13. Whipple TL: Arthroscopic surgery of the wrist. Operative Orthopaedics. Philadelphia, JB Lippincott Co. In press.
14. Watson KH, and Ryu J: Degenerative Disorders of the Carpus. Orthop Clin North Am 15:337–354, 1984.

PART III

Trauma-Related Conditions and Their Treatment

CHAPTER 10

Acute Fractures and Dislocations of the Carpus

EUGENE T. O'BRIEN, M.D.

The majority of carpal injuries consist of a spectrum of bone and ligamentous damage resulting from loading the wrist in extension. Prompt and accurate diagnosis of the acute injury is the prime prerequisite for restoring function to this most complicated joint in the body. Special roentgenograms, including distraction views and stress views, as well as, occasionally, trispiral tomography, may be required to make an accurate diagnosis. Early precise reduction and continuous maintenance of the reduced position until ligamentous and bone healing is complete provide the best chance of achieving a satisfactory restoration of function. With the exception of bone grafting for an ununited scaphoid fracture, the late treatment of carpal fractures and dislocations that have been undetected or improperly treated is often not very satisfactory. The results of ligamentous reconstruction for chronic carpal instabilities have been disappointing, and the long-term results of intercarpal fusions for this problem are not yet known.

In this chapter, emphasis is placed on making the proper diagnosis in the acutely injured wrist and on the technique of obtaining and maintaining a satisfactory reduction.

THE FRACTURED SCAPHOID
Mechanism of Fracture
The unique position of the scaphoid in bridging the two rows of carpal bones makes it more susceptible to injury than any of the other carpal bones. Elucidation of the mechanism of fracture has provided rational basis for determining the position of immobilization most conducive to union. Weber and Chao[184] produced experimental scaphoid waist fractures by loading the radial aspect of the palm of fresh cadaver specimens, with the wrist in 95° to 100° of dorsiflexion. Mathematical analysis of the forces about the scaphoid showed that the waist fracture resulted from bending forces applied to the distal pole of the scaphoid as the proximal pole was strongly stabilized against the radius by the radiocapitate and the radioscaphoid ligaments. Because tension in the radial collateral ligaments causes displacement of the distal pole, they recommended immobilizing waist fractures in slight radial deviation and slight palmar flexion to relax this ligament.

Experimental scaphoid fractures were also produced by Mayfield.[103] He loaded fresh cadaver wrists in nonphysiologic hyperextension and ulnar deviation, noting that the dorsal aspect of the scaphoid engaged the dorsal rim of the radius, thus creating an anvil effect leading to fracture. Fractures of the proximal pole resulted when the scaphoid first subluxated dorsally before being fractured over the dorsal rim of the radius. He concluded that the position of immobilization for these injuries should be the reverse of their mechanism of production, that is, flexion, radial deviation, and intercarpal pronation.

Vascularity

Three extraosseous vascular systems were noted by Taleisnik and Kelly[165] in their injection studies: a predominant laterovolar group entering the scaphoid volar and lateral to its radial articular surface, a dorsal group penetrating the narrow grooved dorsal surface of the scaphoid, and a distal group supplying a circumscribed area in the tuberosity. Gelberman and Menon[64] also performed injection studies and noted two major blood vessel systems, both usually derived from the radial artery, entering the scaphoid. Dorsal ridge vessels, entering dorsally between the articular surfaces for the scaphoid and for the trapezium and trapezoid, supply the proximal 70 to 80 percent of the scaphoid. The other 20 to 30 percent of the internal vascularity of the bone, all in the region of the distal pole, is supplied by branches entering the scaphoid tubercle. Gelberman and Menon felt that their dorsal ridge vessels were analogous to Taleisnik and Kelly's laterovolar vessels. Both studies failed to find any blood supply entering through the proximal pole of the scaphoid, confirming the anatomic basis for the clinically noted high incidence of delayed healing and avascular necrosis of proximal pole scaphoid fractures.

Diagnosis

The diagnosis of acute fracture of the scaphoid is still occasionally missed. Clinically, in addition to checking for snuffbox tenderness, one should look for swelling causing the obliteration of the normal concavity of the snuffbox. Pain elicited on resisted pronation is also a useful clinical sign.[176] Bone scan findings are nonspecific, since soft tissue injury or other adjacent bony injury may cause increased activity. A negative bone scan 72 hours after injury, however, effectively rules out an occult fracture of the scaphoid.[60, 125, 155, 160] Russe[140] recommended four roentgenographic views: 20° supination, 20° pronation, a neutral posteroanterior view, and a lateral view. Many authors have recommended taking posteroanterior and oblique roentgenograms with the patient making a fist in some degree of ulnar devia-

tion, so that the scaphoid profile is maximal and the beam will be more apt to parallel the fracture line. Trispiral tomography is very helpful in delineating hard-to-visualize fractures and is quite valuable in assessing the presence or absence of healing.[93]

Terry and Ramin[168] noted a normal triangular or linear fat collection located between the radial collateral ligament and the tendon sheaths of the abductor pollicis longus and the extensor pollicis brevis. They coined the term navicular fat stripe (NFS) for this finding and noted its absence or displacement in 29 of 33 acute scaphoid fractures. They believed the NSF to be a useful roentgenographic sign, alerting one that the presence of an underlying scaphoid fracture is likely.[32]

Fractures of the scaphoid in children are uncommon and differ significantly from adult scaphoid fractures.[60, 74, 76, 122, 172] Children's scaphoid fractures more commonly involve the distal pole, and small avulsion fractures of the dorsoradial aspect of the bone are frequent. Proximal pole fractures are not seen. Healing is the rule, but nonunion of a child's scaphoid fracture is not unknown.[132, 150]

Classification

Fractures can be classified as to location—tuberosity, distal pole, waist, and proximal pole; and as to direction of the fracture line—horizontal oblique, vertical oblique, transverse.[140]

Recently, several authors have attempted to classify scaphoid fractures according to stability.[36, 85, 103, 183] Displacement implies instability, and these fractures most often result from incomplete or spontaneously reduced perilunate dislocation, as evidenced by the frequently associated dorsiflexion instability of the lunate. In fact, Cooney and associates[36] define a displaced unstable fracture as one having more than 1 mm offset, or more than 15° of lunocapitate angulation, or more than 45° of scapholunate angulation. Weber[183] added the concept of an angulated scaphoid fracture hinged open dorsally on the intact volar lateral ligament, associated with mild dorsiflexion instability of the lunate.

Uncorrected displacement is associated with a marked increase in the rate of pseudoarthrosis. Eddeland and associates[46] noted failure of union in 23 of 25 scaphoid frac-

Table 10–1. **HEALING IN FRESH FRACTURES OF THE SCAPHOID**

Author(s)	Year	Number of Cases	Percent Healed
Shands[146]	1944	198	98.5
Stewart[158, 159]	1954	323	95
Böhler et al[14, 15]	1954	734	96.6
Russe[140]	1960	220	98.5
Eddeland et al[46]	1975	92	95
Cooney et al[36]	1980	32	94
Morgan and Walters[118]	1984	100	96

tures (92 percent) in which the displacement exceeded 1 mm. In their study, delay in treatment of over four weeks and location of the fracture in the proximal pole were the other two factors adversely affecting healing.

Uncomplicated scaphoid fractures have a union rate approaching 95 percent when diagnosed promptly and properly immobilized* (Table 10–1).

Treatment

IMMOBILIZATION

Every conceivable position of the wrist has at one time or another been recommended as the best position for immobilization to achieve union of a scaphoid fracture.[8, 23, 42, 56, 89, 152] Cadaver studies[169, 176, 177] do seem to demonstrate that passive pronation and supination of the forearm result in motion of

*References 14, 36, 46, 94, 118, 140, 146, 158.

the two fragments of an artificially created scaphoid fracture. Theoretically then, an above-elbow cast should improve the rate of union of scaphoid fractures, particularly those fractures that are unstable. Several studies have been performed comparing healing times using a long-arm cast versus a short-arm cast in comparable types of scaphoid fractures.[4, 24, 68] No study has yet shown any statistical evidence of superiority of the long-arm cast. In spite of this, it seems reasonable to use a long-arm thumb spica cast for the first six weeks in treating a patient with a displaced or angulated fracture that has been reduced by manipulation.[36, 38, 118]

Influenced by the work of Vichick and Dehne,[178] Weber and Chao,[184] Mayfield,[103] and Johnson,[85] I have been using a short-arm cast with the wrist in slight palmar flexion (10° or so) and radial deviation (the metacarpal of the middle finger aligned with the radial shaft) to close any palmar fracture gap (Fig. 10–1). The thumb is placed in full palmar abduction, and its distal joint is left free. The cast must be snugly applied and well molded between the thenar and the hypothenar eminences. It is changed every four to six weeks, until union is achieved. The average healing time is 12 weeks. Three to four weeks after immobilization is discontinued, another roentgenogram is obtained to confirm bone union. If there is any question of whether or not the fracture is healed, trispiral tomography is performed.[93]

If, on serial roentgenograms, progress toward union is lacking or ceases, considera-

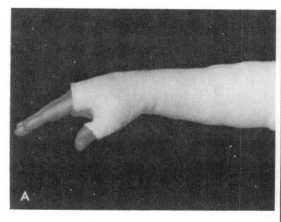
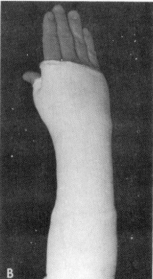

Figure 10–1. A and B, Position of immobilization for fracture of the scaphoid. (From O'Brien ET: Orthop Clin North Am 15:237–258, 1984.)

tion must be given to bone grafting or electrical stimulation[18, 19, 58, 191] between three and four months after injury. Patients who have a persistent fracture line despite adequate immobilization should not be subjected to bone grafting without a clinical trial out of the cast or a fluoroscopic examination demonstrating motion of the fracture. Fisk[52] coined the term "peanut fracture" for those asymptomatic, radiologically ununited fractures that have united centrally by fibrous tissue and are surrounded by a shell of healed articular cartilage. Operative treatment under these circumstances is not indicated. Avascular necrosis of the proximal pole certainly delays the union of the fracture but is not an indication for bone grafting as long as there is evidence of progress toward union.[140]

MANAGEMENT OF DISPLACED SCAPHOID FRACTURES

Displaced scaphoid fractures are uncommon and require accurate reduction by either the closed or the open method. Closed reduction by employing traction on the thumb while molding the snuffbox was advised by Soto-Hall.[148] Cooney and associates[36] attempted closed reduction of a displaced scaphoid fracture by longitudinal traction combined with manual pressure on the proximal carpal row, with the wrist in flexion to reduce the proximal scaphoid fragment and the malrotated lunate. A long-arm cast with the wrist in flexion and radial deviation was used to maintain the reduction. Four of the seven displaced fractures in their series that healed had been reduced and immobilized in a long-arm cast. Two other fractures that were initially undisplaced became displaced during treatment. They recommended obtaining radioulnar deviation stress views and traction oblique views if there was doubt initially about the stability of the fracture. King and associates[89] compared the trapezium and distal radius, which are connected by the radial collateral ligament, to a carpenter's C clamp holding the scaphoid. By positioning the wrist in mid-dorsiflexion, full ulnar deviation, and full supination, the "clamp" tightens and the scaphoid fragments are reduced. Union was achieved within four to six weeks in 22 out of 23 scaphoid fractures treated using this method.

Weber[183] attempted closed reduction of a dorsally angulated fracture of the scaphoid by maximal radial deviation of the wrist in neutral flexion. This abolished the mild accompanying dorsiflexion instability of the lunate by causing the lunate to palmar flex, and the scaphoid angulation was corrected.

Securing and maintaining a satisfactory reduction of a displaced scaphoid fracture are quite difficult using closed methods, and open reduction is usually necessary. Accurate reduction and secure fixation enhance healing and early revascularization of the often avascular proximal fragment. Displaced fractures without significant associated dorsiflexion instability of the lunate can be satisfactorily reduced and fixed with one or two Kirschner wires through a volar approach radial to the flexor carpi radialis tendon. The Kirschner wires should be passed through the distal fragment, from distal to proximal, to emerge at the fracture surface prior to reduction, in order to ensure their accurate placement. The fixation wire is cut off outside the skin and bent over on itself to prevent migration, and a thumb spica cast is applied. An excellent though more technically demanding method of fixation is the Herbert screw.[79] Compression can be achieved, and prolonged plaster immobilization can often be avoided. Healing was achieved in 19 of 22 cases of acute displaced fractures in which Herbert and Fischer employed the double-threaded compression screw. Displaced scaphoid fractures with significant associated dorsiflexion instability of the lunate should be approached dorsally so that the lunocapitate joint can be reduced and pinned along with the scaphoid fracture. Kirschner wires, a cancellous screw,[78, 102, 109] or the Herbert screw used without the guide can be used to fix the scaphoid fracture through this approach.

OTHER CARPAL BONE FRACTURES

The Hamate

Fractures of the body of the hamate are unusual. Milch[112] classified them into fractures medial or lateral to the hook. Coronal fractures involving the dorsal surface are hinged proximally[20] and may be associated with a dorsal dislocation of the fourth and fifth metacarpal bones, which remain attached to the dorsal fragment.[99, 170]

Hook fractures are usually more common than body fractures and more apt to be missed (Fig. 10–2). These fractures occur

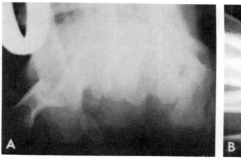
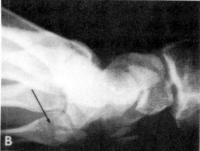
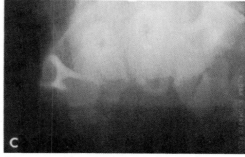

Figure 10–2. Roentgenograms had been made on several occasions in this 31-year-old man who had hypothenar pain for two years after injuring his wrist playing racquetball, but they were interpreted as normal. *A,* An ununited fracture of the hook of the hamate can be seen on the carpal tunnel and oblique views. *B, C,* Excision of the ununited fragment relieved the patient's pain. (*A* and *C* from Kane WJ [ed.]: Current Orthopaedic Management. New York, Churchill Livingstone Inc, 1981. *B* from O'Brien ET: Orthop Clin North Am 15:237–258, 1984.)

most commonly at or near the base of the hook and result from a fall or, more commonly, from the direct force of the handle of a racket, club, or bat.[153] Persistent pain and tenderness in the hypothenar eminence result. The chronic case is easily diagnosed radiologically by a carpal tunnel view, and the results of excision of the ununited fragment are excellent.[30, 153] Attritional rupture of the flexor tendons to the ring and little fingers[33, 41, 126, 153, 162] and neuropathy of the deep branch of the ulnar nerve[5, 26, 81] occur occasionally in the long-standing case. Obtaining a diagnostic carpal tunnel view in the acute case may be difficult because of pain. An oblique view with the forearm in mid-supination and the wrist in some degree of dorsiflexion and radial deviation may permit diagnosis of a fresh fracture. Lateral tomography,[12, 30] trispiral tomography of the carpal tunnel,[75] and computerized tomography[47, 133] have also been utilized to diagnose a fracture of the hook of the hamate. Lateral tomographs and sagittal CT scans have been utilized to delineate dorsal fracture dislocation of the hamatometacarpal joint.[99] Healing of the acute hook fracture, even with open reduction and Kirschner wire fixation,[12] is very unusual. Schlosser and associates[143] reported one patient with spontaneous healing of a hamate hook fracture 22 months after injury with no treat-

ment. Even so, if the diagnosis is made acutely, a trial cast immobilization for six weeks seems reasonable.

Displaced fractures of the body of the hamate should be reduced anatomically, and open reduction is usually necessary. Internal fixation with Kirschner wires is indicated whether reduction is achieved by closed or open means. Marck and Klasen[99] accomplished internal fixation of a dorsal fracture dislocation of the hamatometacarpal joint with a small T plate and 2.7 mm cancellous screws. Treatment of an old unrecognized dorsal fracture dislocation of the hamatometacarpal joint requires reduction and an arthrodesis of the joint (Fig. 10–3).

The Trapezium

In 1960 Cordrey and Ferrer-Torells[39] reviewed 75 trapezial fractures in the literature, added five new cases, and noted the incidence to be about 5 percent of all carpal bone fractures. The recent literature has focused on two main fracture types: a split fracture of the trapezium with lateral subluxation of the first metacarpal, which remains attached to the lateral trapezial fragment, and a fracture of the trapezial ridge (base or tip). An isolated trapezial fracture results from a direct blow on the abducted thumb or from a fall on the hyperextended

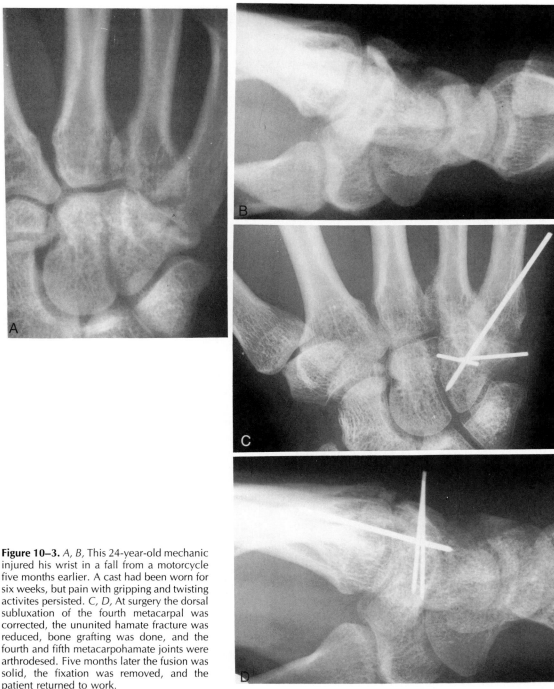

Figure 10–3. *A, B,* This 24-year-old mechanic injured his wrist in a fall from a motorcycle five months earlier. A cast had been worn for six weeks, but pain with gripping and twisting activites persisted. *C, D,* At surgery the dorsal subluxation of the fourth metacarpal was corrected, the ununited hamate fracture was reduced, bone grafting was done, and the fourth and fifth metacarpohamate joints were arthrodesed. Five months later the fusion was solid, the fixation was removed, and the patient returned to work.

hand in radial deviation, which compresses the trapezium between the first metacarpal and the radial styloid.[26] A fall on the outstretched hand results in a fracture of the trapezial ridge either by direct trauma or through tension applied through the attached transverse carpal ligament as the thenar and hypothenar eminences diverge.[128]

Trapezial fractures can best be visualized in the oblique roentgenogram obtained with the ulnar border of the hand on the cassette and with the forearm pronated 20°.[39] Trapezial ridge fractures, like fractures of the hook of the hamate, are more apt to be missed, as they can be seen only on the carpal tunnel view (Fig. 10–4).[108]

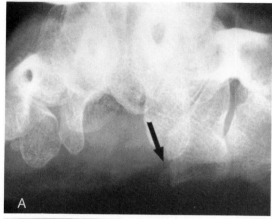

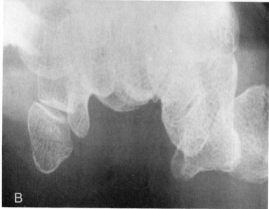

Figure 10–4. *A*, This 61-year-old professor sustained a trapezial ridge fracture in a fall onto her outstretched hand two months earlier. Volar wrist pain was present, but there were no symptoms or signs of carpal tunnel syndrome. *B*, Follow-up roentgenograms six months later showed apparent healing despite the lack of any immobilization.

Clinically, ridge fractures are characterized by localized tenderness at the base of the thenar eminence and pain elicited on resisted wrist flexion; associated carpal tunnel syndrome is frequent.

Displaced vertical fractures of the trapezium with lateral subluxation of the first metacarpal require accurate reduction and internal fixation, as does a Bennett's fracture dislocation (Fig. 10–5). Cordrey and Ferrer-Torells[39] achieved excellent results in five such injuries treated by open reduction and Kirschner wire fixation. The first Kirschner wire was introduced into the lateral fragment and used to manipulate it and to hold the reduction, while a second wire was drilled through both fragments. Normal function was noted by Freeland and Finley[55] after open reduction and cancellous lag screw fixation in one patient who had a

vertical trapezial fracture with lateral subluxation of the first metacarpal.

As in fractures of the hamate hook, healing of ridge fractures is uncommon. Palmer[128] recorded one case of a fracture through the wider base of the trapezial ridge that healed after thumb spica immobilization. Excision of the ununited fragment, with release of the carpal tunnel if necessary, usually relieves the patient's symptoms, but the recovery is often prolonged.[108]

The Capitate

A fracture of the capitate is similar in several ways to a fracture of the scaphoid. The blood supply enters mainly through the waist, so avascular necrosis and nonunion of proximal fractures occur rather frequently. Undisplaced fractures may also be missed initially, so follow-up roentgenograms and perhaps even lateral tomography[2] may be necessary to make the diagnosis. The incidence of capitate fracture varies in the literature from 1.3 percent[137] to 14 percent[11] of carpal fractures. Capitate fractures have been classified by Rand and associates[137] into isolated fractures, fractures associated with perilunate dislocation (scaphocapitate syndrome), and fractures associated with other carpal injury. The mechanism of injury may be direct violence to the dorsal wrist, dorsiflexion in neutral or ulnar deviation, dorsiflexion in radial deviation (scaphocapitate syndrome), or trauma to the heads of the second and third metacarpals with the wrist palmar flexed.[2]

Displaced capitate fractures require open reduction and internal fixation with Kirschner wires. This is best accomplished through a dorsal incision (Fig. 10–6). Transient avascular changes are common in proximal pole fractures, but collapse and resorption after fracture seem to be quite unusual.[137] Most reported cases of avascular necrosis of the capitate have involved the proximal end and were not associated with a definite fracture.* The report by Vander Grend and associates[174] is an exception: they reported nonunion and proximal avascular necrosis in four patients. Only two of them, however, could recall a specific injury. Curettage with cancellous grafting was successful in achieving union in the three patients in whom nonunion was amenable to this

---

*References 16, 84, 88, 121, 124, 136.

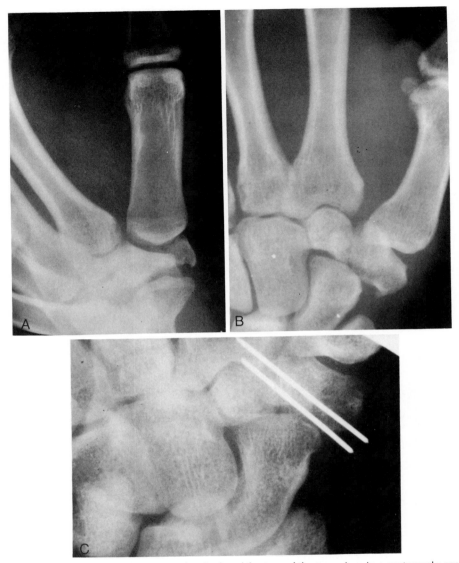

Figure 10–5. *A, B,* This 20-year-old man sustained a displaced fracture of the trapezium in a motorcycle accident. *C,* An open reduction and internal fixation carried out three days after injury restored the articular surface of the trapezium, and healing was noted 10 weeks later.

treatment. Rand and associates[137] achieved union in two patients with nonunion of the capitate and emphasized the need for an intercalary bone graft to restore the length of the shortened bone. They noted a significantly high incidence of arthrosis in the late follow-up of isolated capitate fractures as well as those associated with a trans-scaphoid perilunate dislocation.

The Pisiform

Fractures of the pisiform usually result from direct trauma to the volar ulnar aspect of the wrist. The fracture line may be transverse (usually a chip fracture of the distal end of the bone) or longitudinal; occasionally the bone is comminuted. The fracture is best visualized in the 30° supination palm up view, or the carpal tunnel view. Displacement of the fracture fragments is rare, and Vasilas and associates[175] noted healing after three to six weeks of immobilization in all but one of the 13 patients having pisiform fractures on whom they reported. Nonunion or malunion with post-traumatic arthritis is an indication for excision, as is an acute fracture involving the articular surface, in which there is significant displacement.[76]

The Triquetrum

Small avulsion fractures of the dorsal aspect of the triquetrum are commonly seen after hyperextension injury of the wrist. These fractures are best seen in lateral or oblique roentgenograms. Three weeks of immobilization in a short-arm cast or splint usually relieves the patient's pain, and even though nonunion of the small fragment is common,[17] it is rarely of clinical significance.[6] Most fractures of the main body of the triquetrum, especially if displaced, are associated with perilunate dislocations or with other associated carpal injuries. They require accurate reduction and internal fixation. Avascular necrosis of the triquetrum has not been reported.

INTERCARPAL DISLOCATIONS AND FRACTURE-DISLOCATIONS

The contributions of Mayfield and associates[103–106] and Taleisnik[163, 164] have helped to clarify the mechanism and sequence of injury in carpal dislocations. Tanz[167] first pointed out the importance of intercarpal rotation in determining the direction of displacement of the distal carpal row. Mayfield and associates[106] defined four stages of increasing perilunar instability (PLI) when cadaver wrists were experimentally loaded in extension, ulnar deviation, and intercarpal supination. Scapholunate instability is the first stage, dorsal perilunate dislocation the second, dorsal perilunate dislocation with triquetrolunate diastasis the third, and volar dislocation of the lunate is the fourth and final stage. Because of its strategic position, when a perilunate dislocation occurs, the scaphoid either fractures or tears loose its proximal ligamentous connection to the lunate and the radius.

The exact mechanism of loading that results in volar perilunate dislocation and dorsal dislocation of the lunate has not been

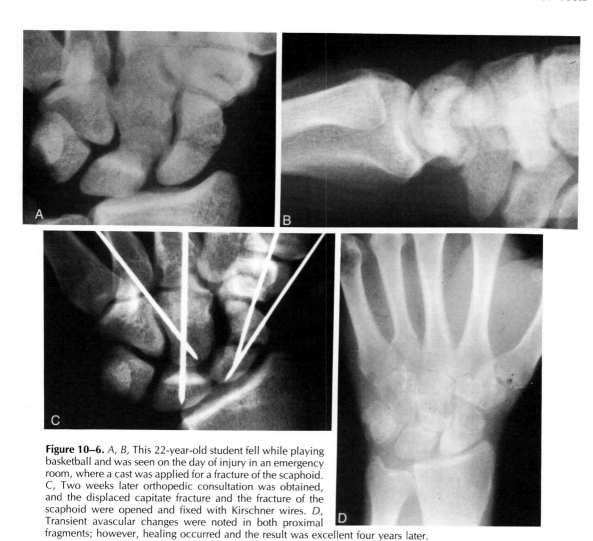

Figure 10–6. *A, B,* This 22-year-old student fell while playing basketball and was seen on the day of injury in an emergency room, where a cast was applied for a fracture of the scaphoid. *C,* Two weeks later orthopedic consultation was obtained, and the displaced capitate fracture and the fracture of the scaphoid were opened and fixed with Kirschner wires. *D,* Transient avascular changes were noted in both proximal fragments; however, healing occurred and the result was excellent four years later.

defined. Forced hyperflexion from a fall on the back of the hand has been proposed as the mechanism of injury by Aitken and Nalebuff.[3] Two of the patients whom I have seen, however, were quite certain that they fell with the wrist in dorsiflexion. One patient died of other injuries two weeks after his volar perilunate dislocation. Postmortem manipulation of the dissected segment showed that the midcarpal displacement could be recreated by pronating and extending the distal fragment on the fixed proximal segment (with rotation occurring around the triquetrum). A fall on the hyperextended wrist with supination of the forearm and the proximal carpal row on the fixed hand and distal row (intercarpal pronation) appears to be the likely mechanism for this injury.

Intercarpal dislocations and fracture-dislocations can be conveniently classified as follows:

1. Scapholunate dissociation (rotatory subluxation of the scaphoid).
2. Dorsal perilunate dislocation.
3. Volar lunate dislocation.
4. Dorsal trans-scaphoid perilunate dislocation.
5. Volar perilunate dislocation.
6. Dorsal lunate dislocation.
7. Volar trans-scaphoid perilunate dislocation.
8. Trans-scaphoid perilunate variants:
   a. Scaphocapitate syndrome.
   b. Transtriquetrial trans-scaphoid perilunate dislocation.
   c. Volar dislocation of proximal scaphoid fragment with or without the lunate.
9. Total dislocation of the scaphoid with or without the lunate.
10. Other individual carpal bone dislocations (trapezoid, trapezium, pisiform, hamate, triquetrum, and capitate).
11. Other intercarpal dislocations:
    a. Scaphotrapezial—trapezoid dislocation (triscaphoid dislocation).
    b. "Crush injury of the carpus"—dislocation of capitohamate and pisotriquetral joints.

Diagnosis

Clinically, the patient with an acute scapholunate dissociation (rotatory subluxation of the scaphoid) presents with a "sprained wrist." After a fall on the outstretched hand, he or she complains of pain, particularly over the dorsoradial aspect of the wrist, that is accentuated by dorsiflexion. Swelling, if present, is minimal. Tenderness is present dorsally over the scapholunate joint, and pressure over the scaphoid tuberosity may be painful.

Early diagnosis is essential for successful treatment, and the six views of the wrist (motion study) recommended by Dobyns and coworkers[43] are useful in evaluating the "sprained wrist." These include posteroanterior and lateral views in neutral, lateral views in maximum dorsiflexion and in palmar flexion, and posteroanterior views in maximum radial and in ulnar deviation. If scapholunate dissociation is suspected, an anteroposterior (not posteroanterior) view in supination and in ulnar deviation with the patient making a tight fist is also obtained. Supination and longitudinal compression across the wrist accentuate and make fully apparent any scaphoid subluxation. Moneim[115] has found that a tangential posteroanterior view with the ulnar border of the hand elevated 20° off the cassette is particularly helpful in demonstrating the scapholunate gap in the patient who cannot cooperate. Scapholunate dissociation is diagnosed when the following features are present in the anteroposterior or posteroanterior view: a gap greater than 2 mm between the scaphoid and the lunate (the "Terry Thomas" sign),[54] a foreshortened appearance of the scaphoid, and a double-density projection of the cortical waist of the scaphoid (the "ring" sign). In the lateral view, the scaphoid assumes a more vertical orientation, and the proximal pole is dorsal to the lunate. Taleisnik[164] has described a "V sign." In the lateral view, the normal, wide C-shaped line along the volar margins of the scaphoid and the radius becomes a sharper V-shaped pattern when the scaphoid is subluxated. Scapholunate angles in excess of 70° are said to be diagnostic of scapholunate dissociation. Wrist arthrography, cineradiography and trispiral tomography are sometimes useful adjuvant diagnostic techniques in the more chronic carpal instabilities. These studies are less helpful and not often indicated in the acutely injured wrist.

Patients with a dorsal perilunate dislocation have considerable swelling, and a mini silver fork deformity is often present. If the swelling is not too great, it may be possible to palpate the edge of the capitate dorsally. Dislocation of the lunate causes volar swelling, and two-point discrimination is frequently diminished in the median nerve distribution, secondary to acute carpal tunnel syndrome. The patient holds his or her fingers in semiflexion, and active and passive extension of the fingers is incomplete and painful. Both perilunate and trans-scaphoid perilunate dislocations have recently been reported to occur in children.[65, 129]

In a dorsal perilunate dislocation, the lateral roentgenogram shows the longitudinal axis of the capitate dorsal to the longitudinal axis of the radius, and the proximal scaphoid is rotated dorsally. In the anteroposterior projection, the carpus is foreshortened, with overlapping of the proximal capitate and distal lunate margins, and there is an abnormal gap between the scaphoid and the lunate. In a dorsal trans-scaphoid perilunate dislocation, the proximal scaphoid fragment remains with the lunate, while the distal fragment is displaced dorsally with the distal carpal row. There is often considerable radial displacement of the scaphoid fracture and the distal carpus in the anteroposterior view. The proximal scaphoid fragment and the lunate often tend to slide toward the ulna under these circumstances. Concomitant avulsion fractures involving the radial styloid process and the triquetrum are often present.

In a lunate dislocation, the longitudinal axis of the capitate tends to be colinear with that of the radius, and the lunate is displaced volarly, with its cup tilted forward (the "spilled teacup" sign). In the anteroposterior view, the lunate assumes a triangular shape instead of its normal quadrilateral shape (the "piece of cheese" sign).[182] Occasionally, the entire lunate may be displaced volarly and proximally under the anterior margin of the distal radius (Fig. 10–7).

In both perilunate and trans-scaphoid perilunate dislocations, there is also an intermediate stage of injury, in which the carpal displacements are halfway between a perilunate and a lunate dislocation. The capitate is slightly dorsal to the longitudinal axis of the radius, and the lunate is tipped volarly but has not fully dislocated. Distraction views made during finger-trap traction are often helpful in determining the degree of ligamentous damage and the presence of associated fractures in patients having perilunate or lunate dislocations.

Treatment

SCAPHOLUNATE DISSOCIATION

Scapholunate dissociation results when the scapholunate interosseous and radioscaphoid ligaments are torn. Prompt diagnosis, along with reduction and internal fixation to allow ligamentous healing, results in a high degree of success. Unfortunately, the diagnosis is often missed, and the golden opportunity for restoring function is lost. Reduction, however, is feasible with some hope of ligamentous healing[21, 38] even as late as five to six weeks after injury.

If the injury is very fresh (within the first few days), it is sometimes possible to close the scapholunate gap and to restore the colinear alignment of the lunate and capitate by dorsiflexing and radially deviating the wrist. Two 0.045-in Kirschner wires are then inserted laterally through the scaphoid, one into the lunate and one into the capitate, using the image intensifier. The wires, which are cut off outside the skin and bent over, are left in place for eight weeks. A short-arm cast is worn full time for the first eight weeks, and then a removable splint (with the wrist in radial deviation and dorsiflexion) is worn for an additional four weeks. If

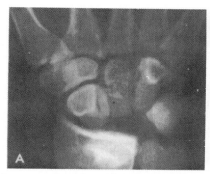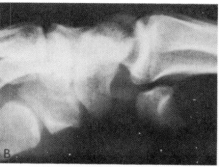

Figure 10–7. Posteroanterior (A) and lateral (B) roentgenograms showing complete volar dislocation of the lunate. (From O'Brien ET: Orthop Clin North Am 15:237–258, 1984.)

there is any question about the adequacy of reduction or if the injury has been present for more than a few days, an open reduction is performed. Recently, I have begun almost exclusively to use primary open reduction, as I think the final results are more predictable. The wrist is opened dorsally through an oblique incision between the radial and ulnar styloid processes. The skin flaps are undermined, with care being taken to avoid injury to the branches of the superficial radial nerve. The joint is entered through a longitudinal incision between the third and fourth extensor compartments. Blood clot is removed from the scapholunate space, and the proximal pole of the subluxated scaphoid is reduced by pushing it volarly using a Freer elevator. At the same time, the dorsiflexion instability of the lunocapitate joint is corrected by palmar flexing the lunate and dorsiflexing the capitate. It is often helpful to insert a 0.045-in threaded Kirschner wire into the waist of the scaphoid for use as a lever to reduce the scapholunate joint. While the surgeon holds the reduction, an assistant drills the Kirschner wires across the scapholunate and scaphocapitate joints. It is often possible in a fresh injury to tack the short ligamentous tags of ruptured scapholunate interosseous ligament together dorsally with 4-0 or 5-0 nonabsorbable suture material using a small needle. The postoperative course is the same as that for closed reduction and pinning. The treatment of a missed chronic scapholunate dissociation after five to six weeks is covered in Chapter 19.

DORSAL PERILUNATE AND VOLAR
LUNATE DISLOCATIONS

If the hyperextension force continues, the radiocapitate ligament tears (or an avulsion fracture of the radial styloid occurs), and the capitate dislocates dorsally from the lunate (Stage II perilunate instability). Further hyperextension and intercarpal supination tear the dorsal and volar radiotriquetral ligaments, and volar dislocation of the lunate results when the distal carpus spontaneously reduces, pushing the lunate volarly (Stage IV perilunate instability). Acute perilunate and lunate dislocations are usually relatively easy to reduce if the patient is seen early. After a thorough neurovascular evaluation of the extremity, closed reduction of the dislocation is attempted. After adequate anesthesia (axillary block or general anesthesia), finger-trap traction is applied

with 10 to 15 pounds of counterweight across the upper arm and left undisturbed for about five minutes. Anteroposterior and lateral distraction views are obtained during this time. Supplemental manipulation, consisting of dorsiflexion followed by gradual palmar flexion and pronation to reduce the capitate back into the cup of the lunate, is then performed. If the lunate is dislocated volarly, the operator's thumb stabilizes the lunate as the capitate is brought over into palmar flexion. Often, the initial stages of reduction of the lunate will reproduce the dorsal perilunate stage prior to final reduction. With traction maintained, the reduction is checked with anteroposterior and lateral roentgenograms. Rarely, the dislocation is completely reduced, and there is no residual scapholunate dissociation. If this is the case, the hand and wrist are prepped and the scapholunate and scaphocapitate joints are fixed in the reduced position with percutaneously inserted 0.045-in Kirschner wires, using the image intensifier. Under no circumstances should one rely on a cast alone to maintain the reduction.

The postoperative course is the same as that described previously for the closed or open pinning of scapholunate dissociation. After pinning of the perilunate dislocation, however, the cast is applied with the wrist palmar flexed about 30°, so that the torn volar ligaments are approximated. Any associated carpal tunnel syndrome usually resolves rather promptly after the reduction, and formal carpal tunnel release is not usually necessary. Commonly, residual scapholunate dissociation is present after reduction of the perilunate displacement. Reduction of the gap and correction of the dorsiflexion instability of the lunate can sometimes be accomplished by slight dorsiflexion and maximal radial deviation of the wrist. If reduction is achieved, closed pinning is performed. Usually, however, the gap cannot be closed or dorsiflexion will cause a recurrence of the perilunate displacement (the "paradox of reduction").[103] Open reduction and pin fixation through a dorsal approach, as described previously, are therefore necessary (Fig. 10–8). The dorsiflexion instability of the lunate is often greater than that in an isolated scapholunate dissociation. A second threaded Kirschner wire, drilled into the dorsal nonarticular surface of the lunate to pull the lunate dorsally while the capitate is pushed volarly, is helpful. With this "han-

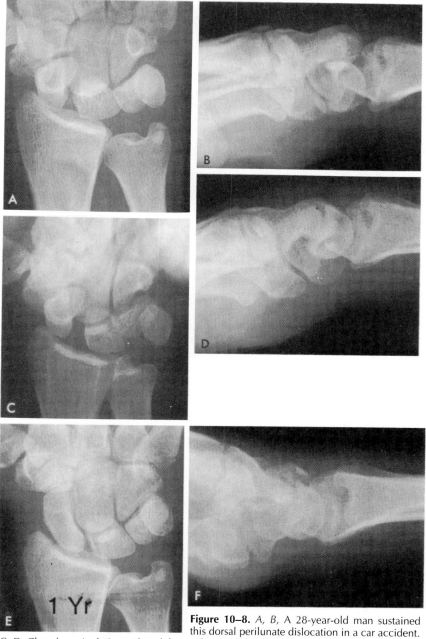

Figure 10–8. *A, B,* A 28-year-old man sustained this dorsal perilunate dislocation in a car accident. *C, D,* Closed manipulation reduced the perilunate dislocation, but an obvious scapholunate dissociation is present. Open reduction and Kirschner wire fixation were performed through a dorsal approach, and the pins were left in for eight weeks. *E, F,* Function was excellent at one year, and the roentgenograms were normal. (From O'Brien ET: Orthop Clin North Am 15:237–258, 1984.)

dle" and the vertical scaphoid Kirschner wire, the reduction can be obtained and held, while Kirschner wires are drilled transversely through the scaphoid and lunate and the scaphoid and capitate.

After closed reduction of a volar lunate dislocation or an intermediate dislocation (halfway between a perilunate and lunate dislocation), residual scapholunate dissociation as well as considerable dorsal instability of the lunate may be present. Open reduction through a dorsal approach, utilizing the temporary Kirschner wire handles in the scaphoid and the lunate, is often successful in restoring normal carpal alignment. Internal fixation and plaster immobilization with the wrist in 30° of volar flexion then achieves satisfactory ligamentous healing. Occasionally, since this injury involves more ligamentous damage and tends to be quite unstable, a second incision volarly is necessary to achieve reduction of the lunate and restoration of a colinear lunocapitate joint. This is especially true if the reduction has been delayed. The volar approach, an expanded standard carpal tunnel incision, reveals a transverse tear in the volar capsule with the lunate volarly subluxated or dislocated through it into the carpal canal. Unsuspected osteochondral fractures, usually of the capitate and the lunate, are sometimes found and require removal. Utilizing both incisions, the lunate is reduced and the volar capsular rent is repaired with nonabsorbable sutures. Through the dorsal exposure, the lunocapitate relationship is restored and maintained with a longitudinal 0.045-in Kirschner wire inserted from distal (between the bases of the third and fourth metacarpals) to proximal. The dorsally subluxated scaphoid is reduced and held, while a Kirschner wire is drilled through the scaphoid and the lunate. The postoperative management is the same as that outlined for other carpal dislocations.

DORSAL TRANS-SCAPHOID PERILUNATE DISLOCATION

In this injury, the midcarpal dislocation is accompanied by a fracture through the waist of the scaphoid, and the distal scaphoid fragment is displaced dorsally with the rest of the carpus, leaving the proximal fragment attached to the lunate. The initial clinical evaluation and closed reduction techniques are identical to those described previously for patients with a perilunate dislocation without fracture. Again, reduction of the midcarpal dislocation is usually easily accomplished, but residual scaphoid malalignment is the rule rather than the exception. The oblique roentgenograph best shows the displacement. Even if perfect alignment of the fractured scaphoid is achieved by closed reduction, it is very difficult to maintain with plaster immobilization in these inherently unstable injuries. Adkinson and Chapman[1] noted that 13 of 19 trans-scaphoid perilunate dislocations that were initially anatomically reduced by closed methods subsequently lost position and required late open reduction. Satisfactory closed pinning of the scaphoid fracture is difficult, and distraction may result. For these reasons, I now prefer to reduce and fix the scaphoid by open means.* Prompt accurate reduction and internal fixation also seem to speed healing, and revascularization of the commonly associated avascular necrosis of the proximal scaphoid fragment is more rapid.

The open reduction of the scaphoid fracture can be performed either through a dorsal or a volar incision. If the perilunate dislocation is well reduced, as it often is, the fracture can be approached volarly using the Russe incision paralleling the flexor carpi radialis tendon. Fixation can be accomplished with Kirschner wires or with the Herbert screw; the latter achieves excellent fixation with some compression of the fragments (Fig. 10–9). Union was achieved with the screw in all 15 acute fracture-dislocations treated by Herbert and Fisher.[79] It is a demanding technique to master, requires a significant exposure of the normal scaphotrapezial joint, and, as Herbert and Fisher noted themselves, unstable fractures associated with midcarpal dislocations are technically the most difficult ones to fix. Herbert screw fixation does allow earlier discontinuance of the cast immobilization (at six weeks when ligamentous healing is satisfactory) than does Kirschner wire fixation.

If difficulty is experienced in inserting the screw, one should not hesitate to abandon it in favor of Kirschner wire fixation. Two 0.045-in Kirschner wires are drilled percutaneously in a parallel manner through the distal fragment, so that their position can be checked prior to reduction. The fracture is then reduced and held with a towel clip or reduction clamp, while the wires are ad-

---

*References 1, 54, 80, 116, 117, 130, 190.

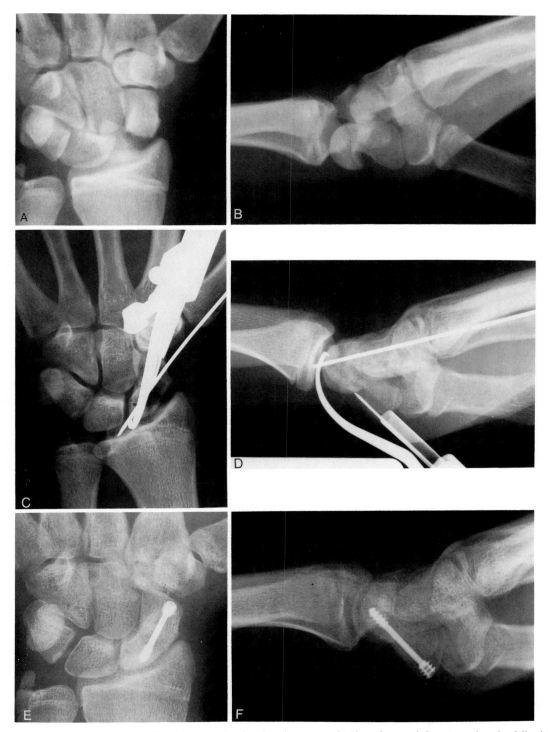

Figure 10–9. *A, B,* This 17-year-old student sustained a dorsal trans-scaphoid perilunate dislocation when he fell while playing baseball. Closed reduction was successful in reducing the perilunate dislocation. *C, D,* Through a volar Russe approach, the scaphoid was reduced and temporarily fixed with a Kirschner wire, and a Herbert screw was inserted. Plaster immobilization was continued for only six weeks. *E, F,* Three and a half months after injury, the patient had regained most of his wrist motion, and union was almost complete.

vanced into the proximal fragment as far as the subchondral bone. The Kirschner wires, which are cut off and bent over outside the skin, are left in place for eight weeks or so, but the thumb spica cast immobilization is continued until union is achieved. If serial roentgenograms fail to show progress toward union by about four months, consideration should be given to bone grafting or to electrical stimulation. Supplemental bone grafting is indicated during the initial open reduction only for the rare, markedly comminuted fracture that has no stability.[72, 79]

Open reduction of the scaphoid fracture can also be performed through the dorsal interstyloid incision. This approach is especially indicated when the perilunate dislocation is incompletely reduced and lunate dorsiflexion instability is present in addition to the malaligned scaphoid. Two parallel Kirschner wires are inserted percutaneously through the distal fragment until they appear at the fracture site. The wrist is distracted, and a Freer elevator is inserted into the lunocapitate joint to assist in reducing this joint. The wires are then drilled across the fracture while the reduction is maintained with a towel clip or a reduction clamp. Firm fixation of the scaphoid restores the stability to the midcarpal joint, and supplemental fixation is usually unnecessary. The Herbert screw can also be utilized by those familiar with its use, through the dorsal approach, but it must be inserted freehand without the aid of the alignment jig.

VOLAR PERILUNATE AND VOLAR TRANS-SCAPHOID PERILUNATE DISLOCATION

Only a few isolated cases of this rare injury have been reported in the literature.[3, 50, 134, 142, 189] Volar perilunate dislocation, like its more common dorsal counterpart, is always accompanied by either a fracture or dorsal subluxation of the scaphoid. The lunate is palmar flexed, and the capitate is displaced volarly. Because of the rarity of this injury, the proper diagnosis is liable to be missed.

Forced hyperflexion from a fall on the back of the hand has been proposed as the mechanism of injury by Aitken and Nalebuff.[3] Based on the histories obtained from several of my patients and the manipulation of a postmortem wrist specimen from a patient who had a volar trans-scaphoid perilunate dislocation, I believe the injury results from hyperextension and intercarpal pronation.

Closed reduction of a volar perilunate dis-

location utilizing finger-trap traction, with supination of the hand and distal carpal row on the fixed forearm and proximal row, is sometimes successful. Correction of the residual scapholunate dislocation should be performed through a dorsal approach. Kirschner wire fixation must be maintained for eight weeks.

A volar trans-scaphoid perilunate dislocation is apt to be widely displaced and may be more unstable[142] than the more common dorsal variety. Open reduction and internal fixation of the scaphoid fracture can be accomplished either through a volar Russe incision or through a dorsal approach, once the perilunate dislocation is reduced (Fig. 10–10).

DORSAL DISLOCATION OF THE LUNATE

Dorsal dislocation of the lunate is even more uncommon than volar perilunate dislocation (Fig. 10–11). Fisk[53] postulated that the injury resulted from forced palmar flexion, but the mechanism is unknown. Seidenstein[144] reported that a patient with a dorsal dislocation of the lunate was treated by delayed excision of the bone at two weeks and had a satisfactory result one year after surgery. Bilos and Hui[10] reported on two patients with dorsal dislocation of the lunate, both of whom were treated by open reduction and pin fixation. Each achieved a satisfactory clinical result, although increased density of the lunate without collapse was noted in one of the patients at one year.

TRANS-SCAPHOID PERILUNATE VARIANTS

Scaphocapitate Syndrome. In this relatively uncommon variation of trans-scaphoid perilunate dislocation, the head of the capitate is fractured and rotated 180°. The squared-off contour of the proximal end of the capitate, best seen in a distraction view, is the key to making the proper diagnosis.[186] Fenton[49] coined the term "naviculocapitate syndrome" in 1956, postulating that the fracture resulted from a force transmitted from the radial styloid through the waist of the scaphoid. Stein and Seigel[156] presented what appears to be the most logical mechanism of injury, that is, direct compression of the proximal end of the capitate against the dorsal lip of the radius with the wrist in acute hyperextension. The proximal capitate fragment is rotated 90° secondary to its dorsiflexion, and return of the hand to the neutral position completes the 180° rotation.

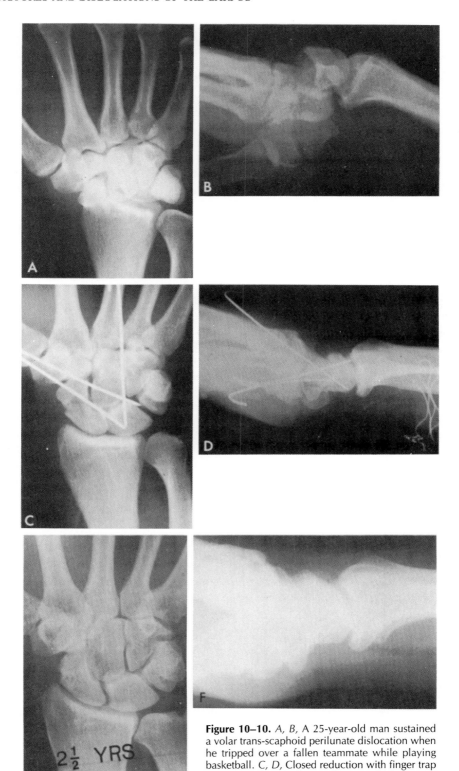

Figure 10–10. *A, B,* A 25-year-old man sustained a volar trans-scaphoid perilunate dislocation when he tripped over a fallen teammate while playing basketball. *C, D,* Closed reduction with finger trap traction reduced the perilunate displacement; however, residual displacement of the scaphoid fracture necessitated open reduction and Kirschner wire fixation through a volar Russe approach. The pins were left in place for eight weeks, and plaster immobilization was continued for 13 weeks. *E, F,* Two and a half years after injury, he had 90 percent of normal wrist motion and only a 20-lb diminution of grip strength. (From Kane WJ [ed]: Current Orthopaedic Management. New York, Churchill Livingstone Inc, 1981.)

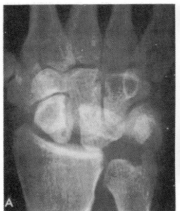
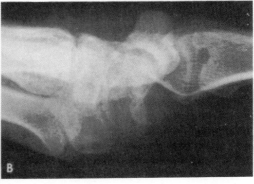

Figure 10–11. *A, B,* This dorsal dislocation of the lunate resulted from a fall from a wheelchair. The patient, who suffered from a paralytic neuromuscular disorder, eventually had the lunate excised because of a long delay in diagnosis. (Case courtesy of Richard Eaton, M.D.)

At least one half of the reported cases have been associated with a dorsal trans-scaphoid perilunate dislocation, and two cases of volar trans-scaphoid perilunate dislocation with fracture of the proximal capitate have been reported.[110, 114] When a scaphocapitate syndrome is seen without a perilunate dislocation, diagnosis of the capitate fracture is often missed. Presumably, perilunate dislocation occurred at the time of injury and spontaneously reduced.[86]

Fenton[49] advocated excision of the proximal pole as primary treatment because he believed that avascular necrosis and nonunion were inevitable. Although Jones,[86] and Adler and Shaftan[2] have reported cases in which the fragment healed in its malrotated position, Marsh and Lampros[100] subsequently demonstrated that the fragment may undergo necrosis if left unreduced. Healing of the capitate fracture with good restoration of function has been achieved by open reduction and internal fixation.[48, 110, 138, 173, 186] Transient avascular changes are usually seen, but collapse and nonunion are unusual (Fig. 10–12).[137] Even late reduction and fixation of a capitate fracture that was initially missed can be done if the articular cartilage looks healthy.

Transtriquetral Trans-scaphoid Perilunate Dislocation. Small avulsion fractures from the dorsal aspect of the triquetrum are seen fairly commonly in association with perilunate dislocations. A transverse or oblique fracture through the bone is occasionally seen in conjunction with a trans-scaphoid perilunate dislocation or a scaphocapitate syndrome.[186] The line of cleavage separating the midcarpal joint extends through the trique-

trum, leaving its proximal half attached to the lunate and allowing the distal fragment to be displaced with the capitate. The fracture fragments may reduce nicely as the perilunate dislocation is reduced. If open reduction and fixation are required for persistent displacement, the slightly oblique dorsal incision that is usually employed needs to be made more distal and transverse, so that the triquetrum can be exposed through a separate longitudinal capsular incision medial to the extensor digitorum communis.

Volar Dislocation of the Proximal Scaphoid Fragment (With or Without Dislocation of the Lunate). Weiss and associates[185] reported treating a patient with a dorsal trans-scaphoid perilunate dislocation that could not be reduced because the proximal fragment was dislocated anteriorly and rotated 180°. The displaced proximal scaphoid fracture had a circumferential appearance in the posteroanterior view. Open reduction through a volar Russe approach was followed by union without evidence of avascular necrosis. This injury most likely results when a scapholunate dissociation and a waist fracture of the scaphoid occur together. The displaced bone should be approached volarly to avoid injuring any remaining soft tissue attachment (Fig. 10–13). O'Carroll and Gallagher[127] reported a patient with an irreducible dorsal trans-scaphoid perilunate dislocation, in which the proximal scaphoid was displaced dorsally and rotated 180°. Open reduction through a dorsal incision five days after injury was followed by healing.

A fractured scaphoid is rarely encountered in association with a volar dislocation of the

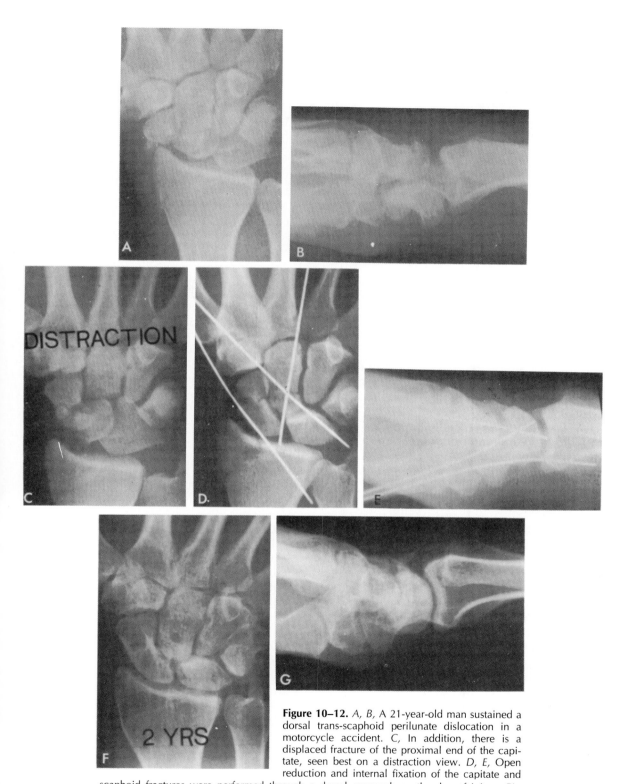

Figure 10–12. *A, B,* A 21-year-old man sustained a dorsal trans-scaphoid perilunate dislocation in a motorcycle accident. *C,* In addition, there is a displaced fracture of the proximal end of the capitate, seen best on a distraction view. *D, E,* Open reduction and internal fixation of the capitate and scaphoid fractures were performed through a dorsal approach on the day of injury. Pin fixation was continued for eight weeks, and plaster immobilization was discontinued at 20 weeks. *F, G,* Two years later, roentgenograms showed good healing of the scaphoid and capitate fractures, and function was good. (From Kane WJ [ed]: Current Orthopaedic Management. New York, Churchill Livingstone Inc, 1981.)

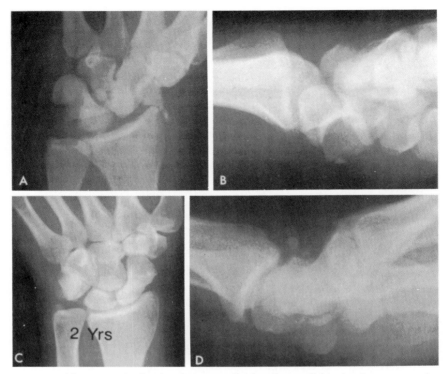

Figure 10–13. A 23-year-old man sustained a dorsal trans-scaphoid perilunate dislocation in a motorcycle accident. *A,* In the posteroanterior view, the proximal scaphoid fragment is displaced and overlapped by the capitate. *B,* In the lateral view, the proximal scaphoid fragment is volarly displaced and rotated forward. Closed reduction failed, so open reduction was performed through a volar incision. Casting was continued for six months. *C, D,* At two years, the scaphoid fracture was well healed, and function was excellent. (From Kane WJ [ed]: Current Orthopaedic Management. New York, Churchill Livingstone Inc, 1981.)

lunate. When these injuries coexist, the proximal scaphoid fragment is apt to be displaced volarly with the lunate as a single unit. The injury is more likely to be open than is the usual trans-scaphoid perilunate or lunate dislocation.[73] As Russell[141] noted in the six cases he reported, reduction is more difficult than in the routine case, and in two of his cases, the displaced lunate and scaphoid fragment were excised when reduction failed. Unsatisfactory results (nonunion and avascular necrosis of the proximal scaphoid) followed open reduction and fixation in both patients with this injury, as cited in the report by Green and O'Brien.[72] Stern,[157] however, achieved satisfactory results in two patients with this injury treated by immediate open reduction and internal fixation.

Dislocation of the Scaphoid (With or Without Dislocation of the Lunate). Dislocation of the scaphoid can occur alone* or in association with a volar dislocation of the lunate.[25, 28, 34, 91] If both bones are dislocated, they may

*References 27, 51, 92, 98, 120, 171, 180.

have done so as a unit or separately. The mechanism of injury is unknown, but loading in dorsiflexion and ulnar deviation seems most likely.

In isolated dislocations of the scaphoid, the bone dislocates radially, and often there is an accompanying fracture of the radial styloid (Fig. 10–14). The scaphoid may dislocate without any intercarpal displacement, but often there is a radial displacement of the distal carpal row, with the head of the capitate displaced between the dislocated scaphoid and the lunate. Closed reduction using longitudinal traction and radial deviation often successfully reduces the scaphoid, but a residual scapholunate dissociation is often present. Avascular necrosis following replacement of the scaphoid is usually transient, if it occurs at all.[188]

Taleisnik and associates[166] reported treating a patient with simultaneous volar dislocation of the scaphoid and lunate as a unit. Closed reduction was successful, but lunotriquetral dissociation and palmar flexion instability of the lunate were noted six weeks after injury. They collected five sim-

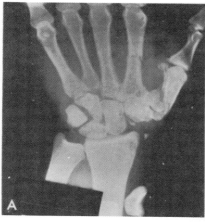
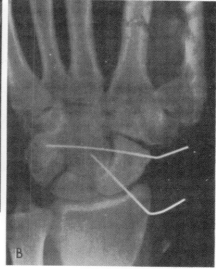

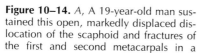

Figure 10–14. *A*, A 19-year-old man sustained this open, markedly displaced dislocation of the scaphoid and fractures of the first and second metacarpals in a motorcycle accident. The capitate is displaced proximal and radial to the lunate. The scaphoid was replaced and fixed with Kirschner wires. *B*, Two months later, there is slightly increased density of the scaphoid. The pins were removed at this time, and unfortunately, the patient was lost to follow-up. (From Orthop Clin North Am 15:237–258, 1984.)

ilar cases from the literature, but only one had an adequate follow-up. This patient, as reported by Dunn,[45] had a good result two years after open reduction and Kirschner wire fixation. In Küpfer's patient,[91] a dorsiflexion intercalated segment instability followed an open reduction and internal fixation performed 90 days after volar dislocation of the scaphoid and the lunate as a unit. Cleak[34] and Küpfer[91] both emphasized the need for early reduction and internal fixation of this injury.

Gordon[71] described a patient who had simultaneous volar dislocation of the scaphoid and the lunate, but the bones were dissociated from each other. Open reduction and cast immobilization for four weeks were followed by chronic rotatory subluxation of the scaphoid a year after injury (Fig. 10–15).

OTHER INDIVIDUAL CARPAL BONE DISLOCATIONS

The Trapezoid

Twenty cases of trapezoid dislocation (16 dorsal and four volar) have been recorded.[90] Volar dislocations are commonly associated with metacarpal injuries. Open reduction of the volarly dislocated trapezoid is usually necessary because of its wedge shape, the palmar surface area being over one half that of the dorsal surface.[154] Open reduction may require only a dorsal incision, but late volar

dislocation of the trapezoid requires both dorsal and volar incisions. Acute dorsal dislocations of the trapezoid can usually be reduced by closed manipulation.[7, 111] Avascular necrosis may follow open reduction of either type of dislocation;[139, 154] anticipating this problem, Goodman and Shankman[69, 70] performed a primary limited arthrodesis after relocation of a volarly dislocated trapezoid and reduction of an associated index and middle carpometacarpal dislocation.

The Trapezium

Complete dislocation of the trapezium is a rare injury that is usually produced by direct trauma. Volar dislocations[22, 67, 145, 147] predominate over dorsal dislocations,[13, 45] and open injury is common. Several methods of treatment have been reported, including acceptance of the dislocation,[141] closed reduction,[45] and primary excision.[67, 131] Open reduction and internal fixation of the displaced trapezium may be followed by complete loss of thumb carpometacarpal motion.[145, 147] Good results, however, have been achieved by open reduction,[13, 22] and it is the method of choice when closed reduction is unsuccessful.

The Pisiform

Dislocation of the pisiform is an uncommon injury, usually resulting from sudden violent

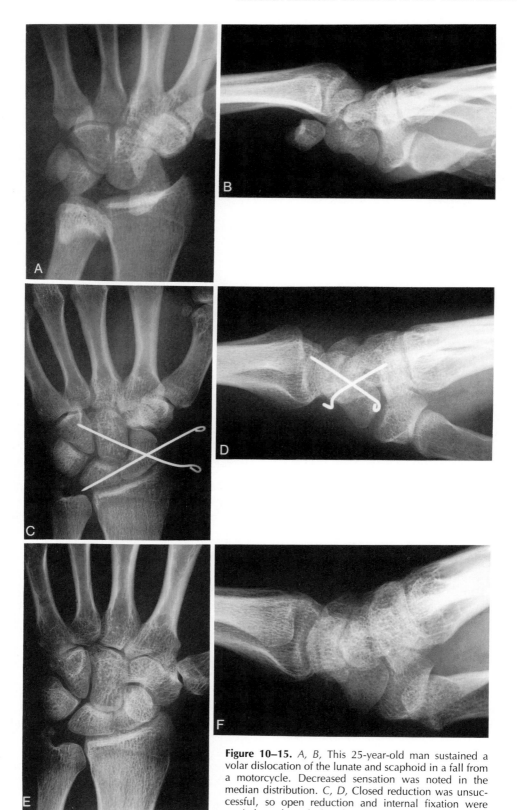

Figure 10–15. *A, B,* This 25-year-old man sustained a volar dislocation of the lunate and scaphoid in a fall from a motorcycle. Decreased sensation was noted in the median distribution. *C, D,* Closed reduction was unsuccessful, so open reduction and internal fixation were carried out through dorsal and volar incisions. *E, F,* Four months later, bone density was unchanged, but early narrowing of the lunocapitate and scapholunate joints was present. The patient regained full sensibility, had no pain, and returned to work.

contraction of the flexor carpi ulnaris muscle and only occasionally from direct injury. Proximal,[101] distal,[113] ulnar,[59] and volar[35] dislocations have been reported. Closed reduction may be successful but is likely to be followed by persistent or recurrent dislocation after removal of the cast.[82, 101] Redisplacement has resulted even after open reduction and pin fixation for eight weeks.[113] Excision of this expendable bone is the best treatment for an acute or recurrent dislocation.

The Hamate

Dislocation of the hamate is an exceedingly rare injury. In the nine published cases in which the direction of dislocation is known, five were volar and four dorsal. Duke[44] achieved a stable closed reduction of a volarly dislocated hamate by pronating the forearm without anesthesia. If closed reduction fails, open reduction and temporary Kirschner wire fixation should yield a satisfactory result.[59, 63, 77]

The Triquetrum

Only three cases of isolated triquetral dislocation have been reported, two volar[57, 149] and one dorsal.[9] Both volar dislocations were missed initially (one was discovered seven weeks and one four months later) and required late excision. The chronic median compression was relieved, and essentially full motion was restored 19 months and 34 months, respectively, after excision. Open reduction of a dorsal triquetral dislocation seven days after injury was followed by full return of motion and grip strength eight months later in the patient reported by Bieber and Weiland.[9]

The Capitate

Russell[141] reported a patient who had an open dorsal dislocation of the capitate with the third and fourth metacarpals and a dorsal dislocation of the trapezoid with the second metacarpal. Open reduction and plaster immobilization for 10 weeks were followed six months later by a return of one third of normal wrist motion and a powerful grip. Two total volar dislocations of the capitate have been reported, both associated with other carpal injuries. Open reduction was carried out in both patients, and carpometacarpal degenerative changes were noted 10 months[96] and 20 months[45] later.

OTHER INTERCARPAL DISLOCATIONS

Scaphotrapezial-Trapezoid Dislocations

Gibson[66] reported a patient with a dorsal dislocation of the scaphotrapezial-trapezoid joint in which full motion was restored by open reduction and Kirschner wire fixation for six weeks. He made reference to a patient reported by Tachakra[161]—a 13-year-old boy with a diastasis of the scaphotrapezial joint that closed spontaneously after four weeks of plaster immobilization. Two patients having chronic (six months and eight months) dorsal dislocation of the trapezium and trapezoid with their attached first and second metacarpals on the scaphoid ("radial hand dislocation") were reported by Watson and Hempton.[181] Satisfactory function was restored in both cases by triscaphoid arthrodesis.

Crush Injury of the Carpus

Garcia-Elias and associates[61] coined the term "crush injury of the carpus" to describe an injury characterized by disruption of the carpal arch through the capitohamate joint distally and the pisotriquetral joint proximally. Nine similar cases from the literature[2, 135] were reviewed, and the details and outcomes of four new cases were added. Disruption of the capitohamate joint distally with medial and volar dislocation of the hamate and its attached fourth and fifth metacarpals, with disruption of the pisotriquetral joints proximally results from a severe crush with flattening of the carpal arch. Clinically, the ring and little finger are ulnar-deviated and malrotated, and there is often an associated bursting type laceration of the thenar eminence. Three different variations of medial capitohamate dislocation were described by Garcia-Elias and associates:[61] fracture of the hamate with pisotriquetral dislocation, dislocation of the capitohamate and pisotriquetral joints without fracture, and dislocation with a displaced fracture of the triquetrum. Closed reduction may be successful if done early; however, the initial diagnosis is apt to be missed, necessitating open reduction and internal fixation (Fig. 10–16).[135]

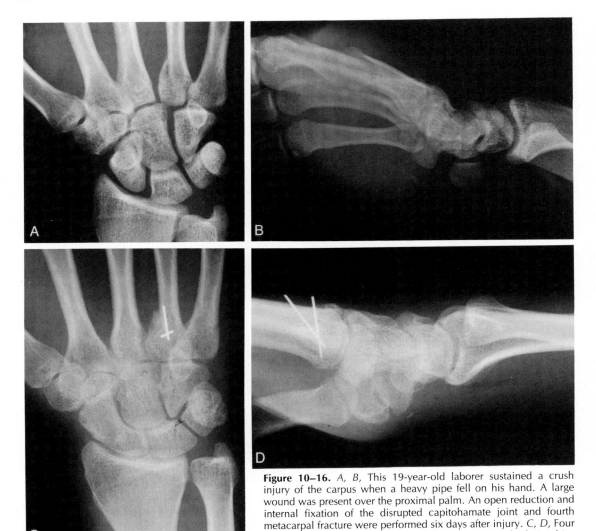

Figure 10–16. *A, B,* This 19-year-old laborer sustained a crush injury of the carpus when a heavy pipe fell on his hand. A large wound was present over the proximal palm. An open reduction and internal fixation of the disrupted capitohamate joint and fourth metacarpal fracture were performed six days after injury. *C, D,* Four months later, the fracture had healed, and intercarpal relationships were normal (Case courtesy of William E. Sanders, M.D.)

Late Treatment of Missed Dislocations

Intercarpal dislocations continue to be missed despite the fact that the patient usually presents for treatment shortly after injury and wrist radiographs are ordered. Scapholunate dislocation is the most commonly missed acute intercarpal injury, and its late management is discussed in Chapter 19.

Volar dislocation of the lunate is the next most frequently missed carpal dislocation. Fortunately, the dislocated bone can usually be replaced with a fair chance of success up to six months[28] and possibly even up to a year[15] after injury. Campbell and associates[28] reported satisfactory results in three late open reductions of the lunate done six weeks, three and a half months, and six months after injury. They emphasized the rarity of avascular necrosis following this injury and believed strongly that replacement gives a more satisfactory result than excision.

In this procedure, the median nerve is released and the lunate is inspected through a volar modified carpal tunnel incision. If the bone is not damaged and its cartilage surfaces appear healthy, the lunate is carefully mobilized using a Freer elevator, with care taken not to disrupt the consistently intact volar radiolunate ligament. An auxiliary dorsal incision is required to clean the fibrous tissue from the space between the radius and capitate formerly occupied by the lunate. The lunate is then replaced by means of longitudinal traction, utilizing the two incisions to gently effect reduction without traumatizing the bone or compromising its blood supply. Kirschner wire fixation of the scapholunate and scaphocapitate joints is maintained for six weeks (Fig. 10–17). If the lunate cartilaginous surfaces are not healthy and too much time has elapsed since the dislocation occurred, excision of the bone[159] without the insertion of a Silastic implant still yields an acceptable result.

Late open reduction of a neglected perilunate dislocation can be attempted up to six or eight weeks after injury, if the cartilage covering the displaced bones is healthy. Through a dorsal incision, a Freer elevator is used to carefully dissect around the capitate, lunate, and proximal pole of the scaphoid. Temporary Kirschner wire handles in the scaphoid and lunate are useful in secur-

ing and maintaining the reduction while the internal fixation is inserted. After four to six weeks of delay, consideration should be given to triscaphoid fusion at the same time that the reduction is performed. Pin fixation is continued for eight weeks. If the reduction is delayed more than six to eight weeks, or if the condition of the bones precludes reduction, then proximal row carpectomy is an excellent salvage procedure.[28, 40, 83, 87, 123] Pain relief is good, and instability has not been a problem. Motion and grip strength are surprisingly good, and the results do not seem to deteriorate with time (Fig. 10–18). If arthritis has occurred in both the radiocarpal and intercarpal joints, a radiocarpal arthrodesis should be performed, correcting the deformity at the same time.

The same principles apply to the neglected trans-scaphoid perilunate disloca-

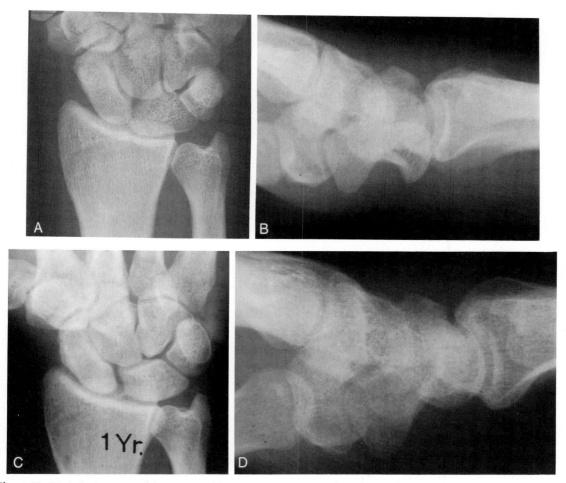

Figure 10–17. *A, B,* A 21-year-old man injured his wrist in a fall from a motorcycle. This volar lunate dislocation remained undiagnosed for four months. Open reduction through dorsal and volar incisions was done. *C, D,* At one year, motion had almost returned to normal, and grip strength was equal to that of the uninjured side. (From Kane WJ [ed]: Current Orthopaedic Management. New York, Churchill Livingstone Inc, 1981.)

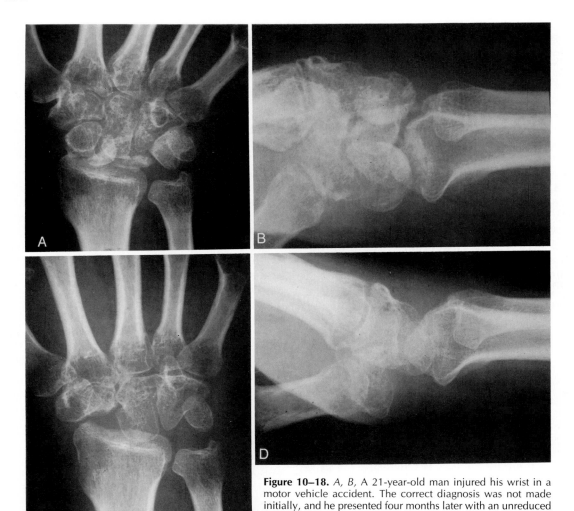

Figure 10–18. *A, B,* A 21-year-old man injured his wrist in a motor vehicle accident. The correct diagnosis was not made initially, and he presented four months later with an unreduced dorsal perilunate dislocation. A proximal row carpectomy was performed. *C, D,* At one year, dorsiflexion was 40°, palmar flexion was 50°, and grip strength was two-thirds normal. Symptoms were minimal. (From Kane WJ [ed]: Current Orthopaedic Management. New York, Churchill Livingstone Inc, 1981.)

tion; however, success in reducing and obtaining union of the displaced scaphoid fracture and in achieving a good result is less likely than for neglected lunate and perilunate dislocations. If delayed open reduction is performed, bone grafting of the scaphoid should be done at the same time. The indications for proximal row carpectomy and radiocarpal arthrodesis are the same as for perilunate dislocations. Both fragments of the scaphoid should be excised if proximal row excision is performed.

Complications of Intercarpal Dislocations and Fracture-Dislocations

Scaphoid nonunion, delayed union, and avascular necrosis of the proximal fragment of the scaphoid are more commonly encountered with trans-scaphoid perilunate dislocations than with simple scaphoid fractures. Their management has been discussed under "Treatment." Scaphoid malunion usually results in subsequent painful arthritis and must be avoided by maintaining accurate reduction until healing is complete. Ostectomy can occasionally save the day in a malunited scaphoid fracture.[50]

Recurrence of scapholunate dissociation following closed or open reduction and fixation is sometimes noted after the fixation is removed and mobility of the wrist is regained. Its management is discussed in Chapter 19. Instances of patients with recurrent dorsal trans-scaphoid perilunate dislocation were reported by Lowdon and asso-

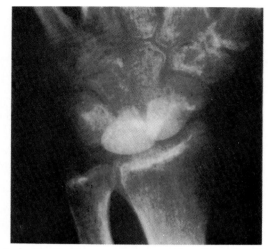

Figure 10–19. This roentgenogram, taken 12 weeks after closed reduction of a dorsal trans-scaphoid perilunate dislocation, shows increased density of the lunate and proximal pole of the scaphoid. Healing occurred without collapse or fragmentation of either bone, and function was good. (From Orthop Clin North Am 15:237–258, 1984.)

ciates.[95] A 20-year-old man had a closed reduction of a dorsal trans-scaphoid perilunate dislocation, and the wrist was immobilized for three months. Nonunion was noted eight months after injury, and five years later, after another dorsiflexion injury, recurrent closed trans-scaphoid perilunate dislocation occurred through the nonunion. Open reduction and scaphoid bone grafting corrected the deformity, but union was not achieved.

Avascular necrosis of the lunate is rarely encountered following closed or open reduction of dislocations of this bone. Wagner[179] and Cave[31] each reported a single case of avascular necrosis of the lunate following closed reduction, but neither case had the collapse and fragmentation typical of Kienböck's disease. A peculiar type of avascular necrosis involving the lunate and the proximal pole of the scaphoid has been seen in several cases of trans-scaphoid perilunate dislocation reported in the literature[187] and in this series. The changes do not seem to be progressive, and revascularization occurs (Fig. 10–19).

Median neuritis accompanying perilunate and lunate dislocations has a good prognosis if the dislocation is reduced early. Delayed treatment may result in persistent symptoms, even if a carpal tunnel release is performed. Sympathetic dystrophy is a rare complication of intercarpal dislocations.[107]

References

1. Adkinson JW, and Chapman MW: Treatment of acute lunate and perilunate dislocations. Clin Orthop 164:199–207, 1982.
2. Adler JB, and Shaftan GW: Fractures of the capitate. J Bone Joint Surg 44A:1537–1547, 1962.
3. Aitken AP, and Nalebuff EA: Volar transnavicular perilunar dislocation of the carpus. J Bone Joint Surg 42A:1051–1057, 1960.
4. Alho A, and Kanhaanjää U: Management of fractured scaphoid bones. A prospective study of 100 fractures. Acta Orthop Scand 46:737–743, 1975.
5. Baird DB, and Friedenberg ZB: Delayed ulnar nerve palsy following fracture of the hamate. J Bone Joint Surg 570–572, 1968.
6. Bartone NF, and Grieco RV: Fracture of the triquetrum. J Bone Joint Surg 38A:353–356, 1956.
7. Bendre DV, and Baxi VK: Dislocation of trapezoid. J Trauma 21:899–900, 1981.
8. Berlin D: Position in the treatment of fracture of the carpal scaphoid. N Engl J Med 201:574, 1929.
9. Bieber EJ, and Weiland AJ: Traumatic dorsal dislocation of the triquetrum: a case report. J Hand Surg 9A:840–842, 1984.
10. Bilos J, and Hui PW: Dorsal dislocation of the lunate with carpal collapse. J Bone Joint Surg 63A:1484–1486, 1981.
11. Bizairo AH: Traumatology of the carpus. Surg Gynecol Obstet 34:574–588, 1922.
12. Blair WF, Kilpatrick WC, and Over GE: Open fracture of the hook of the hamate: a case report. Clin Orthop 163:180–184, 1982.
13. Boe S: Dislocation of the trapezium (multangulum majus). Acta Orthop Scand 50:85–86, 1979.
14. Böhler L, Trojan E, and Jahna H: Die Behandlung sergebnisse von 734 frischen bruchen des kahnbein korpers der hand. Widerherst, Traumatology 2:86–111, 1954.
15. Böhler L: The Treatment of Fractures. New York, Grune & Stratton, Inc, 1956.
16. Bolton-Maggs BG, Held BH, and Ravell PA: Bilateral avascular necrosis of the capitate: a case report and a review of the literature. J Bone Joint Surg 66B:557–559, 1984.
17. Bonnin JG and Greening WP: Fractures of the triquetrum. Br J Surg 31:278–283, 1943.
18. Bora FW, Osterman AL, and Brighton CT: The electrical treatment of scaphoid non-union. Clin Orthop 161:33–38, 1981.
19. Bora FW Jr, Osterman AL, Woodbury DF, et al: Treatment of non-union of the scaphoid by direct current. Orthop Clin North Am 15:107–112, 1984.
20. Bowen TL: Injuries of the hamate bone. Hand 5:235–238, 1973.
21. Boyes JG: Subluxation of the carpal navicular bone. South Med J 69:141–144, 1976.
22. Brewood AFM: Complete dislocation of the trapezium: a case report. Injury 16:303–304, 1985.
23. Brittain HA: Fracture of the carpal scaphoid. Br Med J 2:671–673, 1938.
24. Broomé A, Oedell CA, and Coléen S: High plaster immobilization for fracture of the carpal scaphoid bone. Acta Chir Scand 128:42–44, 1964.
25. Brown RHL, and Muddu BN: Scaphoid and lunate dislocation: a report on a case. Hand 13:303–307, 1981.
26. Bryan RS, and Dobyns JH: Fractures of the carpal bones other than lunate and navicular. Clin Orthop 149:107–111, 1980.

27. Buzby BF: Isolated radial dislocation of carpal scaphoid. Ann Surg 100:553–555, 1934.

28. Campbell RD Jr, Lance EM, and Yeoh CB: Lunate and perilunar dislocations. J Bone Joint Surg 46B:55–72, 1964.

29. Campbell RD Jr, Thompson TC, Lance EM, et al: Indications for open reduction of lunate and perilunate dislocations of the carpal bones. J Bone Joint Surg 47A:915–937, 1965.

30. Carter PR, Eaton RG, and Littler JW: Ununited fracture of the hook of the hamate. J Bone Joint Surg 59A:583–588, 1977.

31. Cave EF: Fractures and Other Injuries. Chicago, Year Book Medical Publishers Inc, 1958, p 388.

32. Cetti R, and Christensen SE: The diagnostic value of displacement of the fat stripe in fracture of the scaphoid bone. Hand 14:75–79, 1982.

33. Clayton ML: Rupture of the flexor tendon in carpal tunnel (non-rheumatoid) with specific reference to fracture of the hook of the hamate. J Bone Joint Surg 51A:798–799, 1969.

34. Cleak DK: Dislocation of the scaphoid and lunate bones without fractures: a case report. Injury 14:278–281, 1982.

35. Cohen I: Dislocation of the pisiform. Ann Surg 75:238–239, 1922.

36. Cooney WP, Dobyns JH, and Linscheid RL: Fractures of the scaphoid: a rational approach to management. Clin Orthop 149:90–97, 1980.

37. Connell MC, and Dyson RP: Dislocation of carpal scaphoid. Report of a case. J Bone Joint Surg 37B:252–253, 1955.

38. Cope JR: Rotatory subluxation of the scaphoid. Clin Radiol 35:495–501, 1984.

39. Cordrey LJ, and Ferrer-Torells M: Management of fracture of the greater multangular. J Bone Joint Surg 42A:1111–1118, 1960.

40. Crabbe WA: Excision of the proximal row of the carpus. J Bone Joint Surg 46B:708–711, 1964.

41. Crosby EB, and Linscheid RL: Rupture of the flexor profundus tendon of the ring finger secondary to ancient fracture of the hook of the hamate. Review of the literature and report of two cases. J Bone Joint Surg 56A:1076–1078, 1974.

42. Dehne E, Deffer PA, and Feighney RE: Pathomechanics of the fracture of the carpal navicular. J Trauma 4:96–114, 1964.

43. Dobyns JH, Linscheid RL, Chao EYS, et al: Traumatic instability of the wrist. American Academy of Orthopaedic Surgeons Instructional Course Lectures 24:182–199, 1975.

44. Duke R: Dislocations of the hamate bone. J Bone Joint Surg 45B:744, 1963.

45. Dunn AW: Fractures and dislocations of the carpus. Surg Clin North Am 52:1513–1538, 1972.

46. Eddeland A, Eiken O, Hellgren E, et al: Fractures of the scaphoid. Scand J Plast Reconstr Surg 9:234–239, 1975.

47. Egawa M, and Asai T: Fractures of the hook of the hamate: report of six cases and the suitability of computerized tomography. J Hand Surg 8:393–398, 1983.

48. ElKhoury G, Usta HY, and Blair WF: Naviculocapitate fracture-dislocation. AJR 139:385–386, 1982.

49. Fenton RL: The naviculo-capitate fracture syndrome. J Bone Joint Surg 38A:681–684, 1956.

50. Fernandes HJA Jr, Köberle G, Ferreira GHS, et al: Volar trans-scaphoid perilunar dislocation. Hand 15:276–280, 1983.

51. Fishman MC, Dalinka MK, and Osterman L: Case report 309. Skeletal Radiol 13:245–247, 1985.

52. Fisk GR: An overview of injuries of the wrist. Clin Orthop 149:137–144, 1980.

53. Fisk GR: The Wrist. J Bone Joint Surg 66B:396–407, 1984.

54. Frankel VH: The Terry-Thomas sign. Clin Orthop 129:321–322, 1977.

55. Freeland AE, and Finley JS: Displaced vertical fracture of the trapezium treated with a small cancellous lag screw. J Hand Surg 9A:843–845, 1984.

56. Friedenberg ZB: Anatomic considerations in the treatment of carpal navicular fractures. Am J Surg 78:379–381, 1949.

57. Frykman E: Dislocation of the triquetrum. Scand J Plast Reconstr Surg 14:205–207, 1980.

58. Frykman G: Pulsing electromagnetic field treatment of nonunion of the scaphoid: a preliminary report. Orthop Trans 6:160, 1982.

59. Gainor BJ: Simultaneous dislocation of the hamate and pisiform: a case report. J Hand Surg 10A:88–90, 1985.

60. Gamble JG, and Simmons SC III: Bilateral scaphoid fractures in a child. Clin Orthop 162:125–128, 1982.

61. Garcia-Elias M, Abanco J, Salvador E, et al: Crush injury of the carpus. J Bone Joint Surg 67B:286–289, 1985.

62. Ganel A, Engel J, Oster Z, et al: Bone scanning in assessment of fractures of the scaphoid. J Hand Surg 4:540–543, 1979.

63. Geist DG: Dislocation of the hamate bone. J Bone Joint Surg 21:215–217, 1939.

64. Gelberman RH, and Menon J: The vascularity of the scaphoid bone. J Hand Surg 5:508–513, 1980.

65. Gerard FM: Post-traumatic carpal instability in a young child: a case report. J Bone Joint Surg 62A:131–133, 1980.

66. Gibson PH: Scaphoid-trapezium-trapezoid dislocation. Hand 3:267–269, 1983.

67. Goldberg I, Amit S, Bahar A, et al: Complete dislocation of the trapezium (multangulum majus). J Hand Surg 6:193–195, 1981.

68. Goldman S, Lipscomb PR, and Taylor WF: Immobilization for acute carpal scaphoid fractures. Surg Gynecol Obstet 129:281–284, 1969.

69. Goodman ML, and Shankman GB: Palmar dislocation of the trapezoid: a case report. J Hand Surg 8:606–609, 1983.

70. Goodman ML, and Shankman GB: Update: palmar dislocation of the trapezoid: a case report. J Hand Surg 9A:127–131, 1984.

71. Gordon SL: Scaphoid and lunate dislocation: report of a case in a patient with peripheral neuropathy. J Bone Joint Surg 54A:1769–1772, 1972.

72. Green DP, and O'Brien ET: Open reduction of carpal dislocations: indications and operative techniques. J Hand Surg 3:250–265, 1978.

73. Green DP, and O'Brien ET: Classification and management of carpal dislocations. Clin Orthop 149:55–72, 1980.

74. Green MH, Hadied AM, and LaMont RL: Scaphoid fractures in children. J Hand Surg 9A:536–541, 1984.

75. Greenspan A, Posner MA, and Tucker M: The value of carpal tunnel trispiral tomography in the diagnosis of fracture of the hook of the hamate. Bull Hosp Joint Dis Orthop Inst 45:74–79, 1985.

76. Grundy M: Fractures of the carpal scaphoid in children. Br J Surg 56:523–524, 1969.

77. Gunn RS: Dislocation of the hamate bone. J Hand Surg 10B:107–108, 1985.

78. Heim U, and Pfeiffer KM, in collaboration with Meuli HC: Small Fragment Set Manual. Technique recommended by the ASIF Group (Swiss Association for Study of Internal Fixation). New York, Springer-Verlag, 1974.

79. Herbert TJ, and Fisher WE: Management of the fractured scaphoid using a new bone screw. J Bone Joint Surg 66B:114–123, 1984.

80. Hill NA: Fractures and dislocations of the carpus. Orthop Clin North Am 1:275–284, 1970.

81. Howard FM: Ulnar nerve palsy in wrist fractures. J Bone Joint Surg 43A:1197–1201, 1961.

82. Immerman EW: Dislocation of the pisiform. J Bone Joint Surg 30A:489–492, 1948.

83. Inglis AE, and Jones EC: Proximal row carpectomy for diseases of the proximal row. J Bone Joint Surg 59A:460–463, 1977.

84. James ETR, and Burke FD: Vibration disease of the capitate. J Hand Surg 9B:169–170, 1984.

85. Johnson RP: The acutely injured wrist and its residuals. Clin Orthop 149:33–44, 1980.

86. Jones GB: An unusual fracture-dislocation of the carpus. J Bone Joint Surg 37B:146–147, 1955.

87. Jorgensen EC: Proximal row carpectomy. An end result study of twenty-two cases. J Bone Joint Surg 51A:1104–1111, 1969.

88. Kimmel RB, and O'Brien ET: Surgical treatment of avascular necrosis of proximal pole of capitate: a case report. J Hand Surg 7:284–286, 1982.

89. King RJ, Machenney RP, and Elnur S: Suggested method for closed treatment of fractures of the carpal scaphoid: hypothesis supported by dissection and clinical practice. J R Soc Med 75:860–867, 1982.

90. Kopp JR: Isolated palmar dislocation of the trapezoid. J Hand Surg 10A:91–93, 1985.

91. Küpfer K: Palmar dislocation of scaphoid and lunate as a unit: case report with special reference to carpal instability and treatment. J Hand Surg 11A:130–134, 1986.

92. Kuth JR: Isolated dislocation of the carpal navicular. J Bone Joint Surg 21:479–483, 1939.

93. Linscheid RL, Dobyns JH, and Younge DK: Trispiral tomography in the evaluation of wrist injury. Bull Hosp J Dis Orthop Inst 44:297–308, 1984.

94. London PS: The broken scaphoid bone. The case against pessimism. J Bone Joint Surg 43B:237–244, 1961.

95. Lowdon IMR, Simpson AHRW, and Burge P: Recurrent dorsal trans-scaphoid perilunate dislocation. J Hand Surg 9B:307–310, 1984.

96. Lowrey DG, Moss SH, and Wolff TW: Volar dislocation of the capitate. J Bone Joint Surg 66A:611–613, 1984.

97. Lowry WE, and Cord SA: Traumatic avascular necrosis of the capitate bone: a case report. J Hand Surg 6:245–248, 1981.

98. Maki NJ, Chuinard RG, and D'Ambrosia R: Isolated, complete radial dislocation of the scaphoid. J Bone Joint Surg 64A:615–616, 1982.

99. Marck KW, and Klasen HJ: Fracture-dislocation of the hamatometacarpal joint: a case report. J Hand Surg 11A:128–130, 1986.

100. Marsh AP, and Lampros PJ: The naviculo-capitate fracture syndrome. AJR 82:255–256, 1959.

101. Mather JH: Dislocation of the pisiform bone. Br J Radiol 29:17–18, 1924.

102. Maudsley RH, and Chen SC: Screw fixation in the management of the fractured scaphoid. J Bone Joint Surg 54B:432–441, 1972.

103. Mayfield JK: Mechanism of carpal injuries. Clin Orthop 149:45–54, 1980.

104. Mayfield JK, Johnson RP, and Kilcoyne RF: The ligaments of the human wrist and their functional significance. Anat Rec 186:417–428, 1976.

105. Mayfield JK, Johnson RP, and Kilcoyne RF: Carpal dislocations: pathomechanics and progressive perilunar instability. J Hand Surg 5:226–241, 1980.

106. Mayfield JK: Patterns of injury to carpal ligaments. Clin Orthop 187:36–42, 1984.

107. McBride ED: An operation for late reduction of the semilunar bone. South Med J 26:672–676, 1983.

108. McClain EJ, and Boyes JH: Missed fracture of the greater multangular. J Bone Joint Surg 48A:1525–1528, 1966.

109. McLaughlin HL, and Parkes JC: Fracture of the carpal navicular (scaphoid) bone. Gradations in therapy based upon pathology. J Trauma 9:311–319, 1969.

110. Meyers MH, Wells R, and Harvey JP Jr: Naviculocapitate fracture syndrome: review of the literature and a case report. J Bone Joint Surg 53A:1383–1386, 1971.

111. Meyn MA Jr, and Roth AM: Isolated dislocation of the trapezoid bone. J Hand Surg 5:602–604, 1980.

112. Milch H: Fracture of the hamate bone. J Bone Joint Surg 16:459–462, 1934.

113. Minami M, Yamazaki J, and Ishii S: Isolated dislocation of the pisiform: a case report and review of the literature. J Hand Surg 9A:125–127, 1984.

114. Monaham PRW, and Galasko CSB: The scaphocapitate fracture syndrome: a mechanism of injury. J Bone Joint Surg 54B:122–124, 1972.

115. Moneim MS: The tangential posteroanterior radiographs to demonstrate scapholunate dissociation. J Bone Joint Surg 63A:1324–1326, 1981.

116. Moneim MS, Hofammann KE III, and Omer GE: Trans-scaphoid perilunate fracture-dislocation. Results of open reduction and pin fixation. Clin Orthop 190:227–235, 1984.

117. Morawa LG, Ross PM, and Schock CC: Fracture and dislocation involving the navicular-lunate axis. Clin Orthop 118:48–53, 1976.

118. Morgan DAF, and Walters JW: A prospective study of 100 consecutive carpal scaphoid fractures. Aust NZ J Surg 54:233–241, 1984.

119. Munck JT, Andresen JH, Thommesen P, et al: Scanning and radiology of the carpal scaphoid bone. Acta Orthop Scand 50:663–665, 1979.

120. Murakami Y: Dislocation of the carpal scaphoid. Hand 9:79–81, 1977.

121. Murahami S, and Nakajima H: Aseptic necrosis of the capitate bone in two gymnasts. Am J Sports Med 12:170–173, 1984.

122. Müssbichler H: Injuries of the carpal scaphoid in children. Acta Radiol (Stockh) 56:316–368, 1961.

123. Neviaser RJ: Proximal row carpectomy for posttraumatic disorders of the carpus. J Hand Surg 8:301–305, 1983.

124. Newman JH, and Watts I: Avascular necrosis of the capitate and dorsiflexion instability. Hand 12:176–178, 1980.

125. Nielsen PT, Hedeboe J, and Thommesen P: Bone scintigraphy in the evaluation of fracture of the carpal scaphoid bone. Acta Orthop Scand 54:303–306, 1983.

126. Okuhara T, Matsui T, and Sugimoto Y: Spontaneous rupture of flexor tendons of a little finger due to projection of the hook of the hamate. Hand 14:71–74, 1982.

127. O'Carroll PF, and Gallagher JE: Irreducible trans-scaphoid-perilunate dislocation. IJMS 152:424–427, 1983.

128. Palmer AK: Trapezial ridge fractures. J Hand Surg 6:561–564, 1981.

129. Peiró A, Martos F, Mut T, et al: Trans-scaphoid perilunate dislocation in a child. A case report. Acta Orthop Scand 52:31–34, 1981.

130. Pellegrino EA, and Peterson ED: Trans-scaphoid perilunate dislocation of the wrist. J Bone Joint Surg 55A:1319, 1973.

131. Peterson CL: Dislocation of the multangulum majus or trapezium and its treatment in two cases with extirpation. Arch Chir Neerl 2:369–376, 1950.

132. Pick RY, and Segal D: Carpal scaphoid fracture and non-union in an eight-year-old child. J Bone Joint Surg 65A:1188–1189, 1983.

133. Polivy KD, Millender LH, Newberg A, et al: Fractures of the hook of the hamate: a failure of clinical diagnosis. J Hand Surg 10A:101–104, 1985.

134. Pournaras J, and Kapas A: Volar perilunar dislocation: A case report. J Bone Joint Surg 61A:625–626, 1979.

135. Primiano GA, and Reef TC: Disruption of the proximal carpal arch of the hand. J Bone Joint Surg 56A:328–332, 1974.

136. Rahme H: Idiopathic avascular necrosis of the capitate bone: a case report. Hand 15:274–275, 1983.

137. Rand J, Linscheid RL, and Dobyns JH: Capitate fractures. A long term follow-up. Clin Orthop 165:209–216, 1982.

138. Resnik CS, Gilberman RH, and Resnick D: Trans-scaphoid-transcapitate, perilunate fracture dislocation (scaphocapitate syndrome). Skeletal Radiol 9:192–194, 1983.

139. Rhoades CE, and Reckling FW: Palmar dislocation of the trapezoid: a case report. J Hand Surg 8:85–88, 1983.

140. Russe O: Fracture of the carpal navicular. J Bone Joint Surg 42A:759–768, 1960.

141. Russell TB: Inter-carpal dislocations and fracture-dislocations: a review of fifty-nine cases. J Bone Joint Surg 31B:524–531, 1949.

142. Saunier J, and Chamay A: Volar perilunar dislocation of the wrist. Clin Orthop 157:139–142, 1981.

143. Schlosser H, and Murray JF: Fracture of the hook of the hamate. Can J Surg 27:587–589, 1984.

144. Seidenstein H: Two unusual dislocations of the wrist. J Bone Joint Surg 38A:1137–1141, 1956.

145. Seimon LP: Compound dislocation of the trapezium. J Bone Joint Surg 54A:1297–1300, 1972.

146. Shands AR Jr: Analysis of more important orthopaedic information. Surgery 16:584–586, 1944.

147. Siegel MW, and Hertzberg H: Complete dislocation of the greater multangular (trapezium): a case report. J Bone Joint Surg 51A:769–772, 1969.

148. Soto-Hall R: Recent fractures of the carpal scaphoid. JAMA 129:335–338, 1945.

149. Soucacos PN, and Hartofilakidis-Garafalidis GC: Dislocation of the triangular bone: report of a case. J Bone Joint Surg 63A:1012–1013, 1981.

150. Southcott R, and Rosman MA: Non-union of carpal scaphoid fracture in children. J Bone Joint Surg 59B:20–23, 1977.

151. Speed K: Traumatic Injuries of the Carpus. New York, D Appleton and Co, 1929.

152. Squire M: Carpal mechanics and trauma. J Bone Joint Surg 41B:210, 1959.

153. Stark HH, Jobe FW, Boyes JH, et al: Fracture of the hook of the hamate in athletes. J Bone Joint Surg 59A:575–582, 1977.

154. Stein AH: Dorsal dislocation of the lesser multangular. J Bone Joint Surg 53A:377–379, 1971.

155. Stein F, Miale A, and Stein A: Enhanced diagnosis of hand and wrist disorders by triple phase radionuclide bone imaging. Bull Hosp J Dis Orthop Inst 44:477–484, 1984.

156. Stein F, and Seigel MW: Naviculo-capitate fracture syndrome: a case report. J Bone Joint Surg 51A:391–395, 1969.

157. Stern PJ: Trans-scaphoid-lunate dislocation: a report of two cases. J Hand Surg 9A:370–373, 1984.

158. Stewart MJ: Fractures of the carpal navicular (scaphoid): a report of 436 cases. J Bone Joint Surg 36A:998–1006, 1954.

159. Stewart MJ, and Cross H: The management of injuries in the carpal lunate with a review of sixty cases. J Bone Joint Surg 50A:1489, 1968.

160. Stordahl A, Schjoth A, Woxholt G, et al: Bone scanning of fractures of the scaphoid. J Hand Surg 9B:189–190, 1984.

161. Tachakra SS: A case of trapezio-scaphoid subluxation. Br J Clin Pract 31:162, 1977.

162. Takami H, Takahashi S, and Ando M: Rupture of flexor tendon associated with previous fracture of the hook of the hamate. Hand 15:73–76, 1983.

163. Taleisnik J: The ligaments of the wrist. J Hand Surg 1:110–118, 1976.

164. Taleisnik J: Wrist: anatomy, function and injury. American Academy of Orthopaedic Surgeons Instructional Course Lectures 27:61–87, 1978.

165. Taleisnik J, and Kelly PJ: The extraosseous and intraosseous blood supply of the scaphoid bone. J Bone Joint Surg 48A:1125–1137, 1966.

166. Taleisnik J, Malerich M, and Prietto M: Palmar carpal instability secondary to dislocation of scaphoid and lunate: report of a case and review of the literature. J Hand Surg 7:606–612, 1982.

167. Tanz SS: Rotation effect in lunar and perilunar dislocations. Clin Orthop 57:147–152, 1968.

168. Terry DW Jr, and Ramin JE: The navicular fat stripe. A useful roentgen feature for evaluating wrist trauma. Am J Roentg Radium Ther and Nucl Med 124:25–28, 1975.

169. Thomaidis V Th: Elbow-wrist-thumb immobilization in the treatment of fractures of the carpal scaphoid. Acta Orthop Scand 44:679–689, 1973.

170. Thomas AP, and Birch R: An unusual hamate fracture. Hand 15:281–286, 1983.

171. Thomas HO: Isolated dislocation of the carpal scaphoid. Acta Orthop Scand 48:369–372, 1977.

172. Vahvanen V, and Westerlund M: Fracture of the carpal scaphoid in children. Acta Orthop Scand 51:909–913, 1980.

173. Vance RM, Gelberman RH, and Evans EF: Scapho-capitate fractures. J Bone Joint Surg 62A:271–276, 1980.

174. Vander Grend R, Dell PC, Glowczewskie BS, et al: Intraosseous blood supply of the capitate and its

correlation with aseptic necrosis. J Hand Surg 9A:677–680, 1984.

175. Vasilas A, Grieco RV, and Bartone NF: Roentgen aspects of injuries to the pisiform bone and piso-triquetral joint. J Bone Joint Surg 42A:1317–1328, 1960.

176. Verdan C: Fracture of the scaphoid. Surg Clin North Am 40:461–464, 1960.

177. Verdan C, and Narakas A: Fractures and pseu-doarthrosis of the scaphoid. Surg Clin North Am 48:1083–1095, 1968.

178. Vichick DA, and Dehne E: Fractures of the carpal scaphoid: an akinetic approach. Paper presented at Society of Military Orthopaedic Surgeons Meeting, San Antonio, Texas, November, 1977.

179. Wagner CJ: Perilunar dislocations. J Bone Joint Surg 38A:1198–1230, 1956.

180. Walker GBW: Dislocation of the carpal scaphoid reduced by open operation. Br J Surg 30:380–381, 1943.

181. Watson HK, and Hempton RF: Limited wrist arthrodesis. I. The triscaphoid joint. J Hand Surg 5:320–327, 1980.

182. Watson-Jones R: Fractures and Joint Injuries. 3rd ed. Edinburgh, E & S Livingstone, 1943.

183. Weber ER: Biomechanical implications of scaphoid waist fractures. Clin Orthop 149:83–89, 1980.

184. Weber ER, and Chao EYS: An experimental approach to the mechanism of scaphoid waist fractures. J Hand Surg 3:142–148, 1978.

185. Weiss C, Laskin RS, and Spinner M: Irreducible trans-scaphoid perilunate dislocation: a case report. J Bone Joint Surg 52A:565–568, 1970.

186. Weseley MS, and Barenfeld PA: Trans-scaphoid trans-capitate, transtriquetral, perilunate fracture-dislocation of the wrist: a case report. J Bone Joint Surg 54A:1073–1078, 1972.

187. White RE, and Omer GE: Transient vascular compromise of the lunate after fracture-dislocation or dislocation of the carpus. J Hand Surg 9A:181–184, 1984.

188. Walker GBW: Dislocation of the carpal scaphoid reduced by open operation. Br J Surg 30:380–381, 1943.

189. Woodward AH, Neviaser RJ, and Nisefeld F: Radial and volar perilunate trans-scaphoid fracture-dislocation: a case report. South Med J 68:926–928, 1975.

190. Worland RL, and Dick HM: Transnavicular perilunate dislocation. J Trauma 15:407–412, 1975.

191. Zichner L: Repair of non-unions by electrically pulsed current stimulation. Clin Orthop 161:115–121, 1981.

CHAPTER 11

Unstable Fractures of the Distal Radius

CHARLES P. MELONE, JR., M.D., F.A.C.S.

The hallmark of unstable distal radius fractures is comminution. Excessive fragmentation of multiple fracture components creates instability that is often impossible to manage by closed manipulation and immobilization. The problem is axiomatic: Reduction of comminuted fractures is easy to achieve but difficult to maintain. Without supplementary fixation, redisplacement of the fractures—frequently to their prereduction position[18]—is inevitable.

Despite a consensus regarding the need for stabilization of these fractures, the best method of achieving this goal is a topic of considerable controversy. Functional bracing,[32] percutaneous pinning,[6, 12, 13, 35] Rush rod fixation,[26, 31] pins and plaster,[3, 5, 7, 19, 22, 33] external fixators,[2, 10, 21, 40, 42] and even open reduction with internal fixation[11, 14, 17, 23] have been employed for seemingly similar injuries. Much of the confusion can be eliminated if a basic distinction is made between fractures confined to the metaphysis and those involving the distal radial articulations.

Extra-articular injuries, traditionally called Colles' and Smith's fractures, result from tension forces incurred by falls on the outstretched hand. Despite fracture displacement, these relatively low-energy injuries tend to be stable after closed reduction. In contrast, the articular injuries, often termed Barton's fractures, usually occur among physically active persons whose wrists are exposed to violent compression forces (Fig. 11–1). These high-energy injuries are characterized by extensive comminution and profound instability. The articular fractures are frequently associated with injuries to the adjacent nerves and tendons as well as to the carpus and distal ulna. Maximum recovery from these more serious fractures requires a method of treatment that not only ensures skeletal stability but also restores joint congruity and soft tissue integrity.

Rational management of unstable distal radial fractures is based on prompt recognition of the magnitude of injury. The extent of comminution, articular disruption, and periarticular injury must be carefully assessed in the planning of treatment for each injury.

CLASSIFICATION OF DISTAL RADIUS FRACTURES

The classifications commonly employed for distal radius fractures reflect the extent of articular involvement (Table 11–1). Clearly,

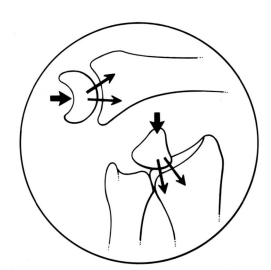

Figure 11–1. "Die punch" mechanism of articular fractures.[33, 36] A compression force, transmitted primarily by the lunate, disrupts the distal radius articular surfaces. The direction and magnitude of force account for predictable patterns of fracture displacement.

Table 11–1. **CLASSIFICATION OF DISTAL RADIUS FRACTURES**

Fracture	Type
Gartland and Werley (1951)[18]	
Extra-articular	I
Articular—undisplaced radiocarpal joint	II*
Articular—displaced radiocarpal joint	III*
Thomas (1957)[38]	
Extra-articular—oblique	I
Articular	II*
Extra-articular—transverse	III
Frykman (1967)[16]	
Extra-articular	I
Extra-articular—distal ulna	II
Articular—radiocarpal (RC)	III*
Articular—RC, distal ulna	IV*
Articular—radioulnar (RU)	V*
Articular—RU, distal ulna	VI*
Articular—RC, RU	VII*
Articular—RC, RU, distal ulna	VIII*

*Articular fractures

the major factor influencing the prognosis of these injuries is disruption of the distal radius articulations. In their evaluation of healed Colles' fractures, Gartland and Werley[18] observed that 88 percent of the fractures involved the radius articular surfaces, and residual displacement of these surfaces consistently led to an unsatisfactory recovery. Significantly, 22 percent of their cases resulted in traumatic arthritis. The authors concluded that closed reduction with cast immobilization was inadequate treatment for displaced articular fractures.

Frykman,[16] like Gartland and Werley, devised a classification system for distal radius fractures based on the differentiation of extra-articular from intra-articular injuries. In a comprehensive analysis of 516 fractures, he reported a 64 percent incidence of articular disruption and, compared with extra-articular injuries, an inferior degree of recovery for the articular group. He also emphasized the frequency of distal radioulnar joint disruption and distal ulna fractures and the serious impairment that can result from radioulnar malalignment. Frykman concluded that articular fractures (Types III to VIII) are prone to complications, which can only be lessened by precision in treatment.

Frykman's series included 17 patients with Smith's fractures; however, no distinction was made between these fractures with anterior displacement and the more frequent Colles' type fractures. In contrast, Lidström,[25] in his extensive review, found a worse prognosis for the Smith's type frac-

tures. Thomas,[38] acknowledging frequent difficulties in management, categorized Smith's fractures into three types. The most unstable injury is the Smith's Type II fracture—an injury identical to Barton's fracture-dislocation. Typically, the plane of injury obliquely traverses the distal end of the radius, displacing its palmar articular surface anteriorly with the carpus. Because of the uniformly poor results of closed reduction and manipulation, open treatment has often been recommended for these unstable articular fractures.[11, 14, 17, 42]

In my experience with 275 consecutive distal radius fractures, radiographic evidence of articular disruption has been present in 237 cases (86 percent). Even minor fracture displacement has resulted in disturbances of the radioulnar joint, and in 99 cases, major displacement has caused serious disruption of both distal radial articulations. In this series of cases, consistent radiographic observations have led to the formulation of a classification of articular fractures that has considerably facilitated their treatment.[28]

Despite frequent comminution, articular fractures comprise four basic components: (1) the radial shaft, (2) the radial styloid, (3) a dorsal medial fragment, and (4) a palmar medial fragment (Fig. 11–2). The key medial fragments with their strong ligamentous attachments to the proximal carpals and to the ulnar styloid are in a pivotal position, forming the cornerstone of the distal radius articulations; they have been designated the *medial complex*. Displacment of this complex causes a serious disruption of both the radiocarpal and the radioulnar joints and is the basis for a classification into four categories of the articular fractures:

Type I fractures are undisplaced or displaced but stable after closed reduction with preservation of the joint surfaces.

Type II fractures are characterized by comminution and instability, with displacement of the medial complex as a unit. In most instances, the dorsal medial fragment—previously termed the "die-punch" fragment[33]—is impacted more than the palmar fragment, and the radiographs demonstrate posterior displacment. Less often, greater compression of the palmar fragment results in anterior displacement of the medial complex—an injury analogous to Smith's Type II or Barton's fracture. Regardless of the direction of displacement, the medial fragments are not widely separated.

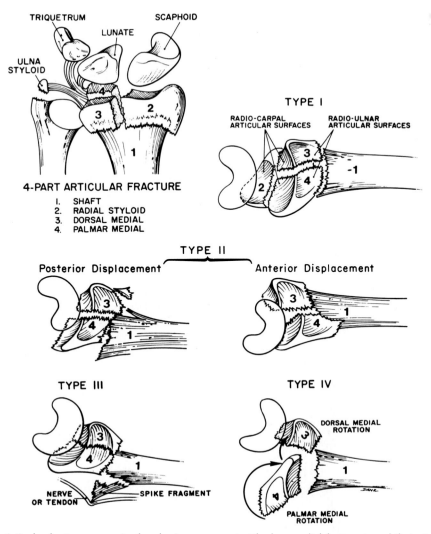

Figure 11–2. Articular fractures comprise four basic components. The key medial fragments and their strong ligamentous attachments to the carpals and ulnar styloid have been termed the medial complex. Displacement of this complex is the basis for classification of articular fractures into four types. The Type II fracture with anterior displacement is analogous to the Smith Type II or Barton's fracture.

Type III fractures are unstable, with displacement of the medial complex as a unit as well as displacement of an additional spike fragment from the comminuted radial shaft. Typically, the spike projects into the flexor compartment of the wrist, causing injury to the median nerve or to the adjacent tendons.

Type IV fractures demonstrate wide separation or rotation of the dorsal and palmar medial fragments with profound disruption of the distal radial articulations. These injuries are always associated with serious damage to adjacent tissues.

For purposes of clarity, this classification can be correlated with those previously mentioned. The *Type I injuries* in this classification of articular fractures are analogous to the Group II fractures of Gartland and Werley and to the Types III to VI fractures of Frykman. The unstable *Type II articular fractures* are analogous to the Group III fractures of Gartland and Werley and to the Types VII and VIII fractures of Frykman. Also, the *Type II articular fractures with anterior displacement* are comparable to the majority of Smith's Type II (Barton's) fractures described by Thomas. *Types III and IV articular fractures* have not been previously specified.

PRINCIPLES OF MANAGEMENT

The fundamental goal of treatment is an accurate and stable reduction—a seemingly simple objective, but one that is difficult to achieve for unstable fractures of the distal radius. Successful treatment requires a method of reduction that restores anatomic relationships between the fractured radius and the adjacent ulna and carpus and maintains this alignment until the healing process is completed. For articular fractures, precise restitution of the *medial complex* is essential for the preservation of the distal radius articulations, and this occasionally requires open treatment. Also, because the unstable fractures are frequently complicated by serious concomitant soft tissue and skeletal damage, optimal treatment requires prompt repair of many of these injuries.

Accuracy of Reduction

The success of recovery consistently parallels the accuracy of reduction. Lidström,[25] in a radiographic review of distal radius fractures, has demonstrated that residual radial shortening of only 6 mm is prone to compromise wrist function, and Palmer and Werner[30] have indicated that even smaller discrepancies in radial and ulnar length may cause serious alterations in load-bearing leading to derangement of the wrist. Although an unsatisfactory reduction is occasionally followed by satisfactory function, malunion must be recognized as the common factor predisposing to poor results. Clearly, complications are lessened by precision in fracture reduction.

The accuracy of reduction is usually assessed by restoration of radial length on the posteroanterior radiograph and of radial palmar tilt on the lateral radiograph. Radial length is the vertical distance between the distal ends of the radial styloid and the ulna and normally ranges between 9 and 14 mm. Palmar tilt, the angle which the radial articular surface projects from the long axis of the shaft, measures 10° to 14°. Unstable comminuted fractures typically demonstrate a 10 mm or more loss of length as well as a marked reversal of the palmar tilt. Postreduction radiographs showing less than 6 mm of shortening on the frontal view and restoration of the radial articular surface to a neutral plane on the lateral view have often been correlated with a successful recovery and are generally considered reliable criteria for an accurate reduction.*

Undoubtedly, measurements of radial length and palmar tilt have proved useful as guidelines for treatment of distal radial fractures. However, the major disturbance in articular fractures occurs between the medial corner of the radius—not the radial styloid—and the ulnar head. Displacement of the medial complex resulting in serious disruption of the radial articular surfaces may neither affect the distance between the radial styloid and the ulnar head nor cause a significant alteration in palmar tilt. Therefore a more precise measurement of the accuracy of reduction for articular fractures is restoration of ulnar length: the vertical distance between the distal ends of the medial corner of the radius and the ulnar head (Fig. 11–3). Since supination creates an illusory shortening of the ulna and pronation projects an image of increased ulnar length,

---

*References 7, 10, 12, 16, 22, 25, 26, 32, 40.

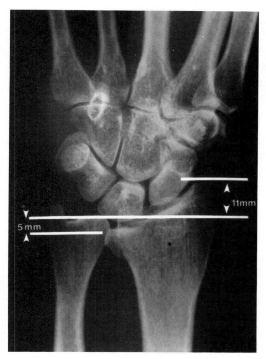

Figure 11–3. The accuracy of reduction. Restoration of radial length is usually measured from the radial styloid to the ulnar head. However, a more precise measurement of the accuracy of reduction for articular fractures is the vertical distance between the distal ends of the medial corner of the radius and the ulnar head. This fracture resulted in significant shortening of the medial complex (5 mm), but, typically, it did not affect the radial styloid–ulnar head distance, which is a normal 11 mm.

inspection of comparable views of the un-injured wrist is necessary to determine normal ulnar length and to avoid misinterpretations due to variations in radiographic techniques.

An alteration in normal ulnar length, termed ulnar variance, is recognized as an important causative factor in both radioulnar and carpal derangements.[20, 30] Any abnormality in length should also be recognized for its deleterious effect on recovery after articular fractures. Before injury, the distal ulna and medial corner of the radius are usually at the same level (neutral variance); after fracture, compression of the medial complex results in relative lengthening of the ulna, so-called positive variance. Since any change in ulnar length can profoundly affect wrist function, and inasmuch as several millimeters of collapse is unavoidable as a result of impaction of comminuted fragments, an accurate reduction should restore the preinjury relationships between the medial complex and the ulnar head.

Methods of Reduction

Closed Reduction

The majority of unstable distal radius fractures can be reduced by closed manipulation. The reduction is performed after the administration of a regional anesthetic, usually an axillary block. If additional analgesia is necessary, aspiration of the fracture hematoma under sterile conditions and local infiltration of 3 to 5 ml of 2 percent lidocaine provides a safe and effective adjuvant method of anesthesia.

The reduction is essentially a reversal of the mechanism of injury. Usually a hyper-extension-compression force applied to the pronated wrist results in posterior displacement with relative supination of the distal fragments; thus, the reduction is achieved by axial traction on the wrist, followed by palmar flexion, ulnar deviation, and pronation of the displaced fragments. Although pronation is a controversial position for immobilization,[10, 12, 32, 43] its efficacy in reduction is twofold: first, it approximates the supinated distal fragments to the pronated proximal radius; second, it relocates the posteriorly displaced medial complex with the anteriorly positioned ulnar head, thereby facilitating restoration of radioulnar congruity.

Stability of unstable fractures can be achieved only by restoration of a buttress provided by at least one radial cortex. Invariably, the dorsal cortex is severely comminuted and stability hinges on accurate apposition of a relatively intact anterior cortex. If both cortices are extensively comminuted, preservation of the reduction demands immediate skeletal fixation (Fig. 11–4). It is important to remember that extreme positioning of the wrist does not enhance stability and should be avoided. For example, immobilization in excessive palmar flexion—the so-called Cotton-Loder position—is notorious for causing median nerve compression and joint contractures.[1, 9]

Smith's fractures are usually caused by a severe compression force transmitted to the supinated wrist; the result is anterior displacement and relative pronation of the distal fragments. Thus, the reduction maneuver consists of traction and supination.[14, 38] Satisfactory alignment can often be achieved for extra-articular fractures, whereas manipulation of the more unstable articular fractures, particularly their palmar medial component, is extremely difficult and seldom successful. It needs to be emphasized that dorsiflexion of the wrist does not correct the anterior displacement of these articular fractures; instead, it increases lunate compression of the medial complex, resulting in persistent anterior displacement.

Open Reduction

Because of the difficulties encountered with closed reduction, open reduction has been advocated and used in conjunction with buttress plate fixation for Smith's Type II fractures.[11, 14, 17, 42] There is also increasing awareness of the occasional need for open reduction of Colles' type fractures. Frykman[16] employed open reduction for seven cases in which closed reduction failed to correct severe articular displacement; Kristiansen and Gjersøe[23] reported 17 cases of open reduction for unstable Colles' fractures demonstrating displacement after closed reduction. Cooney et al,[9] after reviewing the complications of 565 Colles' fractures, suggested that open reduction be carried out for young patients with significant articular disruption that cannot be corrected by closed techniques.

In my experience, two indications for open treatment have become apparent: first, the displaced spike fragment characteristic of Type III articular fractures requires reduc-

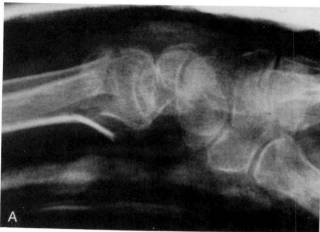

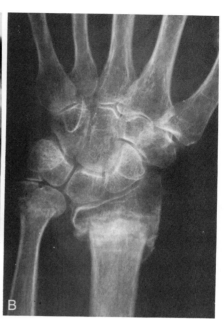

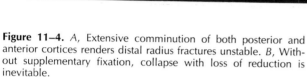

Figure 11–4. A, Extensive comminution of both posterior and anterior cortices renders distal radius fractures unstable. B, Without supplementary fixation, collapse with loss of reduction is inevitable.

tion or excision in conjunction with repair of any nerve or tendon injury (see Fig. 11–12); second, the widely separated or rotated medial fragments of the Type IV fracture necessitate open reduction for precise restitution of the severely disrupted radius articulations (see Fig. 11–13). Chapman et al,[5] in a review of 80 comminuted fractures, noted the frequent concurrence of a persistently displaced palmar fragment and median nerve compression. They advised prompt reduction of these palmar fragments. Others[1, 9, 45] have observed similar fractures causing both median and ulnar neuropathy. Displaced palmar fragments have also been implicated in attrition rupture of adjacent flexor tendons.[4, 9, 34] These displaced fragments are undoubtedly analogous to the spike fragments of Type III fractures or the palmar medial fragments of Type IV fractures. Without precise open reduction of the displaced fragments and repair of the frequent concomitant injuries, these articular fractures are prone to cause a major impairment.

Fracture Stabilization

EXTERNAL FIXATION

A review of the references at the end of this chapter clearly indicates that the majority of unstable distal radius fractures are comminuted articular Type II injuries. After an accurate reduction of these fractures, the use of some method of stabilization is essential to prevent redisplacement. Experience confirms that a stable reduction is best maintained by continuous skeletal traction, using either pins and plaster or external fixators. Other methods, such as percutaneous pin fixation,[6, 35] ulnar pinning,[12, 13] and Rush rod fixation,[26, 31] have been used for similar injuries, but their application is limited by the presence of comminuted articular surfaces.

The strong ligament component of the medial complex is the basis for successful traction. This intricate capsular-ligamentous structure has been described in detail by Taleisnik,[37] and is schematically depicted in Figure 11–5. Basically, the medial fragments are connected to the ulnar styloid by the triangular fibrocartilage and to the carpus by the ulnocarpal ligaments. DePalma[12] has demonstrated experimentally that, regardless of the severity of fracture, these ligaments remain intact—an observation that has been substantiated by clinical experience. Traction maintains the critical soft tissues under constant tension, aligning and stabilizing the attached articular fragments (Fig. 11–6).

Traditionally, pins and plaster has been the preferred method of traction for comminuted articular fractures.[3, 7, 19, 22, 33] The quality of recovery achieved with this method is still the standard by which other treatments are judged. One pin is placed distal to the wrist joint through the metacarpals, and a second pin is placed proximally through

THE MEDIAL COMPLEX

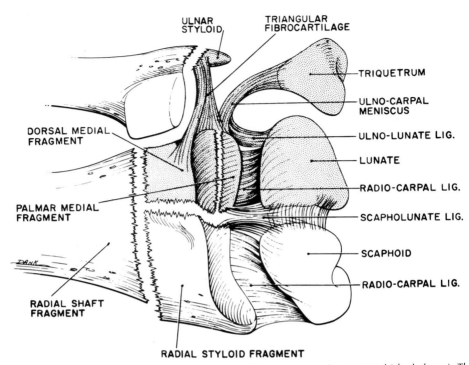

Figure 11–5. The skeletal and soft tissue components of the medial complex are demonstrated (*shaded area*). The successful use of traction for articular fractures depends on the strength of the ligament component, which remains intact regardless of the severity of the fracture. Maintenance of the critical soft tissues under constant tension affords stability to the attached articular fragments.

either the radius or the ulna. Traction is applied to the wrist and maintained by incorporating the pins in a well-molded plaster cast.

Despite variations in procedure, the common factor for success is precision in technique; hence, one should not be misled by the apparent simplicity of pin fixation. Failure to observe technical details can result in a complication rate as high as 33 percent.[5, 22] Pin loosening, pin tract infection, pin site fracture, and osteomyelitis must be recognized as potentially serious problems that can be prevented only by skillful pin placement.

The major criticism of the pins and plaster method has been its inability to achieve rigid fixation. The fracture fragments tend to rotate on the distal pin, frequently causing failure to maintain normal palmar tilt.[5, 7, 22, 33] A minor reversal of tilt may occur with no appreciable effect on wrist function, but occasionally a significant deformity develops that does compromise recovery. Once the pins are incorporated in plaster, no correction in fracture alignment is possible.

In an effort to improve the accuracy and stability of reduction, external fixation systems have been advocated as an alternative to pins and plaster.[2, 10, 21, 40, 42] This treatment of articular fractures with external fixators is now commonly called ligamentotaxis[42]—a term synonymous with traction. Following radiographic confirmation of an accurate reduction, multiple skeletal fixation pins are attached to a metal frame that maintains constant tension on the soft tissues traversing the wrist, thereby stabilizing the fracture components (Fig. 11–7). Adjustable clamps and sliding connecting bars permit continual correction of fracture alignment during the healing process. In contrast to pins and plaster, the external fixator has the capacity to permit secondary corrections in fracture reduction.

Clinical use of the external fixator is enhanced by the observation of several key technical points.[8, 41] First, fracture stability requires a sturdy frame. Bilateral, quadrilateral, circular, and triangular configurations have proved mechanically sound. Second, stability also requires at least two pins,

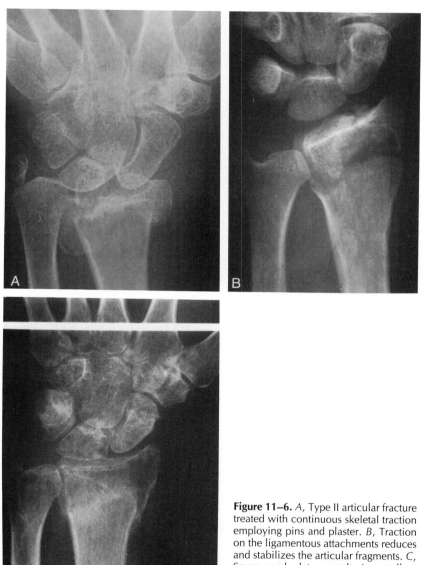

Figure 11–6. *A*, Type II articular fracture treated with continuous skeletal traction employing pins and plaster. *B*, Traction on the ligamentous attachments reduces and stabilizes the articular fragments. *C*, Seven weeks later, results in excellent restoration of the radiocarpal and radioulnar joints.

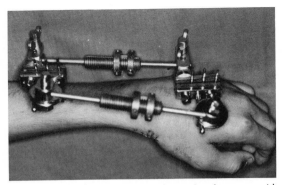

Figure 11–7. The treatment of articular fractures with external fixators has been termed ligamentotaxis.[42] The ideal system provides rigid fixation and versatility in fracture management. Multiple pins, inserted both proximal and distal to the wrist, are attached to a sturdy but adjustable frame that maintains continuous traction.

both proximal and distal to the fracture. Three millimeter half-threaded pins are preferred, and bicortical purchase is essential for secure fixation. Finally, pin insertion must be precise. An open technique through small incisions that provide direct exposure of bone avoids injury to the vulnerable extensor tendons and the sensory branch of the radial nerve. Insertion with a high-torque

low-speed drill, or preferably by first predrilling and then by manual introduction with a hand drill, decreases thermal necrosis and reaming at the pin holes and lessens the incidence of pin-site loosening, infection, and fracture. Employment of a strong but lightweight frame and the appropriate number, size, and configuration of pins has steadily improved the results of treatment with external fixation.

Despite refinement in designs and techniques of external fixators, these complex systems, with their considerable risk for serious complications, should not be used indiscriminately for treatment of distal radius fractures. In the majority of cases, simpler and less invasive methods achieve an equivalent, if not superior, recovery with less morbidity and are better tolerated by the patient than the constantly exposed and often bulky external apparatus. External fixators have unequivocally proved most beneficial for the following distal radius injuries (Fig. 11–8):

1. Severely comminuted fractures with loss of bone substance.

2. Open fractures requiring meticulous wound care or resurfacing procedures.

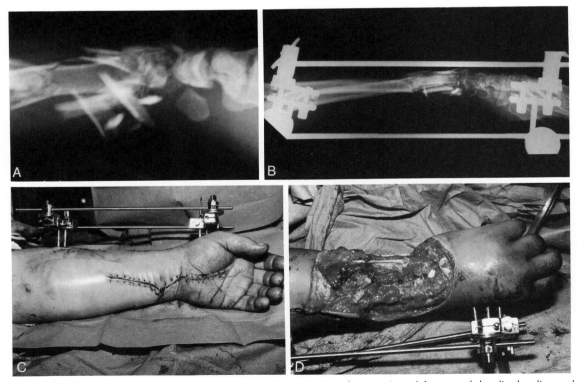

Figure 11–8. Principal indications for external fixators. *A, B, C,* Severely comminuted fracture of the distal radius and concomitant nerve and tendon injuries. *D,* Open fracture of the distal radius with substantial soft tissue loss. In these cases, external fixation restores skeletal alignment and stability in preparation for extensive osseous and soft tissue repairs.

3. Limb salvage situations necessitating revascularization as well as staged soft tissue and skeletal reconstruction.

In these cases usually caused by massive trauma, the external fixator provides excellent provisional stability for extensive primary and reconstructive surgery.

INTERNAL FIXATION

Displaced fractures with wide separation of their articular fragments (Type IV fractures) require open reduction and internal fixation for restitution of joint congruity. Occasionally, small cancellous screws (3.5 mm) or small screws inserted through T plates can secure the fracture fragments; however, excessive comminution usually precludes techniques of rigid fixation for articular fractures. Buttress plates provide no fixation of the unstable medial fragments and in my experience have not been applicable to most fractures requiring open reduction. Stabilization with a minimum of three 0.045 or 0.062 Kirschner wires has been the most successful method of internal fixation.

Concomitant Injuries

A force that is great enough to cause distal radius articular disruption is also likely to result in injury to the adjacent nerves and tendons as well as to the distal ulna and the carpus.* In such cases maximum recovery requires both precise treatment of the fracture and prompt recognition and repair of concomitant soft tissue and skeletal damage.

The following discussion is based on personal experience with 99 patients with unstable articular fractures (Table 11–2).

---

*References 1, 4, 5, 9, 15, 24, 26–29, 34, 39, 44, 45.

NERVE INJURY

Careful examination at the time of injury, prior to the administration of an anesthetic, is necessary to detect nerve injury, which should be suspected with all displaced fractures. Median or ulnar neuropathy (often in combination) has occurred in 55 percent of the unstable articular injuries. In all but one case, nerve contusion by a displaced bone fragment resulted in a neuropraxia with loss of sensibility immediately after injury. The one exception was a complete transection of the median nerve, occurring with a Type IV fracture.

Open reduction of four Type III and 17 Type IV fractures has provided the opportunity to define the neuropathology more precisely. The median nerve is injured either by a displaced spike fragment or by the sharp edge of the radial shaft just proximal to the carpal tunnel; the ulnar nerve is compressed by a displaced palmar medial fragment at the level of Guyon's canal. The contused nerves have been grossly edematous and, on microscopic inspection, have consistently demonstrated subepineurial and intraneural hemorrhage. Occasionally, partial disruption of the epineurium has been noted.

Treatment of nerve injury is guided by the concurrent type of fracture. For Type II fractures with neuropathy, an accurate closed reduction maintained by traction has invariably been followed by complete recovery of nerve function over a period of several months. Nerve transection did not occur with Type II fractures, and no case required primary or secondary nerve surgery. Thus, one can expect Type II fracture neuropathy to improve spontaneously with successful fracture treatment.

In contrast, neuropathy associated with Type III and IV fractures requires a prompt

Table 11–2. **UNSTABLE FRACTURES: CONCOMITANT INJURIES**

Fracture Type	II	III	IV	Total
Number of Fractures	78	4	17	**99**
Concomitant Injury				
Median Nerve Contusion	14	4	14	**32**
Median Nerve Laceration	0	0	1	**1**
Ulnar Nerve Contusion	4	0	7	**11**
Flexor Pollicis Longus Laceration	0	0	4	**4**
Arterial Laceration	0	0	2	**2**
Scapholunate Dissociation	3	0	1	**4**
Scaphoid Fracture	3	0	2	**5**
Ulnar Head Fracture	4	0	0	**4**

neurolysis and possibly even nerve suturing, in conjunction with open reduction and internal fixation of the fracture. The nerve must be thoroughly decompressed from the distal forearm to the palm in order to prevent the occurrence of a secondary compression neuropathy.

OTHER SOFT TISSUE INJURIES

The flexor pollicis longus tendon is prone to injury with Type IV fractures. In four cases, the tendon had been lacerated at the sharp edge of the radial shaft fragment and was repaired primarily at the time of fracture treatment. All of these tendon injuries were associated with contusions of the adjacent median nerve, and in one case both the radial and the ulnar arteries were lacerated. In this case, microvascular repairs as well as a fasciotomy were necessary to restore circulation to the ischemic hand.

The flexor pollicis longus, like the median nerve, is also prone to injury with Type III fractures. Although acute disruption has not yet been observed, delayed rupture has occurred at unreduced spike fragments in cases of malunion (Fig. 11–9). In these instances of attrition rupture, tendon transfers have been necessary to improve thumb motion.

It is important to recognize that every structure traversing the wrist is vulnerable to disruption with displaced articular fractures. Obviously, repair of these critical soft tissues is essential to optimal management. One must also realize that the excessive trauma causing these fractures is apt to result in profound edema within the flexor compartment of the wrist. Like neuropathy, compartmental ischemia must always be suspected and, if present, alleviated promptly by fasciotomy. Unstable articular fractures should not be considered simple Colles' fractures; they are violent injuries that can seriously threaten survival of the damaged tissues.

ASSOCIATED SKELETAL INJURIES

Unstable scaphoid fractures occurring with Type II articular fractures create a dilemma: Traction is necessary for stability of the articular fracture but detrimental to healing of the scaphoid. The problem is solved by open reduction and internal fixation of the scaphoid through a small anterior incision. The operation stabilizes the scaphoid so that traction can be continued. Displaced scaphoid fractures associated with Type III or IV fractures require open reduction and internal fixation in conjunction with open treatment of the articular fractures.

Scapholunate ligament disruption has occurred with severely displaced articular fractures (Fig. 11–10). Because of strong soft tissue attachments, the lunate displaces along with the medial complex, whereas the scaphoid remains with the radial styloid. Restoration of the medial complex corrects the carpal diastasis, and maintenance of the reduction permits successful ligamentous healing and preservation of carpal stability.

The most frequent concomitant skeletal injury is fracture of the ulnar styloid. Stevens[36] has stated that the fracture results from a force transmitted through an intact

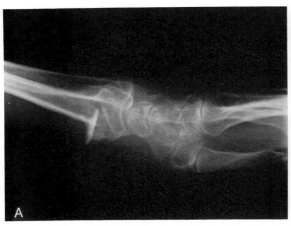
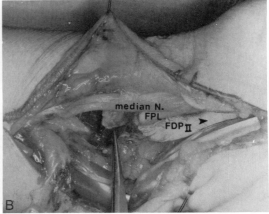

Figure 11–9. *A,* Malunited Type III articular fracture. *B,* Persistent displacement of the spike fragment (at the tip of the forceps) resulted in chronic median neuropathy and attrition ruptures of the flexor pollicis longus tendon (FPL) and flexor digitorum profundus tendon of the index finger (FDP II). These soft tissue injuries could have been prevented by an accurate reduction at the time of injury.

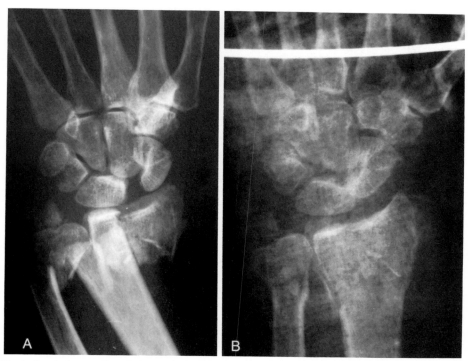

Figure 11–10. *A,* Scapholunate dissociation and ulnar head displacement occurred with this markedly displaced Type II articular fracture. *B,* Continuous skeletal traction restored radiocarpal, radioulnar, and intercarpal stability.

triangular fibrocartilage and occurs secondarily to the major fracture of the radius. This concept is substantiated by continuing experience with articular fractures in which the tip of the ulnar styloid has been avulsed in almost 90 percent of the cases. Neither the ulnar styloid fracture nor its frequent failure to unite appreciably influences recovery, provided the radial articular surfaces are successfully restored.

Rehabilitation

Attainment of maximum recovery after fracture depends largely on a carefully planned and executed program of therapy. Patients should be cautioned that a perfect reduction does not ensure a satisfactory recovery; they should also be reassured that a motivated patient working with a skilled therapist can often convert a fair anatomic result into an excellent functional result.

Rehabilitation starts immediately after fracture reduction and stabilization; digital, elbow, and shoulder motion is encouraged and must not be impaired by faulty techniques of immobilization. Mobilization of the uninjured finger joints can be enhanced by static and dynamic splinting, massage, anti-inflammatory medication, and a variety of other therapeutic modalities commonly used by the hand therapist. With early, aggressive therapy, the disastrous complications of digital joint contractures and reflex sympathetic dystrophy rarely develop.

After the fracture is healed, the pins are removed in the physician's office, a protective splint is provided, and mobilization of the wrist is begun. Over a period of several months, the patient progresses from active exercises to increasingly resistive activities with weights. Steady improvement is expected for at least eight months after cast removal.

Assessment of Results

A thorough evaluation of treatment should include a review of operative complications; measurement of recovery of wrist motion, of grip and pinch strength, of preservation of nerve, tendon, and adjacent joint function; radiographic analysis of articular restoration; consideration of the duration of impaired activity; and the patient's appraisal of function. The McBride system of disability evaluation and the Lidström classification of radiographic results incorporate these parameters and are the standard methods of analyzing recovery* (Table 11–3). In the vast majority of cases a high level of function can be expected to follow an accurate reduction.

Based on the McBride and Lidström criteria, a personal review of 99 unstable articular fractures leads to several conclusions: First, the classification described herein provides a useful guide for successful treatment; second, an accurate and stable reduction of

*References 7, 10, 13, 16, 18, 25, 26, 32, 40.

the medial complex consistently results in satisfactory function; third, the more complex Types III and IV articular fractures are optimally managed by open treatment.

THE AUTHOR'S PREFERRED METHODS OF TREATMENT

Pins and Plaster (Fig. 11–11)

This method of continuous skeletal traction is indicated principally for Type II articular

Table 11–3. **EVALUATION OF TREATMENT OF UNSTABLE DISTAL RADIUS FRACTURES**

Modified McBride Demerit Point System[32]*		Lidström Radiographic Classification[25]
Points		
Residual Deformity		Grade 1‡: No deformity, no dorsal angulation beyond neutral, 3 mm or less of shortening
Prominent ulnar styloid	1	
Residual dorsal tilt	2	
Radial deviation of hand	2 to 3	Grade 2‡: Slight deformity, 1 to 11 degrees of dorsal angulation, 3 to 6 mm of shortening
Point range: 0 to 3		
Subjective Evaluation		Grade 3: Mild to moderate deformity, 11 to 15 degrees of dorsal angulation, 6 to 12 mm of shortening
Excellent: no pain, disability, or limitation of motion	0	
Good: Occasional pain, slight limitation of motion, no disability	2	Grade 4: Severe deformity, more than 15 degrees of dorsal angulation, more than 12 mm of shortening
Fair: Occasional pain, some limitation of motion, feeling of weakness in wrist, no particular disability if careful, activities slightly restricted	4	
Poor: Pain, limitation of motion, disability, activities more or less markedly restricted	6	
Point range: 0 to 6		
Objective Evaluation†		
Loss of dorsiflexion	5	
Loss of ulnar deviation	3	
Loss of supination	2	
Loss of palmar flexion	1	
Loss of radial deviation	1	
Loss of circumduction	1	
Pain in distal radioulnar joint	1	
Grip strength—60 per cent or less of opposite side	1	
Loss of pronation	2	
Point range: 0 to 5		
Complications		
Arthritic change		
Minimum	1	
Minimum with pain	3	
Moderate	2	
Moderate with pain	4	
Severe	3	
Severe with pain	5	
Nerve complications (median)	1 to 3	
Poor finger function due to cast	1 to 2	
Point range: 0 to 5		
End-Result Point Ranges		
Excellent	0 to 2	
Good	3 to 8	
Fair	9 to 20	
Poor	21 and above	

*Modified from Sarmiento A, Pratt GW, Berry NC, et al: J Bone Joint Surg 57A:313, 1975.
†Points are deducted for ranges of motion less than 45° dorsiflexion, 30° palmar flexion, 15° radial deviation, 15° ulnar deviation, 50° pronation, 50° supination. In this system, these are the minimum motions considered consistent with normal functions.
‡Grades 1 and 2 are considered consistent with satisfactory (good to excellent) function.

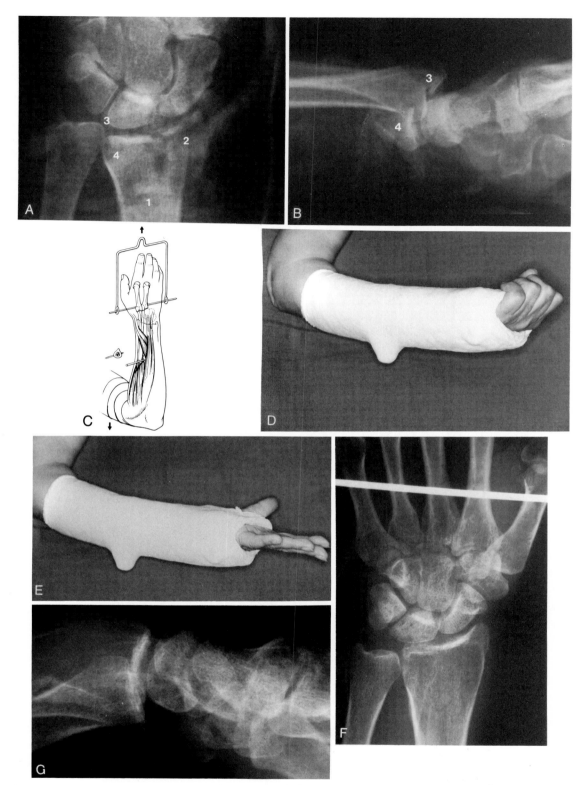

Figure 11–11. Type II articular fracture treated with pins and plaster. Preoperative radiographs demonstrating *A*, disruption and collapse of the articular surface and *B*, anterior displacement of the palmar medial fragment. 1 = radial shaft; 2 = radial styloid; 3 = dorsal medial fragment; 4 = palmar medial fragment. *C*, The distal pin passes through the base of the index and middle metacarpals, and the proximal pin passes through the radius at the "bare bone interval." The wrist is suspended by a traction bow, and a countertraction weight is applied to the padded arm. *Inset*, the radial pin must achieve bicortical purchase but avoid the critical soft tissue of the forearm. *D, E*, After an accurate reduction, the pins are incorporated in a short arm cast that permits immediate active motion of the fingers and thumb. *F, G*, Postoperative radiographs illustrating uncomplicated fracture union with excellent preservation of the joint surfaces.

fractures and occasionally for extra-articular fractures with extensive comminution.

The technique employs two percutaneous 3/32-in smooth Steinmann's pins incorporated in a short arm cast. A high-torque, variable-speed power drill facilitates accurate pin placement and undoubtedly lowers the incidence of pin complications. The distal pin is inserted transversely through the base of the index and long finger metacarpals, with the thumb and fingers held in maximum abduction. Careful positioning of the digits maintains the normal transverse arch of the hand and prevents the development of web space contractures.

The radius, rather than the ulna, is preferred for placement of the proximal pin because pin insertion at this site affords better control of the fracture and causes less interference with elbow function. The forearm is pronated and the pin is inserted just proximal to the abductor pollicis longus muscle in the "bare bone interval" between the wrist and the finger extensors. The radial pin, placed perpendicular to the distal pin,

must achieve bicortical purchase for secure fixation but should not pass more than several millimeters beyond the anterior cortex so as to avoid the critical soft tissues of the forearm.

The wrist is suspended by a traction bow that is first attached to the distal pin and then to an overhead bar. Avoidance of Chinese finger traps or similar devices eliminates unnecessary trauma to the digits. With the elbow flexed, a 2 to 3 kg weight suspended from the well-padded arm provides sufficient countertraction. The wrist is gently manipulated, usually by flexion and pronation; after operative radiographs confirm an accurate reduction, the pins are incorporated in a plaster cast, leaving the fingers free for immediate active exercises. The cast may be trimmed to allow full digital motion, but the pins are not disturbed for six weeks or until radiographic union is clearly demonstrated.

This method proved consistently successful for 78 consecutive Type II fractures, including 11 with anterior displacement (Bar-

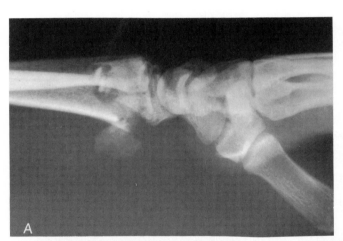

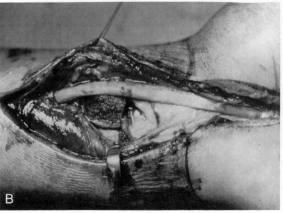

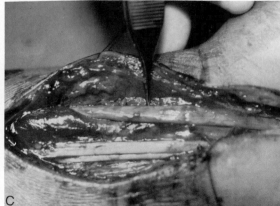

Figure 11–12. *A*, Type III fracture with displacement of the characteristic spike fragment causing *B*, contusion of the median nerve. *C*, The injury required reduction of the fragment (at the tip of the forceps) and median nerve neurolysis. The fragment was stabilized with a Kirschner wire, whereas the radius articular surfaces were stabilized with traction.

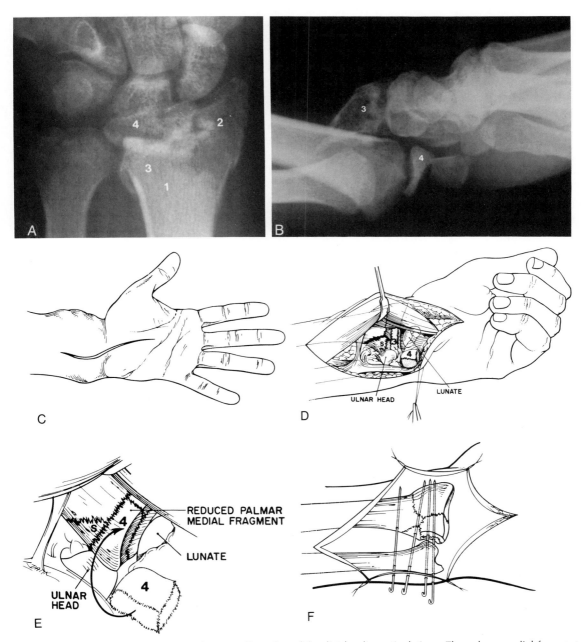

Figure 11–13. *A, B,* Type IV fracture with severe disruption of the distal radius articulations. The palmar medial fragment (4) is rotated 180° so that its articular surface faces the radial shaft rather than the lunate. *C,* Open reduction through an anterior approach to the wrist reveals *D,* compression of the ulnar neurovascular bundle by the palmar medial fragment (4) and contusion of the median nerve at the comminuted edge of the radial shaft(s). *E,* The key step for articular restoration is the derotation and reduction of the palmar medial fragment so that it lies in apposition with the dorsal medial (3), radial shaft(s), and radial styloid fragments. *F,* Fracture stability is achieved with multiple Kirschner wires.

ton's type fractures). According to the Mc-Bride and Lidström criteria, the results in 71 of these cases (91 percent) were rated good to excellent. Radial shortening averaged 3.5 mm and palmar tilt averaged 5° (a loss of 5°). The complication rate was 6 percent: two patients developed disabling digital joint contractures and three patients had loosening of their proximal pins. Significantly, no instance of pin site fracture or infection was encountered, and 18 concomitant neuropraxias resolved completely during the course of fracture treatment. It is emphasized that precision—in reduction, pin placement, and cast application—is the key to successful treatment.

Open Reduction and Internal Fixation

Open treatment is indicated for Type III and Type IV articular fractures. In the majority of cases, an anterior approach extending from the ulnar aspect of the distal forearm across the carpal tunnel to the proximal palm provides excellent exposure of the displaced fragments and the damaged soft tissues.

In Type III fractures (Fig. 11–12), the spike fragment must be accurately reduced (or occasionally excised) and fixed with Kirschner wires, but the articular fragments that are not widely separated do not require internal fixation and can be stabilized by continuous traction.

In contrast, traction cannot correct the severe articular displacement of Type IV fractures (Fig. 11–13). The key step for articular restoration is precise reduction of the medial fragments. Usually the palmar medial fragment is displaced most severely and must be derotated, reduced, and stabilized with Kirschner wires to the dorsal medial fragment. These fragments, as a unit, are then reduced and fixed to the radial shaft, restoring radioulnar joint congruity, and to the radial styloid, reconstituting the radiocarpal joint. If excessive comminution causes a major bone defect between the medial fragments and the radial shaft, a corticocancellous strut graft, obtained from the ilium and inserted into the defect, prevents articular collapse.

Optimal management of these articular injuries requires accurate reduction of the medial complex, adjunctive grafting for bone loss, stable fixation with a minimum of three

Kirschner wires, and prompt repair of concomitant soft tissue and skeletal injuries. Postoperatively, the wrist is immobilized in a cast incorporating the thumb metacarpal and humeral epicondyles. Except in cases requiring tendon repair, the digits are free for immediate active motion.

Fifteen type IV articular fractures treated by these techniques were recently analyzed.[29] The results of these cases can be summarized as follows: Recovery was rated good to excellent in 12 cases and fair in three cases. Loss of radial length averaged 3.2 mm, and residual palmar tilt averaged 1.5°—anatomic results comparable to those reported for less serious injuries treated by traction. On follow-up evaluation ranging from 18 months to eight years, no functional or radiographic deterioration was observed.

SUMMARY

Unstable fractures of the distal radius are characterized by extensive comminution, severe articular disruption, and frequent concomitant soft tissue and skeletal injury. These fractures should be differentiated from the less serious extra-articular Colles' and Smith's injuries and recognized for their greater magnitude of damage and their frequent need for external or internal fixation.

The articular fractures, which invariably disrupt both the radiocarpal and radioulnar joints, comprise four basic parts: (1) the radial shaft, (2) the radial styloid, (3) a dorsal medial fragment, and (4) a palmar medial fragment. Displacement of the key medial fragments is the basis for classification into four types of articular fractures; reduction of these fragments restores biarticular congruity and is the basis for successful treatment.

Most unstable fractures can be managed by closed methods of reduction and fixation, but those fractures with marked joint displacement require open treatment for repair of the articular surfaces as well as any associated nerve, tendon, or skeletal injuries. For all cases, an accurate and stable reduction, followed by thorough rehabilitation of the injured wrist, its usually rewarded by a superior recovery of function.

References

1. Abbott LC, and Saunders JB de CM: Injuries of the median nerve in fractures of the lower end of the radius. Surg Gynecol Obstet 57:507, 1933.

2. Anderson R, and O'Neill G: Comminuted fractures of the distal end of the radius. Surg Gynecol Obstet 78:434, 1944.

3. Böhler L: The Treatment of Fractures. 5th ed, Vol 1. New York, Grune & Stratton Inc, 1956.

4. Broder H: Rupture of the flexor tendons, associated with a malunited Colles' fracture. J Bone Joint Surg 36A:404, 1954.

5. Chapman DR, Bennett JB, Bryan WJ, et al: Complications of distal radial fractures: pins and plaster treatment. J Hand Surg 7:509, 1982.

6. Clancey GJ: Percutaneous Kirschner wire fixation of Colles' fractures. A prospective study of thirty cases. J Bone Joint Surg 66A:1008, 1984.

7. Cole JM, and Obletz BE: Comminuted fractures of the distal end of the radius treated by skeletal transfixation in plaster cast. An end-result study of thirty-three cases. J Bone Joint Surg 48A:931, 1966.

8. Cooney WP: External fixation of distal radial fractures. Clin Orthop 180:44, 1983.

9. Cooney WP III, Dobyns JH, and Linscheid RL: Complications of Colles' fracture. J Bone Joint Surg 62A:613, 1980.

10. Cooney WP III, Linscheid RL, and Dobyns JH: External pin fixation for unstable Colles' fractures. J Bone Joint Surg 61A:840, 1979.

11. DeOliveira JC: Barton's fractures. J Bone Joint Surg 55A:586, 1973.

12. DePalma AF: Comminuted fractures of the distal end of the radius treated by ulnar pinning. J Bone Joint Surg 34A:651, 1952.

13. Dowling JJ, and Sawyer B Jr: Comminuted Colles' fractures: evaluation of a method of treatment. J Bone Joint Surg 43A:657, 1961.

14. Ellis J: Smith's and Barton's fractures. A method of treatment. J Bone Joint Surg 47B:724, 1965.

15. Engkvist O, and Lundborg G: Rupture of the extensor pollicis longus tendon after fracture of the lower end of the radius—a clinical and microangiographic study. Hand 2:76, 1979.

16. Frykman G: Fracture of the distal radius including sequelae—shoulder-hand-finger syndrome, disturbance in the distal radioulnar joint, and impairment of nerve function: a clinical and experimental study. Acta Orthop Scand (Suppl) 108:1–153, 1967.

17. Fuller DJ: The Ellis plate operation for Smith's fracture. J Bone Joint Surg 55B:173, 1973.

18. Gartland JJ Jr, and Werley CW: Evaluation of healed Colles' fractures. J Bone Joint Surg 33A:895, 1951.

19. Geckeler EO: Treatment of comminuted Colles' fractures. J Int Coll Surg 20:596, 1953.

20. Gelberman RH, Salamon PB, Jurist JM, et al: Ulnar variance in Kienböck's disease. J Bone Joint Surg 57A:674, 1975.

21. Grana WA, and Kopta JA: The Roger Anderson device in the treatment of fractures of the distal end of the radius. J Bone Surg 61A:1234, 1979.

22. Green DP: Pins and plaster treatment of comminuted fractures of the distal end of the radius. J Bone Surg 57A:304, 1975.

23. Kristiansen A, and Gjersøe E: Colles' fracture. Operative treatment, indications and results. Acta Orthop Scand 39:33, 1968.

24. Lewis MH: Median nerve decompression after Colles' fracture. J Bone Joint Surg 60B:195, 1978.

25. Lidström A: Fracture of the distal end of the radius. A clinical and statistical study of end results. Acta Orthop Scand (Suppl) 41:1–118, 1959.

26. Lucas GL, and Sachtjen KM: An analysis of hand function in patients with Colles' fractures treated by Rush rod fixation. Clin Orthop 155:172, 1981.

27. McMaster PE: Late ruptures of extensor and flexor pollicis longus following Colles' fracture. J Bone Joint Surg 14:93, 1932.

28. Melone CP Jr: Articular fractures of the distal radius. Orthop Clin North Am 15:217, 1984.

29. Melone CP Jr: Open treatment for displaced articular fractures of the distal radius. Clin Orthop 202:103–111, 1986.

30. Palmer AK, and Werner FW: The triangular fibrocartilage complex of the wrist—anatomy and function. J Hand Surg 6:153, 1981.

31. Rush LV: Closed medullary pinning of Colles' fracture. Clin Orthop 3:152, 1954.

32. Sarmiento A, Pratt GW, Berry MC, et al: Colles' fractures. Functional bracing in supination. J Bone Joint Surg 57A:311, 1975.

33. Scheck M: Long-term follow-up of treatment of comminuted fractures of the distal end of the radius by transfixation with Kirschner wires and cast. J Bone Joint Surg 44A:337, 1962.

34. Southmayd WW, Millender LH, and Nalebuff EA: Rupture of the flexor tendons of the index finger after Colles' fracture. Case report. J Bone Joint Surg 57A:562, 1975.

35. Stein AH, and Katz SF: Stabilization of comminuted fractures of the distal inch of the radius: percutaneous pinning. Clin Orthop 108:174, 1975.

36. Stevens JH: Compression fractures of the lower end of the radius. Ann Surg 71:594, 1920.

37. Taleisnik J: The ligaments of the wrist. J Hand Surg 1:110, 1976.

38. Thomas FB: Reduction of Smith's fracture. J Bone Joint Surg 39B:463, 1957.

39. Vance RM, and Gelberman RH: Acute ulnar neuropathy with fractures at the wrist. J Bone Joint Surg 60A:962, 1978.

40. Vaughan PA, Spenser ML, Harrington IJ, et al: Treatment of unstable fractures of the distal radius by external fixation. J Bone Joint Surg 67B:385, 1985.

41. Vidal J: External fixation. Yesterday, today, and tomorrow. Clin Orthop 180:7, 1983.

42. Vidal J, Buscayret C, Paran M, et al: Ligamentotaxis. In Mears: External skeletal fixation. Baltimore/London, Williams & Wilkins, 1983.

43. Wahlstrom O: Treatment of Colles' fracture. A prospective comparison of three different positions of immobilization. Acta Orthop Scand 53:225, 1982.

44. Younger CP, and DeFiore JC: Rupture of the flexor tendons to the finger after a Colles' fracture. A case report. J Bone Joint Surg 59A:828, 1977.

45. Zoëga H: Fractures of the lower end of the radius with ulnar nerve palsy. J Bone Joint Surg 48B:514, 1966.

CHAPTER 12

The Trapeziometacarpal Joint: Basic Principles of Surgical Treatment

RICHARD M. BRAUN, M.D.

INTRODUCTION

The trapeziometacarpal joint located at the base of the thumb determines the functional range of motion, strength, and prehensile prowess of the thumb. This joint does not communicate with the intercarpal or radiocarpal joints and serves as a transitional articulation between the wrist and the most powerful digit in the hand. The general alignment of the joint places the thumb in between zero and 45° of angulation in its orientation with respect to the plane of flexion of the fingers.

Strength, range of motion, and joint surface quality deteriorate in some patients, owing to arthritis, imbalance, or deformity. A basic understanding of the anatomy, biomechanics, and pathologic conditions associated with the trapeziometacarpal joint will serve to introduce the significant aspects of treatment by repair or by replacement.

FUNCTIONAL ANATOMY

The shape of the trapeziometacarpal joint has caused it to be characterized as a "saddle joint." It is preferable, in this era of scientific nomenclature, to refer to this joint surface as resembling a hyperbolic paraboloid. The "hypar" shape is well known to mathematicians, architects, and engineers. It is a mathematical form that has been used in creating large surfaces and can be seen in peripherally supported ceilings and in building designs, including their reflective surfaces. Its mathematical essence is as follows: Straight lines traveling across the surface of a hypar form a tangential alignment that does not require a method of rolling to minimize friction, to permit displacement, or to provide support. Each hypar has a longitudinal focal axis along which any hypothetical body may move and still maintain constant contact with the surface below.

The opposing surface of the metacarpal is relatively flat. This permits rotation of the metacarpal while it is gliding in the plane already determined by the surface of the trapezium. This relationship gives this unconstrained joint the ability to abduct from the palm and to rotate and elevate from the surface of the hand simultaneously. The system allows for combined movements of divergence from the palm in abduction-extension-supination and for convergence toward the fingers in flexion-adduction-pronation (Fig. 12–1).[1, 2]

The entire system would lose stability without strong ligaments permitting a cam effect in purposeful movement of the thumb metacarpal. The relatively inelastic ligament at the deep volar surface of the joint tethers this apical area in abduction and forces the thumb metacarpal to diverge with angulation from the mid-plane of the palm (Fig. 12–2). This movement constitutes true abduction in the palmar plane. It moves the metacarpal away from the palm, while holding the proximal apex of the joint in secure stable alignment. Loss of this deep ligament results in an imbalance of the thumb, which in turn results in displacement of the metacarpal proximally. This leads to adduction of the distal metacarpal, owing to attachment of the adductor muscle-tendon unit in the

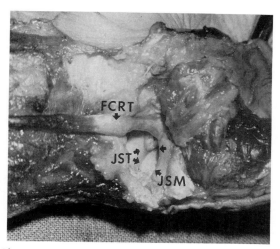

Figure 12–1. A cadaver dissection shows the relationship of the curved metacarpal (JSM) and trapezium (JST) joint surfaces. The cam effect of the curved articular surfaces allows rotation of the metacarpal in the middle position during normal thumb function. In maximal angulation, the shift of the metacarpal on the surface cam produces tension in the ligaments, stabilizes the joint, and prevents rotation or displacement during stress. The flexor carpi radialis tendon (FCRT) lies adjacent to the joint and may be used in reconstruction of the deep ligament system.

region of the metacarpophalangeal joint. The resultant collapse deformity is frequently seen in arthritic thumbs.

The ligaments are not taut when the thumb lies against the palm in a relaxed attitude. Manipulation of the thumb during muscle relaxation indicates that passive rotation and displacement are easily accomplished. This means that dynamic force acting on the thumb is also required for stability. When thenar muscles function, impaction across the joint results in stability as the surfaces are forced together under

pressure. Thumb mobility then occurs because of the joint surfaces and the modulated muscle forces applied to the system. Functional anatomy of this joint depends on a balance between the intrinsic thenar musculature and the extrinsic muscles found in the forearm that affect the thumb through tendons crossing the trapeziometacarpal joint. Normal trapeziometacarpal joint motion requires a congruous articular surface, an appropriate structural design of the surface, a cam effect of the surface-ligament relationship, and balanced motor power. These concepts must be thoroughly understood by the surgeon attempting to restore thumb function.[3, 4]

It is impossible to comprehend the anatomy of the trapeziometacarpal joint without consideration of the functional and dynamic balance of the motor system. Divergence of the thumb from the palm requires that an articular surface be available to allow for sliding of the metacarpal away from the midpoint of the palm. This slide excursion must be limited by an appropriate, deep volar ligament, which causes an impaction cam effect on the joint.[5] The travel of the metacarpal away from the deep volar ligament places the ligament on load. Excessive strain and resultant ligament laxity permit deformity and prevent appropriate tracking. Imbalance and excessive wear may be anticipated under these circumstances.

In normal situations, the cam effect of the taut ligament and the double curvature of the articular surfaces allow impaction loading at the base of the thumb and abduction of the metacarpal away from the midline. This motion must be balanced so that the

Figure 12–2. The inelastic volar ligament system stabilizes the unconstrained joint surfaces. All muscles and tendons that cross the joint produce forces that cause the metacarpal to displace proximally. Angulatory displacement in abduction and in elevation from the palm occurs because the volar apex of the joint is a stable, fixed fulcrum. Incompetence of the deep ligament results in proximal displacement of the metacarpus and resultant collapse deformity of the thumb.

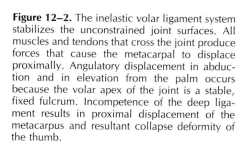
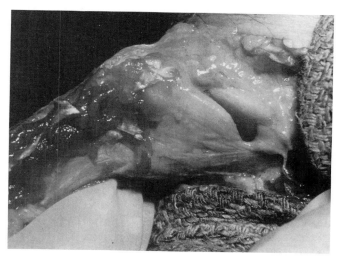

short abductor and the extrinsic abductor-extensor tendons work in concert to permit angular displacement of the thumb away from the palm. Appropriate balanced restraint is provided by those muscles on the opposite side of this axis of movement. The nervous system allows for modulated function so that fibers of the abductor brevis muscle that are closest to the mid-palm fire initially and then phase into less electrical activity as those fibers closest to the forearm become more responsible for divergence of the thumb from the palm.

In the reverse maneuver—that of pinch—the motor balance shifts in favor of those muscles producing convergence. The adductor (ulnar innervated) muscle performs in concert with the convergence-oriented short flexor and opponens fibers to produce the complex movement of adduction-flexion pronation. The antagonist group of muscles that provides strong active divergence from the palm shows little clinical or electrical activity in pinch or adduction. The reader is instructed to perform a strong pinching motion between the thumb and index finger while palpating the long abductor tendon. There is no activity in the abductor tendon during pinch, but immediate activity in this tendon is clinically evident with release and extension of the thumb.

Biomechanical and functional anatomic data of this type are useful in considering reconstructive procedures. Surgical migration of a muscle that is functionally inactive during pinch phase cannot be expected to provide dynamic support to the trapeziometacarpal joint during strong pinch. An experienced surgeon will rely on this tendon for tenodesis but not for dynamic enhancement of joint stability, that is, the long abductor tendon does not function during pinch and cannot be expected to change phase. This example is given to illustrate the point that the functional anatomy and biomechanics of the trapeziometacarpal joint relate directly to the planning of reconstructive surgical procedures.

BIOMECHANICS

A reasonable understanding of the kinematics of the thumb facilitates the solving of problems involving imbalance and deformity. It should be noted that paralysis itself does not produce deformity. A fixed contracture or similar deformity occurs only when imbalance in muscle forces occurs over a prolonged period of time. This imbalance may be corrected in several ways, but a basic understanding of the cause of the imbalance is essential.

In the thumb, three separate segments are longitudinally aligned on the trapeziometacarpal joint. Angulation of this joint with appropriate sensory feedback and muscle control permits a bridge of balance in the remainder of the thumb. This allows appropriate management of stress forces applied to the system. The strain pattern present in the thumb is determined by the articular surfaces, ligament stability, and balanced motor function available in this mechanical system. It has been estimated that eight to 10 times' magnification of force occurs in this system. Pinch with 1 lb at the tip of the thumb may result in a force of 8 lb across the trapeziometacarpal joint. It is, therefore, extremely important to maintain this system in balance in order to prevent these forces, which are always applied in the direction of impaction loading, from destroying the system. Equilibrium means the balance of forces, and this can only be preserved by articular surfaces that are congruous, by ligament systems that forcefully maintain appropriate alignment, and by proper motor balance.[6, 7]

A biomechanical analysis of the injured thumb can be made quickly and effortlessly by the experienced surgeon. This permits evaluation of the stress-strain relationship in the system. Initial questions of importance include:

1. Is a congruous joint surface present?
2. Is long bone alignment appropriate?
3. Is capsular stability present?
4. Is motor power balanced or available through transfer?

These four basic questions provide the substance for thinking about reconstructive surgery. They completely avoid the simplistic question, "What operation that I know how to do can be used in this situation?" In addition, the experienced surgeon must have some idea of the amount of work that is done by the patient's thumb and the time that is required for the performance of that work. Some operations are better designed for patients who do light repetitive work, while other procedures allow the patient to do powerful, prolonged grasping of tools or objects in the workplace. In addition, the performance of multiple repetitive tasks leads to problems of wear and deterioration. The same pathologic findings of an injured articular surface on clinical and radiographic examination may require different operative procedures based on the work required of the thumb or performed by the patient; e.g., a 38-year-old migrant farm worker with a post-traumatic arthritis of the trapeziometacarpal joint has a different work profile and thus different operative requirements from those of an urban attorney of similar age and body build with the same pathologic condition.

Consideration must also be given to the mechanics and balance of the metacarpophalangeal and interphalangeal joints in the thumb. These joints contribute directly to the stress loading of the trapeziometacarpal joint. For example, a rupture of the volar ligament of the metacarpophalangeal joint with resultant hyperextension of the joint puts excessive stress on the deep volar ligament of the trapeziometacarpal joint. Subsequent strain patterns may lead to laxity at the base of the thumb, with resultant displacement of the trapeziometacarpal joint. Inappropriate sliding over the surface of the trapeziometacarpal joint may then lead to the development of chondrolysis and arthritis, despite the absence of direct injury to this joint. This initial pathologic disorder—instability of the metacarpophalangeal joint—leads to ligamentous laxity and arthritic degenerative disease at a more proximal level. The astute clinician will, therefore, insist on providing stability and balance of the metacarpophalangeal joint before considering reconstruction at the trapeziometacarpal level. It is important to understand the inter-relationships among these three bones in a digit that requires mobility and strength, dexterity and durability, and range and balance.

PATHOLOGIC CONDITIONS

The trapeziometacarpal joint can be affected by trauma, inflammatory arthritis, congenital disorders, and many other medical conditions that adversely affect the functional anatomy and biomechanical properties noted previously in this chapter. Direct trauma may certainly destroy articular surface, ligaments, capsule, long bones, and muscles (Fig. 12–3). Extent of injury to each of these tissues must be determined individually when treating trauma to a given area.

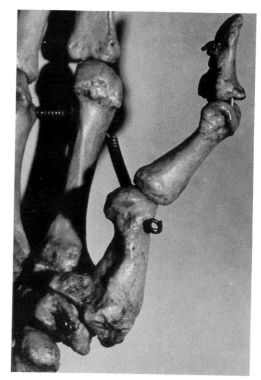

Figure 12–3. Fracture and collapse deformity of the thumb are seen in this skeleton. Loss of stability resulted from the traumatic separation of the fractured joint surface. The proximal and medial fragment remained stable in its anatomic position, owing to deep ligament competence. Proximal migration and adduction of the metacarpal shaft resulted in the typical intercalated segment collapse pattern.

Thus, a small chip fracture at the base of the thumb may not endanger surface congruity, since only a small portion of the joint surface has been injured; nevertheless, loss of ligament function in cases of Bennett's fracture results in instability, subluxation, and premature degenerative arthritis.

Major soft tissue trauma may result from an inappropriate focus of attention on significant muscle injury, while capsule repair is ignored. Again, the resultant instability will lead to joint demise unless corrected (Fig. 12–4). In many cases, direct comminuted fractures of joint surfaces have not resulted in major functional impairment, if the joint has been properly protected during the period of healing. Following bone union, appropriate balance is maintained. Stress loading is distributed according to the original design. In an area of major mobility such as the trapeziometacarpal joint, surface contact stress points change rapidly as the thumb passes through its conical range of motion. If the surface is relatively smooth and the loading is appropriate, it can be anticipated that the healed irregular areas will both load and unload rapidly, and thus the development of prolonged local stress risers leading to chondrolysis may be avoided. The formula for management of direct joint trauma in this area appears to be similar to that in other articular injuries, i.e., alignment of articular surfaces, reconstruction of capsular stability, appropriate protection from stress while healing occurs, and balanced early mobilization when possible. Under ideal circumstances, internal fixation would provide stability and alignment so that motion could begin as soon as possible. In actual experience, however, it is rare that this can be accomplished with comminuted fractures. A reasonable period of three to six weeks of immobilization does not appear to lead to irreparable contracture if the joint is fixed in a balanced position of abduction and elevation from the palm. Results are invariably poor when fixation and immobi-

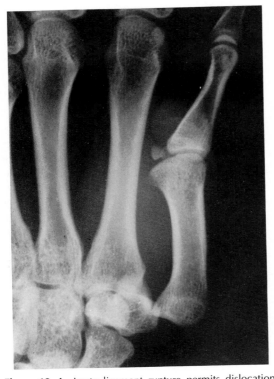

Figure 12–4. Acute ligament rupture permits dislocation and resultant imbalance of the joint to occur. Surgical reconstruction of the stabilizing ligament system will be necessary if conservative treatment fails to restore a fixed fulcrum to the joint. Chronic subluxation or instability will lead to excessive wear of the trapeziometacarpal joint cartilage surface. Subluxation also places excessive stress on the volar ligament of the metacarpophalangeal joint.

lization permit adduction of the joint and adduction-supination of the metacarpal. Thumb-index web space contracture can obviously occur without direct articular injury, but, when superimposed on articular derangement, it presents a more difficult reconstructive problem for the attending surgeon. Clearly, contracture of the thumb-index web space is best prevented.[8]

Arthritic involvement of the trapeziometacarpal joint is common. The most frequently encountered situation involves a middle-aged woman with erosive osteoarthritis. This is frequently associated with partial joint subluxation. It has yet to be determined whether imbalance and loss of ligament stability at the apex of the joint lead to the arthritis or are part of the degenerative process. Early realignment of the joint through ligament reconstruction has been proposed by Littler and Eaton.[9, 10] Despite early criticism of this concept, it is appropriate to consider restoration of alignment in arthritic conditions of other joints, and it would seem reasonable that realignment of the trapeziometacarpal joint would deter the development of erosive arthritic conditions. Osteotomy of the metacarpal has been proposed but has not been popular in actual practice, despite experience in other joints such as the knee, in which correction of weight-bearing forces by appropriate osteotomy prolongs joint serviceability. The concept that inappropriate shear stress at the joint surface produces cartilage debris leading to inflammatory joint destruction is basic in orthopedic surgery, and there is no reason to believe that this does not occur at the trapeziometacarpal joint.

Inflammatory arthritis—usually rheumatoid disease—also appears to affect the trapeziometacarpal joint. Early synovitis may lead to ligament and capsular laxity. This produces further mechanical instability of the joint, which enhances the destructive properties of proliferative synovium and leads to joint destruction. A prolonged synovitis may also lead to joint contracture in an adducted position, which complicates surgical repair. The presence of rheumatoid arthritis in this joint precludes serious consideration of capsular stabilization, because of the laxity of the tissues present. Nevertheless, synovectomy and reconstruction of volar ligaments with free tendon grafts have resulted in reasonable results, especially when associated with surface replacement arthroplasty.[11, 12] At times, subluxation of the metacarpophalangeal joint in rheumatoid arthritis can lead to secondary imbalance of the trapeziometacarpal joint, as noted above. In these instances, correction of the metacarpophalangeal joint imbalance must precede or accompany proximal joint reconstruction. The thumb must be considered as a structural unit, dependent on the mechanical stability of all of its integral segments.

Bacterial infection is rarely seen in the trapeziometacarpal joint.

SURGICAL TREATMENT

The goals of surgical treatment for disorders of the carpometacarpal joint of the thumb are similar to those for other abnormal joints. These goals include the maintenance or restoration of painless function and the prevention of further deterioration. The surgical procedures available may be generally described as those that attempt to repair the joint, those that propose replacement or reconstruction of the surface and periarticular structures, and procedures that assist thumb function by joint ablation.

Considerations for Derangement of the Trapeziometacarpal Joint

Reparative operations may be organized toward a specific tissue system, for instance, osteotomy to realign a malarticulation or a malunion of a fracture on the surface of the joint. Capsular stability may be repaired following reduction of chronic dislocation. Capsuloplasty procedures may stabilize the joint and prevent the development of erosive arthritis due to inappropriate tracking on the surface. Long bone alignment may be corrected either by changing the static shape of the bone through osteotomy, by reconstructing the capsule, or by applying dynamic procedures to restore motor balance. Restoration of motor balance in cases of nerve injury or direct muscle trauma may prevent deterioration of the joint or may correct alignment so that further deterioration will not occur, and thus further reconstructive procedures may not be necessary.

In most clinical cases, however, reconstruction of the joint surface is required. The operating surgeon should carefully review the basic problem before selecting the procedure of choice. An evaluation of articular surfaces, capsular stability, long bone align-

ment, and motor balance should be performed. All of these factors must be considered and integrated when choosing a reconstructive plan. In some operations, an implant will fulfill virtually the entire reconstructive requirement. It is essential that the operating surgeon be aware of other possibilities in which the implant serves as only a part of a reconstructive operation. Consideration of a complex procedure involving the implant, soft tissue repair, and bone and tendon balance may be required to realistically confront a difficult clinical situation.

Clinical Correlation

Several available procedures will be reviewed to provide clinical correlation with basic principles presented. Specific operative technique is described in Chapter 13. Technical variations exist in each of the major operative categories, but basic surgical alternatives remain constant. These include (1) fusion, (2) trapezectomy with or without implant arthroplasty, (3) spacer implant arthroplasty with small or large spacer implants, and (4) total joint replacement.

Fusion. Joint ablation and arthrodesis of the metacarpal to the trapezium has long been recommended for patients requiring strength and extended durability. Despite the theoretical advantages of retaining mobility, a patient rarely complains about a thumb that has been made strong and painfree. The arthrodesis procedure has several disadvantages, however, including a prolonged period of postoperative immobilization, excessive stress transfer to the metacarpophalangeal and scapho-trapezio-trapezoidal joints and a relatively high incidence of failure of fusion, requiring additional procedures. Nevertheless, in selected patients, it remains the procedure of choice in producing a joint that is pain-free, serviceable, reliable, and—following solid arthrodesis—rarely in need of revision.[13–15] Solid arthrodesis may not occur after the initial operation despite primary bone grafting. Further grafting may be necessary through the area of fibrous union. This should be explained to the patient so he or she is not excessively disappointed when initial arthrodesis requires a secondary procedure.

An appropriate angle of thumb placement is that degree of abduction and palmar elevation that allows the distal digital touch pad of the thumb to intercept the radial border of the index finger at the level of the distal interphalangeal joint. This will usually produce an angle of about 35° of abduction and similar palmar elevation with appropriate pronation, to bring the distal digital touch pad into a good position for distal key pinch. It should be noted that arthrodesis is usually recommended for those individuals who require extremely strong, repetitive grasp and pinch prehension. Key pinch produces stronger function than tip or three-point chuck-key pinch; therefore, thumb orientation toward the distal portion of the index finger for key pinch is reasonable in patients requiring arthrodesis. As in all fusion procedures, a preoperative trial may define an optimal position for arthrodesis. It is not unreasonable to place the thumb metacarpal in a position that is considered appropriate for fusion and to introduce a transarticular K wire across the joint or into the adjacent index metacarpal for trial placement. The procedure may be performed under local anesthesia with some input from the patient, who is then asked to carry out a series of activities with the joint immobilized in the predetermined position. If there is an adjustment to be made in the position that would be better for a particular patient, it can be considered in the preoperative planning phase of treatment rather than during the surgical procedure. It is better to make a basic plan for the position of arthrodesis with the patient awake and cooperative during the pre-operative period than to rely on some arbitrary value found in a text; each patient will have needs that vary, and arthrodesis is the least forgiving of all the surgical procedures considered in this region. In addition, the preoperative plan must consider the stability of the metacarpophalangeal joint that will receive much of the excess stress in proximal joint arthrodesis.

A patient who will require 20 years or more of durability in this area should also be informed that gradual laxity in the metacarpophalangeal joint may be expected when this joint attempts to perform a circumduction type movement for which it has not been designed. It is not uncommon to see a patient in whom arthrodesis was successfully performed 20 years earlier, who now complains of instability at the metacarpophalangeal joint level. This problem is usually tolerable and occurs after the end of the period in the patient's life in which

extremely strenuous work is required. An arthrodesis is particularly well suited to a person who is young, engages in extremely strenuous activity, and will not be available for frequent revision procedures. Successful arthrodesis in a farmer, dock worker, or similarly employed individual may provide decades of pain-free use of a powerful thumb without the need for revision.

Trapezectomy. Excision of the trapezium has proved to be a reliable procedure for arthritic disease at the base of the thumb.[16–18] This operation may cause a shortening of the thumb ray with some resultant imbalance; however, techniques have been devised to prevent this outcome through the use of a tendon graft interposition to substitute for the trapezium. The loss of the trapezium, however, does present a problem in revision procedures, should instability or weakness of pinch appear after trapezectomy. In general, excisional arthroplasty is best reserved for patients who will not place significant stress demands on their thumbs but who require adequate mobility.

Spacer Implant Arthroplasty. Spacer arthroplasty has been successful in providing relatively pain-free mobility at the trapeziometacarpal joint.[19, 20] However, soft spacer material provides no inherent stability for a joint that requires stable capsular integrity. It is, therefore, important for any surgeon contemplating soft spacer arthroplasty to carefully consider the need for a soft tissue reconstructive procedure in association with the implant insertion. Subluxation of spacer implants at the base of the thumb is common and has led to the development of modifications in the spacer itself and in the surgical technique designed to stabilize the area. Careful study of the surgical literature provides numerous methods available for stabilization. The operating surgeon should become comfortable with these methods and should apply them with each soft spacer arthroplasty. This will drastically reduce the problem of subluxation and will provide the patient with a more fixed fulcrum for retaining balanced and appropriate mobility in this active joint.

Implant modification can afford a reasonable solution to the problem of instability; e.g., a central hole placed through the trapezium replacement spacer allows for reconstruction of a ligament to keep the implant securely fixed in the area previously occupied by the trapezium. Howard[11] and

Swanson[12] have also described procedures to stabilize implants that are smaller than those spacers used after trapezectomy, in which soft tissue reconstruction for spatial security is still required. It is a basic premise that stability of this joint is required for appropriate pinch strength. Unstable motion is unacceptable and leads to weakness, pain, and architectural collapse.

Recent data suggest that some individuals may develop cystic degenerative changes in bone following Silastic implant arthroplasty.[21] This usually appears in areas where implants slide, roll, twist, or face compressive forces from bone. These changes in bone have not appeared to be associated with flexible hinges or implant arthroplasty at the base of the thumb as much as with carpal implant procedures. Nevertheless, several years of experience in this area will be required before final statements can be made regarding "silicone synovitis" and cyst formation. Fracture of Silastic implants has also been carefully studied by clinical investigators and implant manufacturers. At present, it appears that an acceptable fracture rate—

below 5 percent—is associated with implants in this area. The patient should be informed of the possibility of wear, erosion, and fracture in any implant arthroplasty procedure. Operations at the base of the thumb are no exception to this rule.

Total Joint Replacement. Total joint replacement at the base of the thumb has been studied over the last decade. The implant system usually favored is that of a semiconstrained ball and socket. Reasonable success can be anticipated including restoration of a full range of motion and a joint that is stable and pain-free.[22–24] The long-term results of the bone-cement interface have yet to be determined. The wear and breakage rate seems to be reasonable and probably lies just under 10 percent. The advantages of total joint replacement are that it does provide immediate mobility in the area and relies only minimally on soft tissue reconstruction. It is not appropriate for young, active patients or for patients with insufficient bone stock. In patients with an adequate skeletal system, total joint replacement does retain reasonable stock for later reconstructive pro-

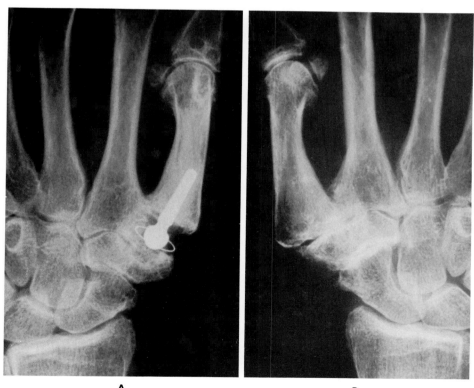

A   B

Figure 12–5. This patient underwent successful total joint replacement (TJR) eight years previously (A). She requested a similar TJR procedure on her opposite hand (B). Her pain was produced by thumb and wrist movement. Total joint replacement was not offered despite her request. Symptomatic pantrapezial arthritis was treated with trapezectomy and Silastic spacer arthroplasty. A mobile, stable, pain-free joint was created utilizing this alternative procedure.

cedures necessary if the operation is followed by a serious complication. Developments in metal technology and implant fabrication have allowed for the design of total joint replacements that do not necessarily rely on bone cement. These procedures should be considered experimental and evolutionary, since insufficient time has elapsed to evaluate the use of total joint replacement without cement in the base of the thumb.

CONCLUSION

Each of the procedures discussed in this presentation requires careful preoperative planning, knowledge of appropriate surgical technology, and thorough study of the response and functional needs of the patient (Fig. 12–5). There is no simple algorithmic program that will guarantee a successful operation in every case. Various factors influence the surgical decision. All of the decisions are based on a thorough understanding of the anatomy and the biomechanics of the area as well as the specific surgical materials and procedures mastered by the operating surgeon. Each operation must be assessed and the patient followed over a long period of time in order for the surgeon to derive meaningful data from the experience. One single operative procedure obviously cannot provide a successful solution for every patient with problems related to the base of the thumb. In addition, it is quite likely that two surgeons will propose different operations for the same patient, based on their experience, technical expertise, and overall clinical assessment of patient need. The applicability, reliability, and durability of the procedure will be determined as time passes and by professional scrutiny. Each operation should meet the challenge of appropriate restoration of function and should also answer questions related to future retrievability, if further surgical treatment should be necessary.

References

1. Hains RW: The mechanism of rotation at the first carpometacarpal joint. J Anat 78:44–46, 1944.
2. Kaplan EB: Functional and surgical anatomy of the hand. 2nd ed. JB Lippincott Co, Philadelphia, 1965.
3. Napier JR: The form and function of the carpometacarpal joint of the thumb. J Anat 89:362–369, 1955.
4. Pieron AP: The mechanism of the first carpometacarpal (CMC) joint. An anatomical and mechanical analysis. Acta Orthop Scand (Suppl) 148, 1973.
5. Braun RM: Stabilization of silastic implant arthroplasty at the trapeziometacarpal joint. Clin Orthop 119:273, 1976.
6. Cooney WP, Lucca MJ, and Chao EY: The kinesiology of the thumb trapeziometacarpal joint. J Bone Joint Surg 63A:1371–1381, 1981.
7. Cooney WP, and Chao EY: Biomechanical analysis of static forces in the thumb during hand function. J Bone Joint Surg 59A:27–36, 1977.
8. Sandzen SC: Thumb web reconstruction. Clin Orthop 195:66–82, 1985.
9. Littler JW: The prevention and correction of adduction contracture of the thumb. Clin Orthop 13:182, 1959.
10. Eaton R, and Littler JW: Ligament reconstruction for the painful thumb carpometacarpal joint. J Bone Joint Surg (Am) 55:1655, 1973.
11. Howard FM, Simpson LA, and Belsole RJ: Silastic condylar arthroplasty. Clin Orthop 195:144–150, 1985.
12. Swanson AB, and Swanson G: Arthroplasty of the thumb basal joints. Clin Orthop 195:151–160, 1985.
13. Eaton RG, and Littler JW: A study of the basal joint of the thumb. Treatment of its disabilities by fusion. J Bone Joint Surg 51A:661–668, 1969.
14. Caroll R, and Hill N: Arthrodesis of the carpometacarpal joint of the thumb. J Bone Joint Surg (Br) 55:292, 1973.
15. Stark H, Moore J, Ashworth C, et al: Fusion of the first metacarpotrapezial joint for degenerative arthritis. J Bone Joint Surg (Am) 59:22, 1977.
16. Carroll RR: Fascial arthroplasty for carpometacarpal joint of the thumb. Orthop Trans 1:15, 1977.
17. Froimson A: Tendon arthroplasty of the trapeziometacarpal joint. Clin Orthop 70:191, 1970.
18. Millender L, Nalebuff E, and Amadio P: Interpositional arthroplasty for rheumatoid carpometacarpal joint disease. J Hand Surg 3:533, 1978.
19. Swanson AB, Swanson G, and Watermeir JJ: Trapezium implant arthroplasty: long term evaluation of 150 cases. J Hand Surg 6(2):125, 1981.
20. Eaton R: Replacement of the trapezium for arthritis of the basal articulations. A new technique with stabilization by tenodesis. J Bone Joint Surg (Am) 61:76, 1979.
21. Smith RJ, Atkinson R, and Jupiter J: Silicon synovitis of the wrist. J Hand Surg 10A:47, 1985.
22. de la Caffinière J, and Aucouturier P: Trapeziometacarpal arthroplasty by total prosthesis. Hand 11:41, 1979.
23. Braun RM: Total joint replacement at the base of the thumb—preliminary report. J Hand Surg 7:245, 1982.
24. Braun RM: Total joint arthroplasty at the carpometacarpal joint of the thumb. Clin Orthop 195:161–167, 1985.

The Carpometacarpal Joint of the Thumb: Practical Considerations

STEPHEN FLACK GUNTHER, M.D.

The great range and complexity of motion of the first metacarpal have been described in the previous chapter. Suffice it to repeat here that the metacarpal is relatively loosely and therefore precariously perched on the trapezium. It has been likened to the boom of a sailboat, in that it attaches near the base of the rigid, mainmastlike second carpometacarpal (C-MC) complex and is suspended by shrouds of ligament and muscle.[12] Stability and alignment of the joint can be disrupted by one or more events and factors that include trauma, osteoarthritis, rheumatoid arthritis, physiologic muscle forces, and use over time. The volume of literature describing different variations in surgical management of the first C-MC joint is large. Because space does not permit a detailed review of all or even most procedures, those that the author prefers are discussed here.

TRAUMATIC DISLOCATIONS

Pure dislocation of the first metacarpal (Fig. 13–1A) is quite rare. As far as the author knows, there are no published series or papers dealing specifically with this subject, and there is only brief mention of it in most textbooks. The mechanism probably includes longitudinal compression of the flexed metacarpal against the trapezium,[9] with perhaps an adduction force distally or an abduction force proximally or both. The cause of the dislocation can range from a simple fall to a severe crush injury (Fig. 13–1B). All ligaments are torn, and there is no inherent stability after closed reduction. Since healing of the strong ulnovolar liga-

ment* to the bony beak at the base of the metacarpal is essential to restoration of stability, anatomic reduction should be fixed with a Kirschner wire for at least six weeks. The wire can be passed either from the first metacarpal into the second[18] (Fig. 13–1C) or from the first metacarpal into the trapezium.[28] The former is more easily done and does not violate the joint surface. It is important that the metacarpal be pinned in proper position and not left in external rotation (supination) relative to the palm. The wire serves as a good handle with which to manipulate the bone, but it must be inserted accurately at the beginning, so that it is aimed at the second metacarpal when the first is properly positioned. It is important to use a smooth Kirschner wire, because false passage across the palm with a threaded pin can damage important soft tissues; the author has seen a woman in whom the motor branch of the ulnar nerve was destroyed in this way. Although local anesthesia is sufficient for most patients, the procedure should be carried out under full surgical skin preparation and radiologic control. The thumb must be protected in a spica cast for as long as the Kirschner wire is in place in order to prevent metal fatigue and breakage at this very mobile articulation.

Careful x-ray examination may demonstrate that tiny bits of bone have been avulsed from the metacarpal base by the ulnovolar ligament. This is a good sign, since bone-to-bone healing is then possible if re-

---

*This has been called the ulnar ligament by Kaplan[19] and the volar ligament by Eaton and Littler.[11]

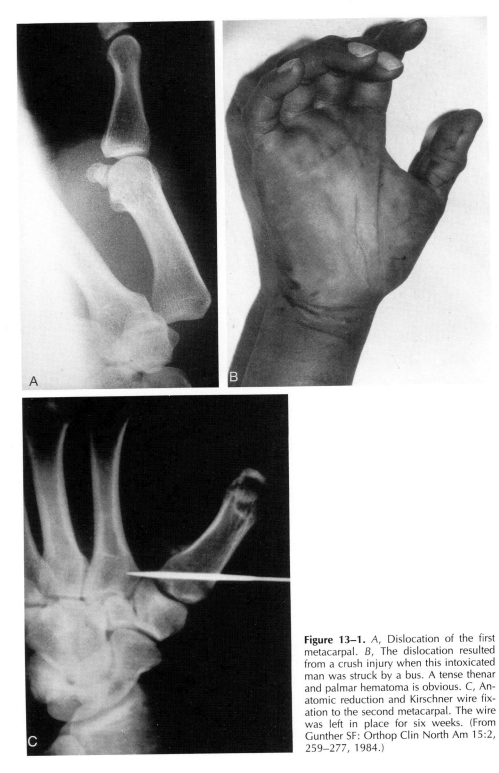

Figure 13–1. *A*, Dislocation of the first metacarpal. *B*, The dislocation resulted from a crush injury when this intoxicated man was struck by a bus. A tense thenar and palmar hematoma is obvious. *C*, Anatomic reduction and Kirschner wire fixation to the second metacarpal. The wire was left in place for six weeks. (From Gunther SF: Orthop Clin North Am 15:2, 259–277, 1984.)

duction is adequate. Ligament-to-bone healing is less reliable.

If a good closed reduction cannot be accomplished, or if time reveals the metacarpal to be unstable, open reduction and ligament reconstruction are indicated. Eaton and Littler[9, 11] have described a procedure that entails passing a partial-thickness strip of distally based flexor carpi radialis (FCR) tendon through a hole drilled in the base of the metacarpal. The tendon enters the bone at the ulnovolar beak and emerges on the opposite radial surface, from which it is led back around the volar capsule under the first extensor compartment tendons to the remaining FCR, through which it is passed and sutured. This re-establishes the strong ulnovolar ligament to bone and creates a new radiovolar ligament with a tendency to hold the thumb metacarpal bone in a position of opposition. The metacarpal is pinned in position for at least six weeks, as previously described. If painful arthritis has already developed, it is better to perform arthrodesis (described later in this chapter) than to attempt ligament reconstruction.

BENNETT'S FRACTURE

Bennett's fracture is really a fracture-dislocation of the metacarpal base. It is more common than pure dislocation and most often occurs in falls or during fisticuffs.[8, 24] The mechanism of the two injuries is similar, and the difference between them is that in Bennett's fracture an avulsed piece of metacarpal, including the ulnovolar beak and up to one third of the articular surface, remains in place with the ligament, whereas the remaining metacarpal dislocates radially (Fig. 13–2A).

Closed reduction of the metacarpal onto the trapezium can usually be accomplished with the help of local anesthesia if pressure is applied to the dorsum of the metacarpal base, while axial traction is applied to the thumb phalanges. Unfortunately, reduction is difficult to maintain. The abductor pollicis longus and the other dorsoradial tendons exert a dislocating force proximally and radially at the base of the metacarpal, and the adductor pollicis and flexor pollicis brevis augment this tendency by their ulnar pull distally. The traditional position in plaster after closed reduction has been radial abduction of the thumb with careful molding of the cast over a felt pad at the base of the metacarpal.[4, 8] In the past, some have felt that dynamic traction should be added.[5] Others have felt that it is better to hold the metacarpal in a position of flexion and internal rotation (opposition), in line with the

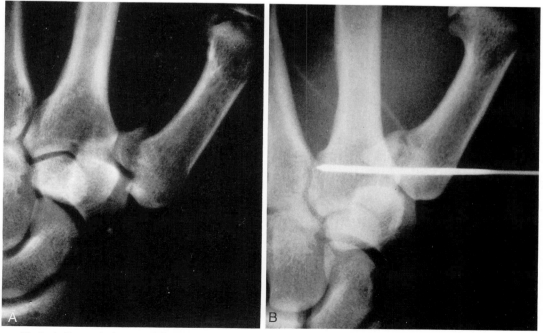

Figure 13–2. *A*, Bennett's fracture-dislocation. *B*, Percutaneous pin fixation after closed reduction. The metacarpal must be replaced in anatomic position on the trapezium. (From Gunther SF: Orthop Clin North Am 15:2, 259–277, 1984.)

second metacarpal when the hand is viewed on its palmar aspect.[16] They feel that this more accurately matches the metacarpal to the avulsed piece. Whichever method is used, frequent x-ray checks must be made, since initial reduction is frequently lost over the ensuing weeks. In addition, the surgeon must be wary of causing pressure necrosis of the skin at the point of plaster molding at the base of the metacarpal.

A preferable alternative to uncertain closed reduction is percutaneous pin fixation (Fig. 13–2B), as described in the previous section. It is not necessary that the pin traverse the avulsed piece, although that is helpful when the piece is large enough. The metacarpal should be anatomically positioned on the trapezium, but a 1 or 2 mm step-off of the smaller fragment is not significant, provided that the piece is apposed to the metacarpal, where it can heal and provide stability. This is especially true when the piece is small and does not constitute a major portion of the articulation. Displacement is usually away from the joint surface and therefore should not cause arthritis. Some authors disagree with this and feel that any recognizable incongruity of the joint surface is reason to perform open reduction and pinning.[14, 23] The proponents of nonoperative treatment point out that there is no long-term study of Bennett's fracture results that indicates that surgery is justified more than rarely, if ever.[8, 16, 24] Although they surely exist, the author has never seen a patient who complained of arthritic pain years after Bennett's fracture, treated or untreated, and it is common to find old unreduced and asymptomatic Bennett's fractures in hand x-rays that are done for other reasons (Fig. 13–3).

If open reduction is required, it can be accomplished through a transverse incision around the base of the metacarpal from the dorsal to the volar aspect, extending approximately 1 cm onto the palmar skin over the thenar muscles. An alternative is the less cosmetic longitudinal incision along the subcutaneous border of the metacarpal, between the thenar muscles and the extensor pollicis brevis tendon. Through either incision, the thenar muscles can be elevated from bone and capsule volarly, allowing inspection of the fracture and reduction under direct vision. Both the fracture and the joint are pinned. Postoperative treatment is essentially the same as for the percutaneous procedure and for dislocation.

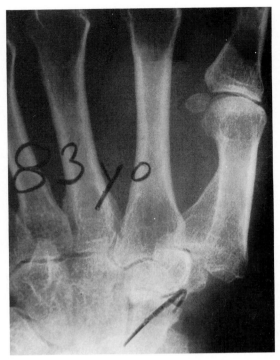

Figure 13–3. An untreated Bennett's fracture that occurred during the youth of this 83-year-old man. He continues to be asymptomatic and was asymptomatic all his working life. The hand looks remarkably good. (From Gunther SF: Orthop Clin North Am 15:2, 259–277, 1984.)

OTHER FRACTURES

Markedly displaced and angulated fractures may occur in the proximal metaphysis of the metacarpal (Fig. 13–4). Complete x-ray examination is important. Films should be ordered of the thumb specifically, and they should include three views, since major displacements can otherwise be overlooked (Fig. 13–4B). When a fracture spares the joint, it can usually be handled nonsurgically. Closed reduction provides at least a general restoration of alignment, and the fracture will heal despite a disquieting degree of displacement. The great range of motion at the C-MC joint makes a moderate residual displacement and even angulation insignificant.

Rolando's T-condylar or other comminuted fractures into the joint frequently do require reduction and pinning (Fig. 13–5). This is particularly true when the joint surface is broken into two or more pieces, none large enough to serve alone as a satisfactory articulation for the metacarpal. Although small plates and screws are available for this purpose, simple pinning with Kirschner wires is almost always preferable for its

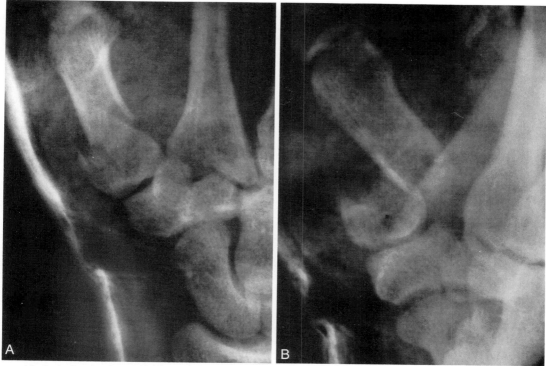

Figure 13–4. *A,* Proximal metaphyseal fracture of the thumb metacarpal. *B,* Anteroposterior view of the same thumb (lateral view of the hand) demonstrates the necessity for complete x-ray studies. This fracture is not uncommon. The position of the thumb can usually be improved by closed manipulation, and only rarely is open reduction or internal fixation necessary.

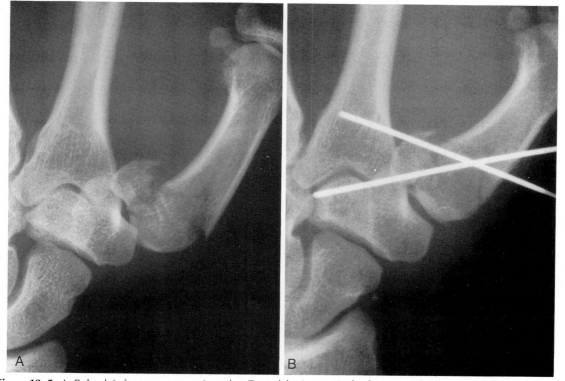

Figure 13–5. *A,* Rolando's fracture, a comminuted or T-condylar intra-articular fracture at the base of the first metacarpal. *B,* An excellent result was obtained by manipulation and percutaneous pin fixation. (X-rays courtesy of Captain HJ Kimmich, MC, USNR, National Naval Medical Center, Bethesda, MD.)

simplicity and for ease of hardware removal later on. Plaster protection should be provided for approximately six weeks, but the pins can be left in place a few weeks longer if they do not penetrate the joint and if they are cut off beneath the skin.

Fractures of the trapezium are extremely rare. These are usually comminuted fractures, which are best left alone. Reconstruction can be accomplished later on by arthroplasty or arthrodesis, if necessary.

OSTEOARTHRITIS

Osteoarthritis of the thumb C-MC joint is a common malady. The average patient is a woman in her 50s or 60s, who presents with pain and deformity at the base of the thumb. She may know exactly where the pain is, or its location may be vague. The duration has usually been several months or even years, and the pain has steadily increased up to the time of presentation. She knows that opening jars and turning keys cause pain. Physical examination reveals swelling or prominence at the joint. The base of the metacarpal may be luxated radially, and the

thumb may be limited in its ability to abduct. Coincident with adduction deformity of the metacarpal, there is compensatory hyperextension of the MP joint in severe cases. This may also be painful. Along with point tenderness over the C-MC joint, there is usually some crepitation during motion and examination. Distraction and twisting of the metacarpal may elicit pain; longitudinal compression most definitely does. X-rays show loss of joint space, subchondral sclerosis, and generally some degree of subluxation of the metacarpal on the trapezium (Fig. 13–6).

It would seem obvious that the heavy stresses imposed on this relatively loosely constrained joint by pinching and grasping are responsible for the fact that it requires surgical intervention for osteoarthritis more often than any other hand joint; however, it ranks only seventh among hand joints in incidence of arthritis, as determined by general radiographic screening of the population at large.[1] Some patients have severe symptoms with moderate arthritic changes, while others are asymptomatic with advanced arthritic changes demonstrated on x-ray films.

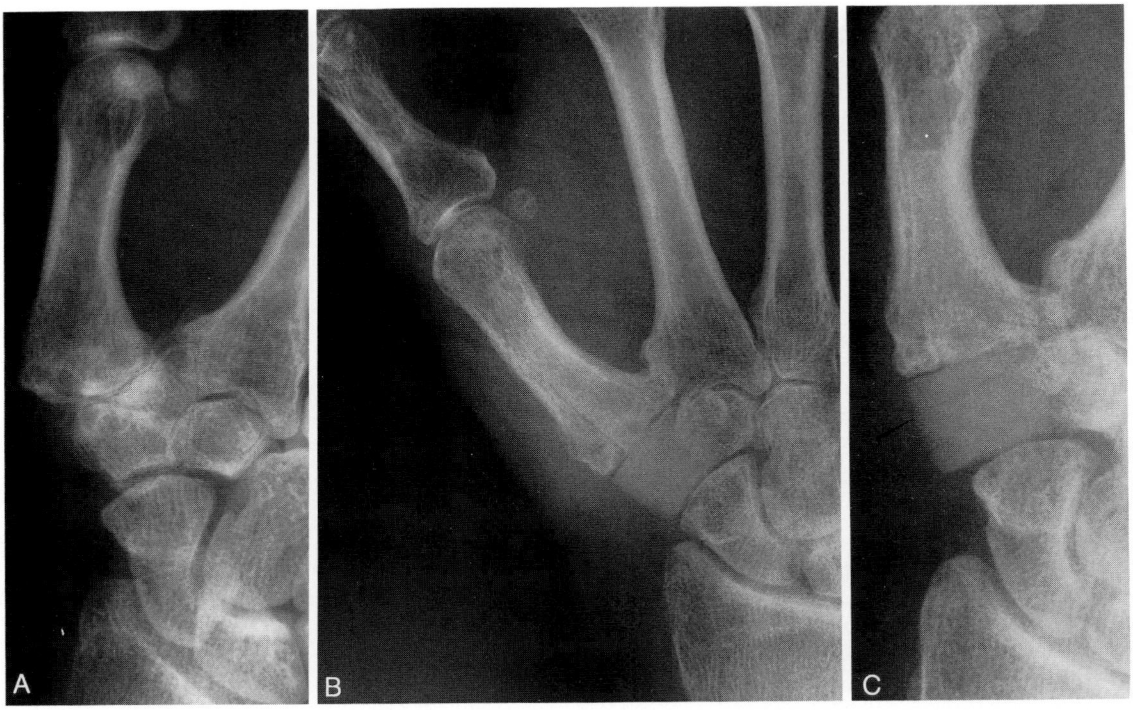

Figure 13–6. A, This 62-year-old woman had experienced pain at the base of the first metacarpal for over two years. An injection of triamcinolone brought relief for only a few months. Subluxation of the metacarpal base is obvious. B, Radiograph taken 11 weeks after Swanson Silastic trapezium arthroplasty was performed as described in the text. C, Minimal change in position of the prosthesis on the scaphoid is seen at four years.

Conservative Management

When the patient presents with pain, the initial treatment should be rest and injection of a cortisone analog. The injection serves two purposes. The first is diagnostic, since local anesthetic in the joint gives complete temporary relief if the pain truly comes from the joint. The second is therapeutic, since the pain is almost always relieved for some period of time. It will return anywhere from two to six months after injection in most patients, but it can be relieved for a much longer time (Fig. 13–7). Accurate placement of the injection is easily accomplished by the experienced surgeon but may be difficult for the beginner. I prefer to introduce a 25-gauge needle from the dorsoradial aspect of the joint. The needle is angled distally and can be walked proximally along the metacarpal shaft until it falls into the joint. Simultaneous distraction of the thumb is helpful. A simple test for position is removal of the syringe while leaving the needle in the joint. If the joint has been distended with anesthetic, the fluid will flow backward out of the needle in drops. This will not occur

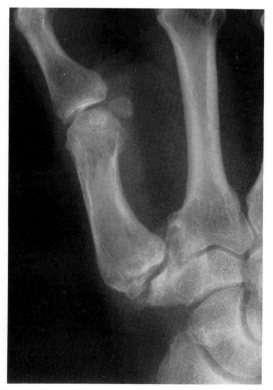

Figure 13–7. This 67-year-old man with advanced C-MC arthritis has been asymptomatic for four years following injection of triamcinolone into the C-MC joint.

if the needle is in soft tissue. Approximately 0.4 ml of triamcinolone is injected with a second syringe. A week or two of immobilization in a plaster splint may be helpful as well. Oral anti-inflammatory drugs have only a partial effect, and it does not seem to be worth risking the occurrence of potential side effects on the stomach.

Selection of Surgical Procedure

If pain persists or recurs within a few months after injection and it is severe enough to require medications and to alter the patient's everyday activities, surgery is recommended. Deformity is a relative indication, but surgery is almost never performed for deformity alone. There are far more people in the population at large with asymptomatic deformities than there are patients with pain.

A number of different operations can be successful, and there is no consensus among hand surgeons today as to which is the best. As for treatment of most joints, the two general categories of operation are *resection arthroplasty* and *arthrodesis*.

RESECTION ARTHROPLASTY

Resection includes procedures that entail removal of the base of the metacarpal,[20, 29] part of the trapezium,[3] or the whole trapezium.[15, 17, 22, 25, 27] The space that remains can be left empty,[15, 17, 22] it can be filled with a biologic spacer of tendor or fascia,[10, 13, 29] or it can be filled with any of a number of different kinds of implants.[2, 3, 6, 23, 25, 27] The proponents of resection alone or resection followed by use of a biologic spacer argue that their procedure is simple, sure to relieve pain, and not subject to implant dislocation, implant failure, or silicone synovitis. The proponents of silicone rubber implants of one sort or another argue that their operation is safe, that it reliably relieves pain, and that it maintains the length of the first ray and thereby gives a mechanically better thumb. It is the author's practice to replace the trapezium with a Swanson silicone rubber implant (Figs. 13–6A and B) in most patients and to perform arthrodesis in the few who have very heavy work requirements or severe deformity.

The early complication associated with trapezium replacement arthroplasty is dislocation of the prosthesis from the scaphoid. The amount of pre-operative subluxation and the joint angle at the base of the metacarpal vary considerably from patient to patient (Fig. 13–8), so careful pre-operative assessment of the patient and of the x-rays is necessary. Several techniques and their modifications have been described for reinforcing the capsule between the scaphoid and the metacarpal base. It is my contention that this procedure is generally not as important as correct preparation of the base of the metacarpal and alignment of the prosthesis within it. McGrath and Watson[21] published a series of 37 cases in which Swanson's trapezium replacement was performed without capsular reinforcement and in which there were no dislocations. They stressed the importance of resecting the radial border of the trapezoid.

The author feels that proper fashioning of the base of the first metacarpal is equally important. The prosthesis should be aligned in the first metacarpal in such a way that it faces into the wrist and not down the lateral border of the radius (Fig. 13–9). While it is tempting to use the line of the radial cortex of the first metacarpal as a guide, to do this would be a mistake. If the prosthesis is generally aligned with this cortex, it does not naturally aim in toward the scaphoid. To prevent this, the proximal 2 mm or so of

the metacarpal should be cut with either a small saw or rongeur, and the surface at the base should form an acute angle with the lateral cortex once this is done. A line drawn perpendicular to this surface does not pass straight up the medullary shaft. It angles from the ulnar aspect to the radial, becoming tangential to the proximal portion of the ulnar cortex. Thus, the biconcave proximal surface of the metacarpal is transformed into a flat, cancellous surface that is approximately perpendicular to the longitudinal axis of the distal half of the scaphoid. It has the appearance of facing 15° or 20° into the wrist.

A channel is then made in the medullary cavity perpendicular to this flat surface. This is begun with a small curette and finished with a power-driven blunt-tipped bur. The sizers are used to find the prosthesis that can fill the space without being at all tight. A slightly small one is preferred to a slightly large one. Since the medullary canal fashioned in the way described here does not correspond exactly to the natural medullary canal, the stem may be a bit too long. If so, it can be cut shorter. The prosthesis should fit flush on the proximal surface of the metacarpal, and it should be fairly stable on the scaphoid prior to any capsular closure.

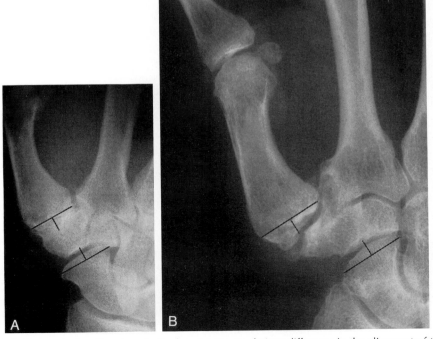

Figure 13–8. A, B, Two patients with osteoarthritis demonstrate an obvious difference in the alignment of the metacarpal base relative to the scaphoid. Stable silicone arthroplasty can be achieved more easily in A than in B.

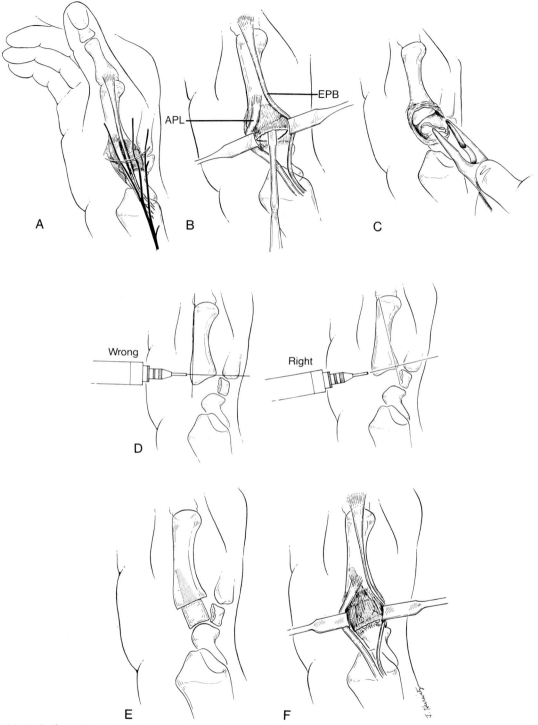

Figure 13–9. Outline of the author's technique for Swanson Silastic trapezium arthroplasty. *A,* A transverse skin incision allows good exposure and is cosmetically inconspicuous after healing. The sensory branches of the radial nerve are identified in the subcutaneous tissue and are retracted. *B,* The joint capsule is incised transversely between the retracted abductor pollicis longus (APL) and the extensor pollicis brevis (EPB) tendons. The capsule is elevated from the trapezium and is left attached to the scaphoid proximally and to the metacarpal distally. *C,* The trapezium is removed piecemeal. Small pieces of bone can be left rather than risk damage to the volar capsule. *D,* The wrong and right ways to cut the base of the metacarpal (see text). *E,* The prosthesis should be fairly stable on the scaphoid before capsular closure. The radial one third of the trapezoid has been removed to provide room for the prosthesis. *E,* The prosthesis should be fairly stable on the scaphoid before capsular closure. The radial one third of the trapezoid has been removed to provide room for the prosthesis. *F,* The capsule is closed. The APL tendon can be incorporated in the closure if the capsule is deficient.

The capsule is then closed transversely. Tendon reinforcement is not employed unless the capsule is clearly deficient. The abductor pollicis longus tendon can be incorporated into the closure if necessary. The thumb is casted in comfortable extension and abduction, roughly the position of the thumb when the hand is closed in a fist. It is judicious to leave the cast on for six weeks. The patient can then begin exercising, but heavy activity and sports should be avoided for another three months.

If a biologic spacer is preferred to the silicone prosthesis, a rolled-up tendon can be put into the defect after removal of the trapezium. Surgeons most often use half the thickness of the flexor carpi radialis or the full thickness of the palmaris longus. Other tendons or fascia may be used with equal success. Amadio et al[2] found no significant difference in the results after two years in 25 silicone arthroplasties and 25 resection arthroplasties. Pain relief, motion, strength, and appearance were essentially the same according to this report, although the x-ray of a resection case did show settling of the metacarpal base towards the scaphoid. This settling has been noted in other studies.[15, 22]

Ancillary Surgical Procedures. These procedures alone may not be sufficient in the face of severe deformity. The combination of advanced subluxation of the metacarpal base, fixed adduction of the metacarpal, adduction contracture of the web fascia, and compensatory hyperextension of the metacarpophalangeal joint (Fig. 13–10A) carries a high risk of persistent deformity and prosthetic dislocation. Additional steps can be taken to prevent this. In the rare case in which there is a true soft tissue contracture, the fascia in the thumb-index web can be released and a formal recession of the adductor pollicis muscle can be carried out at either its origin or its insertion. The hyperextensible metacarpophalangeal joint can be pinned in slight flexion for six weeks, and in the most severe cases, a surgical tightening or free tendon graft substitution of the volar plate is indicated. The metacarpal base can be shortened slightly more than usual during fashioning of the proximal surface. The capsule around the trapezial implant can be reinforced with a half-section of the flexor carpi radialis tendon, which is left attached to the second metacarpal, and the abductor pollicis longus tendon can be advanced distally. The first metacarpal can be pinned to the second for six weeks.

ARTHRODESIS

Each of these steps should be considered prior to surgery and during surgery, although it is extremely unlikely that all of them would ever be employed in one case. A patient who would require all of these procedures would be a good candidate for arthrodesis, which permanently rids the patient of pain and restores normal posture of the thumb (Fig. 13–10B and C). Arthrodesis can be performed through the same incision that is used for arthroplasty. The cartilage surfaces and subchondral bone plates are removed from each side of the C-MC joint, and cancellous bone graft from either the ilium or the distal radius is packed into the space. At least two Kirschner wires are placed through the joint, cut off below the skin, and left in place for 12 weeks. The proper position of the metacarpal is roughly that which it naturally assumes in the making of a fist, that is, 25° palmar abduction, 25° extension, and mild rotation toward opposition. Secondary procedures are not necessary because proper positioning of the metacarpal restores tendon balance, and the thumb MP will naturally return to a resting position of slight flexion. Although most hand surgeons today do few arthrodeses, published series show excellent functional results and patient satisfaction.[7, 26] Arthrodesis of the trapeziometacarpal joint surely increases the daily stress at the scaphotrapezial joint, but this is unlikely to ever pose a problem in patients who undergo this operation after 50 years of age.

RHEUMATOID ARTHRITIS

Rheumatoid arthritis presents special problems. Although it affects the basal joint of the thumb, this is rarely an isolated problem as it is so often in the case of osteoarthritis. Deformity, instability, and pain are frequently present at the MP and the IP joints as well, and this may necessitate arthrodesis of one or both of these joints. This potential makes arthrodesis at the C-MC joint unwise in most cases. Silicone arthroplasty can be done, but resection should always be considered, especially when there is poor seating for a prosthesis owing to wrist collapse or a partially destroyed scaphoid.

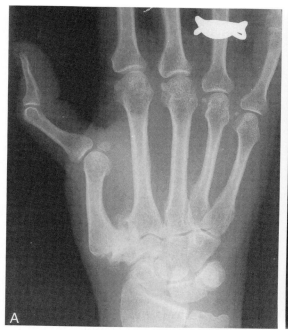

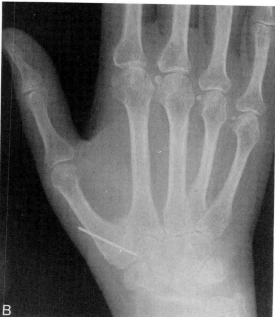

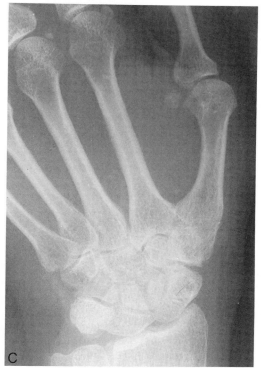

Figure 13–10. *A,* Severe deformity in a 57-year-old nurse who presented with pain, adduction contracture of the metacarpal, and compensatory hyperextension deformity of the metacarpophalangeal joint. *B,* Arthrodesis of the C-MC joint has completely relieved pain and has restored normal thumb posture without any procedure being done at the MP joint. The patient returned to full-time work at four months. *C,* The opposite thumb is asymptomatic 16 years after arthrodesis. Note that there is some degenerative change at the scaphotrapezial joint.

References

1. Acheson RM, et al: New Haven survey of joint diseases. XII. Distribution and symptoms of osteoarthritis in hands. Ann Rheum Dis 29:275–286, 1970.

2. Amadio PC, Millender LH, and Smith RJ: Silicone spacer or tendon spacer for trapezium resection arthroplasty—comparison of results. J Hand Surg 7:237–244, 1982.

3. Ashworth CR, Blatt G, Chuinard RG, et al: Silicone-rubber interposition arthroplasty of the carpometacarpal joint of the thumb. J Hand Surg 2:345–357, 1977.

4. Barton NJ: Fractures and joint injuries of the hands. In Wilson JN (ed): Watson-Jones, Fractures and Joint Injuries. 6th ed. Edinburgh, Churchill Livingstone Inc, 1982, pp 739–788.

5. Bradford CH, and Dolphin JA: Fractures of the hand and wrist. In Flynn JE (ed): Hand Surgery. Baltimore, Williams & Wilkins, 1966, pp 142–143.

6. Braun RM: Total joint replacement at the base of the thumb—preliminary report. J Hand Surg 7:245–251, 1982.

7. Carroll RE, and Hill NA: Arthrodesis of the carpometacarpal joint of the thumb. J Bone Joint Surg 55B:292–294, 1973.

8. Charnley J: The Closed Treatment of Common Fractures, 2nd ed. Edinburgh, ES Livingstone Ltd, 1957, pp 125–130.

9. Eaton RG: Joint Injuries of the Hand, Springfield, Charles C Thomas, 1971, pp 66–69.

10. Eaton RG, Glickel SZ, and Littler JW: Tendon interposition arthroplasty for degenerative arthritis of the trapeziometacarpal joint of the thumb. J Hand Surg 10A:645–654, 1985.

11. Eaton RG, and Littler JW: Ligament reconstruction for the painful thumb carpometacarpal joint. J Bone Joint Surg 55A:1655–1666, 1973.

12. Flatt AE: The Care of Minor Hand Injuries. 3rd ed. St Louis, CV Mosby Co, 1972, pp 3–5.

13. Froimson AI: Tendon arthroplasty of the trapeziometacarpal joint. Clin Orthop 70:191–199, 1970.

14. Gedda KO, and Moberg E: Open reduction and osteosynthesis of the so-called Bennett's fracture in the carpo-metacarpal joint of the thumb. Acta Orthop Scand 22:249–257, 1953.

15. Goldner JL, and Clippinger FW: Excision of the greater multangular bone as an adjunct to mobilization of the thumb. J Bone Joint Surg 41A:609–625, 1959.

16. Harvey FJ, and Bye WD: Bennett's fracture. Hand 8:48–53, 1976.

17. Jervis WH: A review of excision of the trapezium for osteoarthritis of the trapeziometacarpal joint after 25 years. J Bone Joint Surg 55B:56–57, 1973.

18. Johnson EC: Fracture of the base of the thumb—a new method of fixation. JAMA 126:27–28, 1944.

19. Kaplan EB: Functional and Surgical Anatomy of the Hand. 2nd ed. Philadelphia, JB Lippincott Co, 1965, pp 88, 94–98.

20. Kessler I: Silicone arthroplasty of the trapeziometacarpal joint. J Bone Joint Surg 55B:285–291, 1973.

21. McGrath MH, and Watson HK: Arthroplasty of the carpometacarpal joint of the thumb in arthritis—an emphasis of bone configuration. Orthop Rev 8:127–131, 1979.

22. Murley AHG: Excision of the trapezium in osteoarthritis of the first carpometacarpal joint. J Bone Joint Surg 42B:502–507, 1960.

23. O'Brien ET: Fractures of the metacarpals and phalanges. In Green DP (ed): Operative Hand Surgery, New York, Churchill Livingstone Inc, 1982, pp 583–635.

24. Pollen AG: The conservative treatment of Bennett's fracture-subluxation of the thumb metacarpal. J Bone Joint Surg 50B:91–101, 1968.

25. Poppen NK, and Niebauer JJ: "Tie-in" trapezium prosthesis: long-term results. J Hand Surg 3:445–450, 1977.

26. Stark HH, Moore JF, Ashworth CR, et al: Fusion of the first metacarpotrapezial joint for degenerative arthritis. J Bone Joint Surg 59A:22–26, 1977.

27. Swanson AB: Disabling arthritis of the base of the thumb. Treatment by resection of the trapezium and flexible silicone implant arthroplasty. J Bone Joint Surg 54A:456–471, 1972.

28. Wagner CJ: Method of treatment of Bennett's fracture-dislocation. Am J Surg 80:230, 1950.

29. Wilson JN: Arthroplasty of the trapeziometacarpal joint. Plast Reconstr Surg 49:143–148, 1972.

CHAPTER 14

The Medial Four Carpometacarpal Joints

STEPHEN FLACK GUNTHER, M.D.

INTRODUCTION

Compared with the many articles, chapters, and symposia devoted to the wrist and basal thumb joints during the past 15 years, very little has been written about the medial four carpometacarpal (C-MC) joints. The obvious reasons are that clinical problems are uncommon, and their consequences are not devastating, but the unhappy result of this inattention is that many surgeons who treat the hand are incompletely trained in this area. Architectural integrity and painless stability of the C-MC joints and the bones that form them are essential to good hand and wrist function, especially in power grip and in activities that involve torque.

The following paragraphs outline the anatomy and both degenerative and traumatic disorders of these joints. Infections and tumors are not covered here since they are exceedingly rare, and their treatment is not specific to this anatomic area.

ANATOMY

Eleven joints lie between the bones of the distal carpal row and the metacarpal bases. Each is invested with a heavy capsule and many well-defined capsular ligaments (Fig. 14–1A and B). In general, the second and third metacarpals are rigidly fixed to the trapezoid and captitate bones, giving the hand a stable base around which the thumb, the phalanges, and the ulnar two metacarpals rotate during hand motion. With the help of the transverse carpal ligament, this central fixed unit maintains both the longitudinal and the transverse arches of the hand.[28] The second C-MC joint is capable of only 1° or 2° of motion, and the third allows no more than 3°. The normal motion is so

slight that arthrodesis of either of these joints has no deleterious effect at all and is good treatment for traumatic disruption or for painful arthrosis. Different sources quote different figures, but my own observations during fresh cadaver dissection indicate that the fourth C-MC joint allows some 8° to 10° of flexion-extension, and the fifth allows in excess of 15°. Flexion-rotation of the ulnar metacarpals is most obvious when the hand is cupped and is important for making a tight fist as well, although I am not aware of any studies showing that arthrodesis of these C-MC joints reduces grip strength or leads to any clinical problem.

The joint surfaces of the second and third metacarpal bases interlock with those of the trapezoid and capitate (Fig. 14–1B). In addition to these matched joint surfaces and the heavy ligamentous capsules, stabilizers of the second and third metacarpals include the radial wrist flexor and extensor tendons.

DEGENERATIVE AND INFLAMMATORY DISORDERS

Arthritis

Although rarely mentioned, rheumatoid destruction of the medial four carpometacarpal joints is more common than many realize (Fig. 14–2). Loss of stability and shortening of the fixed C-MC unit contribute to weakness and pain. Because this occurs without great deformity and usually as a part of an overall wrist destruction that tends to capture the physician's attention, surgical stabilization is rarely done. Nevertheless, it is worth consideration at the time of arthroplasty in the treatment of some wrist disorders.

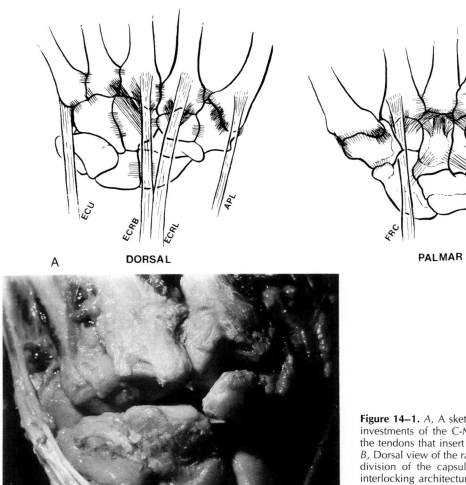

ECU   ECRB   ECRL   APL

A   DORSAL

FRC   FCU

PALMAR

B

Figure 14–1. *A*, A sketch of the ligamentous investments of the C-MC joints, along with the tendons that insert in proximity to them. *B*, Dorsal view of the radial C-MC joints after division of the capsules and tendons. The interlocking architecture of the bones is obvious. (*A*, From Gunther SF: Orthop Clin North Am 15:2, 259–277, 1984.)

Osteoarthritis without antecedent injury does not seem to be a problem in these joints, but gout and other crystal deposition arthritides can present as acute inflammation. The principal differential is infection, and the treatment is in the form of anti-inflammatory medication and immobilization.

Acute overuse in manual work or sports can cause C-MC joint pain severe enough to require treatment. The author has seen this at the fourth C-MC joint in a golf professional who was hitting practice balls for many hours a day. The same thing can happen in racquet sports. Immobilization and rest are the treatment for this disorder.

Fracture and fracture-dislocation can lead to degenerative arthritis in the C-MC joints (Fig. 14–3). The incidence and severity of this are undefined in the literature, but patients do gradually develop enlargement of these joints during the years following com-plete dislocation, and they can retain some symptoms with either prolonged or very heavy use.[16] It is uncommon that pain and disability are sufficient to warrant arthrodesis.

The architecture of the fifth C-MC joint allows more motion than the other joints, while providing less intrinsic stability. The joint is gently slanted from radial to ulnar aspect. The extensor carpi ulnaris muscle is a deforming force, since it tends to pull the metacarpal base proximally and in an ulnar direction. Fracture-subluxation of the fifth metacarpal base is the ulnar counterpart of Bennett's fracture of the thumb (Fig. 14–4), and traumatic arthritis will surely follow if the need for anatomic reduction and pinning is overlooked (Fig. 14–5).[4, 35, 36, 39, 40] Nonoperative treatment of such arthritis with splintage and corticosteroid injection may control the symptoms, but the definitive treatment

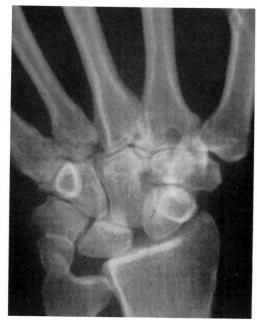

Figure 14–2. A 45-year-old rheumatoid patient with the incidental finding of C-MC arthritis in her wrist, which was being examined for radiocarpal pain.

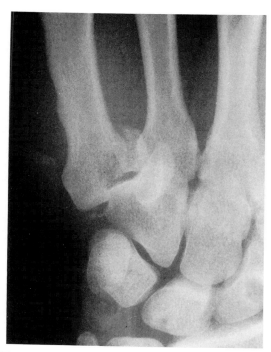

Figure 14–4. A 25-year-old man sustained this fracture-subluxation by punching another man's forehead.

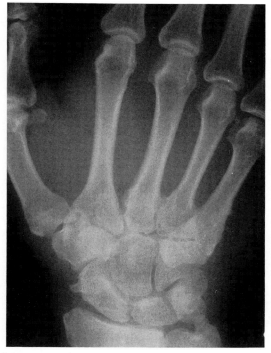

Figure 14–3. This x-ray was taken seven and a half years after this 37-year-old police officer dislocated all four C-MC joints. He was treated initially by open reduction and pinning. He is back on full-time duty and has mild symptoms only in bad weather or after very heavy use of the hand. The joints are mildly prominent dorsally, both on observation and on palpation. They are not tender. (From Gunther SF: J Hand Surg 10A:2, 197–201, 1985.)

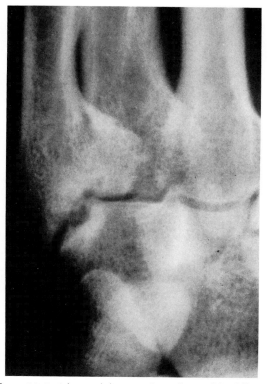

Figure 14–5. Advanced degenerative arthritis of the fifth C-MC joint only two years after fracture-subluxation. (From Gunther SF: Orthop Clin North Am 15:2, 259–277, 1984.)

is either by interposition arthroplasty or arthrodesis. Different Silastic prostheses have been modified for interposition in this joint, and good results have been reported.[13] There are no long-term studies, however. Interposition of rolled-up tendon or other biologic spacer is another option. As mentioned previously, there is little in the literature about arthrodesis of the mobile fourth and fifth C-MC joints, but anecdotal experience indicates that patients suffer no loss of strength and no disability from loss of motion in those joints.[22, 23, 31, 35]

In the absence of data from comparative studies in the literature, treatment should be individualized to the patient, with the expectation that arthrodesis is a permanent remedy that will stand up to heavy use over time.

Carpal Boss

The term carpal boss describes a bony prominence of unknown etiology on the dorsal aspect of either the second or third C-MC joint (Fig. 14–6A). These prominences do not usually occur before early adulthood. Most are noticed as incidental findings on a hand being examined for something else,[2]

since only a small percentage are painful. The bump is a buildup of new bone on both the metacarpal and the carpal bones (Fig. 14–6B). Radiographically, it suggests osteophyte formation as in osteoarthritis, and its gross appearance is similar to that of degenerative arthritis of these joints; however, there is no joint space narrowing and no subchondral bony sclerosis that one would expect in arthritis. It has been suggested that the bossing is sometimes an anomaly of an accessory ossification center in the styloid process of the third metacarpal base,[3, 9] and it has also been suggested that it is the result of a periostitis initiated by some unknown form of microtrauma.[6, 25]

When patients do come for treatment of a carpal boss, it is generally because of the unsightly swelling. In about one third of cases that are severe enough to warrant surgery, the appearance is made worse by the presence of a sessile ganglion in addition to the bony prominence.[9] If the appearance is unsightly enough, or if the boss is chronically painful, surgery is the only effective treatment. As already mentioned, both the metacarpal base and the carpal bone contribute to the rounded prominence, so the protuberant portions of each bone must be re-

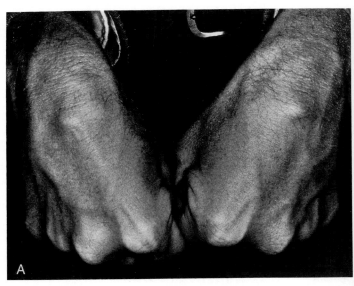
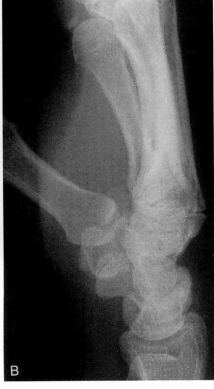

Figure 14–6. A, This middle-aged man had no pain whatsoever associated with bilateral carpal bosses at the second C-MC joints. B, In this case of a carpal boss, the x-ray suggests an accessory ossification center or an ossicle at the base of the metacarpal.

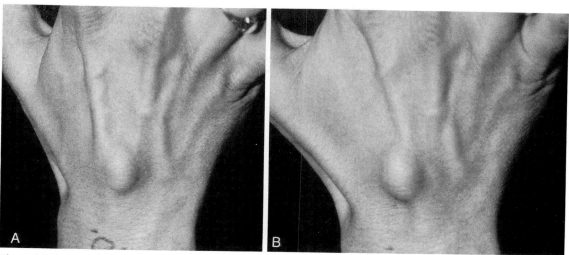

Figure 14–7. A, B, This 24-year-old woman complained that the index extensor tendons snapped back and forth over this large ganglion when she moved the finger in certain ways. The ganglion overlay a small carpal boss. (From Gunther SF: Orthop Clin North Am 15:259–277, 1984.)

moved by generous wedge resection that enters the joint well into its cartilaginous surface. Early reports indicated a high rate of recurrence after surgical excision,[7] but one recent study showed no recurrence in 16 patients treated as mentioned here.[9] It has been the author's experience that some of these recur partially, even after a generous excision. As in other problems of the C-MC joints, arthrodesis is a good solution for persistent problems if simpler surgery fails.

Ganglia

Prominent dorsal ganglia sometimes arise over the second or third C-MC joints, but usually the second. They are clearly different from the far more common dorsal wrist ganglia that arise from the scapholunate ligament. They are frequently multilobulated and emerge from both sides of the adjacent radial wrist extensor tendon. These ganglia are firmly anchored to the joint beneath, and they can become large enough to interfere with normal tracking of the index extensor tendons (Fig. 14–7). Sometimes they coexist with a carpal boss, as mentioned previously, and sometimes they occur alone. In either case, because they originate in the joint, they are very likely to recur unless a wedge resection of the dorsal portion of the C-MC joint is carried out. Use of appropriate surgical technique is essential, since an adequate amount of bone must be excised, while the important lateral ligaments must be left in place. A case in point is that of a young woman with instability of the second car-

pometacarpal joint following ganglion excision (Fig. 14–8). Whether the instability existed prior to surgery is unknown, but the patient did require arthrodesis for pain relief two years after the initial ganglionectomy.

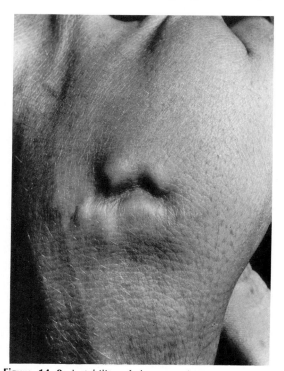

Figure 14–8. Instability of the second C-MC joint was obvious when the examiner forced the metacarpal into flexion. This is the hand of an 18-year-old girl who had undergone ganglionectomy two years previously. At surgery, there were no dorsal ligaments and no evidence of the extensor carpi radialis longus tendon. Arthrodesis cured the pain that she had experienced with writing and any other prolonged activity.

TRAUMATIC DISORDERS

Sprains

Both acute and chronic sprains can be recognized by the physician. These seem to occur mostly in the second and third C-MC joints, probably because these joints are loaded during almost any hand function. Acute sprains are evidenced by pain, diffuse swelling, and ecchymosis on both the dorsal and the palmar aspects of the hand (Fig. 14–9). There is local tenderness on palpation and pain when the examiner stresses the injured joints. The mechanisms of injury are similar to those that cause fracture-dislocations. After a thorough radiologic examination to rule out subluxation of the metacarpal bases, the acute sprain is treated with plaster immobilization until the pain subsides—generally for about six weeks.

Chronic sprains of the second and third C-MC joints are far more common than has been recognized. The diagnosis being used here includes those patients with ongoing pain following significant injury as well as those more common patients with pain after seemingly trivial injury or even no injury at all. Chronic sprain is clearly different from carpal boss and arthritis; patients have nagging pain deep in the hand during or after prolonged and repetitive use, as in writing, or during more strenuous activities. The pain may be poorly localized by the patient, but the diagnosis is not difficult if the examiner looks specifically for this problem. Diagnostic injection of local anesthetic into the involved joint or joints is helpful in the evaluation. Joseph et al[22] reported a series of 28 chronic sprains that were treated successfully by arthrodesis. During the time period in which these cases were collected, the authors recognized 20 other chronic sprains that were not severe enough to warrant surgery and, interestingly, only 10 acute sprains.

Arthrodesis is a reliable and apparently innocuous remedy for this problem. It can be accomplished through a dorsal approach with an inlay bone graft (Fig. 14–10). The author has inserted tricortical iliac grafts oriented transversely, much like anterior interbody fusion in the cervical spine. Joseph and associates used a longitudinally oriented graft. In either case, it is desirable that the graft be fashioned and inserted in such a way as to maintain the normal length of the ray. Kirschner wires should be inserted for fixation and kept in place long enough for the graft to become incorporated, i.e., about 12 weeks. The wires should fix only the carpometacarpal joints and should not extend into the scaphoid proximally. Of course, the wrist extensor tendon insertions should be preserved. Results have been excellent.

Fractures and Fracture-Dislocations

Although uncommon, fractures and fracture-dislocations do compose the majority of clinical problems at the C-MC joints. Great and sudden force is required to disrupt the strong joint capsules. Multiple C-MC dislocations are usually the result of motorcycle accidents, during which the victim was gripping

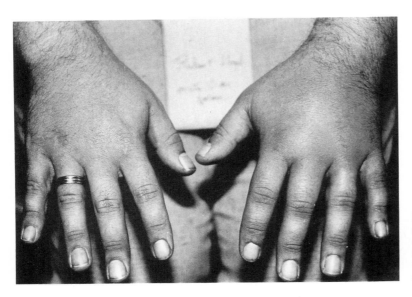

Figure 14–9. This man had normal x-rays, but he had all the signs and symptoms of acute sprain of the second and third carpometacarpal joints in the involved left hand. The sprain did well with plaster immobilization.

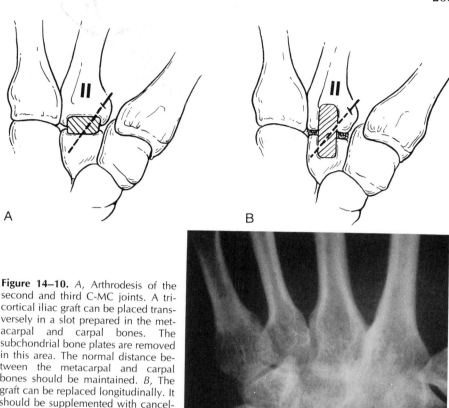

Figure 14–10. *A,* Arthrodesis of the second and third C-MC joints. A tricortical iliac graft can be placed transversely in a slot prepared in the metacarpal and carpal bones. The subchondral bone plates are removed in this area. The normal distance between the metacarpal and carpal bones should be maintained. *B,* The graft can be replaced longitudinally. It should be supplemented with cancellous packing on either side. *C,* This 22-year-old policewoman presented with pain and an unsightly ganglion that had recurred after two separate surgical excisions. Preoperative grip strength was 57 percent that of the opposite, nondominant hand. She returned to full-time duty six months after surgery and by one year the grip strength had improved to 127 percent of the opposite hand. (From Gunther, SF: Orthop Clin North Am 15:2, 259–277, 1984.)

the handlebars at the moment of impact. Injuries limited to the ulnar side are more often from fist fights and falls. Early papers on the subject concentrated on dorsal dislocation of all four metacarpals simultaneously,[37, 42, 43] but it now appears that the most common variant is dorsal or volar dislocation of the fifth metacarpal alone (Fig. 14–11).[4, 14, 15, 35] Next in frequency are the fourth and fifth together (Fig. 14–12), but just about every conceivable pattern of dorsal and volar dislocations of any or all metacarpals has been described.* For example, the fifth metacarpal may dislocate dorsally,[8, 18, 20, 21] volar radially,[23, 29, 32] or volar ulnarly.[33, 34, 39] There are even rotary injuries

in which some metacarpals translate dorsally, while others go in a volar direction.[16, 17] Pure dislocation without fracture is rare. The heavy capsular ligaments usually avulse pieces of bone from the carpus as the metacarpals dislocate, and sometimes the metacarpal bases themselves are fractured.

The importance of a complete x-ray work-up cannot be overstated. Anteroposterior projection alone may be misleading, in that the dislocation may be poorly shown, whereas a good oblique or lateral film makes it very obvious (Fig. 14–12).[4, 27] It is not uncommon for traumatic subluxations to be missed.

It is the author's opinion that, for almost all cases, the best treatment is by open reduction and internal fixation with Kirschner

*References 15, 17–19, 26, 37, 41–43, 45–47.

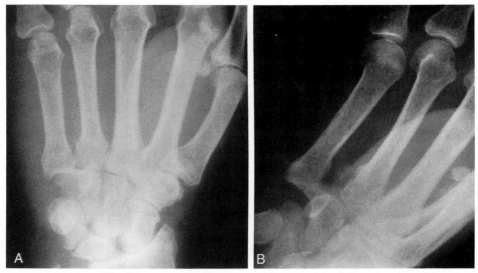

Figure 14–11. *A,* Dislocation of the fifth metacarpal. An 80-year-old man sustained this volar-ulnar dislocation of the fifth metacarpal base in a fall. Treatment was by open reduction and pinning for eight weeks. *B,* The oblique view demonstrates the severity and nature of the dislocation far better than the anteroposterior view seen in Figure 14–11A. (From Gunther SF: Orthop Clin North Am 15:2, 259–277, 1984.)

wires (Fig. 14–13). Closed reduction is usually accomplished easily, but in most cases it is immediately obvious that the reduction is unstable. Even when reduction can be maintained temporarily by careful cast molding, it is difficult to sustain for the full recovery period. Surgical visualization allows anatomic reduction of both the metacarpals and the avulsed carpal fragments. Since these fragments are attached to the capsular ligaments, bone healing should result in nearly normal ligament function. Some surgeons prefer closed reduction and percutaneous pinning,[14, 33, 40] but this method runs the risk of less precise reduction and offers little advantage to the patient, since the hand and arm must be anesthetized anyway.

A dorsal approach is easily made through a transverse skin incision. Mobilization and retraction of the extensor tendons give ready access to the metacarpal bases. It is frequently not necessary to place a Kirschner wire in each dislocated metacarpal, because a pin across one joint will stabilize the adjacent one if the interosseous ligaments at the metacarpal bases are intact (Fig. 14–13C).

The appropriate number of pins is easily determined during surgery. Major carpal fragments can also be reattached by pinning. The pins should be positioned so as to avoid

the extensor tendons, and they should be cut off well below the skin. They can be left in place for 12 weeks, although plaster immobilization should be discontinued after six weeks. Several years' follow-up has demonstrated that this treatment results in excellent hand function. Grip strength returns to normal, and the only residual symptoms are usually mild aching during changes of weather or during extremely heavy work.

C-MC subluxation and even frank dislocation may be overlooked in the setting of multiple injuries from trauma. Appropriate treatment for old injuries is arthrodesis, but of course this is done only if there is enough pain to warrant an operation. An occasional patient has done sufficiently well with no treatment at all (Fig. 14–14).

Fractures of either the metacarpal bases or the carpal bones may predominate over dislocation as the most obvious injuries. Severely comminuted fractures may do best with simple splinting, but major displacements or angulations should be corrected and pinned. There have been many case reports and short series of exceedingly rare fractures and dislocations in the distal carpal row (Fig. 14–15).[24, 30, 44] It is important to know that these fractures may be difficult to define on plain radiographs and that tomograms may be necessary to fully outline the injuries. For example, the hamate bone is

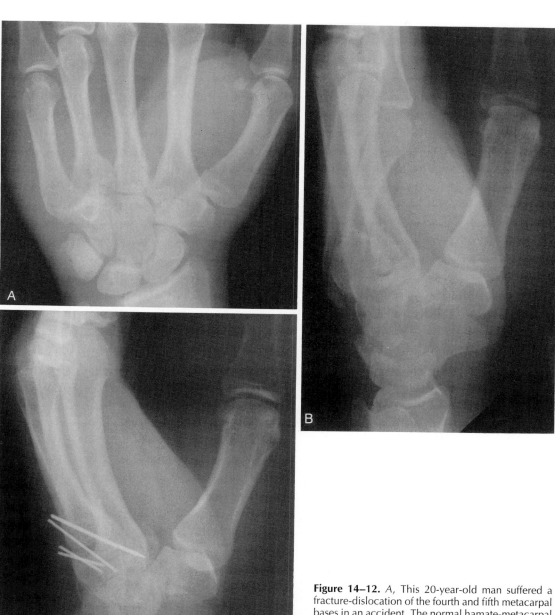

Figure 14–12. *A,* This 20-year-old man suffered a fracture-dislocation of the fourth and fifth metacarpal bases in an accident. The normal hamate-metacarpal joint spaces are not seen on this anteroposterior view. *B,* A lateral view makes the pathology much clearer. Note that a large piece of bone has been avulsed from the dorsal surface of the hamate. *C,* Both the metacarpal bases and the avulsed fragment of the hamate have been pinned back with Kirschner wires. (From Gunther, SF: Orthop Clin North Am 15:2, 259–277, 1984.)

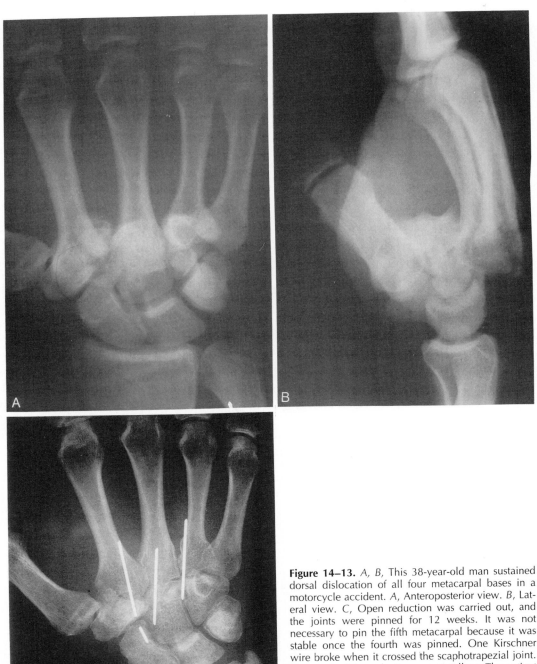

Figure 14–13. A, B, This 38-year-old man sustained dorsal dislocation of all four metacarpal bases in a motorcycle accident. A, Anteroposterior view. B, Lateral view. C, Open reduction was carried out, and the joints were pinned for 12 weeks. It was not necessary to pin the fifth metacarpal because it was stable once the fourth was pinned. One Kirschner wire broke when it crossed the scaphotrapezial joint. The result of the reduction was excellent. The patient was followed off and on for other reasons, until he was killed in another motor vehicle accident five years later. (From Gunther SF: Orthop Clin North Am 15:2, 259–277, 1984.)

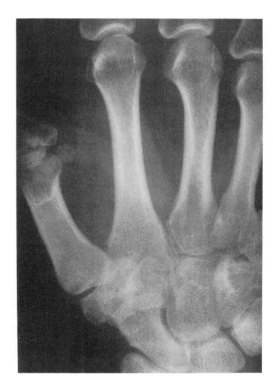

Figure 14–14. This 39-year-old multiple trauma victim from a motor vehicle accident was too sick to complain of hand pain. When this dorsal dislocation of the trapezoid and trapezium was discovered six weeks later, it was irreducible by closed means. The patient did not seem to have pain sufficient to warrant open reduction. Nine months after injury, there was no residual pain whatsoever, but there was an obvious dorsal bump, and grip strength was reduced to 63 percent of that of the uninjured wrist.

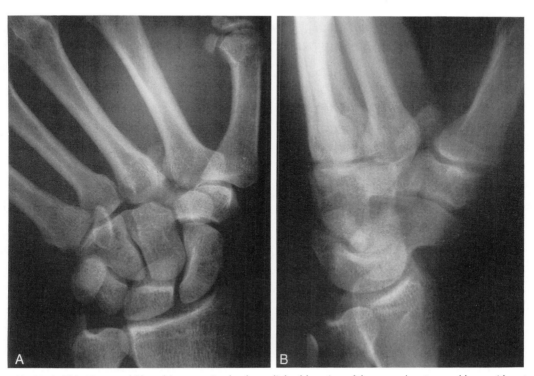

Figure 14–15. *A*, This 35-year-old bus driver sustained volar-radial subluxation of the second metacarpal base with anterior extrusion of a large portion of the articular surface when his steering wheel jolted in an accident and impacted forcibly against the hand. Because the articular surface was severely disrupted, primary arthrodesis was carried out with distal radius bone graft. He returned to bus driving four months later, and continues with an excellent result 39 months later. *B*, Oblique view of the same injury.

References

1. Andress MR, and Peckar VG: Fracture of the hook of the hamate. Br J Radiol 43:141–143, 1970.
2. Artz TD, and Posch JL: The carpometacarpal boss. J Bone Joint Surg 55A:747–752, 1973.
3. Bassoe E, and Bassoe H: The styloid bone and carpe bossu disease. Am J Roentgenol 74:886–888, 1955.
4. Bora FW, and Didizian NH: The treatment of injuries to the carpometacarpal joint of the little finger. J Bone Joint Surg 56A:1459–1463, 1974.
5. Bowen TL: Injuries of the hamate bone. Hand 5:235–238, 1973.
6. Boyes JH: Bunnell's Surgery of the Hand. Philadelphia, JB Lippincott Co, 1964, pp 292–293.
7. Carter RM: Carpal boss: a commonly overlooked deformity of the carpus. J Bone Joint Surg 23:935–940, 1941.
8. Clement BL: Fracture-dislocation of the base of the fifth metacarpal. J Bone Joint Surg 27:498–499, 1945.
9. Cuomo CB, and Watson HK: The carpal boss. Surgical treatment and etiological considerations. Plast Reconstr Surg 63:88–93, 1979.
10. Duke R: Dislocation of the hamate bone: report of a case. J Bone Joint Surg 45B:744, 1963.
11. Gainor BJ: Simultaneous dislocation of the hamate and pisiform: a case report. J Hand Surg 10A:88–90, 1985.
12. Geist DC: Dislocation of the hamate bone. J Bone Joint Surg 21:215–217, 1939.
13. Green WL, and Kilgore ES Jr: Treatment of fifth digit carpometacarpal arthritis with Silastic prosthesis. J Hand Surg 6:510–514, 1981.
14. Greene TL, and Strickland JW: Carpometacarpal dislocations. In Strickland JW, and Steichen JB (eds): Difficult Problems in Hand Surgery. St Louis, CV Mosby Co, 1982, pp. 189–195.
15. Gunther, SF: The carpometacarpal joints. Orthop Clin North Am 15:259–277, 1984.
16. Gunther, SF, and Bruno PD: Divergent dislocation of the carpometacarpal joints: a case report. J Hand Surg 10A:197–201, 1985.
17. Hartwig RH, and Louis DS: Multiple carpometacarpal dislocations. A review of four cases. J Bone Joint Surg 61A:906–908, 1979.
18. Harwin SF, Fox JM, and Sedlin ED: Volar dislocation of the base of the second and third metacarpals. J Bone Joint Surg 57A:849–851, 1975.
19. Hazlet JW: Carpometacarpal dislocations other than the thumb. A report of 11 cases. Can J Surg 11:315–323, 1968.
20. Helal B, and Kavanagh TG: Unstable dorsal fracture-dislocation of the fifth carpometacarpal joint. Injury 9:138–142, 1977.
21. Hsu JD, and Cursti RN: Carpometacarpal dislocations on the ulnar side of the hand. J Bone Joint Surg 52A:927–930, 1970.
22. Joseph RB, Linscheid RL, Dobyns JH, et al: Chronic sprains of the carpometacarpal joints. J Hand Surg 6:172–180, 1981.
23. Ker HR: Dislocation of the fifth carpo-metacarpal joint. J Bone Joint Surg 37B:254–256, 1955.
24. Kopp JR: Isolated palmar dislocation of the trapezoid. J Hand Surg 10A:91–93, 1985.
25. Lamphier TA: Carpal bossing. Arch Surg 81:1013–1015, 1960.
26. Lewis HH: Dislocation of the second metacarpal: report of a case. Clin Orthop 93:253–255, 1973.
27. Lewis RW: Oblique views in roentgenography of the wrist. Am J Roentgenol 50:119–121, 1943.

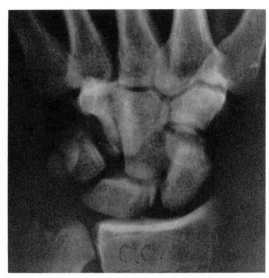

Figure 14–16. The hamate was fractured in the coronal plane and dislocated volarly when this 24-year-old lacrosse player was struck with a stick. He returned to lacrosse nine months after open reduction and pinning of both the hamate and the scapholunate injuries. He is asymptomatic at 7 years.

rarely injured, but it can be dislocated either volarly or dorsally, and it can be fractured in a number of ways (Fig. 14–16).[1, 5, 10–12, 38]

Aside from small dorsal avulsion fractures coincident with metacarpal dislocations, the hamate may be split in two in either the coronal or sagittal plane, or the hamate hook may be avulsed. In particular, the coronal split is most difficult to recognize and very important to reduce and pin. Sometimes, these injuries are more obvious when x-rays are taken with traction or after closed reduction than they are on the initial films.

CONCLUSION

Architectural integrity and stability of the C-MC joints are essential to normal hand and wrist function. With only a few exceptions, it can be said that fractures and dislocations should be accurately reduced and pinned, whereas arthritic conditions should be treated with arthrodesis. Fascial or Silastic arthroplasties seem to be effective at the fifth C-MC joint, but long-term follow-up is not available yet. Surgical excision of a carpal boss or a symptomatic ganglion should include removal of some bone from both the metacarpal and the subjacent carpal bone. Carpometacarpal arthrodesis is a good salvage procedure after failure of treatment in any of these conditions.

28. Littler JW: Hand structure and function. In Symposium on Reconstructive Hand Surgery. St Louis, CV Mosby Co, 1974, pp 3–12.
29. McWhorter GL: Isolated and complete dislocation of the fifth carpometacarpal joint: open operation. Surg Clin Chicago 2:793–796, 1918.
30. Meyn MA, and Roth AM: Isolated dislocation of the trapezoid bone. J Hand Surg 5:602–604, 1980.
31. Millender L: Joint injuries. In Lamb DW, and Kuczynski K (eds): The Practice of Hand Surgery. St Louis, CV Mosby Co, 1981, pp 211–220.
32. Murless BC: Fracture-dislocation of the base of the fifth metacarpal bone. Br J Surg 31:402–404, 1943.
33. Nalebuff EA: Isolated anterior carpometacarpal dislocation of the fifth finger: classification and case report. J Trauma 8:1119–1123, 1968.
34. North ER, and Eaton RG: Volar dislocation of the fifth metacarpal. J Bone Joint Surg 62:657–659, 1980.
35. O'Brien ET: Fractures of the metacarpals and phalanges. In Green DR (ed): Operative Hand Surgery. New York, Churchill Livingstone Inc, 1982, pp 583–635.
36. Petrie PWR, and Lamb DW: Fracture-subluxation of base of fifth metacarpal. Hand 6:82–86, 1974.
37. Picchio A: Sulie lussazioni carpo-metacarpiale. Minerva Chir 9:43–50, 1954.
38. Polivy KD, Millender LH, Newburg A, et al: Fractures of the hook of the hamate—a failure of clinical diagnosis. J Hand Surg 10:101–104, 1985.
39. Roberts N, and Holland CT: Isolated dislocation of the base of the fifth metacarpal. Br J Surg 23:567–571, 1936.
40. Sandzen SC: Fracture of the fifth metacarpal (resembling Bennett's fracture). Hand 5:49–51, 1973.
41. Schrott E, and Wessinghage D: Behandlungsverlauf einer Luxation in den Karpometakarpalgelenken IV and V unter Hamatumbeteiligung. Handchirurgie 15:25–28, 1983.
42. Shephard E, and Solomon DJ: Carpometacarpal dislocation. Report of four cases. J Bone Joint Surg (Br) 42:771–777, 1960.
43. Shorbe HB: Carpometacarpal dislocations. Report of a case. J Bone Joint Surg 20:454–457, 1938.
44. Stein AH: Dorsal dislocation of the lesser multangular bone. J Bone Joint Surg 53A:377–379, 1971.
45. Waugh RL, and Yancey AG: Carpometacarpal dislocations with particular reference to simultaneous dislocation of the bases of the fourth and fifth metacarpals. J Bone Joint Surg 30:397–404, 1948.
46. Weiland AJ, Lister GD, and Villarreal-Rios A: Volar fracture dislocations of the second and third carpometacarpal joints associated with acute carpal tunnel syndrome. J Trauma 16:672–675, 1976.
47. Whitson RO: Carpometacarpal dislocation. A case report. Clin Orthop 6:189–195, 1955.

CHAPTER 15

Nerve Injuries Associated with Wrist Trauma

H. RELTON McCARROLL, JR., M.D.

INTRODUCTION

Orthopedic surgeons examine and treat many patients with wrist trauma or disease. Only a small percentage of these patients have involvement of a peripheral nerve.

The most common cause of nerve pathology at the wrist is open laceration produced by glass, a knife, or a saw. The structures disrupted are the soft tissues, and the focus of attention is on suture of the tendons and nerves.* This article focuses on peripheral nerve problems associated with closed wrist pathology, including fractures.

ANATOMY

In the distal forearm, the median and ulnar nerves are surrounded by soft tissues and are untethered by bone or dense ligamentous structures. Distal to the sublimis muscle belly, the median nerve lies just deep to the fascia and is protected only by the palmaris longus tendon in those patients who have one. Within the carpal tunnel, the median nerve is located in the most volar layer of structures and is easily compressed by the volar carpal ligament. The four unyielding walls of the carpal tunnel limit its volume and guarantee compression of the contained structures if edema or bone fragments occupy part of the available space.

The ulnar nerve enters the palm from the forearm through Guyon's canal. Although the radial, ulnar, and dorsal walls of the canal are firm and unyielding, the palmar ligament is less substantial. Compression within the ulnar canal is possible but less common than compression in the carpal tunnel. At the base of the palm, the ulnar

*For techniques of nerve suture, see reference 16.

nerve divides into two sensory branches as well as the deep motor branch. The sensory branches are minimally tethered by the palmar fascia and are rarely compressed. The deep motor branch is subject to compression over the distal carpal bones as it courses dorsally between the origins of the hypothenar muscles. In this area, it is tethered by unyielding structures.

The distal radius and ulna are separated from the median and ulnar nerves by several layers of soft tissue, including the pronator quadratus muscle belly. These structures provide considerable protection for the nerve when the bones are fractured. At the level of the carpal tunnel, only the wrist capsule separates the carpal bones from the tunnel. The proximity to the bone injury and the unyielding nature of the tunnel increase the incidence of nerve symptoms with injuries of the carpus. The radial nerve is subcutaneous at the level of the wrist. Although it is in close proximity to the distal radius, it is not commonly injured except by lacerations.[7, 8]

MEDIAN NERVE INJURIES ASSOCIATED WITH COLLES' FRACTURE

Reports of large series of patients with Colles' fractures suggest an incidence of median nerve involvement of approximately 0.2 to 3.2 percent.[2, 9] The rate varies, depending on what level of symptoms is defined as significant and the duration of follow-up.

Median nerve injury occurring with a Colles' fracture (laceration or contusion) is quite rare, but should be considered when the fracture is compounded.[1] Most early me-

212

dian nerve problems are related to the progressive edema and hematoma that follow injury and to reduction of the fracture. During the healing phase, exuberant fracture callus, especially in the presence of persistent bone deformity, can result in median nerve symptoms. The residual scarring and thickening that follow healing can eventually result in a carpal tunnel syndrome at a much later date; this is known as tardy median nerve palsy.[6, 30]

Fracture Treatment

The relationship between median nerve symptoms and the position of immobilization used to maintain reduction of a fracture is of particular relevance in cases involving Colles' fractures. Numerous authors have implicated the use of extreme pronation, ulnar deviation, and palmar flexion (the "Cotton-Loder position") as contributory causes of median nerve compression.[1, 22, 23] This is a major reason orthopedists now use a more moderate degree of wrist flexion in immobilizing Colles' fractures if a good reduction cannot be maintained in a neutral position.

Several experimental studies have demonstrated compression of the median nerve with the wrist flexed or extended.[1, 3] Bauman and associates measured the pressure in the carpal tunnel of a patient with a comminuted Colles' fracture and found it elevated over normal controls, even in neutral position.[3] Indeed, in two of the four Colles' fractures they reported with median nerve symptoms, the fracture was immobilized in a neutral position using a pins and plaster technique. Thus, although the trend away from extreme positions of immobilization should decrease the incidence of early median nerve symptoms, it is unlikely to eliminate the problem.

If significant neurologic symptoms are present following closed reduction and plaster cast immobilization, the surgeon's first response should be to split the cast and ensure that the dressings are not too tight. If this does not improve the neurologic symptoms, the wrist should be brought to a neutral position. It is unwise to treat the fracture while ignoring the risk of a prolonged median nerve palsy.[31] Carpal tunnel release may be indicated for profound symptoms that do not respond to the preceding measures.

Gelberman and associates have recommended use of wick catheter pressure measurements to differentiate between median nerve symptoms secondary to compression and symptoms caused by nerve contusion or laceration.[11] Although the technique provides a quantitative measure of the degree of compression, it has not been proved to have predictive value for the future clinical course. The clinician needs to know whether the elevated pressure and the associated symptoms will persist and produce major functional problems in spite of nonsurgical treatment. Thus, the clinician must still use his judgment to decide whether carpal tunnel release is indicated. Whether this technique will become part of accepted clinical practice remains to be determined.

CASE REPORT

Neurologic symptoms can also result from displacement of the fracture fragments, compounded by surrounding hematoma and swelling.

A 42-year-old, right-handed attorney fell forcefully on his outstretched left hand (Fig. 15–1A). Paresthesias were immediately felt in the median nerve distribution. Sensation was impaired but not lost, and thenar muscle function remained intact. Roentgenograms of the affected wrist showed a very distal fracture of the radius, with the distal bone fragment displaced in the direction of the median nerve.

Open reduction, internal fixation, and release of the carpal tunnel were performed four days after the injury (Fig. 15–1B). The median nerve paresthesias resolved immediately following surgery. Although the pins were inserted through a volar incision, their greater length was left on the dorsal aspect, and they were removed at six weeks after surgery through a dorsal incision. The patient's fracture healed, and he has normal median nerve function.

Associated Sudeck's Atrophy

Although Sudeck's atrophy can occur after many different injuries, it is relatively common after Colles' fractures and accounts for some of the most troublesome management problems after that injury. Several authors have commented on an apparent connection between numbness, pain, prolonged disability and a poor functional result or the possibility that median nerve compression may be a precursor of Sudeck's atrophy.[22, 23] The clearest exposition of this thesis is

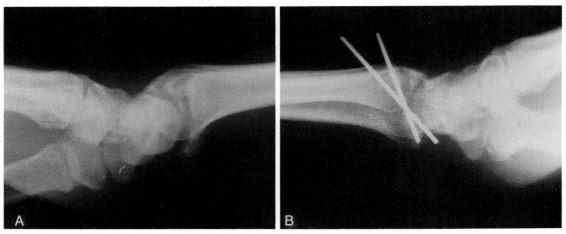

Figure 15–1. *A,* Displaced fracture of the volar lip of the radius. The displaced fragment and associated hematoma compressed the median nerve, producing paresthesias. *B,* Following open reduction and internal fixation of the fracture fragment and carpal tunnel release, the paresthesias resolved promptly. (Case courtesy of Dr. H. Edward Cabaud.)

Stein's report of six patients (four with Colles' fractures) with signs of Sudeck's atrophy, who demonstrated definite improvement after decompression of the median nerve at the carpal tunnel.[32] Although this relationship is not universally accepted, it is certainly worth examining patients for signs of nerve compression at the carpal tunnel when they have early complaints and symptoms suggesting Sudeck's atrophy. The severity of the functional deficit that follows Sudeck's atrophy justifies removing the immobilization to obtain an EMG and a nerve conduction study. Although median nerve decompression may not circumvent all incipient cases of Sudeck's atrophy, its performance is worth considering[10] in all patients.

CASE REPORT

A 67-year-old homemaker fell on her outstretched left hand, sustaining a Colles' fracture of the wrist. A closed reduction was performed and the fracture immobilized in a plaster cast. The cast was split at 24 hours after reduction. Nine days after injury, the fracture was well reduced, but the patient had stiffness of the fingers and numbness in the median nerve distribution. In spite of elevation and supervised exercises, pain and numbness persisted.

One month following the fracture, the bivalved cast was removed for an electromyogram (EMG) and a nerve conduction study. These studies documented severe prolongation of the median nerve sensory and motor

latencies and partial denervation of the superficial thenar muscles.

Six weeks following the fracture, a carpal tunnel release was performed. After release of the volar carpal ligament, the median nerve was observed to be slightly flattened and discolored. The skeletal structure of the carpal tunnel was normal on palpation. Although the operative wound and the Colles' fracture healed well, there was poor progress in regaining finger and wrist motion. The severe pain and sensitivity did subside, however, over the two months following carpal tunnel release.

Three months after the carpal tunnel release, custom-made dynamic splints were fabricated, and joint-specific range-of-motion exercises were instituted (Fig. 15–2A and B). This concentrated program of hand therapy produced a gradual improvement in finger motion and an improvement in the subjective complaints of stiffness and pain. After two and a half months of therapy, the patient was able to begin functional use of the involved hand (Fig. 15–2C and D).

This case report emphasizes several important points. My clinical experience with Sudeck's atrophy or sympathetic dystrophy suggests that there is a consistent natural history to this disease process. The patients generally have severe, increasing or stable pain for a period of three to four months, followed by a longer period of decreasing pain and increasing motion. The total clinical course lasts about one year and then stabilizes, leaving a variable degree of permanent stiffness. The rapid improvement in the severe pain and hypersensitivity after the carpal tunnel release suggests that median nerve compression was causally related to the development of the Sudeck's atrophy.

In this case study, the patient's pain improved much more rapidly than I have come to expect with this syndrome. The syndrome is well documented in this case by the positive results of the EMG and by the findings of the nerve conduction study.

A second important point is the difficulty in regaining joint motion once the fingers become stiff as a result of Sudeck's atrophy. The assistance of hand therapists who have specialized training in hand and finger exercises and who are capable of fabricating customized, dynamic splints is invaluable in the rehabilitation of these patients.

TREATMENT OF SUDECK'S ATROPHY

Sudeck's atrophy is also observed after trauma that is unlikely to produce median nerve compression. It is well known that the syndrome can follow blunt trauma without fracture, which produces edema on the dorsal wrist and hand.

A number of therapies have been recommended for breaking the cycle of pain and swelling and allowing resumption of exercise and use of the hand and fingers. These varied approaches are well reviewed by Wilson.[34]

Most therapies are directed toward interruption of the sympathetic nerve pathways that are thought to mediate much of the process. They include stellate ganglion blocks, intravenous guanethidine,[13] oral phenoxybenzamine[12], and surgical sympathectomy. Other methods of pain reduction include injection of local anesthetic at trigger points, desensitization procedures, and use of a transcutaneous nerve stimulator. Reduction of edema is also a major goal.[19]

It is important to recognize that the goal of these therapies is to allow resumption of exercise and functional use of the affected parts. Regardless of the therapeutic approach chosen, a program of active use and exercise is indispensible.

MEDIAN NERVE INJURIES ASSOCIATED WITH CARPAL AND METACARPAL INJURY

Acute compression of the median nerve has been very common in reported series of

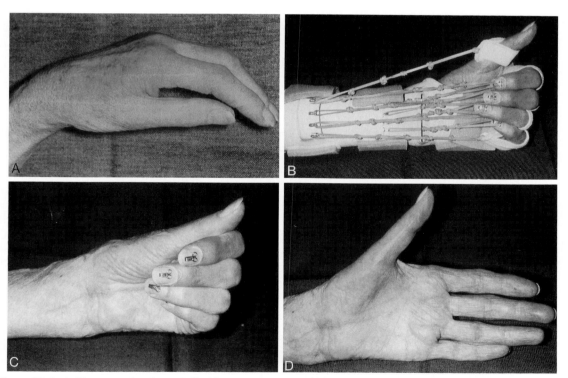

Figure 15–2. *A*, Three months after a Colles' fracture, a 67-year-old homemaker had severe restriction of finger motion. The photograph demonstrates maximum active and passive finger flexion. *B*, A custom dynamic splint facilitated return of motion at all finger joint levels. After two and a half months of vigorous hand therapy, the active range of finger motion was markedly improved. *C*, Active flexion. *D*, Active extension.

lunate dislocations.[17, 26] Most of the cases have required treatment of the dislocation only, and the nerve has recovered without specific treatment. Rawlings[26] did point out a relationship between the duration of nerve symptoms and persistent disability.

Carpal injuries are a common precursor of "tardy median nerve palsy." Both the thickening and scarring that follow a carpal fracture or dislocation and the alteration of the volume of the carpal tunnel that results from imperfect realignment conspire over time to compress the median nerve. In spite of Colles' fractures being more common than carpal injuries, Phalen[25] reported equal numbers of carpal tunnel syndromes resulting from the two types of injuries.

ULNAR NERVE INJURIES ASSOCIATED WITH WRIST INJURIES

Ulnar nerve injury is not commonly associated with fractures and dislocations about the wrist.[14, 18, 33, 35] Both laceration and compression of the ulnar nerve have been reported and are more common with carpal injuries than with distal forearm injuries. Considering the proximity of the nerve to the carpal bones, the rarity of compression problems must relate to the fact that the ulnar nerve is not as firmly tethered as the median nerve is in the carpal tunnel. Despite the fact that many of the cases initially have a complete ulnar nerve palsy, most of those described have shown recovery with treatment of the fracture only.

Ulnar nerve palsy, especially that involving the deep motor branch, has been described as occurring after various vocational and avocational activities. My own experience includes cases related to crutch walking, kayaking, pressing large ledgers on a copy machine, and playing handball. In many instances, the symptoms are acute and the precipitating activity can be eliminated. These patients usually do quite well and do not require surgery but only the elimination of the external pressure. One patient who played handball had had symptoms for a year and a half and continued to play the game regularly. At that advanced stage of repeated injury, neither neurolysis nor changing sports was helpful. At the time of surgery, his nerve was noted to be severely scarred and abnormal over a 2-cm segment.

ULNAR NERVE COMPRESSION BY GANGLIA

Although the ganglion must be one of humankind's most common afflictions, it is a rare cause of nerve compression. Several authors have reported series of ganglia compressing the deep branch of the ulnar nerve as it courses from Guyon's canal to the level of the deep arch.[5, 28, 29] The sensory branches of the ulnar nerve are usually not compressed, resulting in a pure motor lesion. Unlike most ganglia, which are palpable, these are too deep to diagnose pre-operatively. Because this is a curable lesion, patients with an unexplained deep motor branch paralysis should have the base of the palm explored. Successful removal of these ganglia requires reflection of part of the origin of the hypothenar muscles for adequate exposure.

CASE REPORT

A 59-year-old contractor and carpenter sought medical attention because of symptoms in his left hand. He had noted muscle wasting in the left hand over a two- to three-year period, with slow progression of the atrophy. He denied any alteration of sensibility. He finally sought medical attention because the atrophy had progressed to the point that, with firm pinch, the thumb was unstable and the proximal joint hyperextended. He gave a history of a number of minor injuries, but none that seemed likely to have produced a progressive problem. He did not admit to any repetitive activities that seemed likely to compress the motor branch of the ulnar nerve.

Examination was normal except for the muscles innervated by the deep motor branch of the ulnar nerve. The hypothenar muscles functioned normally, but there was complete paralysis of the adductor pollicis and deep head of the short flexor muscle of the thumb. He had a markedly positive Froment's sign, and with firm pinch the proximal joint of the thumb collapsed, causing pain. He was unable to cross the index and long fingers. Key pinch strength was about one third that of the normal right hand.

An EMG and a nerve conduction study showed a severe deficit in the deep motor branch of the ulnar nerve; the other findings were normal. Exploration of Guyon's canal and the base of the palm demonstrated a large ganglion originating from the distal

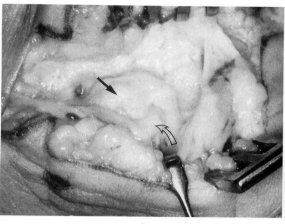 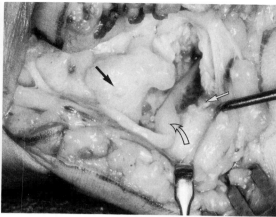

A   **B**

Figure 15–3. *A,* Ganglion from the triquetral-hamate articulation protrudes through the hypothenar muscle origin. The deep motor branch of the ulnar nerve courses around the mass and is compressed as it penetrates the base of the muscle. *Black arrow* = ganglion; *white arrow* = neuroma. *B,* After release of the radial origin of the hypothenar muscles, a neuroma-in-continuity is visible proximal to the tendinous origin. *Black arrow* = ganglion; *open arrow* = neuroma; *white arrow* = tendinous muscle origin. (From McCarroll HR: Orthop Clin North Am 15:279–287, 1984.)

ulnar carpus and compressing the deep motor branch of the ulnar nerve between the heads of the hypothenar muscles (Fig. 15–3A). A large neuroma in continuity was visible proximal to the fascial band compressing the nerve (Fig. 15–3B). The ganglion was excised and the nerve freed.

When the patient was last evaluated seven months following surgery, there had been good return of function in the intrinsic muscles of the fingers, but muscle power had not yet returned to the thumb.

ULNAR ARTERY THROMBOSIS

Trauma to the base of the palm, as can happen when using the hand as a mallet, can result in thrombosis of the ulnar artery as it passes over the carpal bones in Guyon's canal. The resulting symptoms are often a combination of those produced by diminished blood supply and compression of the adjacent ulnar nerve. The standard treatment for this condition has been ligation and resection of the thrombosed segment of the artery. This temporarily sympathectomizes the ulnar portion of the hand, interfering with the vasospastic component of the problem, and also decompresses the ulnar nerve. Reconstruction of the artery using a vein graft is an appealing approach, but has not been shown to improve the result.

RADIAL SENSORY NERVE INJURIES

Most radial sensory nerve problems are related to open injuries, including a number that are iatrogenic in origin.[21]

There are several reports that implicate either a tight wrist watch strap or the application of handcuffs as the cause of a transient neuropathy.[4, 27] Law enforcement officers are not the only ones to use handcuffs. We have seen several cases related to the friendly application of handcuffs by sexual partners. The patients complain of numbness and tingling in the distribution of the radial sensory nerve. All of our cases have resolved completely in about three months without specific treatment other than elimination of the external compression.

Diagnosis

Nerve compression problems that develop long after a wrist injury differ from the idiopathic syndromes only in roentgenographic findings and history. The clinical, EMG, and nerve conduction test findings are well defined and usually allow accurate diagnosis.[25] In the presence of acute trauma and the accompanying pain and swelling plus the often necessary plaster cast, diagnosis of a nerve injury can be very difficult. However, several facts can be very useful.

It is important to include a brief check of nerve function in the initial evaluation. The few patients with laceration of the nerve will have a deficit even if seen very soon after the injury. Nerve laceration will also result in loss of motor as well as sensory function. The loss of sweating that occurs after nerve division is especially useful as an indicator in pediatric cases, since the other tests cannot be performed or the results are unreliable in children. Most patients with compression of the nerve will have intact motor function, at least when tested clinically.[23]

Reduction of a fracture or dislocation can represent a second traumatic event, at least as far as the integrity of the nerve is concerned. A recheck of nerve function will detect those nerves with diminished sensibility because of entanglement at the fracture site.

The number of patients who are categorized as having sensory deficit will depend on the sensory tests used. Sensitive tests such as the plastic ridge device will detect diminished sensibility in the presence of swelling without a fracture or dislocation. Less sensitive tests are more appropriate in the presence of acute trauma.

Two discriminative tests seem to provide useful information and are easily performed. In the initial test, the examiner asks the patient if he or she can tell the *difference* between touch and scratch. The touch is done with the pulp of the examiner's finger and the scratch by light application of the examiner's fingernail. If the patient can tell the difference and the two activities feel normal to him or her, the nerve is probably functioning well. All presently available tests of sensibility are subjective; they require the cooperation of the patient and some will be unable to provide useful answers.

If the fingernail test is abnormal, further testing for sharp and dull discrimination with a safety pin is justified. Patients who cannot differentiate sharp and dull should be considered to have severe nerve impairment.

INDICATIONS FOR EXPLORATION

The surgeon faces an insoluble dilemma when trying to decide whether a particular patient would benefit from exploration of the median or ulnar nerve after wrist trauma. Statistically, most of these lesions resolve with treatment of the bone injury alone. This would suggest caution in undertaking surgery. For a particular individual, however, if the nerve is too damaged or compressed to recover spontaneously, the potential for recovery is better with relatively early surgery. Unfortunately, none of the available tests clearly identify this situation.

Although exploration and decompression of the median nerve at the carpal tunnel is not subject to many complications, it can force a change in the preferred technique of fracture treatment. After opening the volar carpal ligament, the flexor tendons and median nerve must be prevented from bowstringing. This means that the wrist cannot be immobilized in too great a degree of flexion.[15] After decompression, some fractures require pins and plaster or an external fixator for reduction and immobilization, whereas in the absence of nerve decompression, a plaster cast is usually adequate.

The following guidelines are suggested in managing nerve problems associated with wrist trauma:

1. An immediate, complete nerve lesion should be treated by closed reduction of the fracture or dislocation. If the nerve does not show improvement fairly promptly, exploration is justified.

2. If a nerve lesion develops after closed reduction or is much worse after reduction, explore the nerve.

3. If the fracture or dislocation requires open reduction, strongly consider exploration of the nerve at the same time, even with an incomplete nerve lesion.[24]

4. In the presence of disproportionate pain, swelling, and tingling suggesting Sudeck's atrophy, split the cast and padding; in the absence of prompt improvement, change the wrist position to neutral. If symptoms persist, consider carpal tunnel release, even if the clinical picture is not entirely typical of nerve compression.

5. A partial nerve lesion should be treated expectantly. If improvement does not begin in the first week following reduction, consider exploration of the nerve. Exploration is especially relevant if the deficit is in an important sensory or motor area.

Exploration of the ulnar nerve should include Guyon's canal as well as the fracture site. Exploration of the median nerve should include the fracture area as well as the carpal tunnel; compression by proximal hematoma has been described and would be missed if only the carpal tunnel were explored.[20]

CONCLUSION

Nerve injuries are a rare accompaniment of orthopedic wrist problems; however, they can have a profound influence on the functional end result and should, therefore, receive careful attention at all stages of treatment. A guideline for surgical release of the involved nerves is included. When a nerve injury is severe, the final result depends as much on careful management of the nerve problem as on treatment of the underlying orthopedic disorder.

References

1. Abbott LC, and Saunders JB de CM: Injuries of the median nerve in fractures of the lower end of the radius. Surg Gynecol Obstet 57:507–516, 1933.
2. Bacorn RW, and Kurtze JF: Colles' fracture: a study of two thousand cases from the New York State Workman's Compensation Board. J Bone Joint Surg 35A:643–658, 1953.
3. Bauman TD, Gelberman RH, Mubarak SJ, et al: The acute carpal tunnel syndrome. Clin Orthop 156: 151–156, 1981.
4. Braidwood AS: Superficial radial neuropathy. J Bone Joint Surg 57B:380–383, 1975.
5. Brooks DM: Nerve compression by simple ganglia: a review of thirteen collected cases. J Bone Joint Surg 34B:391–400, 1952.
6. Cannon BW, and Love JG: Tardy median palsy; median neuritis; median thenar neuritis amenable to surgery. Surgery 20:210–216, 1946.
7. Cooney WP, Dobyns JH, and Linscheid RL: Complications of Colles' fractures. J Bone Joint Surg 62A:613–619, 1980.
8. Cotton FJ: Wrist fractures: disabilities following restorative operations. Trans Am Surg Assoc 40:289–300, 1922.
9. Frykman G: Fracture of the distal radius including sequelae—shoulder-hand-finger syndrome, disturbance in the distal radio-ulnar joint and impairment of nerve function: a clinical and experimental study. Acta Orthop Scand (Suppl) 108:1–153, 1967.
10. Gaul JS: Letter to the editor. Orthopaedics 1:252, 1978.
11. Gelberman RH, Szabo RM, and Mortensen WW: Carpal tunnel pressures and wrist position in patients with Colles' fractures. J Trauma 24:747–749, 1984.
12. Ghostine SY, Comair YG, Turner DM, et al: Phenoxybenzamine in the treatment of causalgia. J Neurosurg 60:1263–1268, 1984.
13. Hannington-Kiff JG: Intravenous regional sympathetic block with guanethidine. Lancet 1:1019–1020, 1974.
14. Howard FM: Ulnar nerve palsy in wrist fractures. J Bone Joint Surg 43A:1197–1201, 1961.
15. Inglis AE: Two unusual operative complications in the carpal tunnel syndrome. J Bone Joint Surg 62A:1208–1209, 1980.
16. Jewitt DL, and McCarroll HR (eds): Nerve Repair and Regeneration: Its Clinical and Experimental Basis. St Louis, CV Mosby Co, 1980.
17. Jones RW: Primary nerve lesions in injuries of the elbow and wrist. J Bone Joint Surg 12:121–140, 1930.
18. Kornberg M, Aulicino PL, and DuPuy TE: Laceration of the ulnar nerve with a closed fracture of the distal radius and ulna. Orthopaedics 6:729–731, 1983.
19. Leach RE, and Clawson DK: Continuous elevation by spica cast in treatment of reflex sympathetic dystrophy. J Bone Joint Surg 56A:416–418, 1974.
20. Lewis MH: Median nerve decompression after Colles' fracture. J Bone Joint Surg 60B:195–196, 1978.
21. Linscheid RL: Injuries to radial nerve at wrist. Arch Surg 91:942–946, 1965.
22. Lynch AC, and Lipscomb PR: The carpal tunnel syndrome and Colles' fractures. JAMA 185:363–366, 1963.
23. Meadoff N: Median nerve injuries in fractures in the region of the wrist. Calif Med 70:252–256, 1949.
24. Mullen GB, and Lloyd GJ: Complete carpal disruption of the hand. Hand 12:39–43, 1980.
25. Phalen GS: The carpal tunnel syndrome: Seventeen years' experience in diagnosis and treatment of six hundred fifty-four hands. J Bone Joint Surg 48A:211–228, 1966.
26. Rawlings ID: The management of dislocations of the carpal lunate. Injury 12:319–330, 1981.
27. Rayan GM, and Foster DE: Handcuff compression neuropathy. Orthop Rev 13:527–530, 1984.
28. Seddon HJ: Carpal ganglion as a cause of paralysis of the deep branch of the ulnar nerve. J Bone Joint Surg 34B:386–390, 1952.
29. Shea JD, and McClain EJ: Ulnar nerve compression syndromes at and below the wrist. J Bone Joint Surg 51A:1095–1103, 1969.
30. Short DW: Tardy median nerve palsy following injury. Glasgow Med J 32:315–320, 1951.
31. Sponsel KH, and Palm ET: Carpal tunnel syndrome following Colles' fracture. Surg Gynecol Obstet 121:1252–1256, 1965.
32. Stein AH: The relation of median nerve compression to Sudeck's syndrome. Surg Gynecol Obstet 115:713–720, 1962.
33. Vance RM, and Gelberman RH: Acute ulnar neuropathy with fractures at the wrist. J Bone Joint Surg 60A:962–965, 1978.
34. Wilson RL: Management of pain following peripheral nerve injuries. Orthop Clin North Am 12:343–359, 1981.
35. Zoega H: Fracture of the lower end of the radius with ulnar nerve palsy. J Bone Joint Surg 48B:514–516, 1966.

CHAPTER 16

The Distal Radioulnar Joint

ANDREW K. PALMER, M.D.

For some clinicians, the distal radioulnar joint represents the "new frontier" of hand surgery; however, because of the difficulties related to the diagnosis and treatment of a distal radioulnar joint disorder, for most it remains the "low back pain" of upper extremity afflictions. This frustration need not exist. With a clear concept of the normal anatomy and biomechanics of the distal radioulnar joint, the clinical and radiographic evaluations of afflictions of this joint become less arduous, and the diagnosis becomes clearer. Once the diagnosis is made, treatment is frequently relatively straightforward.

ANATOMY

The convex distal ulna is covered with articular cartilage for 270° of its total circumference (Fig. 16–1).[2–4] It varies in proximal to distal height from 5 to 8 mm.[13] It articulates with the sigmoid or ulnar notch of the radius. The concave semicylindrical sigmoid notch has three distinct margins—dorsal, palmar, and distal (Fig. 16–2). Distally, its dorsopalmar distance is 1.5 cm and proximally 1 cm. The sigmoid notch angles distally and ulnarly at approximately 20°. The articular surface (the seat) of the ulnar head correspondingly angles distally and ulnarly at about 20° (Fig. 16–3).[1] Distally, beneath the triangular fibrocartilage complex (TFCC), the flat ulnar head is partially covered with articular cartilage.[29] This articular area is separated from the ulnar styloid by the fovea—an area rich in vascular foramen, around which the TFCC inserts into the distal ulna.

Descriptions of the ligamentous anatomy in the area of the distal radioulnar joint have historically been confusing.* The extensor retinaculum wraps around the distal ulna to insert on the palmar aspect of the carpus and soft tissues but has no real attachment to the ulna itself (Fig. 16–4). The extensor carpi ulnaris tendon lies beneath the retinaculum and is held to the distal ulna not by the retinaculum but by the extensor carpi ulnaris subsheath (Fig. 16–5). The extensor retinaculum provides very little stability to the ulnar head.[20, 21, 32]

The triangular fibrocartilage complex (TFCC) is a term that has been introduced by Palmer and Werner[20] to describe the ligamentous and cartilaginous structure that suspends the distal radius and the ulnar carpus from the distal ulna. The TFCC incorporates the poorly defined dorsal and volar radioulnar ligaments, the ulnar collateral ligament, and the meniscus homologue,

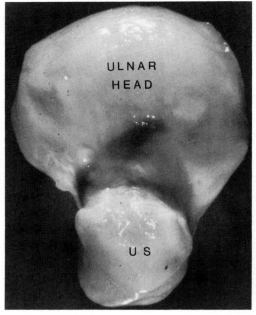

Figure 16–1. The ulnar head is covered with articular cartilage over 270° of its 360° circumference. US = ulnar styloid.

---

*References 2, 6–10, 12, 14, 19, 21, 24, 29, 31–33.

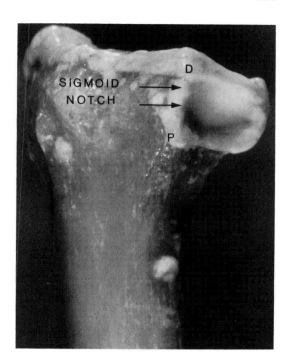

Figure 16–2. The sigmoid notch of the radius has three distinct margins—dorsal, palmar and distal. The proximal margin is indistinct. D = distal; P = proximal.

as well as the clearly defined articular disk and extensor carpi ulnaris sheath (Fig. 16–6). The complex arises from the ulnar aspect of the lunate fossa of the radius (Fig. 16–7). It courses toward the ulna, where it inserts in the fovea at the base of the ulnar styloid. It flows distally, joined by fibers arising from the ulnar aspect of the ulnar styloid (the ulnar collateral ligament), becomes thickened (the meniscus homologue), and inserts distally into the lunate, triquetrum, hamate, and base of the fifth metacarpal. Dorsally, there is a weak attachment of the TFCC to the carpus, except dorsolat-

erally, where the complex incorporates the floor of the sheath of the extensor carpi ulnaris. Volarly, the TFCC is very strongly attached to the lunotriquetral interosseous ligament and to the triquetrum (the ulnotriquetral ligament), with weaker inconstant attachments to the lunate (the ulnolunate ligament), the hamate, and the base of the fifth metacarpal. The dorsal and volar aspects of the horizontal portion of the TFCC are thickened (average, 4 to 5 mm). I believe that these thickenings represent what others have termed the dorsal and volar radioulnar ligaments.[20]

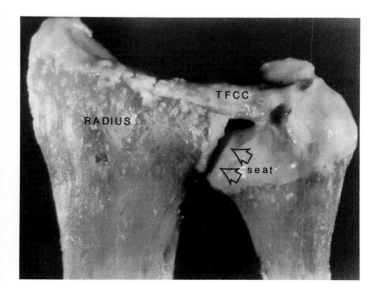

Figure 16–3. The distal radioulnar articulation angles distally and ulnarly at approximately 20°. TFCC = triangular fibrocartilage complex.

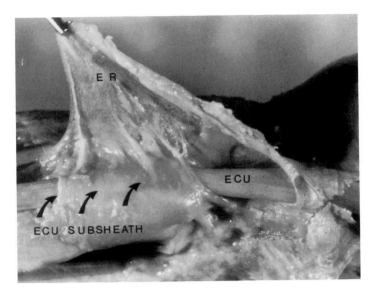

Figure 16–4. The extensor retinaculum (ER) has been reflected, revealing the extensor carpi ulnaris (ECU) held to the distal ulna by the ECU subsheath. (From Palmer AK, Skahen J, Werner FW, et al: J Hand Surg (Brit) 10B:11–16, 1985.)

BIOMECHANICS

Kinematics

Forearm rotation of up to 150° occurs at the distal radioulnar joint, with the distal radius and its fixed distal member (the hand) rotating about the ulnar head.[2, 4, 28, 30] The ulnar head is not, as was once thought, immobile during rotation of the forearm. Modest lateral movement of the ulnar head in a direction opposite that taken by the distal radius of up to 8° or 9° during pronation and supination has been demonstrated by Ray et al.[28] Bunnell[6] and others and, most recently, Ekenstam[1] and Hagert have shown that the ulnar head moves dorsally in the sigmoid notch during pronation and palmarly during supination. This is possible because of the different radii of curvature of the sigmoid notch and the corresponding surface of the ulnar head (the seat). In mid-forearm rotation, there is articular contact between 60° and 80° of the convex ulnar head and the sigmoid notch.[1] In full pronation (Fig. 16–8) as well as in full supination (Fig. 16–9), the ulnar head is nearly completely uncovered, and there is little contact between the ulnar head and the sigmoid notch; contact occurs in full supination on the volar aspect of the sigmoid notch and in full pronation on the dorsal aspect of the sigmoid notch.

Two independent studies by Epner et al[11] and Palmer et al[22] have shown that the ulnar head moves distally in relation to the distal

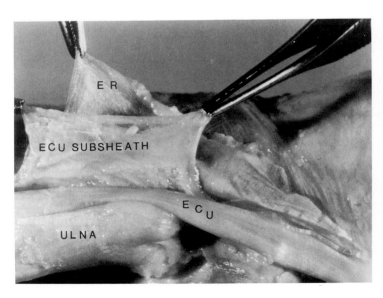

Figure 16–5. The sixth dorsal compartment, containing the extensor carpi ulnaris (ECU), is formed by the ECU subsheath and lies beneath the extensor retinaculum (ER). (From Palmer AK, Skahen J, Werner FW, et al: J Hand Surg (Brit) 10B:11–16, 1985.)

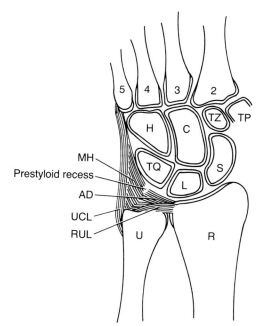

Figure 16–6. The component parts of the TFCC: the meniscus homologue (MH), prestyloid recess, articular disc (AD), ulnar collateral ligament (UCL), and radioulnar ligaments (RUL). H = hamate; C = capitate; TZ = trapezoid; TP = trapezium; S = scaphoid; L = lunate; TQ = triquetrum; R = radius; U = ulna. (From Palmer AK, and Werner FW: J Hand Surg 6:153–162, 1981.)

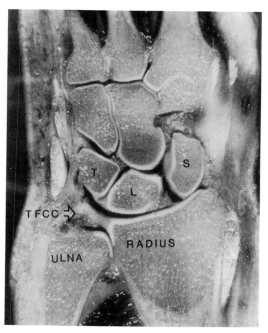

Figure 16–7. The triangular fibrocartilage complex (TFCC) suspends the radius and carpus above the distal ulna. T = triquetrum; L = lunate; S = scaphoid. (From Palmer AK, and Werner FW: J Hand Surg 6:153–162, 1981.)

radius in pronation and proximally in supination, thus altering apparent ulnar variance. For this reason, measurements of ulnar variance should always be performed with the wrist in a standardized position. We have found that x-rays of the wrist in a position of neutral forearm rotation are easy to obtain and reproduce.[22]

In summary, the radius rotates about the distal ulna during forearm rotation as the forearm axis moves laterally in space. The

ulnar head normally glides in the sigmoid notch of the radius from a dorsal distal position to a volar proximal position as the forearm moves from full pronation to full supination.

Kinetics

The exact weights of the loads borne by the normal wrist joint during activities of daily living are not known but are presumed to be great. Brand and colleagues[5] have calculated that the potential tension for producing

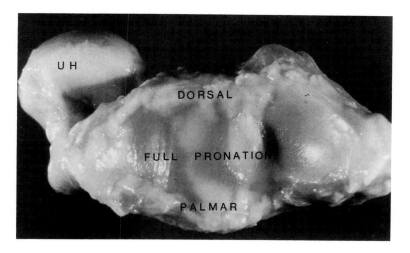

Figure 16–8. In full pronation, the ulnar head becomes nearly totally uncovered dorsally. UH = ulnar head.

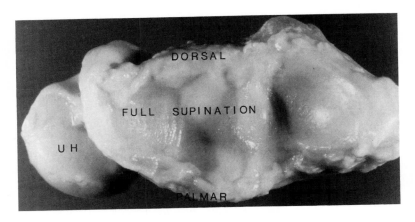

Figure 16–9. In full supination, the ulnar head becomes nearly totally uncovered volarly. UH = ulnar head.

forces of muscles in the arm is approximately 500 kg.

Palmer and colleagues[20, 23, 35] have studied cadaver forearms biomechanically in order to evaluate the role of the distal ulna and the TFCC in load transmission. Approximately 82 percent of the load applied in the experimental model is borne by the distal radius and 18 percent by the distal ulna. Removal of the TFCC decreases the load borne by the distal ulna by approximately 12 percent, and removal of the distal ulna totally unloads the distal ulna (Table 16–1). Radial deviation of the wrist decreases, and ulnar deviation increases, the load borne by the ulna.

These data suggest that the radius carries approximately 80 percent of the axial load of the forearm through its articulation with the lateral carpus, and that the ulna carries approximately 20 percent through its articulation with the medial carpus (via the TFCC). Changes in the forearm-wrist unit of the kind that might been seen if the TFCC or if the distal ulna were excised (Darrach's procedure) could be expected to dramatically and unphysiologically increase radial loading.

Palmer et al[20, 21] have further shown that although the extensor retinaculum, the pro-

nator quadratus, and the geometric shape of the sigmoid notch and the ulnar head all contribute to the stability of the distal radioulnar joint, the TFCC is the major stabilizer of this joint.

Surgically Altered Kinetics

ULNAR VARIANCE

Ulnar lengthening or radial shortening is now commonly used in the treatment of Kienböck's disease, and ulnar shortening is used in the treatment of degenerative perforations of the TFCC.[2, 27] These surgical procedures have been evaluated in terms of their effect on forearm load transmission. The load borne by the ulna was measured as the ulna was lengthened by 2.5 mm at 0.5 mm increments and shortened by 2.5 mm at 0.5 mm increments. Changes in the length of the ulna resulted in dramatic changes in the force borne by the distal ulna. Ulnar shortening of 2.5 mm resulted in a drop of the force borne by the distal ulna from an average of 18 percent of the total force to 4 percent. Ulnar lengthening of 2.5 mm resulted in an increase in the force borne by the distal ulna to 42 percent of the total forearm force (Table 16–2). A similar though less dramatic variation was seen when the ulna was shortened and lengthened in the wrist in which the TFCC had been surgically removed.[35]

The actual pressures between the articular surface of the radius and the ulna (TFCC) and the carpus have been measured by the use of Fuji Pre-Scale Pressure-Sensitive Film (PSF).[23, 34] The average maximum pressures developed at three locations for three ulnar lengths in nine fresh specimens are given in Table 16–3. These locations are the articulations between the ulna and the lunate, the

Table 16–1. **PERCENT AXIAL LOAD***

	Intact Wrist	TFCC Excised	Distal Ulna Excised
Radius (percent)	81.6	93.8	100
Ulna (percent)	18.4	6.2	0

*Axial load borne by the radius and ulna as a percentage of the total load (100 percent), 1983 data. (From Palmer AK, and Werner FW: Biomechanics of the distal radioulnar joint. Clin Orthop 187:26, 1984.)

Table 16–2. **PERCENT AXIAL LOAD WITH ULNAR VARIANCE***

	Intact Wrist			TFCC Excised		
Ulnar Length Variation	− 2.5 mm	0	+ 2.5 mm	− 2.5 mm	0	+ 2.5 mm
Radius (percent)	95.7	81.6	58.1	97	93.8	78.2
Ulna (percent)	4.3	18.4	41.95	3	6.2	21.8

*Percent axial load borne by the radius and ulna as the ulna is lengthened and shortened in the intact wrist and in the wrist after TFCC excision. (From Palmer AK, and Werner FW: Biomechanics of the distal radioulnar joint. Clin Orthop 187:26, 1984.)

radius and the lunate, and the radius and the scaphoid. As can be seen in the Table measurements, lengthening of the ulna produces a dramatic increase in pressure on the ulnar head (the ulnolunate articulation). Removal of the TFCC causes a shifting of pressure centrally to the radiolunate articulation, thus unloading not only the ulnolunate, but the radioscaphoid articulation as well.

In summary, these data illustrate that small changes in relative ulnar length significantly alter load patterns across the wrist. Thus, when a Colles' fracture settles 2.5 mm, one can expect an increase in ulnar axial load of approximately 40 percent. Development of these abnormal load patterns, I believe, greatly increases the risk of secondary degenerative arthrosis at the contact stress point.

ULNOCARPAL IMPINGEMENT SYNDROME

Due to the increased force transmission across the TFCC secondary to actual or relative positive ulnar variance, I believe that several structures may be at risk when the ulna is excessively long. In particular, triangular fibrocartilage complex perforations are more likely to occur under these circumstances. In fact, other than actual traumatic tears (which are very rare), chronic perfora-

tions seem to occur in conjunction with wrists with neutral or positive ulnar variance. Cartilage degeneration of the distal ulna or the proximal lunate articular surfaces or both frequently accompany this condition. It is also likely that triquetrolunate ligament instability will be found in conjunction with late stages of degenerative TFCC perforations and positive ulnar variance. We refer to these associated abnormalities as the "ulnocarpal impingement syndrome." Ulnar shortening has been successful in relieving the ulnar wrist pain that accompanies this syndrome.

TFCC LOAD TRANSMISSION

As partial excision of the TFCC (TFCC débridement) is now recommended by some practitioners for symptomatic TFCC perforations, the effect of the removal of one third, two thirds, and three thirds of the horizontal portion of the TFCC on forearm axial load was studied using the PSF (Fig. 16–10).[15, 20, 25, 27, 32] Using the same experimental model as in the ulnar lengthening/shortening experiment, the percentage of force that was transmitted through the ulna in nine fresh specimens was measured. Measurements were taken with the specimens in the intact state and then after removal of the central

Table 16–3. **PEAK ARTICULAR PRESSURE***

	Ulnolunate Articulation	Radiolunate Articulation	Radioscaphoid Articulation
Ulnar Variance	*Intact Wrist*		
0	1.4	3.0	3.3
+ 2.5 mm	3.3	1.5	3.4
− 2.5 mm	0.34	4.1	3.6
	TFCC Removed		
0	0.76	3.9	2.4
+ 2.5 mm	3.2	3.4	3.6
− 2.5 mm	0.0	3.9	2.5

*Peak articular pressure (N/mm²) at the ulnolunate, radiolunate, and radioscaphoid articulation in the intact wrist and in the wrist after TFCC excision with ulnar length variations, as measured with Fuji Pre-Scale Pressure-Sensitive Film. (From Palmer AK, and Werner FW: Biomechanics of the distal radioulnar joint. Clin Orthop 187:26, 1984.)

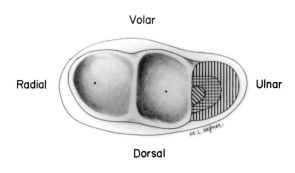

Volar

Radial · · Ulnar

Dorsal

◩ -⅓ Horizontal Portion TFCC

▦ -⅔ Horizontal Portion TFCC

▥ -All Horizontal Portion TFCC

Figure 16–10. An artist's rendering of the experimental removal of one third, two thirds, and finally all of the horizontal portion of the TFCC (triangular fibrocartilage complex).

third of the TFCC, then after enlargement of the hole to remove two thirds of the central portion of the TFCC, and, finally, after the entire horizontal portion of the TFCC was removed. Removal of one third of the TFCC did not significantly alter load transmission through the ulna, but removal of two thirds, and certainly removal of all of the horizontal portion of the TFCC, significantly increased the load through the distal ulna (Fig. 16–11).

In summary, TFCC débridement for the treatment of central perforation of the TFCC

where only the central third of the TFCC is removed insignificantly alters the load patterns on the ulnar aspect of the wrist.

DIAGNOSIS

Diagnostic Problems

At times, it is difficult to specify whether pain on the ulnar aspect of the wrist is related to problems of the distal radioulnar joint or to those of the medial wrist column or the ulnocarpal complex. It is tempting to order an arthrogram in all patients with ulnar wrist pain and, if the arthrogram results are positive for a TFCC perforation, to attribute the patient's symptoms to this abnormality. However, we believe that most arthrographically confirmed TFCC perforations produce no symptoms and are therefore not the cause of the patient's ulnar wrist pain. When evaluating a patient with ulnar wrist pain, the examining physician must review, at least mentally, an algorithm by which a physical finding or ancillary study systematically delineates or excludes an area of abnormality to eventually allow a definitive diagnosis.

Physical Examination

The patient is seated in front of the examiner with the elbow flexed and the hand pointed toward the ceiling. Full passive forearm mo-

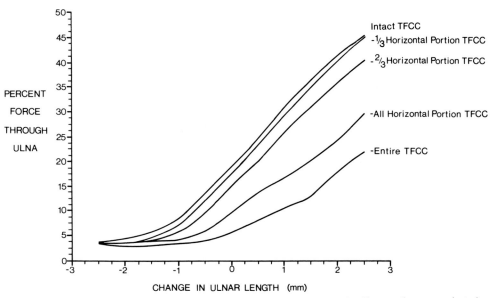

Figure 16–11. Removal of one third of the horizontal portion of the TFCC (triangular fibrocartilage complex) does not, in experimentation, significantly increase load transfer through the ulna. However, removal of two thirds or all of the horizontal portion of the TFCC or the entire TFCC does increase load transfer significantly.

tion is produced by the examiner. Pain in the wrist with forearm motion localizes symptoms to the radioulnar joint. Pain-free forearm motion implies that the patient's symptoms of ulnar wrist pain are of ulnocarpal or carpal origin.

The patient is next asked to perform active forearm rotation as the examiner observes the extensor carpi ulnaris, the distal ulna, and the ulnar carpus for acute subluxation or dislocation. The hand is then examined for point tenderness, with care being taken to palpate each joint or ligamentous complex (Fig. 16–12). The distal radioulnar joint is then stressed, and the examiner notes pain, crepitation, clicking, or subluxation. A standard hand and wrist examination is then additionally performed.

Ancillary Studies

Based on the physical examination, the examiner is often fairly certain of the diagnosis. Further studies, however, are needed for diagnostic confirmation prior to treatment.

Plain Films. These remain the most valuable tool for evaluating ulnar wrist pain.[11, 22] We routinely take posteroanterior, lateral, and oblique views of the wrist with the forearm in neutral rotation. Posteroanterior and lateral pain localizing films are often

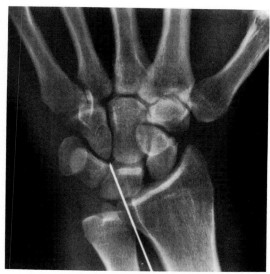

Figure 16–13. At the time that this x-ray was taken, the patient was asked to localize his pain with a metallic pointer. The pointer, in this case, localizes the pain to the junction of the capitate, hamate, lunate, and triquetrum. (From Palmer AK: Orthop Clin North Am 15:2, 321–335, 1984.)

taken as the patient places a metallic marker over the area of greatest pain (Fig. 16–13). Films are reviewed for indications of fracture or dislocation, carpal malalignment, carpal collapse, carpal erosion, localized arthritis (such as pisotriquetral arthritis), and ulnar variance.

CT Scan. We believe that the CT scan is the best way to evaluate the distal radioulnar joint for subluxation or dislocation because it is not only easier to interpret than the lateral film, but it is also easier to perform

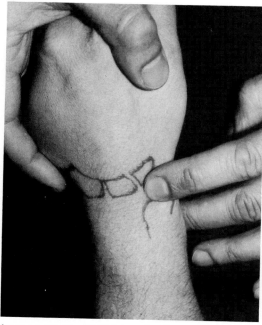

Figure 16–12. The TFCC (triangular fibrocartilage complex) region is palpated for tenderness. (From Palmer AK: Orthop Clin North Am 15:2, 321–335, 1984.)

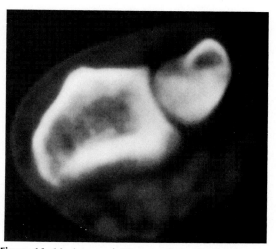

Figure 16–14. A normal CT scan of the distal radioulnar joint, showing the ulnar head located within the sigmoid notch of the radius. (From Palmer AK: Orthop Clin North Am 15:2, 321–335, 1984.)

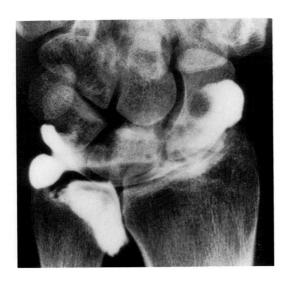

Figure 16–15. An abnormal arthrogram demonstrating communication of the radial and distal radioulnar joints, indicating a perforated TFCC. (From Palmer AK: Orthop Clin North Am 15:2, 321–335, 1984.)

and interpret at a time when the patient's wrist is immobilized in plaster (Fig. 16–14).

Arthrography. Contrast material is introduced slowly into the radiocarpal joint space under fluoroscopy, while the examiner watches for dye leakage into the midcarpal space through the scapholunate or lunotriquetral ligament or into the distal radioulnar joint across the TFCC. We find this study most helpful in identifying lunotriquetral and TFCC abnormalities (Fig. 16–15).[26]

Bone Scan. This study is ordered in patients in whom we suspect Kienböck's disease but in whom the diagnosis cannot be confirmed on plain films (Fig. 16–16).[34]

Wrist Arthroscopy. This modality shows great promise for the diagnosis of wrist disorders, including problems involving the distal radioulnar joint and the TFCC. Its current use in relation to the wrist is discussed elsewhere in this text (see Chapter 9).

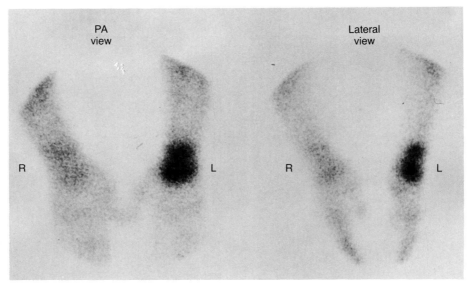

Figure 16–16. A bone scan performed on a patient with Kienböck's disease of the left wrist. (From Palmer AK: Orthop Clin North Am 15:2, 321–335, 1984.)

TREATMENT

Despite a careful and thorough history and physical examination and the use of sophisticated ancillary diagnostic studies, some distal radioulnar joint and ulnocarpal complex problems remain a diagnostic and therefore therapeutic mystery. In these cases, the patients are best followed, for exploratory surgery is rarely satisfying to either the patient or the surgeon. As techniques for wrist arthroscopy are developed, the opportunity for direct visualization and treatment of wrist disorders may greatly expand our therapeutic options. Tears of the TFCC may be particularly amenable to arthroscopic débridement or repair.

For patients in whom the diagnosis is clear, the physician frequently has many acceptable treatment alternatives from which to choose. For example, in order to treat an unstable distal radioulnar joint, one might reconstruct the ligamentous support system, fuse the distal radioulnar joint and create a proximal resection arthroplasty, perform an ulnar shortening, or excise the entire distal ulna. Our methods of treating various maladies of the distal radioulnar joint, both acute and chronic (Tables 16–4 and 16–5) have proved relatively successful.[27]

SUMMARY

The distal radioulnar joint plays an intricate part in the functioning of the wrist and thus in the functioning of the entire upper extremity. The radius and hand move in relation to and function about the distal ulna. Significant loads are transmitted to the forearm unit through the distal ulna via the triangular fibrocartilage complex. The anatomic relationships between the distal radius, the ulna, and the ulnar carpus are precise, and even a minor modification in these relationships leads to significant load changes and resultant pain syndromes. Evaluation of a patient with ulnar wrist pain is, at best, difficult. If the physician has an understanding of the normal anatomy and biomechanics of the distal radioulnar joint, the examination of such a patient and the subsequent treatment should become a challenge that is rewarding for both patient and treating physician.

Table 16–4. **ACUTE MALADIES OF THE DISTAL RADIOULNAR JOINT (DRUJ)***

Diagnosis	Physical Exam	Ancillary Studies	Treatment
Fractures			
Ulnar head	Localized swelling and tenderness	Plain films	Anatomic reduction (ORIF† if necessary)
Ulnar styloid	Localized swelling and tenderness	Plain films	Plaster immobilization (ORIF† if unstable DRUJ)
Radius (involving sigmoid fossa)	Localized swelling and tenderness	Plain films or tomograms	Anatomic reduction (ORIF† if necessary)
Carpal bones	Localized swelling and tenderness	Plain films or tomograms	Anatomic reduction (ORIF† if necessary)
Dislocation or Subluxation			
Distal ulna	Tenderness and deformity	CT scan	Dorsal subluxation—long-arm cast in supination; volar subluxation—long-arm cast in pronation
Carpal bones	Tenderness and deformity	Plain films, CT scan, tomograms	Anatomic reduction (ORIF† if necessary)
Carpal instability	Tenderness and clicking	Plain films, fluoroscopic motion study, arthrogram	ORIF† and ligament repairs
TFCC tear	Swelling, tenderness and click	Plain films, arthrogram	TFCC flap excision
ECU‡ subluxation	Tenderness and swelling	None	Long-arm cast in full supination

*The diagnosis, clinical findings, and treatment of acute problems of the distal radioulnar joint. (Modified from Palmer AK: The distal radioulnar joint. Orthop Clin North Am 15:330, 1984.)
†ORIF = open reduction with internal fixation
‡ECU = extensor carpi ulnaris

Table 16–5. **CHRONIC MALADIES OF THE DISTAL RADIOULNAR JOINT***

Diagnosis	Physical Exam	Ancillary Studies	Treatment
Osseous Nonunion			
Ulnar head	Pain and swelling	Plain films	Limited ulnar head excision (HIT)†
Ulnar styloid (painful)	Pain and occasional swelling	Plain films	ORIF‡ if large; excision if small
Malunion			
Ulnar head	Pain and limited motion	Plain films, tomograms	Limited distal ulnar resection
Distal radius (involving the sigmoid fossa)	Pain and limited motion	Plain films, tomograms	ORIF‡ or distal ulnar resection
Incongruous Wrist Joint			
Subluxated distal ulnar	Pain and swelling, grating and clicking	CT scan	Ulnar shortening or Suavé-Kapandji's (Lauenstein's) procedure
Dislocated distal radioulnar joint	Pain and swelling and limited motion	CT scan	Suavé-Kapandji's (Lauenstein's) or Darrach's procedure
Ulnocarpal region (ulna plus wrist)	Pain and swelling	Plain films	Ulnar shortening
Carpal bones	Pain and swelling	Plain films, wrist motion study, arthrogram	Limited intercarpal fusion
Carpal instability	Pain, swelling, decreased range of motion	Plain films, motion studies, arthrogram	Limited intercarpal fusion
TFCC perforation	Pain, swelling, clicking	Plain films, arthrograms	Flap tear—débridement of the flap Degenerative perforation without ulnar or lunate chondromalacia—limited TFCC débridement Degenerative perforation with ulnar or lunate chondromalacia—ulnar shortening
Localized Arthritis			
Pisotriquetral	Pain and swelling	Oblique films, tomograms	Pisectomy
Lunotriquetral	Pain and swelling	Plain films, tomograms	Lunotriquetral fusion
Localized arthritis of radioulnar joint	Pain and swelling	Plain films, tomograms	Suavé-Kapandji (Lauenstein) HIT†
ECU§ subluxation	Pain, swelling, snapping	None	ECU§ sheath reconstruction

*The diagnosis, clinical findings, and treatment of chronic problems of the distal radioulnar joint. (Modified from Palmer AK: The distal radioulnar joint. Orthop Clin North Am 15:331, 1984.)
†HIT = hemiresection-interposition technique
‡ORIF = open reduction with internal fixation
§ECU = extensor carpi ulnaris

References

1. af Ekenstam FW: The distal radioulnar joint. Doctoral thesis, Uppsala, Acta Universitatis Up Salvensis Uppsala Universitet, 1984.
2. Bowers WH: Distal radioulnar joint. In Green DP (ed): Operative Hand Surgery. New York, Churchill Livingstone Inc, 1982, p 743.
3. Bowers WH: Distal radioulnar joint arthroplasty: the hemiresection interposition technique. J Hand Surg 10A:169, 1985.
4. Bowers WH: Problems of the distal radioulnar joint. Adv Orthop Surg 1:289, 1984.
5. Brand PW, Beach RB, and Thompson DE: Relative tension and potential excursion of muscles in the forearm and hand. J Hand Surg 3:209, 1981.
6. Bunnell S: Surgery of the Hand, 3rd ed. Philadelphia, JB Lippincott Co, 1956.
7. Cooper A, and Bransby B: Treatise of Dislocations, 5th ed. Philadelphia, Lea & Blanchard, 1844, p 417.
8. Dameron TB: Traumatic dislocation of the distal radioulnar joint. Clin Orthop 83:55, 1972.
9. DeSault M: Exrait d'une mémoire de M DeSault sur la luxation de l'extrémité inférieure du radius. J Chir 1:78, 1791.
10. Destot, E: Injuries of the Wrist: A Radiological Study. Atkinson FRB (Trans). New York, Paul B Hoeber Inc, 1926.
11. Epner RA, Bowers WH, and Gailford WB: Ulnar variance: the effect of wrist positioning and roentgen filming techniques. J Hand Surg 7:298, 1982.
12. Hamlin C: Traumatic disruption of the distal radioulnar joint. Am J Sports Med 5:93, 1977.

13. Kaplan E: Functional and Surgical Anatomy of the Hand. Philadelphia, JB Lippincott Co, 1952, p 101.

14. Lewis OJ: Evolutionary changes in the primate wrist and inferior radioulnar joints. Anat Rec 151:275, 1965.

15. Menon J, Wood VE, Schoene HR, et al: Isolated tears of triangular fibrocartilage of wrist: results of partial excision. J Hand Surg 9A:527, 1984.

16. Milch H: So-called dislocations of the lower end of the ulna. Ann Surg 116:282, 1942.

17. Mino DE, Palmer AK, and Levinsohn EM: The role of computerized tomography in the diagnosis of subluxation and dislocation of the distal radioulnar joint. J Hand Surg 8:23, 1982.

18. Mino DE, Palmer AK, and Levinsohn EM: Radiography and computerized tomography in the diagnosis of incongruity of the distal radio-ulnar joint. J Bone Joint Surg 67A:247, 1985.

19. Mohiuddin A, and Janjua MZ: Form and function of radioulnar articular disc. Hand 14:61, 1982.

20. Palmer AK, and Werner FW: The triangular fibrocartilage complex of the wrist—anatomy and function. J Hand Surg 6:153, 1981.

21. Palmer AK, Skahen J, Werner FW, et al: The extensor retinaculum of the wrist: an anatomic and biomechanical study. J Hand Surg (Brit) 10B:11, 1985.

22. Palmer AK, Glisson RR, and Werner FW: Ulnar variance determination. J Hand Surg 7:376, 1982.

23. Palmer AK, and Werner, FW: Biomechanics of the distal radioulnar joint. Clin Orthop 187:26, 1984.

24. Palmer AK, Taleisnik J, Fisk G, et al: Symposium on distal ulnar injuries. Contemp Orthop 7:81, 1983.

25. Palmer AK, and Neviaser RJ: Traumatic perforation of the articular disc of the triangular fibrocartilage complex of the wrist. Bull Hosp Jt Dis Orthop Inst 44:376, 1984.

26. Palmer AK, Levinsohn EM, and Kuzma GR: Arthrography of the wrist. J Hand Surg 8:15, 1982.

27. Palmer AK: The distal radioulnar joint. Orthop Clin North Am 15:321, 1984.

28. Ray RD, Johnson RJ, and Jameson RM: Rotation of the forearm—an experimental study of pronation and supination. J Bone Joint Surg 33A:993, 1951.

29. Rose-Innes AP: Anterior dislocation of the ulna at the inferior radio-ulnar joint. J Bone Joint Surg 42B:515, 1960.

30. Slater N, and Darcus HD: The amplitude of forearm and humeral rotation. J Anat 87:407, 1953.

31. Taleisnik J: The ligaments of the wrist. J Hand Surg 1:110, 1976.

32. Taleisnik J, Gelberman RH, Miller BW, et al: The extensor retinaculum of the wrist. J Hand Surg 9A:495, 1984.

33. Vesely DG: The distal radioulnar joint. Clin Orthop 51:75, 1967.

34. Werner FW, Glisson RR, and Palmer AK: Pressure distribution in the radioulnar carpal joint. Presented at the Second Annual Murray Day, Syracuse, May, 1982.

35. Werner FW, Palmer AK, and Glisson RR: Forearm load transmission: The effect of ulnar lengthening and shortening. In Cracchiolo A (ed): Transactions of the 28th Annual Meeting of the Orthopaedic Research Society, New Orleans, January, 1982, p 273.

CHAPTER 17

Surgical Procedures for the Distal Radioulnar Joint

WILLIAM H. BOWERS, M.D.

INTRODUCTION

Disorders of the ulnar side of the wrist are common, disabling, and difficult to manage. Anatomic information is now available and becoming more uniformly agreed upon.[1-7] Improved methods of diagnosis are helping to identify specific problems that can be effectively treated. This section presents my classification of ulnar wrist disorders and lists the surgical alternatives available for their management (Table 17–1). Anatomy, methods of diagnosis, closed management, and indications are covered elsewhere in this book.

CLASSIFICATION OF ULNAR WRIST DISORDERS

Entries in this classification overlap in one specific area: Acute problems, when untreated, become chronic problems; at times, the treatment for the chronic problem is no different from that of the acute, except for degree of operative difficulty and the extent of the period of postoperative rehabilitation.

In other instances, a reconstructive approach is more direct and effective despite some sacrifice to anatomy. Here judgment and experience become paramount.

SURGICAL PROCEDURES AVAILABLE FOR TREATMENT

Procedure I: Exploration

The intact distal radioulnar joint surfaces and the ulnocarpal joint structures cannot be fully explored by any single approach because of the intimacy of contact between the radius, the ulna, and the triangular fibrocartilage.

DORSAL APPROACH

The dorsal approach (Fig. 17–1) allows visualization of the dorsal 60 percent of the ulnar head and the carpal face of the triangular fibrocartilage, the lunate, the lunatotriquetral ligament, the triquetrum, the meniscus, the prestyloid recess, and most of the distal radioulnar joint synovial cavity. The view one should concentrate on obtaining is seen in Figure 17–1. This sort of exposure requires careful planning of the entry through the dorsal capsular ligaments. I recommend release of the extensor digiti minimi (EDM) from its sheath, subperiosteal reflection of the unviolated sixth dorsal compartment from the styloid and the shaft, and a turning of a 1-cm wide capsular flap from medial to lateral, just at the distal margin of the triangular fibrocartilage and the ulnocarpal joint level. A wide exposure is necessary for complete visualization of the structures mentioned. If the involved structures are carefully dissected and replaced, none of this exposure should alter joint mechanics or stability.

VOLAR APPROACH

A volar approach is possible, which allows the remainder of the articular surface to be seen. This approach is appropriate for release of soft tissue pronation contracture involving the volar capsular structures. The flexor carpi ulnaris and ulnar nerve and artery are retracted ulnarly, and the flexor group is retracted radially. A corner of the pronator quadratus is reflected. In a supinated wrist, the synovial cavity is easily opened for a look (Fig. 17–2). There may be significant scar tissue in this area in a posttraumatic wrist. When joint stability is un-

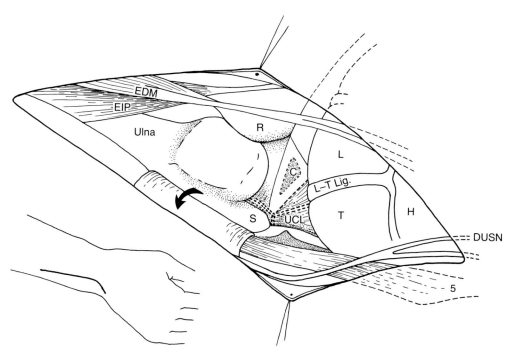

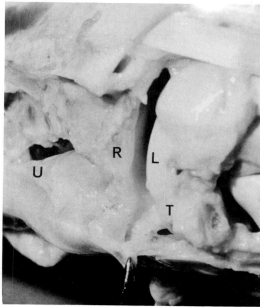

Figure 17–1. Procedure I: Exploration—dorsal approach. TFC = triangular fibrocartilage complex; C = central portion of TFC; H = hamate; L = lunate; R = radius; S = styloid; UCL = ulnocarpal ligaments; EDM = extensor digiti minimi; EIP = extensor indicis proprius; DUSN = dorsoulnar sensory nerve; T = triquetrum; L–T Lig. = lunotriquetral ligament; 5 = fifth metacarpal. The heavy double dotted line around the styloid that extends distally between the ulnolunate and ulnotriquetral ligaments represents the area in which a destabilizing tear of the ulnar wrist ligaments is most often found when the x-ray findings are negative. The same injury pattern may avulse the styloid.

Table 17–1. **CLASSIFICATION OF DRUJ* DISORDERS AND PROCEDURES AVAILABLE FOR THEIR TREATMENT**

Disorder	Procedures Available
I. Fractures	
A. Sigmoid notch–radius	II, III
B. Ulnar articular surfaces	II, X–C
C. Ulnar styloid (see IIB)	II
D. Ulnar shaft	II, IX–A
II. Joint disruption—acute	
A. Partial TFC disruption without instability	I + VII
B. Dislocation—isolated TFC disruption	
1. Dorsal ⎱ (see IC)	IV, V–B, C
2. Volar ⎰	IV
C. Dislocation associated with other injuries (fractures of radius, etc)	II, IV + repair of other injury
III. Joint disruption—chronic—no arthritis	
A. Partial TFC disruption—no instability	VII + IX–A, X–C
B. Recurrent dislocation—instability	IV, V–B, V–C, X–B, X–C + IV
C. Recurrent dislocation—instability associated with shaft deformity	IV + VIII + IX–B, or C
IV. Joint disorders	
A. Ulna—long (Ulnocarpal impingement)	VII + IX–A, X–C, XI
B. Arthritis	
1. Post-traumatic	
a. Stable	X–A, X–B, X–C,† XI
b. Unstable	X–A, X–B,† X–C,† XI†
2. Osteoarthritis	X–A, X–B, X–C,† XI
3. Rheumatoid	
a. Stable	X–A, X–B, X–C†
b. Unstable	X–A, X–B,† X–C
4. Ulnar articular chondromalacia	X–A, X–B, X–C†, XI
C. TFC attritional changes	VII + IX–A, X–C
V. Other problems	
A. Extensor carpi ulnaris subluxation/dislocation	VI
B. Failed Darrach's procedure	X–B + VI,† XII

*DRUJ = distal radioulnar joint
† = plus radiolunate fusion

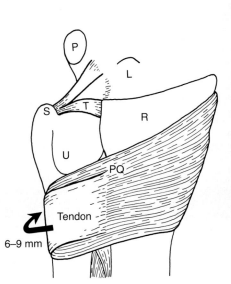 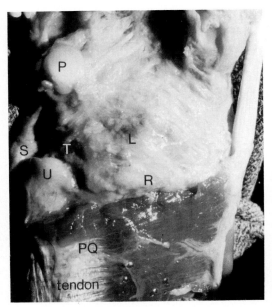

Figure 17–2. The drawing and photograph illustrate the approach to the volar distal radioulnar joint. The pronator quadratus (PQ) muscle-tendon unit as well as the direction and distance for advancement according to Johnson[9] (Procedure V–B) is shown. (See also Fig. 17–4.) P = pisiform; L = lunate; T = triangular fibrocartilage; S = styloid; U = ulna; R = radius; PQ = pronator quadratus.

impaired, release of this scar may be all that is required to relieve a resistant pronation contracture.

Procedure II: Open Reduction, Internal Fixation

The surgical exposures described in Procedure I (Exploration) are adequate for open reduction and internal fixation of the sigmoid notch and the lunate facet in comminuted fractures of this portion of the distal radius; they are also adequate in treatment of styloid fracture and intra-articular fractures of the articular surface of the distal ulna. For distal shaft fractures, exposure of the triangular fibrocartilage complex and the ulnocarpal joint is unnecessary. The exposure can be extended proximally for visualization of the shaft. It is important to visualize the articular surface of the distal radioulnar joint so that internal fixation of the distal shaft will not compromise motion of the distal radioulnar joint itself.

The technique of open reduction and internal fixation of the styloid fracture is not difficult. A compression screw or interosseous wiring technique is recommended. I prefer the latter. The fracture is opened, and under direct visualization, using Kirschner wires for drill points, two drill holes are made proximally from the fracture site to exit opposite the radius at the axilla of the ulnar shaft and its articular surface. An appropriate sized wire is then passed either around the styloid or through it, using similar drill holes, and the two free ends of the wire are then passed proximally through the fracture site into the previously prepared drill holes in the proximal shaft (Fig. 17–3). The wire is then twisted, compressing the styloid to the shaft. Tightening of the wire is done with the patient's forearm in neutral position. The forearm is cast in neutral with the wrist in slight ulnar deviation for a period of four weeks. Limited motion is allowed, using an ulnar gutter splint for an additional two weeks. Unrestricted motion may then be permitted. This procedure is indicated when the styloid fracture is imperfectly reduced and the distal radioulnar joint is unstable following acute injuries. The interosseous wiring technique is also useful when stabilizing repairs of the triangular fibrocartilage complex (TFCC), where this complex has been avulsed from the styloid at its attachment either in acute or

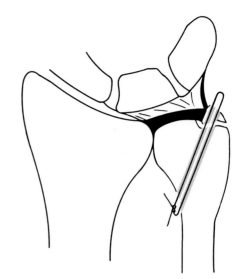

Figure 17–3. Internal fixation using the interosseous wire technique (Procedure II). The same method may be employed to repair a destabilizing tear of the TFCC when no fracture is present or where ulnar shortening is done in conjunction with the hemiresection arthroplasty (Procedure X–C).

recurrent instabilities. This is also my method of choice when shortening of the ulna is done in conjunction with hemiresection arthroplasty (see Procedure X–C).

Procedure III: External Fixation

External fixation is of value when comminuted fractures of the sigmoid notch prevent open reduction and internal fixation. The fixation should be done from radius to metacarpals, allowing forearm rotational motion to mold the fractured surface of the sigmoid notch. This technique alone is *contraindicated* when fractures of the sigmoid notch are associated with instability of the distal radioulnar joint itself. Here external fixation may be employed only after the triangular fibrocartilage complex has been explored and repaired or after the ulnar styloid fracture has been internally fixed (see Procedure II).

Procedure IV: Triangular Fibrocartilage Complex Repair

The exposure described in exploration of the dorsal ulnocarpal area is recommended. With sufficient exposure, disruption of the triangular fibrocartilage or ulnocarpal ligaments can easily be seen. Direct repair of the triangular fibrocartilage and ulnocarpal ligaments when disrupted from the styloid can be accomplished as noted (see Procedure II). I recommend using firm fixation techniques such as the interosseous wire method. Pullout wires may be used, but wire of a sufficient caliber must be employed to achieve firm fixation of the ligament and the fibrocartilage to the bone surfaces. Where tears within the complex are visualized, direct repair may be augmented by locally available tissue. A guide to the location of and some suggestions for harvesting and rerouting this available tissue may be found in Figure 17–4.

Procedure V: Triangular Fibrocartilage Complex Reconstruction or Substitution or Both

There are no excellent procedures available. The functional elements of (1) a smooth carpal articulation, (2) a flexible rotational tether from radius to ulna, (3) suspension of the ulnar carpus from the radius, (4) an ulnocarpal cushion, and (5) ulnar shaft/ulnar carpal connection are difficult to duplicate in any effective fashion. Bunnell-Boyes

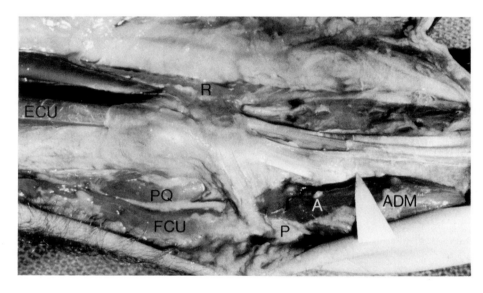

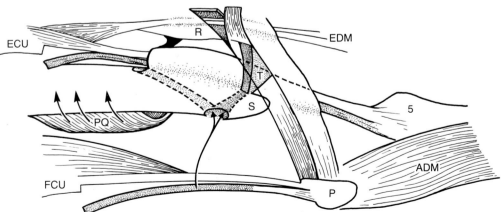

Figure 17–4. A strip of retinaculum, extensor carpi ulnaris (ECU) or flexor carpi ulnaris (FCU) may be dissected distally to be utilized in augmentation or reconstruction of the TFCC. Suggested routes through the ulna allow relatively anatomic reconstruction. If FCU or retinaculum is used, it should be woven through or sutured to firm capsular tissue proximal to the pisotriquetral joint in order to avoid abnormal stress on (and possibly pain from) this joint. The direction of pronator advancement is shown (Procedure V–B). EDM = extensor digiti minimi; PQ = pronator quadratus muscle; ADM = abductor digiti minimi; P = pisiform; R = radius; T = triangular fibrocartilage; S = styloid; 5 = fifth metacarpal.

procedure[8] as a working approach is good but does not attempt to provide elements (1), (3), and (4). If some elements of the triangular fibrocartilage complex are intact, the missing elements may be selectively augmented as mentioned in procedure IV or by reconstruction attempts using this same tissue (distally based portions of ECU, flexor carpi ulnaris, and dorsal retinaculum).

Radioulnar Tether Procedures. These procedures have historically been the approach to this problem.[1] These procedures attempt to resupply one function of the triangular fibrocartilage complex—the radioulnar connection. Each of these procedures approaches the problem at a level proximal to the radioulnar articulation and attempts, by weaving a tendon graft around or through them, to pull the bones together. Each series reports success in a limited number of patients. Follow-up has been insufficient to allow meaningful statements to be made.

Criticism generally reflects that the procedures are ineffective in preventing instability or that rotation is restricted if anteroposterior stability is achieved. A review of some of these procedures may be seen in Figure 17–5. It is my opinion that attempts at achieving stability of the distal radioulnar connection should be directed to repair or reconstruction of the triangular fibrocartilage at its original anatomic site (see Procedures IV and V).

Advancing the Pronator Quadratus. Some support can be given to the rationale of Johnson,[9] who has proposed advancing the pronator quadratus from its normal insertion on the ulna to a more lateral and dorsal insertion. As he postulates, this might increase radioulnar joint stability, particularly in dorsal instability situations. This procedure could additionally be used to augment repair of the triangular fibrocartilage, although he has not proposed its use for treat-

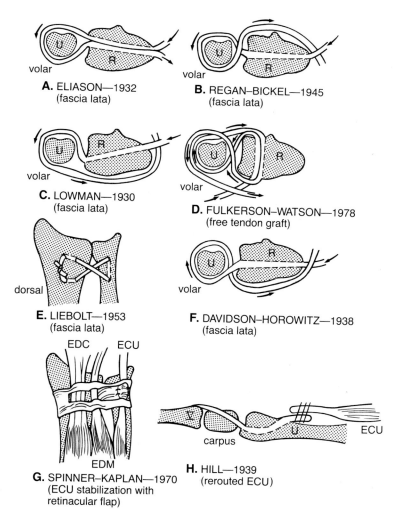

A. ELIASON—1932
(fascia lata)

B. REGAN–BICKEL—1945
(fascia lata)

C. LOWMAN—1930
(fascia lata)

D. FULKERSON–WATSON—1978
(free tendon graft)

E. LIEBOLT—1953
(fascia lata)

F. DAVIDSON–HOROWITZ—1938
(fascia lata)

G. SPINNER–KAPLAN—1970
(ECU stabilization with retinacular flap)

H. HILL—1939
(rerouted ECU)

Figure 17–5. Radioulnar tenodesis procedures (Procedures V–A).

ing that disorder. His method may be conceptualized by a review of Figures 17–2 and 17–4.

Reconstructive Procedures for the Ulnocarpal Ligaments. Two recent reports have described reconstructive procedures for the ulnocarpal ligaments. Both employ distally based portions of the flexor carpi ulnaris tendon, which has been harvested proximally and stripped distally to the pisiform attachment. The concept is an integral part of Bunnell-Boyes procedure and has also been described by Hill.[10] The recent reports emphasize stabilizing the new ligament distally by passing it through the volar ulnocarpal ligaments and then through a drill hole from the ulnar styloid area dorsally and proximally to exit at the axilla of the ulnar articular surface. The repair is then augmented by imbrication of the dorsal capsular ligaments. Both Hui[11] and Tsai[12] comment that their procedure is useful in dorsal subluxation or dislocation of the distal radioulnar joint and contraindicated in volar subluxations. Figure 17–6 indicates the method of Hui. The method of Tsai may also be employed as a modification of Darrach's procedure (see Procedure X). The pronator advancement as described by Johnson may be used alone to correct dorsoulnar instability or as an addition to their techniques.

Procedure VI: Extensor Carpi Ulnaris Stabilization

Spinner and Kaplan[13] stabilize the extensor carpi ulnaris in a retinacular sling created by reversing a flap of extensor retinaculum based in the retinacular septum between the fourth and fifth dorsal compartments. So stabilized, the extensor carpi ulnaris becomes a full-time carpal extensor, losing its

ulnar deviation vector. The procedure is useful in extensor carpi ulnaris subluxation or dislocation from trauma or attrition. The modification as described by Bowers[14] and illustrated in Figure 17–7 is recommended.

Procedure VII: Triangular Fibrocartilage Débridement

The dorsal approach is used for exploration. The pathologic condition is identified and débridement is carried out, leaving as much of the triangular fibrocartilage as possible. There are proponents of total excision who report good results.[15–18]

Recent information on the importance of the TFCC has focused attention on a limited débridement as a more reasonable approach. Results have been equally good, and late problems of destabilization are avoided.[1, 19, 20]

Procedure VIII: Contracture Release

This is mentioned as a separate operative procedure to emphasize the fact that it may occasionally be all that is indicated in relieving a forearm rotational contracture. The volar approach is used, as described in Procedure I. This approach and the release of the volar capsule should not be ignored as useful components of those procedures in which repair of the triangular fibrocartilage complex is attempted in the chronic condition.

Procedure IX: Osteotomy

Osteotomy is an integral part of several procedures involving the distal radioulnar joint.

Ulnar Shortening.[21] This procedure is most often performed by resection of the shaft in

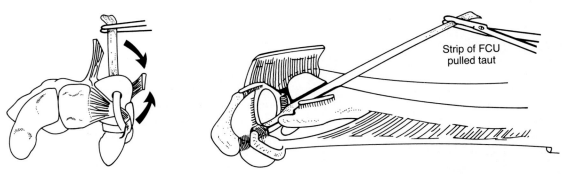

Strip of FCU pulled taut

Figure 17–6. The ulnotriquetral augmentation tenodesis of Hui and Linscheid[11] (Procedure V–C) for dorsal instability. (From Hui FC, and Linscheid RL: J Hand Surg 7:230–236, 1982.)

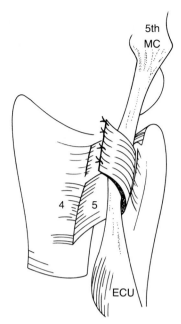

Figure 17–7. Modified retinacular sling stabilization of extensor carpi ulnaris tendon (Procedure VI).

appropriate amounts at 1 to 2 inches proximal to the distal radioulnar joint. Chevron, step-cut, or transverse osteotomies have been used with fixation by wiring, compression screws, or plate (Fig. 17–8). Rotational control must be exact when shortening alone is the intent. Fixation must be secure and left in place for many months. It is useless to do this procedure unless the major functional elements of the triangular fibrocartilage are operative. A preoperative arthrogram is thus necessary. The procedure has its major application in symptomatic ulnar-positive variants with ulnocarpal impingement. It may also be useful in association with limited débridement of the triangular fibrocartilage (Procedure VII) for acute or attritional tears or with the hemiresection interposition technique of arthroplasty (Procedure X–C) to salvage a stable ulnar wrist when the articulation is poor and the ulna is long. Care must be taken to assure that the internal fixation of whatever type employed does not interfere with distal radioulnar joint rotation (Fig. 17–8A).

Rotational Osteotomy of the Ulna. This is a relatively new concept and has been employed by me in several patients in whom radioulnar joint instability has been demonstrated to be related to rotational malalignment of the forearm bones. The presence of this condition is ascertained by comparative CT scans of the distal radioulnar joint in various degrees of rotation. The techniques for rotational osteotomy are similar to those for ulnar shortening. I prefer the transverse osteotomy with plate fixation.

Angular Osteotomy of the Distal Radius. This procedure has been employed to restore stability to the distal radioulnar joint when this instability has been caused by angular malunion of fractures of the distal radius. This osteotomy requires firm plate fixation and, at times, a bone graft.

Procedure X: Arthroplasty

ULNAR HEAD EXTIRPATION
(DARRACH'S PROCEDURE[22-28])

The distal ulnar shaft and head are excised in this procedure. The general indication has been any condition that causes derangement of the joint, interfering with its action and resulting in limited or painful motion. It has also been used in managing painful ulnar wrist instability in rheumatoid arthritis. This procedure has been used for many years and has been a worthy option for surgical treatment. It has become apparent in recent years that the best results are associated with minimal resection and brief immobilization.[28]

The procedure is not without its difficulties; however, two unsubstantiated criticisms are (1) increased ulnocarpal slide, and (2) decreased grip strength. I know of no reports of an ulnar carpal slide after Darrach's procedure in patients who have not also had their radiocarpal ligaments disrupted by trauma or rheumatoid arthritis.

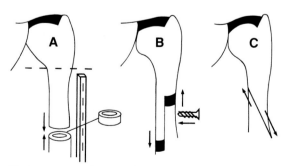

Figure 17–8. Techniques for ulnar osteotomy. The transverse osteotomy (A) may be used for shortening, lengthening (with bone graft), or rotational corrections. The osteotomy should be planned so that the distal end of the plate does not impinge as the forearm rotates. Step-cut (B) and oblique (C) osteotomy techniques are applicable only for shortening. Compression screw or plate fixation can be used.

Thus, the "slide" is not a criticism of Darrach's procedure itself. There are no reports documenting decreased grip strength. I have noted *increased* grip strength in patients in whom the procedure has been appropriately utilized. Darrach's procedure does, however, destroy the bone support for the triangular fibrocartilage complex. In addition to creating ulnocarpal instability, it creates "unstable" rotation of the radiocarpal unit around the ulnar axis. With muscular action, the ulnar stump may abut the radius or fray the overlying tissues. This may be evidenced by symptoms such as painful snapping or rupture of tendons or both.[29-33] If these occur, the temptation to remove more of the ulna must be resisted, as a poor result may be easily converted into a disaster.

There are no excellent salvage procedures for the painful instability of the "too short" Darrach procedure. Some options may be found in the next section. I have found some success by instituting long-term use of the forearm brace (the elbow and the wrist remain free, with the pronounced molding of the interosseous space), a concept borrowed from Sarmiento.[34] For these reasons the use of Darrach's procedure today should be very selective. It may be useful in the ulnocarpal loading syndrome (so-called ulnocarpal impingement), when the distal radioulnar joint surfaces will not permit a successful Milch's shortening osteotomy (see Procedure IX) and also in the advanced rheumatoid group, where it should be combined with a radiolunate fusion[35] or other radiocarpal stabilization procedures.

TECHNICAL MODIFICATIONS TO IMPROVE DARRACH'S PROCEDURE

In order to mitigate the instability created by Darrach's excision, a variety of modifications have been proposed. Swanson[36] has capped the distal ulna with a *silicone implant* that provides a soft end for the stump, maintains its length, and provides a focus around which ligament reconstruction can take place. Although it has theoretical application in traumatic and attritional disorders, its greatest proven application is in the rheumatoid distal radioulnar joint. Disruption and dislocation of the implant are complicating problems. Blatt and Ashworth[29] have sutured a flap of volar capsule to the dorsal ulnar stump to hold it down. Ruby[37] has suggested tethering the distal ulnar stump with a distally based strip of ECU.

The intact portion of the ECU is stabilized in a permanent dorsal position as Spinner and Kaplan[13] have suggested. Kessler and Hecht[31] suggest a dynamic stabilization of the ulnar stump by looping a strip of tendon around the distal ulnar stump and the ECU and tying the two together. Goldner and Hayes[30] have formalized these recommendations by passing a strip of ECU (detached distally) through a drill hole in the ulnar stump with the forearm in supination. Tsai and Stillwell[12] have employed a distally based portion of the *flexor carpi ulnaris* tendon to stabilize the ulnar stump and then looped this tendon to stabilize the extensor carpi ulnaris over the ulnar stump as well (Fig. 17–9). They reported its usefulness in three patients. I have used this procedure with some success in failed Darrach's procedures. A further adjunct in the management of the unstable distal ulnar stump may be the pronator advancement proposed by Johnson[9] (see Procedure V).

THE HEMIRESECTION INTERPOSITION TECHNIQUE OF ARTHROPLASTY (HIT)[14]

This procedure is an outgrowth of what Dingman[28] describes as the "best" Darrach

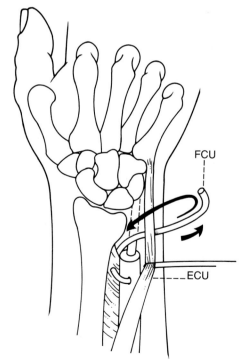

Figure 17–9. Stabilization of the ulnar stump using the flexor carpi ulnaris—a modification of the Darrach procedure (Tsai and Stillwell,[12] Procedure X–B). (From Tsai T, and Stillwell JH: J Hand Surg 98:289–293, 1984.)

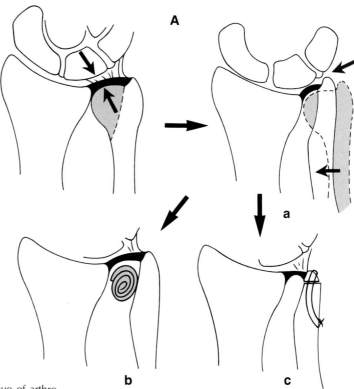

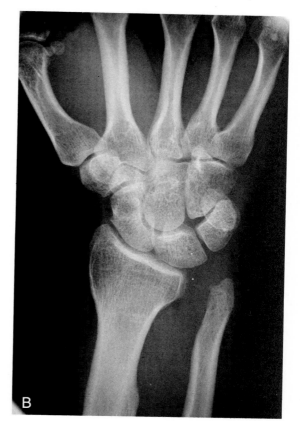

Figure 17–10. *A*, The hemiresection technique of arthroplasty (Bowers: Procedure X–C) employed in the ulnocarpal impingement syndrome. In *a*, the still-too-long ulna produces stylocarpal impingement—a condition caused by the approximation of the radius and ulna that occurs when the articular dome is removed. To obviate this, alternatives *b* (interposition) or *c* (shortening) are necessary. In every instance where this method is employed, intra-operative consideration of this possible complication is mandatory. *B*, This postoperative roentgenogram shows the usual case, i.e., no interposition or shortening is necessary.

procedures, those in which minimal resection was followed by regeneration of the ulnar shaft within the retained periosteal sleeve. The technique involves resection of the ulnar articular head only, leaving the shaft/styloid relationship intact. An interposition "anchovy" of tendon or muscle or capsule[15] was placed in the vacant distal radioulnar joint synovial cavity to limit contact of the radial and ulnar shafts, which tend to approach one another after this procedure. The procedure presupposes an intact or reconstructable triangular fibrocartilage complex. It should not be employed in situations in which ulnar variance is positive, *unless* the ulna is shortened as part of the procedure. Figures 17–10A and B illustrate the use of the procedure and its modifications. The main advantage of the procedure is in the maintenance of both radioulnar and ulnocarpal stability with the deletion of a painful articulation. It is preferred to Darrach's procedure in intra-articular ulnar head fractures, in arthritis, and in ulnocarpal impingement, when the shortening osteotomy (Procedure IX) alone cannot succeed because of arthritic joint surfaces.

Procedure XI: Arthrodesis-Pseudarthrosis Procedure

This procedure either accepts an ankylosis of the distal radioulnar joint (Baldwin) or

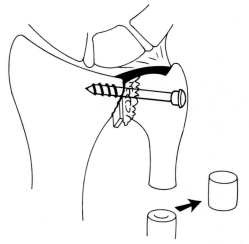

Figure 17–11. The arthrodesis-pseudarthrosis technique attributed to Lauenstein (Procedure XI). Bone graft and a compression screw maintain the ulnar support of the wrist, effectively extending the radius under the entire carpus. Rotation is provided by resection of the proximal ulnar shaft. Interposition of soft tissue helps to maintain the osseous interruption.

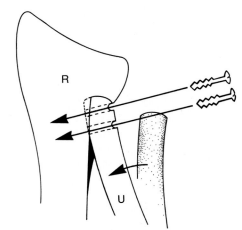

Figure 17–12. Distal radioulnar arthrodesis as described by Carroll and Imbriglia (Procedure XII).

creates one by arthrodesis (Lauenstein*) and then provides forearm rotational potential by creating a pseudarthrosis at a level proximal to the joint. Gonclaves[38] reports in an anecdotal way success in 22 patients with Lauenstein's procedure and in 16 patients with Baldwin's procedure. It has been stated that it provides results that are superior to those of Darrach's procedure in that it is cosmetically preferable and perhaps obviates the supposed complications of ulnocarpal slide and decreased grip strength. Some would use it as an alternative to the shortening osteotomy as well. However, it retains the undesirable characteristic of Darrach's procedure, that of creating an unstable proximal ulnar stump. Reossification of the pseudarthrosis site may also complicate the procedure. A recent discussion by Taleisnik[20] has suggested favorable results. Lauenstein's procedure is graphically presented in Figure 17–11.

Procedure XII: Arthrodesis

If the need for a stable forearm is paramount and rotation can be sacrificed, the technique of Carroll and Imbriglia[40] is trustworthy (successful in 60 of 65 patients). This procedure may be a good choice in the paralytic instability of an otherwise unreconstructable brachial plexus injury or in spastic rotational contractures. The technique of arthrodesis is graphically demonstrated in Figure 17–12.

---

*The correct credit is due Drs. Suavé and Kapandji,[39] although it is still frequently referred to as Lauenstein's procedure.

References

1. Bowers WH: The distal radioulnar joint. In Green DP (ed): Operative Hand Surgery. New York, Churchill Livingstone Inc, 1982, pp 743–769.
2. Hagart CG: Functional aspects of the distal radioulnar joint. J Hand Surg 4:585, 1979.
3. Kapandji IA: The inferior radioulnar joint and pronosupination. In Tubiana R: The Hand. Vol 1. Philadelphia, WB Saunders Co, 1981, p 121.
4. Kauer JMG: The articular disc of the hand. Acta Anat 93:590–605, 1975.
5. Lewis OJ, Hamshere RJ, and Bucknil TM: The anatomy of the wrist joint. J Anat 106:539, 1970.
6. Palmer AK, and Werner FW: The triangular fibrocartilage complex of the wrist: anatomy and function. J Hand Surg 6:153, 1981.
7. Taleisnik J: The ligaments of the wrist. J Hand Surg 1:110, 1976.
8. Boyes JH: Bunnell's Surgery of the Hand. 5th ed. Philadelphia, JB Lippincott Co, 1970, pp 299–303.
9. Johnson RK: Muscle-tendon transfer for stabilization of the distal radioulnar joint. J Hand Surg 10A:437, 1985.
10. Hill RB: Habitual dislocation of the distal end of the ulna. J Bone Joint Surg 21:780, 1939.
11. Hui FC, and Linscheid RL: Unotriquetral augmentation tenodesis. J Hand Surg 7:230, 1982.
12. Tsai T, and Stillwell JH: Repair of chronic subluxation of the distal radioulnar joint (ulnar dorsal) using flexor carpi ulnaris tendon. J Hand Surg 98:289–293, 1984.
13. Spinner M, and Kaplan EB: Extensor carpi ulnaris: its relationship to stability of the distal radioulnar joint. Clin Orthop 68:124–129, 1970.
14. Bowers W: Distal radioulnar joint arthroplasty—the hemiresection interposition technique. J Hand Surg 10A:169–178, 1985.
15. Coleman HM: Injuries of the articular disc at the wrist. J Bone Joint Surg 42B:522–529, 1960.
16. Imbriglia JE, and Boland DS: Tears of the articular disc of the triangular fibrocartilage complex. J Hand Surg 8:620, 1983.
17. Menon J, and Schoene HR: Isolated tears of the triangular fibrocartilage of the wrist joint. J Hand Surg 7:421, 1982.
18. Mossing N: Isolated lesions of the radioulnar disk treated with excision. Scand J Plast Reconstr Surg 9:231–233, 1975.
19. Palmer AK, and Neviaser R: Triangular fibrocartilage complex abnormalities: results of surgical treatment. Second Inter Congress—International Federation of Societies for Surgery of the Hand, Abstract 129, Boston, 1983, p 62.
20. Taleisnik J: Symposium on distal ulnar injuries. Contemp Orthop 7:81–116, 1983.
21. Milch H: Cuff resection of the ulna for malunited Colles' fracture. J Bone Joint Surg 23:311–313, 1941.
22. Darrach W: Forward dislocations at the inferior radioulnar joint with fracture of the lower third of the radius. Ann Surg 56:801, 1912.
23. Darrach W: Anterior dislocation of the head of the ulna. Ann Surg 56:802–803, 1912.
24. Darrach W: Partial excision of lower shaft of ulna for deformity following Colles' fracture. Ann Surg 57:764–765, 1912.
25. Darrach W: Habitual forward dislocation of the head of the ulna. Ann Surg 57:928–930, 1913.
26. Darrach W: Colles' fracture. N Engl J Med 226:594–596, 1942.
27. Darrach W, and Dwight K: Derangements of the inferior radioulnar articulation. Med Rec 87:708, 1915.
28. Dingman PVC: Resection of the distal end of the ulna (Darrach operation). J Bone Joint Surg 34A:893–900, 1952.
29. Blatt G, and Ashworth CR: Volar capsule transfer for stabilization following resection of the distal end of the ulna. Orthop Trans 3:13–14, 1979.
30. Goldner JL, and Hayes MD: Stabilization of the remaining ulna using one half of the extensor carpi ulnaris tendon after resection of the distal ulna. Orthop Trans 3:330–331, 1979.
31. Kessler I, and Hecht O: Present application of the Darrach procedure. Clin Orthop 72:254–260, 1970.
32. Mauer I: Reconstruction following posttraumatic derangement of the distal radioulnar joint. Bull Hosp Jt Dis Orthop Inst 22:95–104, 1961.
33. Newmeyer WL, and Green DP: Rupture of extensor tendons following resection of the distal ulna. J Bone Joint Surg 64A:178–182, 1982.
34. Sarmiento OA, Kiman PB, and Murphy RB: The treatment of ulnar fractures by functional bracing. J Bone Joint Surg 58:1104–1107, 1976.
35. Chaney A, Santa, DD, and Vilaseca A: Radiolunate arthrodesis factor of stability for the rheumatoid wrist. Ann Chir Main 2:5–17, 1983.
36. Swanson AB: Flexible Implant Arthroplasty in the Hand and Extremities. St Louis, CV Mosby Co, 1973, p 275.
37. Ruby LK: Correspondence: Letter 1983–70, Am Soc Surg Hand, 1983.
38. Gonclaves D: Correction of disorders of the distal radioulnar joint by artificial pseudarthrosis of the ulna. J Bone Joint Surg 56B:462–463, 1974.
39. Suavé, and Kapandji IA: Nouvelle technique pour le traitement chirurgical des luxations récidivantes isolées de l'extrémité inférieure du cubitus. J Chir 47:589–594, 1936.
40. Carroll RE, and Imbriglia JE: Distal radioulnar arthrodesis indications and technique. Orthop Trans 3:269, 1979.

CHAPTER 18

Introduction to the Carpal Instabilities

DAVID M. LICHTMAN, M.D.
and ROBERT A. MARTIN, D.O.

The subject of carpal instability has been undergoing constant re-evaluation ever since Navarro attempted to describe carpal mechanics in 1919 with the columnar theory. Since that time, many authors have contributed to the understanding and visualization of carpal kinematics and pathomechanics. This chapter explores and analyzes these theories and presents a new concept for carpal kinematics—the "ring" model. We have outlined a new classification system of carpal instabilities based on this model.

THE WRIST AS A LINK MECHANISM

In 1943, Gilford and colleagues[1] popularized Lambrinudis' concept of the wrist as a "link" mechanism in which the radius, the proximal carpal row, and the distal carpal row constitute the individual links. The link mechanism is stable in tension but collapses with axial compression (Fig. 18–1). In order to explain the deformity noted in certain cases of scaphoid nonunion, Gilford likened the scaphoid to a control rod linking the proximal and distal rows.

The Scaphoid as a Slider-Crank

Later, Linscheid and Dobyns[2] introduced the "slider-crank" analogy to explain the scaphoid's role in preventing intercarpal collapse (Fig. 18–2). According to this theory, the scaphoid acts as a bridge between the two rows controlling intercarpal motion, just as a slider-crank controls motion between piston and drive shaft in an internal combustion engine or between piston and crankshaft in a compressor.

In 1970, Fisk[3] expanded on Gilford's link theory, while stressing the importance of the volar ligamentous structures. He described the intercarpal collapse that occurred after trauma or as a result of Kienböck's disease as a "concertina deformity." Linscheid and Dobyns noted two distinct patterns of intercalary collapse and named them *dorsal intercalary segment instability* (DISI) and *volar intercalary segment instability* (VISI).[2] Their classification was based upon the capitolunate angle seen in the lateral x-ray. In the DISI pattern, the lunate is displaced anteriorly and dorsiflexed (extended) in re-

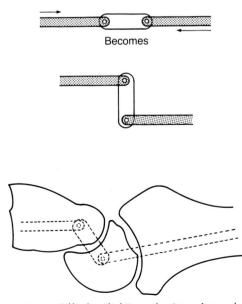

Figure 18–1. Gilford's "link" mechanism of carpal mechanics shows the carpus is stable in tension, but collapses in compression. (Gilford W, Boltar R, Lambrinudi C: Guy's Hospital Report 92:52–59, 1943.)

244

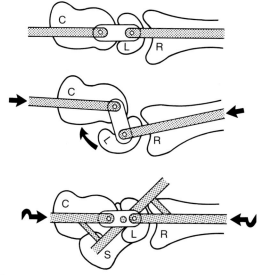

Figure 18–2. The "slider-crank" theory visualizes the scaphoid acting as a bridge between the proximal and distal carpal rows, controlling intercarpal motion much as the piston and crank shaft do in a compressor. (From Linscheid RL, Dobyns JH, et al: J Bone Joint Surg 54A:1612–1632, 1972.)

columnar carpus (Fig. 18–4). The model was amplified in detail by Scaramuzza[4a] in 1969. In 1976, Taleisnik[5] modified Navarro's model in order to accommodate clinically recognized patterns of carpal instability. In Taleisnik's model, the central flexion-extension column consists of the entire distal row and the lunate (Fig. 18–5). The scaphoid is the mobile lateral column, and the triquetrum is the rotatory medial column. This concept has led to the theory that many carpal instabilities occur in columnar or longitudinal patterns, e.g., "radial column instability" and "ulnar column" instability. Consequently, scapholunate dissociation has been classified as a radial instability and triquetrolunate dissociation as an ulnar instability. In many ways this is a useful concept, but it fails to account for the transverse (perilunar) patterns of instability produced in vitro by Mayfield and coworkers[6, 7] as well as for the clinical patterns of transverse midcarpal and proximal carpal instabilities described in several recent papers.[8–11]

lation to the capitate, whereas in the VISI pattern, the lunate is displaced dorsally and palmar flexed (Fig. 18–3). This classification is still a good way to subdivide perilunate instabilities.

THE COLUMNAR WRIST CONCEPT

In 1919, Navarro[4] introduced a model for wrist kinematics based on the concept of a

RECENT PATHOKINEMATIC STUDIES

Perilunate Pattern of Injury

The work of Mayfield and coworkers[6, 7] established the *perilunate pattern of injury* to the volar ligaments of the wrist in an experimentally produced in vitro simulation of a fall on the outstretched hand (Fig. 18–6). As the wrist was forced into progressive dorsi-

DISI—Dorsiflexion Intercalary Segment Instability

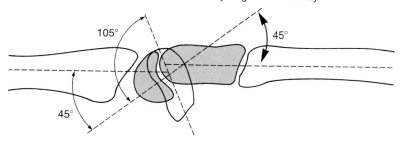

VISI—Volar Flexion Intercalary Segment Instability

Figure 18–3. Dorsiflexion intercalary segmental instability *(top)* shows the lunate displaced anteriorly and dorsiflexed 45°. Volar flexion intercalary segmental instability *(bottom)* shows the lunate dorsal to the capitate and palmar flexed. (From Linscheid RL, Dobyns JH, et al: J Bone Joint Surg 54A:1612–1632, 1972.)

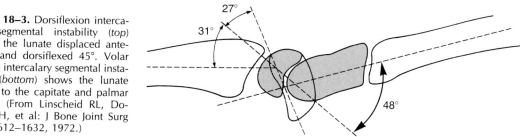

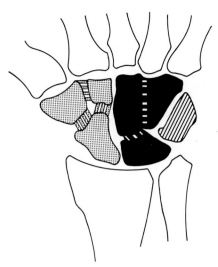

Figure 18–4. The columnar carpus of Navarro, showing three vertical columns: central or flexion-extension column, formed by the lunate, capitate, and hamate; lateral or mobile column, with the scaphoid, trapezium, and trapezoid; medial or rotation column, consisting of the triquetrum and pisiform (see ref. 4).

flexion, ulnar deviation, and intercarpal supination, a reproducible pattern of ligament failure occurred, starting with the radial collateral ligament, progressing to the radio-capitate and the radioscapholunate liga-

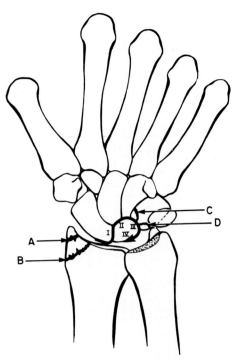

Figure 18–6. The perilunate pattern of injury to the volar ligaments of the wrist is divided into four stages. Stage I is a partial disruption of the scapholunate joint. Stage II is a complete disruption of the scapholunate joint. Stage III is a disruption of the scapholunate, capitolunate, and triquetrolunate joints. Stage IV is a disruption of all the above and the dorsal radiocarpal ligaments, allowing volar lunate dislocation or dorsal perilunate dislocation. Occasionally, radial styloid (A, B) or triquetrum (C, D) fractures accompany perilunate ligament injuries. Other fracture patterns also occur (Fig. 18–8). (From Mayfield JK, Johnson RP, and Kilcoyne RF: J Hand Surg 5:226–241, 1980.)

ments, and then to the scapholunate interosseous ligament. These initial ligament failures were manifested dynamically by scapholunate instability (Stage I). With continued force, the volar radiotriquetral ligament failed, which resulted in triquetrolunate instability (Stage III). Finally, the dorsal radiocarpal ligaments gave way, which permitted volar lunate dislocation or dorsal perilunate dislocation (Stage IV) (Fig. 18–7). Interestingly, it was observed that if the force vector took a wider arc around the lunate, it would create a variety of perilunate fracture dislocations. One example is the transcaphoid transcapitate perilunate dislocation (naviculocapitate syndrome). It has been suggested that a "greater arc" injury is more likely to occur if the hand is radially deviated when the force transmission is initiated.[12] Thus, depending on the relative position of the hand with respect to radial and ulnar deviation at the time of impact, a lesser arc (ligamentous) or greater arc (bone) perilunate instability can be created (Fig. 18–8).

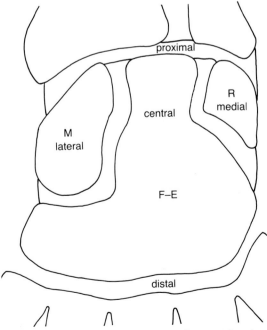

Figure 18–5. Taleisnik's modification of Navarro's columnar model. The entire distal carpal row, along with the lunate, became the central flexion-extension column. The scaphoid forms the lateral mobile column and the triquetrum the medial rotatory column (see ref. 5). R = rotatory column; M = mobile column; F-E = flexion-extension column.

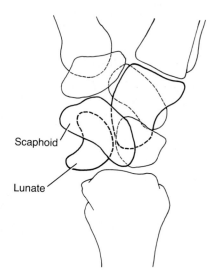

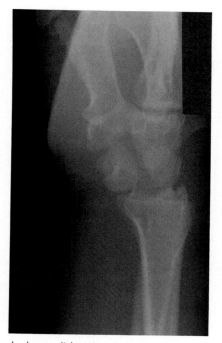

Scaphoid

Lunate

Figure 18–7. A volar lunate dislocation (Stage IV perilunate dissociation) caused by disruption of the radiocarpal ligaments.

NEWLY RECOGNIZED INSTABILITY PATTERNS

Midcarpal Instabilities

In 1980,[13] a series of patients was studied who had palmar subluxation at the midcarpal joint and a painful clunk with ulnar deviation of the wrist. Experimental and

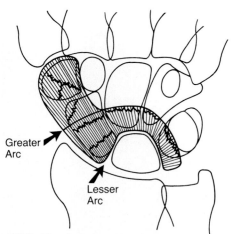

Greater
Arc

Lesser
Arc

Figure 18–8. The greater arc and lesser arc paths of carpal injury. The greater arc injuries tend to occur with the hand radially deviated, transmitting the force through the scaphoid, creating primarily a bony (perilunate) instability. The lesser arc injuries occur with the hand less radially deviated, creating primarily a ligamentous perilunate instability. (From Weber ER, Chao EV: J Hand Surg 3:142–148, 1978.)

clinical studies suggested that the midcarpal subluxation was due to laxity of the ulnar arm of the volar arcuate ligament.[14] Originally, midcarpal instability (MCI) was classified as an ulnar instability, but this led to some confusion, since the ulnar longitudinal column, as described by Taleisnik, is not affected in this type of instability. Instead, it is truly a transverse laxity, the subluxation occurring entirely between the proximal and the distal carpal rows.[15] In addition to the *volar midcarpal pattern*, a few patients have now been identified with the reverse pattern, or *dorsal midcarpal subluxation*.[16] Subsequently, MCI has also been seen following dorsally displaced fractures of the distal radius.[17] In 1984, Taleisnik described this instability, which I call *extrinsic midcarpal instability* to differentiate it from the intrinsic variety described previously. In extrinsic MCI, the dorsally displaced distal radial fracture induces a Z-deformity in the carpus, which eventually results in laxity of the midcarpal ligaments. Correction of the extrinsic instability is achieved by osteotomy of the distal radius.

Proximal Carpal Instabilities

Another group of carpal instabilities occurs at the radiocarpal and ulnocarpal joints. Ulnar translocation of the carpus is the most

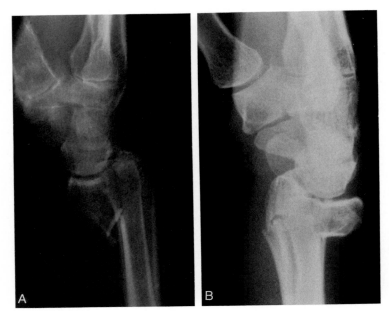

Figure 18–9. *A,* A volar Barton's fracture, showing the carpus in a volar subluxed position. *B,* A dorsal Barton's fracture, showing the carpus in a dorsal subluxated position.

widely recognized entity in this group. It can be due to rheumatoid arthritis or result from surgical resection of the distal ulna.[18, 19] A series of post-traumatic cases has also been described.[20] Other entities in this group include dorsal and palmar carpal dislocations secondary to malunited intra-articular rim fractures of the distal radius (so-called Barton's variants) (Fig. 18–9). Collectively this group is called the *proximal carpal instabilities.*

THE RING CONCEPT

In light of the experimental findings regarding the pathogenesis of perilunar carpal instabilities as well as the clinical recognition of transverse midcarpal and proximal instability patterns, the author finds it difficult to adhere to the columnar wrist concept and the longitudinal classification system of carpal instabilities that derive from it. It is also difficult to continue to visualize the scaphoid as a slider-crank, linking and controlling motion between the proximal and distal rows. Strictly speaking, a slider-crank translates rotary motion into reciprocal motion or reciprocal motion into rotary motion. However, in reality, the entire proximal row—including the scaphoid—moves passively as a unit in response to the resultant compressive and tensile forces acting on its bone surfaces. This motion is guided and restrained by the unique arrangement of bone contacts and ligamentous supports of the wrist. It is well known that radial deviation

of the hand and distal carpus causes palmar flexion of the proximal row and that ulnar deviation of the hand and distal row causes the proximal row to extend (Fig. 18–10). Key components in this reciprocal motion between the carpal rows are the two physiologic "links": the mobile scaphotrapeziotrapezoid (STT) joint and the rotatory triquetrohamate joint. Radial deviation compresses the STT joint, forcing the scaphoid and proximal row into flexion, whereas ulnar deviation forces the triquetrum to glide into its dorsiflexed position against the hamate, carrying the entire proximal row with

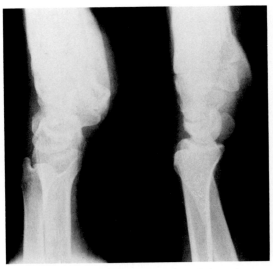

Figure 18–10. In radial deviation (*left*) and ulnar deviation (*right*), the normal wrist displays a "physiologic" VISI and DISI pattern.

it into extension. In neutral deviation, these forces are dissipated if the wrist is relaxed, and they are neutralized by intact bone and ligamentous supports if the wrist is stressed, as by a clenched fist.

By utilizing this transverse "ring" model of carpal kinematics, a clearer visualization of the pathokinematics of perilunate and midcarpal instabilities can be obtained (Fig. 18–11). With a "break" in the ring through the triquetrolunate joint, the proximal carpal row no longer moves as a unit. The lunate palmar flexes with the scaphoid, in response to dynamic forces on the radial side of the carpus, whereas the triquetrum tends to dorsiflex as it is forced ulnarly by the head of the capitate and to assume its low dorsiflexed position in relation to the hamate. Thus, a static VISI deformity (palmar flexion and dorsal translocation of the lunate) will be seen on the routine lateral roentgenograms. With a break in the ring through the scaphoid or the scapholunate joint, the lunate (as well as the proximal scaphoid fragment) is set free to follow the triquetrum as it rotates into its low dorsiflexed position. Even though the scaphoid flexes in response to forces on the radial side, the routine lateral views show a DISI deformity (dorsiflexion and volar translocation of the lunate). In midcarpal instability, laxity of the ulnar arm of the arcuate ligament decreases the influence of the geometric configuration of the triquetrohamate joint on the proximal carpal row. This allows the proximal carpal row to assume a gravity-induced palmarflexed position (VISI), which persists until the last few degrees of ulnar deviation, at which point the proximal row snaps suddenly into its dorsiflexed reduced position, rather than following the normal smooth transition from palmar flexion to dorsiflexion.

Thus, unstable scaphoid fractures or scapholunate ligament disruptions cause a DISI pattern, whereas triquetrolunate injury results in a VISI deformity. If the tear is small or incomplete, the instability may not manifest itself clinically unless significant stress is applied to the wrist. When a DISI or VISI pattern can be seen only with stress views, the pattern has been termed *dynamic instability*, whereas when the pattern is present without additional stress, it is called *static instability*.[21] Static deformities are usually due to unstable complete ligamentous or bone injuries, whereas dynamic instabilities are most likely due to partial ligamentous tears.

CLASSIFICATION OF CARPAL INSTABILITIES

In order to integrate what we have now learned about carpal kinematics, clinical instability patterns, and the pathogenesis of carpal ligament disruptions, a new classification system of carpal instabilities is presented. This system is based on the transverse pattern of carpal instabilities, as visualized by the carpal ring concept, rather than on the more traditional longitudinal or columnar carpus concept. It also assumes that the reader accepts the scaphoid as a full-fledged member of the proximal row rather than as a mechanical linkage between the two.

In the miscellaneous group are trapezioscaphoid and capitolunate instabilities, which are probably subdivisions of midcarpal instability. Sooner or later every articulation of the wrist will have its own reported instability, of either traumatic or congenital origin. However, until these entities can be studied carefully to establish their possible relationship to existing instability patterns, I think that they should remain temporarily in the miscellaneous category.

In the next few chapters, established carpal instability patterns are explored in

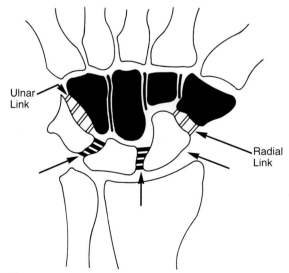

Figure 18–11. The "ring" model of carpal kinematics. The distal arc proximal carpal rows are joined by two physiologic "links," thus allowing reciprocal motion. These links are the mobile scaphotrapezial joint (radial link) and the rotatory triquetrohamate joint (ulnar link).

Ulnar Link

Radial Link

Table 18–1. **CLASSIFICATION OF CARPAL INSTABILITIES**

I. Perilunar instabilities
  A. Lesser arc injuries
    1. Scapholunate instability
      a. Dynamic—partial
      b. Static—complete (DISI)
    2. Triquetrolunate instability
      a. Dynamic—partial
      b. Static—complete (VISI)
    3. Complete perilunate instability
      a. Dorsal perilunate dislocation
      b. Palmar lunate dislocation
  B. Greater arc injury
    1. Scaphoid fracture
      a. Stable
      b. Unstable (DISI)
    2. Naviculocapitate syndrome
    3. Trans-scaphoid transtriquetral perilunate dislocations
    4. Variations and combinations of the above
  C. Inflammatory disorders
    1. Scapholunate
      a. Dynamic—partial
      b. Static—complete (DISI)
    2. Triquetrolunate
      a. Dynamic—partial
      b. Static—complete (VISI)
II. Midcarpal instabilities
  A. Intrinsic (ligamentous laxity)
    1. Palmar midcarpal instability (VISI)
    2. Dorsal midcarpal instability (DISI)
  B. Extrinsic (dorsally displaced distal radial fracture)
III. Proximal carpal instabilities
  A. Ulnar translocation of the carpus
    1. Rheumatoid
    2. Post-traumatic
    3. Iatrogenic (after excision of the ulnar head)
  B. Dorsal instability (after dorsal rim distal radial fracture—dorsal Barton's fracture)
  C. Palmar instability (after volar rim distal radial fracture—volar Barton's fracture)
IV. Miscellaneous

greater depth. The reader is reminded that the classification scheme presented here has evolved from a synthesis of recent experimental studies, case reports, and personal experience. It does not necessarily represent the thought processes of each of our contributors. Dr. Gerald Blatt's chapter (Chapter 19) on scapholunate injuries and the section of Dr. Charlotte Alexander's chapter (Chapter 20) on triquelunate injuries cover the perilunate instabilities. Dr. Alexander's chapter also explores the midcarpal instabilities. The proximal instabilities are discussed individually in several other areas of the book, including Chapter 24 on rheumatoid arthritis by Dr. Donald Ferlic and Chapter 11 on

intra-articular carpal fractures by Dr. Charles Melone.

References

1. Gilford W, Boltan R, and Lambrinudi C: The mechanism of the wrist joint. Guy's Hospital Report 92:52–59, 1943.
2. Linscheid RL, Dobyns JH, et al: Traumatic instability of the wrist. Diagnosis, classification, and pathomechanics. J Bone Joint Surg 54A:1612–1632, 1972.
3. Fisk G: Carpal instability and the fractured scaphoid. Ann R Coll Surg Engl 46:63–76, 1970.
4. Navarro A: Luxaciones del carpo. An Fac Med (Montevideo) 6:113, 1921.
4a. Scaramuzza RFJ: El movimiento de rotation en el carpo y su relacion con la fisiopathologia de sus lesiones traumaticas. Bolentines y trabjos de la Sociedad Argentina de Orthopedia y Traumatologia 34:337, 1969.
5. Taleisnik J: The ligaments of the wrist. J Hand Surg 1:110–118, 1976.
6. Mayfield JK, Johnson RP, and Kilcoyne RF: The ligaments of the human wrist and their functional significance. Anat Rec 186:417–428, 1976.
7. Mayfield JK, Johnson RP, and Kilcoyne RF: Carpal dislocations: pathomechanics and progressive perilunar instability. J Hand Surg 5:226–241, 1980.
8. Jackson WT, and Protas JM: Snapping scapholunate subluxation. J Hand Surg 6:590–594, 1981.
9. Taleisnik J, and Watson K: Midcarpal instabilities caused by malunited fractures of the distal radius. J Hand Surg 9A:350–357, 1984.
10. Lichtman DM, Noble WH, and Alexander CE: Dynamic triquetrolunate instability: case report. J Hand Surg 9A:185–187, 1984.
11. Weeks PM, Young VL, and Gilula LA: A case of painful clicking wrist: a case report. J Hand Surg 4:522–525, 1979.
12. Weber ER, and Chao EY: An experimental approach to the mechanism of scaphoid wrist fractures. J Hand Surg 3:142–148, 1978.
13. Lichtman DM, Swafford AR, and Schneider JR: Midcarpal instability. Presented at the thirty-fifth annual meeting of the American Society for Surgery of the Hand, Atlanta, Feb. 4–6, 1980.
14. Lichtman DM, Schneider JR, Swafford AR, et al: Ulnar midcarpal instability—clinical and laboratory analysis. J Hand Surg 9:350–357, 1981.
15. Alexander CE, and Lichtman DM: Ulnar carpal instabilities. Orthop Clin North Am 15:2, 307–320, 1984.
16. Taleisnik J: Personal communication, 1985.
17. Taleisnik J, and Watson HK: Midcarpal instability caused by malunited fractures of the distal radius. J Hand Surg 9:350–357, 1984.
18. Gainer BJ, and Schaberg J: The rheumatoid wrist after resection of the distal ulna. J Hand Surg 10A:837–844, 1985.
19. Linscheid RL, and Dobyns JH: Radiolunate arthrodesis. J Hand Surg 10A:821–829, 1985.
20. Rayhack JM, Linscheid RL, and Dobyns JH: Post-traumatic ulnar translocation of the carpus. J Hand Surg 12A:180–189, 1987.
21. Lichtman DM, Taleisnik J, and Watson K: Symposium on Wrist Injuries. Contemp Orthop 4:1, 107–144, 1982.

CHAPTER 19

Scapholunate Instability

GERALD BLATT, M.D.

INTRODUCTION

It was only a few years ago that the term carpal instability[10, 59] was essentially synonymous with scapholunate dissociation.[21, 74] In 1980, Lichtman and Schneider[40] presented a series of cases in which a dynamic clunk was attributed to instability at the midcarpal joint. Since then, several types of carpal instabilities have been described.[10, 21, 45, 59, 74] Scapholunate instability—now classified as a radial or a lateral instability by Taleisnik[64, 66, 67] and as one of the perilunate instabilities by Lichtman (see Chapter 18)—still remains the most common of the carpal instabilities. As the classification of scapholunate instability has evolved over the past few years, so has the treatment. This chapter describes the pathomechanics, the diagnosis, and the latest treatment modalities for this complex and dynamic wrist problem.

MECHANISM OF INJURY

The complex support mechanism of the periscaphoid ligamentous system[38, 47–49, 63, 66] has been well described elsewhere in this text, in Chapters 2 and 5. Functioning as the axial link between the proximal and the distal carpal rows,[18, 21, 38] the scaphoid must have a significant range of mobility, while retaining stability in stress and in force loading.[22, 45] With wrist motion (Fig. 19–1), the changing volume of the lateral compartment induces the scaphoid to assume a longitudinal and dorsiflexed stance during ulnar deviation and extension, whereas the compression of the scaphoid space during radial deviation and flexion creates a palmar flexed and more vertical stance.[8, 12, 30, 52, 60, 69, 75]

Most patients describe the mechanism of their injury as a fall on the outstretched hand, usually incurring a compression force at the base of the palm, with the hand in extension.[3, 47] A large percentage of these patients can confirm that the direction of the blow was to the ulnar side of the wrist or hypothenar eminence, often stating that they fell backward, with their hand behind them.[37, 46, 51, 70, 79] Not to be discounted are those descriptions of only a severe twisting injury to the wrist, with significant torque to the carpus. The common denominator appears to be the acute radial deviation of the hand in extension, creating a severe compression of the scaphoid space. This forced vertical alignment of the scaphoid is compounded by the battering-ram effect of the capitate on the scapholunate joint (Fig. 19–2). Often, only very slight alterations in this alignment-force mechanism[47, 49] are required to complete the spectrum of injury, from Colles' fracture to lunate dislocation,[18, 34, 62, 63] perilunate dislocation,[34, 64] fracture of the scaphoid,[10, 21] trans-scaphoid perilunate dislocation,[7, 65] and perhaps even Kienböck's disease.

It is this author's belief that the range of injury involving the scapholunate complex[39] may best be understood by reducing the ligamentous complex to the three major ligaments: the short, tight scapholunate interosseous ligament; the dorsal scapholunate ligament; the large volar radioscapholunate ligament (Fig. 19–3). A series of anatomic studies of cadaveric dissections and in vitro radiographs following sequential ligament division has led to the formulation of a mechanism of progressive ligament incompetence and the associated clinical picture. Division of only the short, tight interosseous ligament retains essential intercarpal stability, and scapholunate dissociation is not demonstrated (Fig. 19–4). When the dorsal scapholunate ligament is divided, an obvious dissociation is seen, with early subclinical rotatory subluxation of the scaphoid (Fig. 19–5). Only after the volar radioscapholunate ligament is divided, however, do we have complete subluxation of the

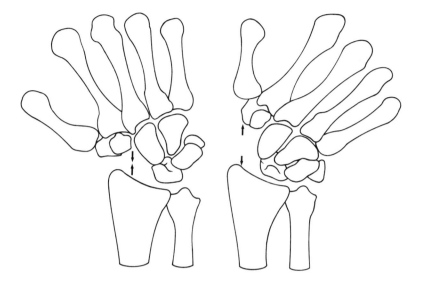

Figure 19–1. On radial deviation, the scaphoid fossa compresses, producing a more vertical alignment. With ulnar deviation, the space elongates and creates a more horizontal scaphoid.

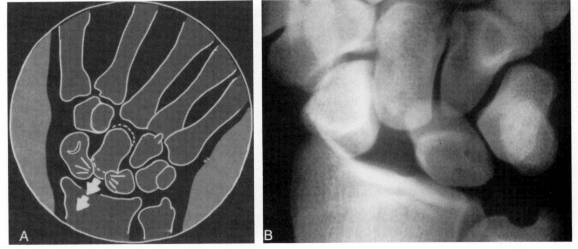

Figure 19–2. *A,* One mechanism of injury is the compressive "battering-ram" effect of the capitate directly into the scapholunate joint. *B,* The capitate is seen acting as a wedge between scaphoid and lunate.

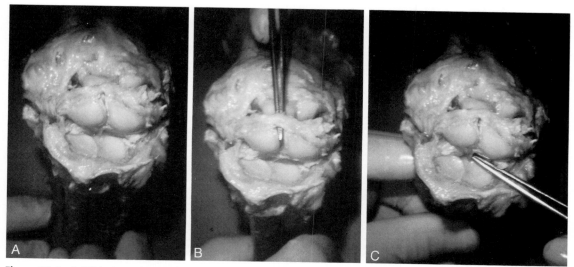

Figure 19–3. *A,* With the radiocarpal joint hinged open, the proximal pole of the scaphoid on the left and the proximal articular surface of the lunate on the right, the short, tight interosseous ligament is noted in between. *B,* The dorsal scapholunate ligament. *C,* The volar radioscapholunate ligament.

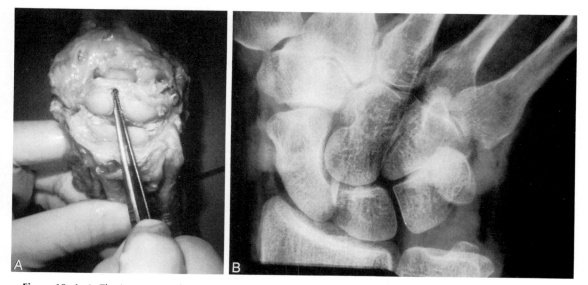

Figure 19–4. *A,* The interosseous ligament is divided. *B,* In vitro radiograph fails to show scapholunate dissociation.

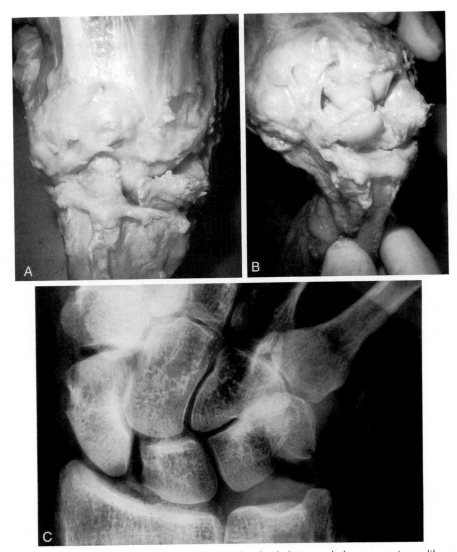

Figure 19–5. *A,* The dorsal scapholunate ligament is now also divided. A scapholunate gap is readily apparent. *B,* A beginning rotatory vertical alignment of the scaphoid is evident. *C,* In vitro radiograph now demonstrates the scapholunate dissociation.

scaphoid and severe (static) carpal instability (Fig. 19–6).

Several conclusions may be drawn from these studies. A rupture of the interosseous ligament alone will yield a negative result in radiographic series and no significant instability. There would most likely be clinical findings of pain and swelling in the area of the "snuffbox." This leads one to speculate on the appropriateness of treatment in suspected fractures of the scaphoid that are initially immobilized[18] but then permitted active range of motion (ROM) when recheck x-rays one week to 10 days later also reveal no fracture; perhaps those patients should still be maintained in a thumb spica cast for

a total of three weeks to permit healing of even this minor ligamentous tear.

It may also be speculated that to have true dynamic scapholunate dissociation, two of the three major ligaments must be compromised; they are the interosseous ligament and either the dorsal scapholunate or the volar radioscapholunate ligament. For the complete picture of static rotatory subluxation to be present all three ligaments would have to be injured, as would occur if the original injury was sufficiently severe. This concept also aids in understanding the reasons for late presentation of the unstable and snapping scaphoid several months after a wrist injury, in which radiographic studies

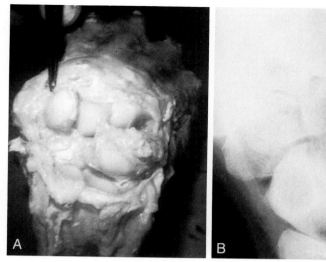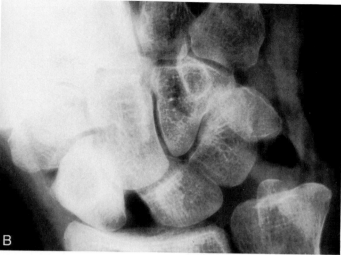

Figure 19–6. *A,* With additional release of the volar radioscapholunate ligament, complete rotatory subluxation of the scaphoid and carpal instability are demonstrated. *B,* Radiograph of the rotated and foreshortened scaphoid.

are deemed negative and no immobilization is initiated. If, at the time of this severe "wrist sprain," the patient had actually torn the dorsal scapholunate and the interosseous ligaments, he or she would be continuing to place excessive loading stress on the remaining volar radioscapholunate ligament, which contains the highest collagen content of the surrounding ligaments[38] and, therefore, the greatest capacity to gradually stretch and become lax. When this last supporting ligament can no longer maintain the alignment of the scaphoid, then the static rotatory subluxation becomes apparent.

These additional concepts should not distract the reader from an understanding of the stages of Mayfield, Johnson, and Kilcoyne's[48, 49] progressive ligamentous disruption and carpal instability; of Fitton's[19] and England's[17] views that rotatory subluxation of the scaphoid is associated with a pronation-subluxation of the midcarpal joint; or of the classic role of the DISI deformity with the dorsal tilt of the lunate as the scaphoid becomes more vertical and more palmar flexed.[17, 42, 43]

DIAGNOSIS

Because the most successful results of treating scapholunate dissociation and rotatory subluxation of the scaphoid are obtained following early diagnosis,[6, 44] awareness and recognition of this entity are imperative. As more attention and education have been devoted to carpal instability patterns and injuries, the probability that the diagnosis will be considered early has been greatly increased.[14, 17]

Pain, swelling, and tenderness over the dorsoradial aspect of the wrist on clinical examination following injury should certainly increase suspicion that injury has occurred at the scapholunate complex (Fig. 19–7). The similarity of these findings to those of an indolent fracture of the scaphoid has been discussed earlier. An additional test for ligamentous disruption has been described by Watson.[76, 79] The examiner places his thumb over the radiovolar aspect of the patient's wrist, palpating the volar tubercle of the scaphoid (Fig. 19–8). As the patient ulnar deviates the hand, the scaphoid elongates and becomes unweighted. However, on radial deviation, there is axial loading as the scaphoid space becomes compressed. The scaphoid begins to move in a more vertical alignment, forcing the volar tubercle against the examiner's thumb. With this additional pressure transmitted to the proximal pole of the scaphoid and to the scapholunate joint, there is increased pain if ligamentous disruption has occurred.

Radiographic examination of the wrist is the most important diagnostic study to be performed in these patients.[3, 13, 15, 16, 23, 32, 33] The evolution of special views, positions, and techniques has greatly increased the possibility for recognition of intercarpal ligamentous disruption.[50] Routine radiographic views of the wrist often do not demonstrate this pathologic condition. In

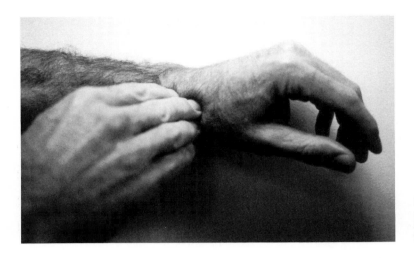

Figure 19–7. Tender swelling in the anatomic "snuffbox" may indicate ligament disruption as well as a possible fractured scaphoid.

particular, the standard PA projection (in pronation) creates a false security in that it gives the impression of normal alignment.[9, 71] Only with the wrist in full supination (AP projection) can the scapholunate dissociation be demonstrated (Fig. 19–9). This gap between the scaphoid and the lunate, at least when it is greater than 2 mm, has become known as the classic Terry-Thomas sign.[20] I concur with the recommendations of Gilula and Weeks[22] that additional information may be obtained from these passive radiographic studies by dynamically loading the carpus. Therefore, the supination views are obtained bilaterally with and without the fist clenched (Fig. 19–10). This maneuver obviously adds a compression-stress load

across the wrist and may further displace carpal alignment where ligamentous laxity (dynamic instability) exists.

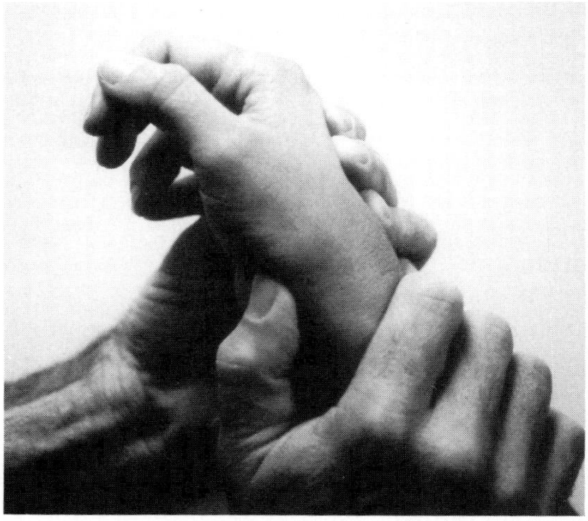

It is important here to reiterate that the presence of a dynamic scapholunate dissociation is not synonymous with a complete static rotatory subluxation of the scaphoid. Although some rotation may coexist, true subluxation with increased vertical alignment of the scaphoid is a more progressive change.[31, 42] There are additional radiographic findings to assist in evaluating the degree of rotation. Again, on the AP projection, as the longitudinal axial alignment of the scaphoid becomes more vertical, there is obvious foreshortening of the axial length.[73] A significant finding is the "ring" sign (Fig. 19–11), which represents the cortical projection of the distal pole of the scaphoid in its vertical alignment. A graphic representation of the formation of the ring sign is given in Figure 19–12A, B, and C.[4, 13, 14, 16] To assess the degree of scaphoid rotation, the lateral radiographic projection of the wrist is essential.[17, 42, 43] The described DISI deformity should be noted with the lunate in dorsiflexion and the long axis of the scaphoid perpendicular to that of the radius (Fig. 19–13). Various studies have provided us with a measurement of 46° for the average scapholunate angle, with a range of 30° to 60°. Abnormal rotation of the scaphoid is confirmed by angles greater than 70°.[16, 42] Considered of benefit by some is the radioscaphoid angle, which ranges between 33° and 73°, with an average of 58°.[27, 64]

However, lateral radiographs of the wrist are often unreliable for so precise an angular measurement. Owing to either poor radiographic quality or technique, the carpal

Figure 19–8. The examiner's thumb is placed over the volar tubercle of the scaphoid with the patient's hand in ulnar deviation. As the wrist is brought into radial deviation, pain is produced in the wrist if there has been ligamentous injury.

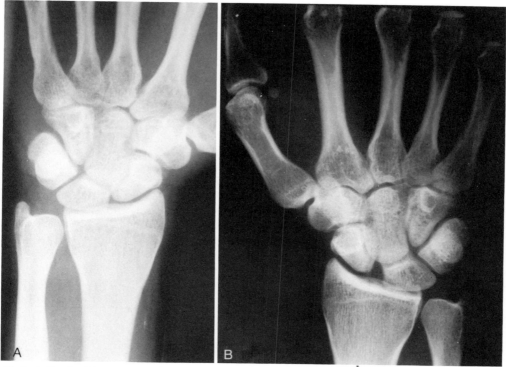

Figure 19–9. *A*, Routine PA projection with the wrist in pronation reveals apparent normal carpal alignment. *B*, The same wrist in supination on AP projection demonstrates scapholunate dissociation, or ''Terry-Thomas'' sign.

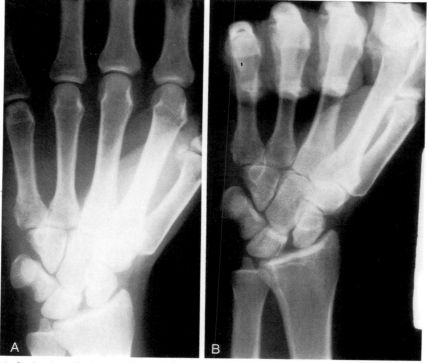

Figure 19–10. *A*, Supination AP view, with scapholunate gap. The hand is relaxed. *B*, A clenched-fist view compresses the carpus and enhances demonstration of the dissociation.

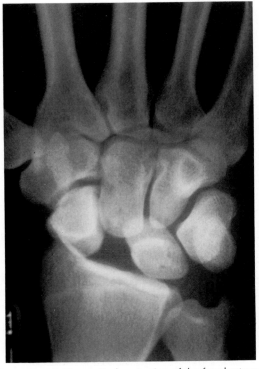

Figure 19–11. The cortical projection of the foreshortened and vertical scaphoid creates the "ring" sign.

bones in question must often be outlined on the x-ray by the examiner, using some degree of artistic license, and then carefully measured at the place where they are supposedly located. I have found a simple, objective measurement obtained from the more reliable frontal projection radiograph to be a consistent indicator of abnormal scaphoid rotation. By combining the presence of the ring sign with the accepted foreshortening of the vertical scaphoid, a measurement of this ring to the proximal pole of the scaphoid indicates degree of rotation (Fig. 19–14). We have found that on bilateral views, with the wrists in neutral, the ring-to-proximal-pole distance is reduced by at least 4 mm, or is no greater than 7 mm, or both. Conversely, when the abnormal scaphoid rotation is corrected and therefore becomes more longitudinal, this ring-to-proximal-pole distance is again increased to equal the greater distance of the normal side (Fig. 19–15).

Of the special studies available to enhance diagnostic evaluation of kinematic disruption, the cineradiograph is the most valuable.[2] It is a simple and noninvasive procedure that can provide significant information

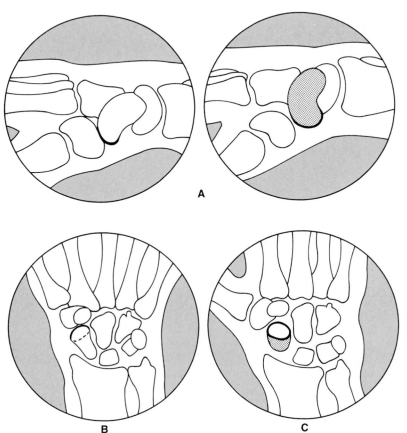

Figure 12. *A,* As the scaphoid rotates, a more tubular projection is created. *B,* Normal alignment in the AP view. *C,* The clearly established "ring" sign.

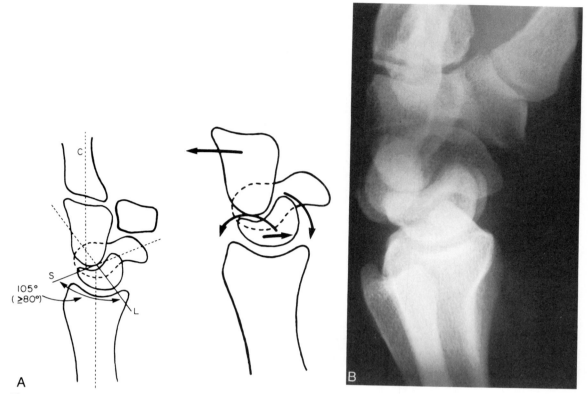

Figure 19–13. *A,* Pathomechanics and technique for measuring scapholunate and radioscaphoid angles in DISI deformity. *B,* Lateral radiograph demonstrating clinical DISI deformity. (*A,* From Gilula LA, Destout JM, Weeks PM, et al: Clin Orthop 187:52–54, 1984.)

about the pattern of instability. Dramatic effects can be demonstrated in both frontal and lateral projections, as the wrist is brought through the full range of flexion and

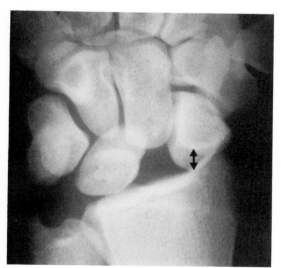

Figure 19–14. The shortened distance from ring to proximal pole (*double-headed arrow*) is noted to be reduced by at least 4 mm and is no greater than 7 mm.

extension as well as radial and ulnar deviation. The obvious instability pattern of a static rotatory subluxation of the scaphoid can be easily differentiated from the more subtle defect of a dynamic scapholunate dissociation.

Although it is rarely indicated, since the diagnosis should have already been well established, mention should be made of the availability of both arthrography and bone scans in the increasingly dimensional perspective employed in diagnostic evaluation.[33, 43, 54]

TREATMENT

As in most ligament injuries, early treatment and repair will yield the best results;[29, 66] consequently, the importance of an accurate diagnosis following wrist trauma is again stressed. The optimum time span acceptable for acute injury to ligament repair is three to five weeks. A review of the broad spectrum of scapholunate injuries and some of the treatment philosophies, all of which depend on the degree and stage of pathologic disorder, are presented.

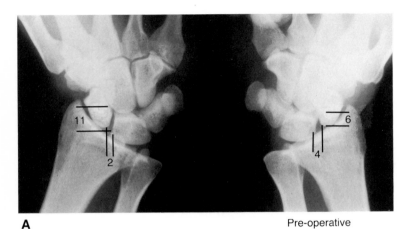

A   Pre-operative

B   One Year Postoperative

Figure 19–15. *A,* Before operation, the distance from ring to proximal pole in this deformity is 6 mm as compared with 11 mm for the normal side. *B,* Postoperative scaphoid derotation and restoration of axial length are confirmed.

The most basic injury to be treated is the painful wrist following trauma, in which the results of x-ray studies, including all special stress views, are completely negative.[14, 23] If a patient has pain and swelling in the "snuff-box"—the area of the scapholunate joint—it is my opinion that the injury is as likely to represent an interosseous scapholunate ligament tear as it is an occult fracture of the scaphoid.[29, 36, 49, 55] Rather than immobilize these patients in a thumb spica cast for one week to 10 days and then recheck for a visible fracture line, I prefer to protect these patients by continuing the cast immobilization for three weeks to allow time for the ligamentous injury to heal.

The next level of severity in this injury presents a similar clinical picture but shows definite evidence of scapholunate gap.[6, 44] As suggested by anatomic studies noted earlier, this would most likely represent a compromise of at least two of the three major support ligaments. Accurate reduction and internal fixation are mandatory. Although it

has been recommended that this may be accomplished by percutaneous technique under cineradiographic control,[57, 64] I feel that the potential severity of this instability warrants the maximum control of open reduction, inspection, and repair (Fig. 19–16). It is only by direct visualization through a dorsal approach that precise carpal alignment can be achieved; use of this technique also assures that portions of torn ligament are not folded into the joint space.[26, 44] Suture approximation, where possible, is desired; but alignment of the ligament fibers with secure intercarpal reduction can only enhance the fibroblastic repair of the capsule. Internal fixation may best be achieved with a smooth 0.045 K wire placed through the distal pole of the scaphoid and into the capitate, and a second K wire placed across the scapholunate joint. Thumb spica cast immobilization is maintained for eight to 10 weeks with the wrist in a neutral to slightly flexed position.

With progression of the degree of trauma,

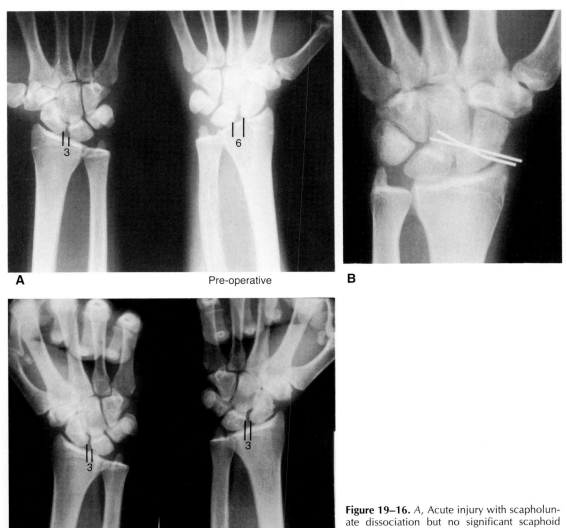

A   Pre-operative   B

C   Postoperative

Figure 19–16. *A*, Acute injury with scapholunate dissociation but no significant scaphoid rotation. *B*, Anatomic alignment following immediate open reduction, ligament repair, and internal fixation. *C*, Postoperative correction and stability on supination clenched-fist view.

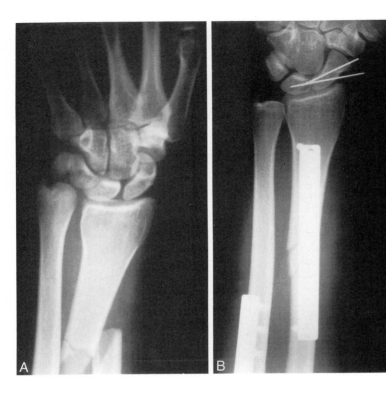

Figure 19–17. *A,* Instability of the scapholunate articulation is seen following a severe fracture of both bones of the forearm. *B,* Radiograph taken following open reduction and internal fixation of fractures of the radius and ulna and disruption of the scapholunate joint.

the severity of associated bone and ligamentous injury is proportionately expanded.[1, 3, 68, 71] In such cases, the scapholunate dissociation and rotatory subluxation of the scaphoid may be overshadowed by severe extracarpal fractures of the wrist and forearm (Fig. 19–17) or other major carpal injuries.[4, 58] In particular, there is a high degree of associated scapholunate ligament disruption with displaced intra-articular fractures of the radial styloid (Fig. 19–18). In young adults, fractures of the styloid with marked scapholunate dissociation should be opened and explored. The styloid can be held in position with K wires and the scapholunate dissociation reduced and fixed as previously described.

Of the other major carpal injuries that require open reduction and repair, the most notable are lunate and perilunate dislocations (Fig. 19–19). Following closed reduction of the acute injury, malrotation of the scaphoid may become evident as the swelling gradually subsides.[26] Because of the obvious volar capsule buttonhole tear produced by the lunate, these injuries require both dorsal and volar surgical approaches (Fig. 19–20). Again, internal K-wire fixation is mandatory to maintain secure alignment during capsular and ligamentous healing.

In cases of late diagnosis, with only radio-graphic evidence of a scapholunate gap with or without applied stress to the wrist,[11, 28, 41] a period of up to six weeks after injury is feasible for open operative intervention and internal fixation, as previously described. If presentation is between six and 12 weeks after injury with no evidence of rotatory

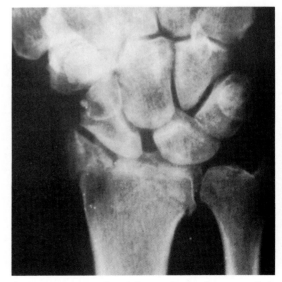

Figure 19–18. Displaced intra-articular fractures of the radial styloid are often associated with scapholunate ligament disruption. (By permission from Taleisnik J: The Wrist. Churchill Livingstone Inc, New York, 1985.)

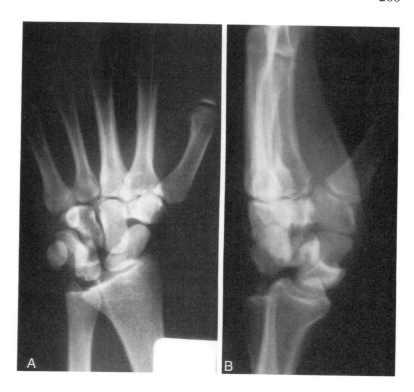

Figure 19–19. *A, B,* Dislocation of the lunate with scaphoid instability due to avulsion of the periscaphoid capsule.

subluxation of the scaphoid (no snap), then cast immobilization for four to six weeks is recommended. After three months past the injury, the patient is cautioned against impaction stress activities to the wrist and is closely observed. The presence of a scapho-lunate gap on x-ray studies is not in itself an indication for surgical correction, unless it is associated with continued pain, discomfort, or a snap.

The next stage in the progression of instabilities is the most problematic and difficult

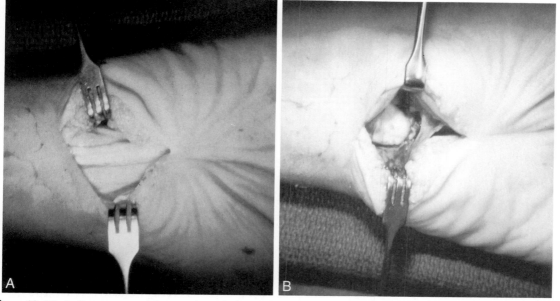

Figure 19–20. *A,* On exposure of the carpal canal, the median nerve is seen to be tented over the bulging flexor tendons. *B,* The median nerve and flexor tendons are retracted to reveal the carpal lunate herniated through the floor of the carpal canal.

to treat: the chronic scapholunate dissociation presenting with a late complete rotatory subluxation of the scaphoid.[1, 3, 68, 71] Patients often relate a history of wrist trauma approximately three to four months before and then note a sudden, loud "snap" or "clunk" over the radial aspect of the wrist on certain reproducible maneuvers. Pain and loss of grip strength are often associated.[66] The cause of the loud snapping sound has been attributed by Howard and coworkers[32] to the penetration of the head of the capitate into the scapholunate space. Because I have found this snap to sometimes occur during palmar flexion as well as during dorsiflexion of the wrist, I ascribe this very disconcerting clinical finding to the proximal pole of the scaphoid impinging upon the dorsal rim of the radius, both as it subluxates and as it reduces. The attempted stabilization of this instability has led to myriad creative surgical procedures.[5, 16, 32, 53, 61, 64, 72] Several recent articles have attested to the progressive de-

generative changes that occur when complete scapholunate instability is left untreated.[66]

An early popularized solution was the use of a free tendon graft[64] laced through drill holes between scaphoid, lunate, and distal radius (Fig. 19–21). Although some limited success was reported, a series of troublesome complications soon became associated with this procedure.[24, 53] If the tendon graft was securely and firmly lashed between radius, scaphoid, and lunate to provide the desired stability, the secondary effect was essentially that of a tenodesis with significant loss of wrist motion. If the graft was tethered in lower tension in order to permit adequate active motion, recurrence of the subluxation was frequently noted. With added reports of complete carpal collapse or disintegration due to the multiple drill holes, the procedure has recently lost considerable favor.

As an alternative to ligamentous repair of chronic scapholunate instability, limited ar-

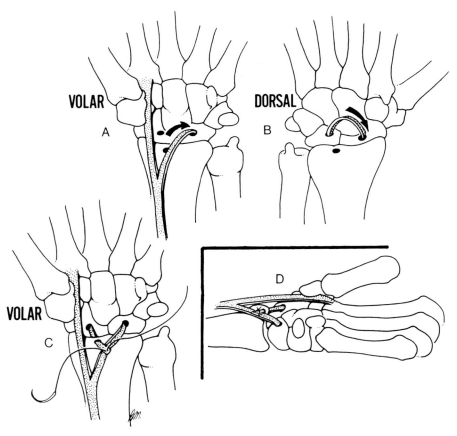

Figure 19–21. Combined volar and dorsal approaches are necessary for this technique (Taleisnik's) of reconstruction of the volar radioscapholunate ligament using a strip of flexor carpi radialis tendon. The multiple drill holes through the carpus and the tenodesis effect have significantly detracted from the popularity of this procedure. (From Green DP: Carpal dislocation. In Green DP (ed): Operative Hand Surgery, Vol I. Churchill Livingstone Inc, New York, 1982.)

throdesis of various carpal bones[56, 61, 72, 76] became the focus of attention. The initial recommendation was to fuse the lunate to the scaphoid.[72] It was soon noted that solid arthrodesis was very difficult to achieve at this articulation because of the limited opposing articular surfaces and the very significant forces applied across this joint.

Fusion of the scaphotrapezial-trapezoid joint, as first proposed by Peterson and Lipscomb[56] in 1967 and more recently popularized by Watson,[76, 79] offers significant advantages (Fig. 19–22). Although this procedure is noted to reduce wrist motion by approximately 50 percent and to add an increased wear component to the radioscaphoid joint,[25, 35] I feel there is indication for its application. Where there is a significant fixed DISI deformity with a marked vertical scaphoid and secondary capsular contracture, restoration of the "lateral column" height with predictable stabilization can be achieved with this procedure.[79] Its applicability as a salvage technique, following failure of any of the soft tissue tendon or capsule procedures, preserves its value as a surgical option. Although intermediate-length follow-up has been promising,[79] the long-term results of limited intercarpal arthrodeses are yet to be determined.[25] The recommended surgical technique, along with indications and contraindications, is presented elsewhere in this text (see Chapter 30).

As an alternative to intercarpal fusion, this author has utilized a technique of dorsal capsulodesis for the past 12 years, with satisfying results.[5] Initially designed for the patient who presents with a late, complete rotatory subluxation of the scaphoid, it is now being applied to all patients with a reducible scapholunate dissociation. It is particularly applicable to the patient with a symptomatic dynamic instability and the early, complete (static) type of deformity.

The principle of the capsulodesis is to stabilize the forceful palmar flexion (volar rotation) of the distal pole of the scaphoid by a proximal checkrein mechanism (Fig. 19–23). The scapholunate gap is essentially ignored, except for its apparent correction once the scaphoid is realigned. Long-term results in 12 patients have been most gratifying, with the recovery of full wrist extension and an average of 80 percent of grip strength, the loss of no more than 20° of wrist flexion, and no recurrent subluxation, except in one patient. A significant feature of this procedure is its ability to anatomically reduce the scaphoid at the time of surgery. A detailed description of the surgical technique is provided (Fig. 19–24).

Through a longitudinal dorsoradial incision, the dorsal wrist capsule is exposed. Next, a longitudinal incision through the capsule in the slightly angulated axis of the scaphoid exposes the full length of the scaphoid. A 1-cm-wide flap of dorsal wrist capsule is then developed from the ulnar side of the capsular incision. This flap is left free on its distal end, while the proximal origin on the dorsum of the distal radius is preserved. The articular cartilage of the proximal pole of the scaphoid is usually visible as the vertical stance is assumed. Confirmation of the rupture of the interosseous and the dorsal scapholunate ligament is made. The scaphoid is reduced by thumb pressure on the volar scaphoid tubercle, as the wrist is brought into slight ulnar deviation and transfixed with a single 0.045 K wire placed at an oblique angle through the distal pole of the scaphoid into the capitate and base of the third metacarpal. A notch is then made in the dorsum of the distal pole of the scaphoid, proximal to the distal articular surface but distal to the mid-axis of rotation of the scaphoid. The dorsal capsuloligamentous flap is now trimmed to the appropriate length and inserted into the distal pole of the scaphoid with a 4–0 stainless steel pull-out wire suture. This is tied over a button on the volar tubercle of the scaphoid. With the dorsal capsulodesis secure, the dorsal wrist capsule may be closed primarily. A secure proximal checkrein

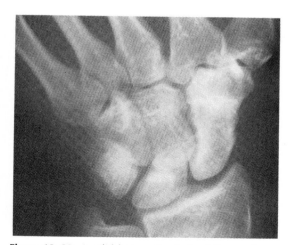

Figure 19–22. A solid bony arthrodesis of the scaphotrapezium-trapezoid joint. (From Kleinman WB, Steichen JB, and Strickland JW: J Hand Surg 7:125, 1982.)

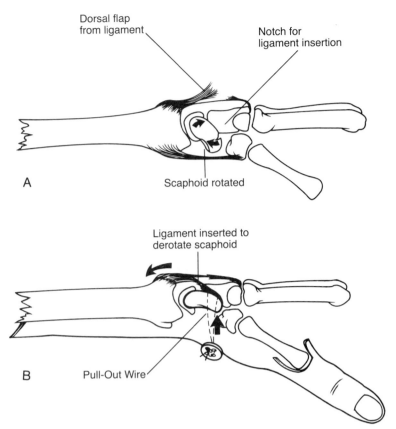

Dorsal flap
from ligament

Notch for
ligament insertion

A

Scaphoid rotated

Ligament inserted to
derotate scaphoid

B   Pull-Out Wire

Figure 19–23. A graphic representation of the technique of dorsal capsulodesis. *A,* A proximally based ligamentous flap is developed from the dorsal wrist capsule. A notch for the ligament insertion is created in the dorsal cortex of the distal pole of the scaphoid, distal to the mid-axis of rotation. *B,* The scaphoid has been derotated and the ligament inserted with a pull-out wire suture.

mechanism to prevent palmar flexion of the distal pole of the scaphoid has been established.

A thumb spica cast is applied for two months. The cast is then removed along with the pull-out wire, but the K-wire fixation remains. A removable splint is applied, and a program of hand therapy for active motion is started. The K wire allows only radiocarpal motion, while still preventing motion between the proximal and distal carpal rows. Three months after operation, the K wire is removed and intercarpal motion is initiated. No forceful stress is permitted for four to six months postoperatively (Fig. 19–25).

The majority of these patients have returned to their preinjury regular work and to unrestricted sports activities (Fig. 19–26). Of particular note is the lack of any attempt to repair or reconstruct the scapholunate joint. It may therefore be concluded that a satisfactory clinical result can be obtained in spite of a persistent scapholunate dissociation by eliminating the dynamic rotatory subluxation. The significant success of this procedure in stabilizing the scaphoid, while still permitting an excellent range of motion

(ROM) as demonstrated by a long-term follow-up study, has encouraged the author to also use this procedure for repair of early, acute subluxation to reinforce the attempted repair of the primary ligaments.

Finally, an even more advanced stage in the untreated scapholunate dissociation with scaphoid malrotation is radioscaphoid arthrosis, which may also be accompanied by degenerative joint changes between the lunate and the capitate. In a patient presenting only with evidence of radioscaphoid arthrosis, my primary choice of procedure is replacement of the scaphoid with an implant (Fig. 19–27). My patients have not experienced the significant problem of silicone synovitis, and I have found this procedure to be extremely satisfactory and durable in relieving pain and in retaining adequate wrist motion.

There are several additional recommendations that may help to minimize the incidence of silicone synovitis: Be sure that the size selected for the implant is not too large; this will avoid increased compression and erosion at the radius-implant interface. It is also imperative to utilize a "no-touch" tech-

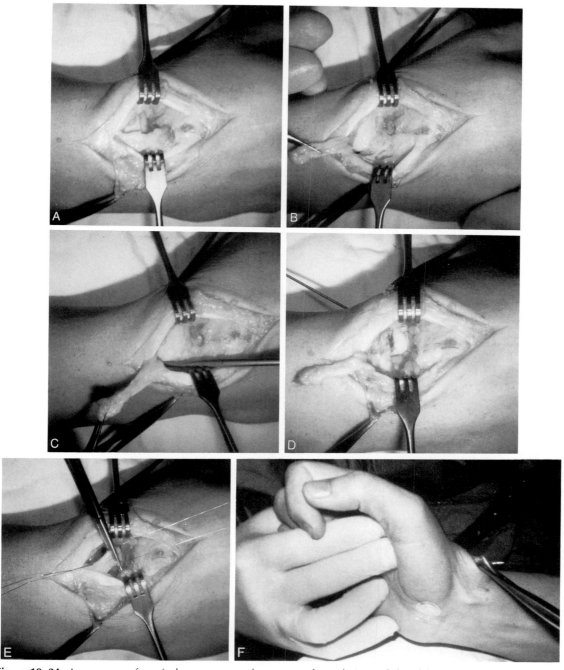

Figure 19–24. A sequence of surgical exposures to demonstrate the technique of dorsal ligament capsulodesis. *A*, A longitudinal dorsoradial incision through the wrist capsule provides exposure of the scaphoid. *B*, A 1-cm-wide flap of the dorsal capsule has been developed and hinged back on its intact origin from the dorsum of the distal radius. The proximal pole of the rotated scaphoid is noted. *C*, A probe is placed into the visible scapholunate gap, confirming disruption of the interosseous and dorsal scapholunate ligaments. *D*, The scaphoid has been reduced and maintained with a 0.045 K-wire. A cortical notch is created in the distal pole of the scaphoid, proximal to the articular surface but distal to the mid-axis of rotation. *E*, Trimmed to the appropriate length, the dorsal ligament is inserted into the fresh bony notch with a wire pull-out suture. The proximal checkrein mechanism has been established. *F*, The wire suture is tied over a button on the radiovolar aspect of the wrist.

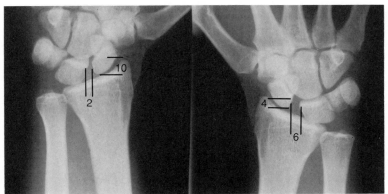

A   Pre-operative

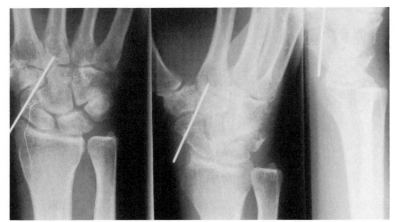

B   Postoperative

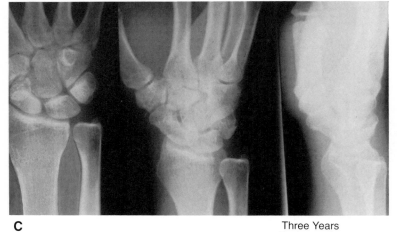

C   Three Years
                                                   Postoperative

Figure 19–25. *A,* Pre-operative radiograph demonstrating scapholunate dissociation, rotatory subluxation of the scaphoid, and shortened ring-to-proximal-pole distance. *B,* Following surgical procedure of dorsal capsulodesis, the reduced scaphoid is maintained by K-wire fixation, while the wire suture keeps the ligament in place. *C,* Long-term follow-up demonstrates continued alignment and stability.

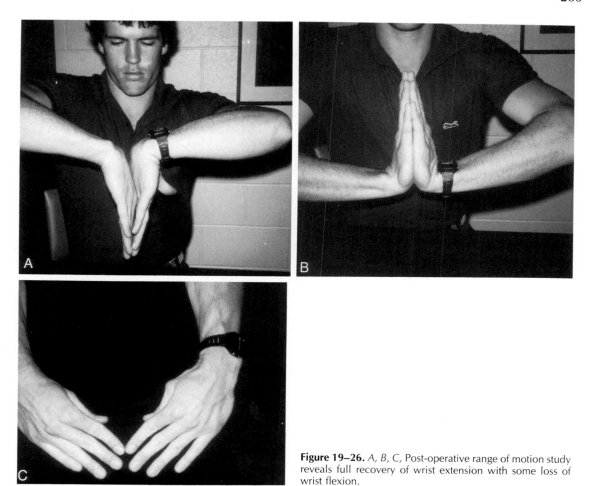

Figure 19–26. *A, B, C,* Post-operative range of motion study reveals full recovery of wrist extension with some loss of wrist flexion.

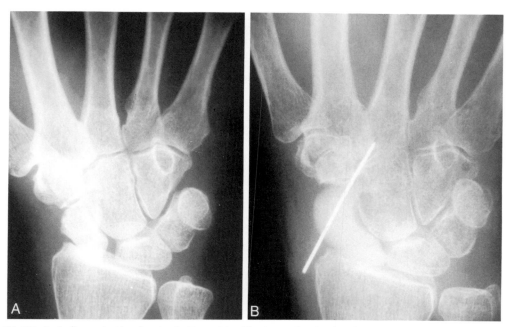

Figure 19–27. *A,* Radioscaphoid arthrosis. *B,* Treated by Silastic scaphoid arthroplasty. Temporary K-wire fixation of the implant is no longer advocated by Dr. Swanson (Chapter 28).

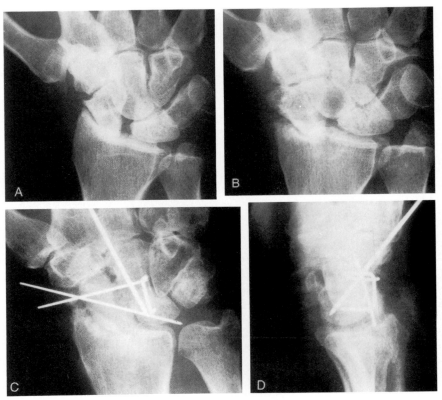

Figure 19–28. As described by Watson and Ballet, the SLAC (scapholunate advanced collapse) wrist includes significant radioscaphoid arthritis with progressive lunocapitate joint degeneration (*A, B*). The recommended treatment is scaphoid implant arthroplasty and lunocapitate arthrodesis (*C, D*). It is currently recommended , however, that K wires not be placed through the silicone prosthesis (see Chapter 28). (By permission from Taleisnik J: The Wrist. Churchill Livingstone Inc, New York, 1985.)

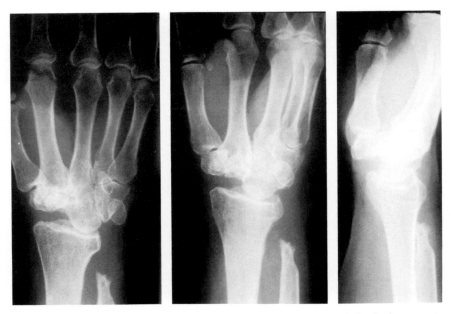

Figure 19–29. Radiograph of wrist eight years after proximal row carpectomy and distal ulna resection. Note well-maintained radiocapitate joint space.

nique when inserting the actual implant. Handling of the trial sizer with latex gloves is acceptable, but the final insertion should be done with instruments only, after the implant has been bathed in a virginal saline solution. As a final precaution, the temporary stabilizing K wire should be left covered beneath the skin and not allowed to penetrate it, because of potential contamination. In fact, there are many who now prefer to avoid K-wire fixation completely (see Chapter 28).

The combination of radioscaphoid and lunocapitate arthrosis meets the criteria for the entity that Watson and Ballet[77, 78] describe as scapholunate advanced collapse—the SLAC wrist (Fig. 19–28). For this more complex involvement, an arthrodesis of the lunocapitate joint is added to the procedure of Silastic scaphoid implant arthroplasty.

Proximal row carpectomy is an excellent procedure that has not been given adequate recognition either as a primary treatment alternative or as a salvage procedure. Although often reported with reassuring conclusions, it has never gained popularity among reconstructive surgeons. Careful excision of the scaphoid, the lunate, and the triquetrum will permit the head of the capitate to articulate with a competent and spherical lunate fossa in the distal radius (Fig. 19–29). By reefing the dorsal capsule, adequate stability is achieved following a six-week course of cast immobilization. Proximal row carpectomy is a procedure with a low morbidity rate, a short postoperative course, and satisfactory reduction of pain with functional wrist ROM and functional grip strength. With advanced destruction and architectural disarray, the possibility of a complete wrist fusion should not be dismissed. Certainly, the proven predictability of the end result and the enduring stability with resistive grip may provide on a long-term basis the strength needed by the heavy laborer.

SUMMARY

Scapholunate injury still remains a significant diagnostic and therapeutic challenge for the orthopedist and hand surgeon. Awareness must be maintained of a minor injury that might later progress to significant instability. As demonstrated in this chapter, it is much easier to treat an acute sprain prophylactically than it is to reconstruct a chronic scapholunate dissociation. Likewise, early surgical repair of the dissociation is preferable to a late salvage operation. Although the long-term results of many of the procedures described in this chapter are still unknown, we have come a long way in recent years in improving results in this difficult therapeutic challenge.

References

1. Adkison JW, and Chapman MW: Treatment of acute lunate and perilunate dislocations. Clin Orthop 164:199, 1982.
2. Arkless R: Cineradiography in normal and abnormal wrists. Am J Roentgenol 96:837, 1966.
3. Armstrong GWD: Rotational subluxation of the scaphoid. Can J Surg 11:306, 1968.
4. Bjelland JC, and Bush JC: Secondary rotational subluxation of the carpal navicular. Ariz Med 34:267, 1977.
5. Blatt G: Dorsal capsulodesis for rotatory subluxation of the carpal scaphoid. Presented at the annual meeting of the American Society for Surgery of the Hand, New Orleans, 1986.
6. Boyes JG: Subluxation of the carpal navicular bone. South Med J 69:141, 1976.
7. Boyes JH: Bunnell's Surgery of the Hand. 5th ed. JB Lippincott Co, Philadelphia, 1970.
8. Buzby BF: Isolated radial dislocation of carpal scaphoid. Ann Surg 100:553, 1934.
9. Campbell RD Jr, Thompson TC, Lance EM, et al: Indications for open reduction of lunate and perilunate dislocations of the carpal bones. J Bone Joint Surg [Am] 47:915, 1965.
10. Cave EF: Retrolunar dislocation of the capitate with fracture or subluxation of the navicular bone. J Bone Joint Surg 23:830, 1941.
11. Collins LC, Lidsky MD, Sharp JT, et al: Malposition of carpal bones in rheumatoid arthritis. Radiology 103:95, 1972.
12. Connell MC, and Dyson RP: Dislocation of the carpal scaphoid. Report of a case. J Bone Joint Surg [Br] 37:252, 1955.
13. Crittenden JJ, Jones DM, and Santerelli AG: Bilateral rotational dislocation of the carpal navicular: case report. Radiology 94:629, 1970.
14. Demos TC: Radiologic case study: painful wrist. Orthopedics 1:151, 1978.
15. Destot E: Traumatismes du Poignet et Rayons x. Masson, Paris, 1923.
16. Dobyns JH, Linscheid RL, Chao EYS, et al: Traumatic instability of the wrist. Am Acad Orthop Surg Instruc Course Lect 24:182, 1975.
17. England JPS: Subluxation of the carpal scaphoid. Proc R Soc Med 63:581, 1970.
18. Fisk GR: Carpal instability and the fractured scaphoid. Ann R Coll Surg Engl 46:63, 1970.
19. Fitton JM: Rotational dislocation of the scaphoid. In Stack GH, and Bolton H (eds): Proceedings of the Second Hand Club, British Society of Surgery of the Hand. Brentwood, Essex, The Westway Press, 1962.
20. Frankel VH: The Terry-Thomas sign. Clin Orthop 129:321, 1977.

21. Gilford WW, Bolton RH, and Lambrinudi C: The mechanism of the wrist joint; with special reference to fractures of the scaphoid. Guy's Hosp Rep 92:52, 1943.
22. Gilula LA, Weeks PM: Post-traumatic ligamentous instability of the wrist. Radiology 129:641, 1978.
23. Gilula LA, Destout JM, Weeks PM, et al: Roentgenographic diagnosis of the painful wrist. Clin Orthop 187:52–64, 1984.
24. Glickel SZ, and Millender L: Results of ligamentous reconstruction for chronic intercarpal instability. Orthop Trans 6:167, 1982.
25. Goldner JL: Treatment of carpal instability without joint fusion—current assessment. J Hand Surg 7:325, 1982.
26. Green DP, and O'Brien ET: Open reduction of carpal dislocations: indications and operative techniques. J Hand Surg 3:250, 1978.
27. Green DP: Carpal dislocation. In Green DP (ed): Operative Hand Surgery. Vol I. Churchill Livingstone Inc, New York, 1982.
28. Hastings DE, and Evans JA: Rheumatoid wrist deformities and their relationship to ulnar drift. J Bone Joint Surg [Am] 57:930, 1975.
29. Hergenröeder PT, and Penix AR: Bilateral scapholunate dissociation with degenerative arthritis. J Hand Surg 6:620, 1981.
30. Higgs SL: Two cases of dislocation of carpal scaphoid. Proc R Soc Med 23:61, 1930.
31. Hockley BJ: Carpal instability and carpal injuries. Aust Radiol 23:158, 1979.
32. Howard FM, Fahey T, and Wojcik E: Rotatory subluxation of the navicular. Clin Orthop 104:134, 1974.
33. Hudson RM, Caragol WJ, and Faye JJ: Isolated rotatory subluxation of the carpal navicular. Am J Roentgenol 126:601, 1976.
34. Kauer JMG: Functional anatomy of the wrist. Clin Orthop 149:73, 1980.
35. Kleinman WB, Steichen JB, and Strickland JW: Management of chronic rotary subluxation of the scaphoid by scaphotrapezio-trapezoid arthrodesis. J Hand Surg 7:125, 1982.
36. Kovalkovits I, and Ficzere O: Habituelle scapholunare Dissoziation. Chirurg 48:428, 1977.
37. Kuth JR: Isolated dislocation of the carpal navicular. A case report. J Bone Joint Surg 21:479, 1939.
38. Landsmeer JM: Studies in the anatomy of articulation. I. The equilibrium of the "intercalated" bone. Acta Morphol Neerl Scand 3:287, 1961.
39. Lewis OJ, Hamshere RJ, and Bucknill TM: The anatomy of the wrist joint. J Anat 106:539, 1970.
40. Lichtman DM, Schneider JR, Swafford AR, et al: Ulnar midcarpal instability—clinical and laboratory analysis. J Hand Surg 6:515, 1981.
41. Linscheid RL: Mechanical forces affecting the deformity of the rheumatoid wrist. J Bone Joint Surg [Am] 51:790, 1969.
42. Linscheid RL, Dobyns JH, Beabout JW, et al: Traumatic instability of the wrist. J Bone Joint Surg [Am] 54:1612, 1972.
43. Linscheid RL, Dobyns JH, Beckenbaugh RD, et al: Instability patterns of the wrist. J Hand Surg 8:682, 1983.
44. Loeb TM, Urbaniak JR, and Goldner JL: Traumatic carpal instability: putting the pieces together. Orthop Trans 1:163, 1977.
45. MacConaill MD: Mechanical anatomy of the carpus and its bearing on some surgical problems. J Anat 75:166, 1941.
46. Maki NJ, Chuinard RG, and D'Ambrosia R: Isolated complete radial dislocation of the scaphoid. A case report and review of the literature. J Bone Joint Surg [Am] 64:615, 1982.
47. Mayfield JK: Carpal injuries—an experimental approach—anatomy, kinematics and perilunate injuries. J Bone Joint Surg [Am] 57:725, 1975.
48. Mayfield JK, Johnson RP, and Kilcoyne RF: The ligaments of the human wrist and their functional significance. Anat Rec 186:417, 1976.
49. Mayfield JK, Johnson RP, and Kilcoyne RF: Carpal dislocations: pathomechanics and progressive perilunar instability. J Hand Surg 5:226, 1980.
50. Moneim MS: The tangential posteroanterior radiograph to demonstrate scapholunate dissociation. J Bone Joint Surg [Am] 63:1324, 1981.
51. Murakami Y: Dislocation of the carpal scaphoid. Hand 9:79, 1977.
52. Nigst H: Luxations et subluxations du scaphoïde. Ann Chir 27:519, 1973.
53. Palmer AK, Dobyns JH, and Linscheid RL: Management of post-traumatic instability of the wrist secondary to ligament rupture. J Hand Surg 3:507, 1978.
54. Palmer AK, Levinsohn EM, and Kuzma GR: Arthrography of the wrist. J Hand Surg 8:15, 1983.
55. Parkes JC, and Stovell PB: Dislocation of the carpal scaphoid: a report of two cases. J Trauma 13:384, 1973.
56. Peterson HA, and Lipscomb PR: Intercarpal arthrodesis. Arch Surg 95:127, 1967.
57. Rask MR: Carponavicular subluxation: report of a case treated with percutaneous pins. Orthopedics 2:134, 1979.
58. Rosenthal DI, Schwartz M, Phillips WC, et al: Fracture of the radius with instability of the wrist. Am J Roentgenol 141:113, 1983.
59. Russell TB: Intercarpal dislocations and fracture-dislocations: a review of fifty-nine cases. J Bone Joint Surg [Br] 31:524, 1949.
60. Schlossbach T: Dislocation of the carpal navicular bone not associated with fracture. J Med Soc NJ 51:533, 1954.
61. Schwartz S: Localized fusion at the wrist joint. J Bone Joint Surg [Am] 49:1591–1596, 1967.
62. Sutro CJ: Hypermobility of bones due to "overlengthened" capsular and ligamentous tissues. Surgery 21:67, 1947.
63. Taleisnik J: The ligaments of the wrist. J Hand Surg 1:110, 1976.
64. Taleisnik J: Wrist: anatomy, function and injury. Am Acad Orthop Surg Instruct Course Lect 27:61, 1978.
65. Taleisnik J: Post-traumatic carpal instability. Clin Orthop 149:73–82, 1980.
66. Taleisnik J: Scapholunate dissociation. In Strickland JW, and Steichen JB (eds): Difficult Problems in Hand Surgery. CV Mosby Co, St Louis, 1982.
67. Taleisnik J: The Wrist. Churchill Livingstone Inc, New York, 1985.
68. Tanz SS: Rotation effect in lunar and perilunar dislocations. Clin Orthop 57:147, 1968.
69. Taylor AR: Dislocation of the scaphoid. Postgrad Med J 45:186, 1969.
70. Thomas HO: Isolated dislocation of the carpal scaphoid. Acta Orthop Scand 48:369, 1977.

71. Thompson TC, Campbell RD Jr, and Arnold WD: Primary and secondary dislocation of the scaphoid bone. J Bone Joint Surg [Br] 46:73, 1964.
72. Uematsu A: Intercarpal fusion for treatment of carpal instability: a preliminary report. Clin Orthop 144:159, 1979.
73. Vance R, Gelberman R, and Braun R: Chronic bilateral scapholunate dissociation without symptoms. J Hand Surg 4:178, 1979.
74. Vaughan-Jackson OJ: A case of recurrent subluxation of the carpal scaphoid. J Bone Joint Surg [Br] 31:532, 1949.
75. Walker GBW: Dislocation of the carpal scaphoid reduced by open operation. Br J Surg 30:380, 1943.

76. Watson HK, and Hempton RF: Limited wrist arthrodesis. Part I: The triscaphoid joint. J Hand Surg 5:320, 1980.
77. Watson HK, Goodman ML, and Johnson TR: Limited wrist arthrodesis. Part II: Intercarpal and radiocarpal combination. J Hand Surg 6:223, 1981.
78. Watson HK, and Ballet FL: The SLAC wrist: scapholunate advanced collapse pattern of degenerative arthritis. J Hand Surg 9A:358, 1984.
79. Watson HK, Ryn J, and Akelman E: Limited triscaphoid intercarpal arthrodesis for rotatory subluxation of the scaphoid. J Bone Joint Surg 68A: 345–349, 1986.

CHAPTER 20

Triquetrolunate and Midcarpal Instability

CHARLOTTE E. ALEXANDER, M.D.
and DAVID M. LICHTMAN, M.D.

Carpal instability represents a spectrum of bone and ligamentous damage. There is an abundance of information in the literature, dealing primarily with carpal instabilities occurring on the radial side of the wrist: scapholunate dissociation, rotatory subluxation of the scaphoid, and radial perilunate instability.* Over the past few years instabilities involving the ulnar aspect of the wrist have become better recognized. These instabilities include several forms of midcarpal instability and triquetrolunate instability. Following increased appreciation of the pathology and clinical nature of the carpal instabilities, triquetrolunate instability is now classified with the perilunate group (see Chapter 18).

Because wrist mechanics are extremely complex, numerous investigators have devoted much effort to the study of carpal kinematics.† Kinematic models have been devised for better understanding of wrist mechanics: the modified columnar model by Taleisnik and the "ring" model proposed by Lichtman (Figs. 20–1 and 20–2). In the author's ring model, the proximal carpal row and the distal carpal row, each of which moves basically as a unit, are connected by two physiologic mobile links—the rotatory triquetrohamate joint and the mobile scaphotrapezial joint. A break in the ring on the ulnar side of the wrist could occur at the triquetrohamate joint, resulting in midcarpal instability, or through the triquetrolunate joint, leading to triquetrolunate dissociation.

In 1934, Mouchet and Belot[28] were the first to report a case of midcarpal subluxation. In 1946, Sutro[37] described two other cases that also had volar intercalated segment instability (VISI) deformities. Lichtman and colleagues[19] reported on a group of patients from their practice who had midcarpal instability and discussed the pathogenesis and pathomechanics of this clinical entity. Recently, Taleisnik[42] reported on another type of midcarpal instability secondary to malunion of distal radial fractures. To avoid confusion, in this chapter midcarpal instability related to distal radial fractures will be referred to as extrinsic midcarpal instability.

Intrinsic midcarpal instability can be either palmar or dorsal in direction. The original series described by Lichtman contained only palmar subluxations, but a few dorsal midcarpal subluxations have subsequently been identified (see Classification, Chapter 18). Dorsal midcarpal instability has not yet been extensively studied.

Recently, other names for midcarpal instability have been introduced. Among them, Carpal Instability, Non-Dissociative (CIND)[4a] and Capitolunate Instability[16a] are well documented with case studies. We believe, however, that with further analysis, these patterns will prove to be similar or identical to those described here.

In palmar midcarpal instability, laxity of the ulnar arm of the arcuate ligament decreases the influence of the geometric configuration of the triquetrohamate joint on the proximal carpal row. This allows the proximal carpal row to assume a gravity-induced palmar-flexed position (VISI) that persists until the last few degrees of ulnar deviation, when the proximal row snaps suddenly into

---

*References 6–8, 21, 22, 25, 26, 30, 35, 39.
†References 1, 2, 6–8, 10, 12, 17, 19–27, 30, 34, 38, 47, 48.

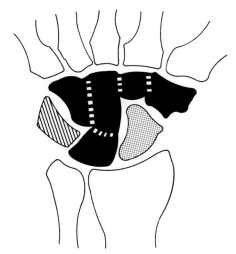

Figure 20–1. Taleisnik's modification of the central (flexion-extension) columnar model. The central column consists of the entire distal row and the lunate; the scaphoid is the lateral column; the triquetrum is the rotatory medial column. (From Lichtman DM, Schneider JR, Swafford AR, et al: J Hand Surg 6:515–523, 1981.)

its dorsiflexed position instead of following the normal smooth transition from palmar flexion to dorsiflexion.

In dorsal midcarpal instability, the capitate is dorsally subluxated upon the lunate in the neutral position. The entire intact proximal carpal row can be seen to be in its low, dorsiflexed attitude (dorsal intercalated segment instability—DISI). The DISI position is maintained in both radial and ulnar deviation; however, in radial deviation, the

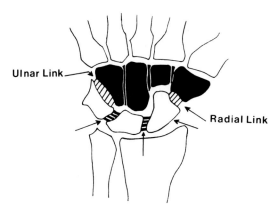

Ulnar Link

Radial Link

Figure 20–2. The "ring" concept of carpal kinematics as proposed by Lichtman. The proximal and distal rows are rigid posts stabilized by interosseous ligaments. Normal controlled mobility occurs at the scaphotrapezial joint and at the triquetrohamate joint. Any break in the ring, either bony or ligamentous (arrows), can produce a DISI or VISI deformity. (From Lichtman, DM, Schneider JR, Swafford AR, et al: J Hand Surg 6:515–523, 1981.)

dislocation may be reduced by a palmar-directed force on the metacarpals.

Reagan and coworkers[32] were the first to describe a series of patients with injuries to the triquetrolunate articulation. Taleisnik[39, 40] attributed the patterns of volar flexion instability (VISI) to disruption of the triquetrolunate ligaments. With a break in the carpal ring through the triquetrolunate joint, the proximal carpal row no longer moves as a unit. The lunate palmar flexes with the scaphoid, in response to dynamic forces on the radial side of the carpus, whereas the triquetrum tends to dorsiflex as it is forced ulnarly by the head of the capitate, and it assumes a dorsiflexed position in relation to the hamate. Thus, a static VISI deformity (palmar flexion of the lunate) may be seen on routine lateral roentgenograms.

In this chapter, we discuss the pathomechanics, clinical presentation, diagnosis, and various types of treatment options for triquetrolunate volar midcarpal and extrinsic midcarpal instability.

PATHOGENESIS

Triquetrolunate Instability. In 1980, Mayfield[25] presented a study dealing with the pathomechanics of perilunar instability. He demonstrated that loading toward maximal extension, ulnar deviation, and intercarpal supination would produce progressive perilunar instability beginning with fractures of the radial styloid or scaphoid or with disruption of the scapholunate joint. It has subsequently been proposed that triquetrolunate instability represents a "forme fruste" of Grade III perilunar instability, in which the scapholunate or trans-scaphoid component has healed, leaving only the triquetrolunate disruption at clinical presentation.[20] It has also been argued that triquetrolunate instability occurs as a result of loading in maximal extension, in radial deviation, and possibly in pronation.[8, 32] Reagan et al[32] suggested that this mechanism may cause perilunar instability in reverse order. They found partial scapholunate tears in two cases of triquetrolunate dissociation. Radial deviation places more tension on the ulnar portion of the arcuate ligament and possibly the triquetrolunate ligaments. Consequently, this force causes disruption of the triquetrolunate ligaments prior to rupture of the radiocapitate or the scapholunate ligaments.

Elsewhere in this text (see Chapter 16) the

ulnocarpal abutment syndrome is discussed. Triquetrolunate ligament injuries may be caused by increased load transmission across the ulnar side of the wrist, in conjunction with an ulnar-positive variant (an excessively long ulna). Ulnar and triquetral chondromalacia, as well as triangular fibrocartilage tears, may frequently accompany triquetrolunate instability when the ulna is longer than the radius.

Midcarpal Instability. In 1981, Lichtman[19] presented a study on midcarpal instability, including laboratory analysis of its pathogenesis. In dissection of fresh cadaver wrists, it was found that the ulnar arm of the arcuate ligament provided the major support for midcarpal stability. Division of the triquetrohamate ligaments alone did not create midcarpal instability; it did not develop until the ulnar limb of the volar arcuate ligament was cut. In most cases of clinical midcarpal instability, the cause is probably attenuation or congenital laxity of the ulnar arm of the arcuate ligament rather than an acute tear.

Triquetrolunate Instability

CLINICAL FINDINGS

Reagan, Linscheid, and Dobyns[32] divided triquetrolunate instability into two groups—triquetrolunate tears (sprains) and triquetrolunate dissociation. Patients with partial disruption of the triquetrolunate interosseous ligaments belong in the first group, and those with complete triquetrolunate ligamentous disruptions belong in the second group. The primary presenting complaint in all of the patients is pain on the ulnar aspect of the wrist. The pain may or may not be associated with a wrist click in radial or ulnar deviation. Some patients complain of stiffness, weakness, or instability. The onset of their symptoms is usually related to a traumatic event described as a fall on the outstretched hand or a twisting or rotatory injury.

On physical exam, there is tenderness over the ulnar aspect of the wrist, particularly at the triquetrolunate joint. Occasionally, a click can be reproduced at the time of exam. Reagan and coworkers[32] have described a lunotriquetral ballottement test that, when positive, can be helpful in diagnosing triquetrolunate instability (Fig. 20–3). This test is performed by stabilizing the lunate with the thumb and index finger of one hand and

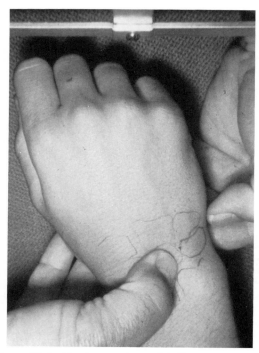

Figure 20–3. The lunate triquetral ballottement test, as described by Reagan, Dobyns, and Linscheid, is used to detect abnormal motion and pain at the triquetrolunate joint. (From Reagan, DS, Linscheid RL, and Dobyns JH: J Hand Surg 9-502–513, 1984.)

attempting to displace the triquetrum and pisiform dorsally, then palmarly, with the other hand. A positive test detects excessive laxity associated with pain and crepitus. Grip strength and range of motion may or may not be altered in these patients.

Triquetrolunate instability may be difficult, in some cases, to differentiate from many other disease entities affecting the ulnar aspect of the wrist. Differential diagnosis should include triangular fibrocartilage complex tears, subluxation or dislocation of the distal radioulnar joint, subluxation of the extensor carpi ulnaris, midcarpal instability, ulnocarpal impingement syndromes, or ulnar head chondromalacia.

RADIOGRAPHIC EVALUATION

Some or all of the carpal instability series of radiographs recommended by Gilula[12] (see Chapter 7) should be obtained on all patients with suspected instability. This series consists of a PA view in neutral, ulnar, and radial deviation; a clenched-fist AP view; an oblique view; a 30° off-lateral oblique to show the pisotriquetral joint; a lateral view with the wrist in neutral and in both extremes of flexion and extension; a lateral

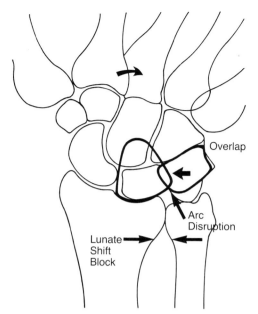

Figure 20–4. Disruption of the smooth convexity of the proximal carpal row is more pronounced with ulnar deviation. Note the overlapping of the lunate and triquetrum. (From Reagan DS, Linscheid RL, and Dobyns JH: J Hand Surg 9:502–513, 1984.)

clenched-fist view. The results of standard static roentgenograms are normal in patients with triquetrolunate tears or sprains. In patients with triquetrolunate dissociation, there is disruption of the normal smooth convexity of the proximal carpal row, with the triquetrum displaced proximally on the AP radiograph. Disruption of the normal arc is particularly pronounced in the presence of ulnar deviation, producing overlapping of the lunate and triquetrum[32] (Fig. 20–4). In some instances, there may be increased distance between the lunate and the triquetrum.[13] On lateral films, the triquetrum may be dorsiflexed in relation to the lunate, when compared with the opposite wrist. The average normal lunotriquetral (LT) angle measurement has been reported by Reagan et al[32] to be +14°. They found that in triquetrolunate dissociation, this angle is less than 0°, with an average of −16°. The LT angle is the angle between the longitudinal axis of the triquetrum and the longitudinal axis of the lunate (Fig. 20–5A and B). A VISI deformity may or may not be present on the lateral radiograph. PA films with the wrist in a neutral position should be checked for ulnar variance.

Arthrography has been advocated by various authors to better evaluate the anatomic abnormalities in patients with symptoms of instability.[11, 18, 29] It is important to obtain serial films or to use fluoroscopy immediately after injection to detect the location of the leak between the radiocarpal and midcarpal rows. Arthrograms are probably the most helpful diagnostic aid in the evaluation of triquetrolunate tears (sprains). When contrast medium is injected into the radiocarpal

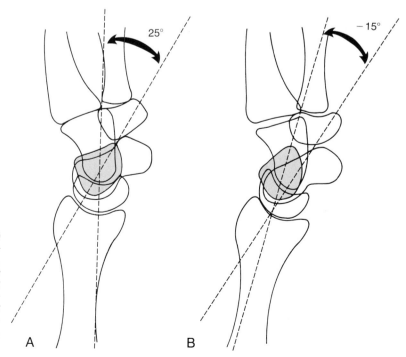

Figure 20–5. The lunotriquetral (LT) angle determination on a lateral x-ray diagram. *A,* Normal LT angle. *B,* In triquetrolunate dissociation, the LT angle is less than zero, secondary to volar flexion of the lunate in relationship to the triquetrum. (After Reagan DS, Linscheid RL, and Dobyns JH: J Hand Surg 9:502–513, 1984.)

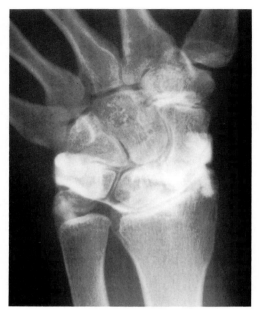

Figure 20–6. Arthrography reveals a dye leak from the radiocarpal to the midcarpal joint through the triquetrolunate joint. (From Lichtman DM, Noble WH, and Alexander CE: J Hand Surg 9:185–187, 1984.)

joint a positive study will demonstrate a dye leak through the triquetrolunate space from the radiocarpal space to the intercarpal space (Fig. 20–6). Injection of dye into the intercarpal space outlines the midcarpal joint first and demonstrates retrograde flow into the radiocarpal joint if a tear is present. Reagan et al[32] found that in 11 surgically treated patients with positive arthrograms, all had significant triquetrolunate ligament tears. We currently prefer intercarpal injection when looking for triquetrolunate or scapholunate tears.

Cineradiographs are usually normal and are therefore helpful in distinguishing between midcarpal instability and triquetrolunate instability.

ARTHROSCOPY

Arthroscopic techniques are now being developed for the wrist, which will undoubtedly enhance our ability to diagnose ulnocarpal disorders. Differentiation of triquetrolunate instability from triangular fibrocartilage tears should be relatively easy with this technique. See Chapter 9 for the current state of this modality.

TREATMENT

All patients with a diagnosis of triquetrolunate tear (sprain) with acute injury should have a trial of immobilization. Surgical treatment should be reserved for those patients with chronic symptoms that have not responded to immobilization or anti-inflammatory agents. Patients with acute triquetrolunate dissociation should have open reduction with internal pin fixation. A trial of immobilization and anti-inflammatory agents may also be used for patients with chronic triquetrolunate dissociation.

Surgical treatment options for chronic tears and chronic triquetrolunate dissociation are repair of the interosseous ligament, reconstruction of the triquetrolunate ligaments, using a free tendon graft, or triquetrolunate arthrodesis. When surgical exploration is undertaken, a dorsal ulnar approach should be used, exposing the wrist capsule between the fourth and fifth dorsal compartments. A second volar incision may be required for ligament repair and reconstruction. For ligament reconstruction, a portion of the extensor carpi ulnaris tendon can be passed through drill holes in the lunate and the triquetrum and sutured to itself.[32] This procedure is technically difficult, and care must be taken to avoid fracture of the bones or damage to the ulnar neurovascular bundle. Ligament repairs are best performed by horizontal mattress sutures through the torn flap of ligament passed into drill holes in the adjacent bone.

When performing an arthrodesis, it is important to maintain the normal external dimensions of the triquetrum and the lunate. A trough is created in the dorsal surface of the triquetrum and the lunate, after stabilizing the two bones with a Kirschner wire. This slot should extend almost to the palmar cortical surface of both bones. A strut of iliac crest bone graft is placed in this trough so that it fits snugly. The cartilaginous surfaces of the triquetrolunate joint should be denuded and the space maintained with cancellous bone graft chips (Fig. 20–7). Arthrodesis should probably be the surgical treatment used in patients with significant triquetrolunate dissociation or in those individuals who perform strenuous activities using the wrist. Varying results have been obtained with all methods of surgical treatment. We, however, prefer arthrodesis to ligament reconstruction.

In patients with a positive ulnar variance and evidence of ulnocarpal abutment syndrome (see Chapter 16), an ulnar shortening procedure should be performed in conjunction with triquetrolunate stabilization.

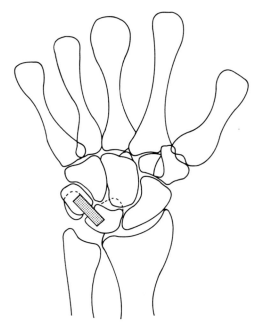

Figure 20–7. Triquetrolunate arthrodesis. An iliac crest strut graft is used, and stabilization is attained with Kirschner wires. After denuding the articular surfaces between the lunate and the triquetrum, the space is maintained using cancellous bone chips.

Palmar Midcarpal Instability

CLINICAL FINDINGS

The presenting complaint in most of these patients is a painful clunk that occurs spontaneously during activities involving ulnar deviation and pronation of the wrist. On inspection of the wrist, an obvious volar sag can be seen at the level of the midcarpal joint. The examiner can reproduce the clunk by gently moving the hand into ulnar deviation from the relaxed neutral position. As the wrist reaches maximal ulnar deviation, a visual and palpable "clunk" is detected, and the volar sag is corrected. There is tenderness over the ulnar aspect of the wrist, particularly at the triquetrohamate joint. Some patients have fullness in the ulnar aspect of their wrist, which suggests localized synovitis. Examination of the nonaffected wrist often reveals increased laxity in response to dorsal palmar translational stress applied to the hand with the forearm stabilized. In many of these patients, a similar clunk can be produced by manipulation on the nonaffected side. However, this clunk is not painful and does not occur spontaneously during activities.

In contrast to individuals with triquetrolunate instability, most of the patients with midcarpal instability cannot relate the onset of symptoms to a specific episode of trauma. Those patients with a history of trauma report either a fall on the outstretched hand or a rotatory injury.

RADIOGRAPHIC EVALUATION

Standard roentgenograms made in neutral, ulnar, and radial deviation may be normal. Most of the patients have a VISI pattern with the wrist in the neutral position on lateral radiograms. The presence or absence of a VISI pattern is probably related to the position of the wrist when the x-ray is taken. Most of these patients would have a VISI deformity if the wrist were unsupported and in neutral deviation or if axial compression were applied to the hand. This VISI deformity corresponds to the volar sag seen clinically.

Cineradiography has been shown to be a valuable aid in evaluating wrist instability and is the most helpful tool in diagnosing midcarpal instability.[1, 31] Motion in flexion and extension is normal. In going from radial to ulnar deviation, the proximal carpal row snaps suddenly from a palmar-flexed position to a dorsiflexed position, instead of making a smooth synchronous transition.

Videotapes made for later study have proved invaluable in most of these cases. Careful review of videotapes reveals the pathomechanics of palmar midcarpal instability. In neutral, the distal row is anteriorly subluxated with a compensatory proximal row VISI deformity. With ulnar deviation, the distal row reduces, causing a clunk as the proximal row suddenly snaps into its physiologic dorsiflexed position.

Arthrograms are usually normal in this condition, a helpful differential consideration. In many instances, however, a positive arthrogram, with dye flow through the triquetrolunate interval, may coexist with midcarpal instability. In these cases, the clinical picture of midcarpal instability overshadows the triquetrolunate instability.

TREATMENT

All patients should have a trial of conservative management, including immobilization, anti-inflammatory agents, and, occasionally, steroid injection in the triquetrohamate joint. For many patients, understanding the problem and avoiding aggravating activities are sufficient.

A splint that pushes dorsally on the pisiform has been helpful for certain individu-

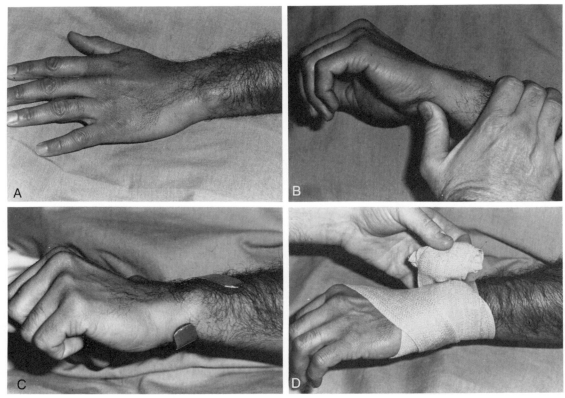

Figure 20–8. A splint for volar midcarpal instability, indicated for individuals who are primarily symptomatic during athletic or other strenuous activities. VISI deformity and midcarpal sag (A) can be reduced by dorsal pressure on the pisiform bone (B). A simple splint (C) that applies continuous dorsal pressure on the pisiform can be held in place by an elastic wrap (D), and the patient can participate in a full range of activities.

als. By reducing the VISI sag of the proximal row, the splint eliminates the "catch-up" clunk in ulnar deviation. The splint (Fig. 20–8) can be worn during athletic activities and does not significantly interfere with wrist motion.

Currently, in those patients in whom conservative measures have failed to relieve symptoms, triquetrohamate arthrodesis is an option. At surgery, the pathologic condition is checked under direct vision. Particular attention is paid to the triquetrohamate, the triquetrolunate, and the distal radioulnar joints. Temporary pinning of the triquetrohamate joint, followed by passive range of motion testing, is done to confirm

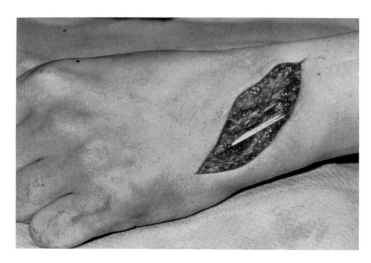

Figure 20–9. Dorsal ulnar approach for triquetrohamate arthrodesis. Access to the wrist capsule should be between the fourth and fifth dorsal compartments.

the preoperative diagnosis. Pinning should eliminate the midcarpal subluxation completely.

Triquetrohamate arthrodesis is performed through a dorsal ulnar incision (Fig. 20–9). The wrist capsule is exposed between the fourth and fifth dorsal compartments, and the triquetrohamate joint is identified. The finding of synovitis or chondromalacia of the articular surfaces of the triquetrum is not uncommon. The normally thin triquetrohamate capsule is usually attenuated. The normal spatial relationship between the triquetrum and the hamate must be maintained. This is done by filling the joint space with cancellous bone chips after denuding subchrondral bone of cartilage. The triquetrohamate joint is stabilized in a reduced position by means of Kirschner wires. The wires should be left long enough to be palpated through the skin. A trough is created in the dorsal surfaces of both bones, which is filled with an iliac crest corticocancellous bone plug (Fig. 20–10A and B). The graft should fit snugly in the trough to prevent

dislodging. The wrist is immobilized for eight to 10 weeks in a short-arm cast. The Kirschner wires are removed at eight weeks.

In the literature, results of ligamentous reconstruction for various types of wrist instability have been variable.[14, 15, 22] In the past, tendon grafts have been used by us to stabilize the triquetrohamate joint. With time, some of these patients have had recurrences of their pre-operative symptoms. Currently, we no longer use this form of soft tissue reconstruction for treating midcarpal instability. Direct advancement and reefing of lax midcarpal stabilizing ligaments are now under investigation.

Watson[44–46] has advocated limited carpal arthrodesis for various types of radial carpal instability and has had some promising results. Uematsu[43] has reported good results with intercarpal arthrodesis in three out of four cases of carpal instability. He found that loss of flexion was greater than loss of extension postoperatively. This is to be expected, as demonstrated by Sarrafian's[34] kinematic study. Postoperative motion in most

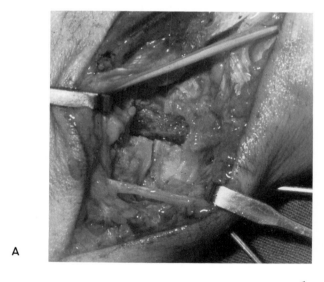

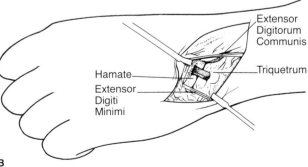

Figure 20–10. Triquetrohamate arthrodesis. *A,* A trough is created on the dorsal surfaces of the triquetrum and the hamate, which is filled with a corticocancellous iliac bone graft. The joint surfaces have been denuded and the spatial relationship maintained by filling the space with cancellous bone chips. *B,* Illustration based on operative photograph.

of our patients after triquetrohamate fusion correlates with that described in Uematsu's report.

Although the loss of motion after intercarpal arthrodesis is significant, most surgeons who perform this procedure note that the majority of patients attain a range of motion well within the functional range reported by Brumfield et al.[2, 16, 36, 40, 42, 44, 45] Using an electrogoniometer to monitor wrist motion, they found that 10° of flexion and 35° of extension are needed for performing most activities of daily living.

Carpal range of motion increases for up to one year after intercarpal arthrodesis.[40, 43–45] This increase in motion may be secondary to the development of compensatory increased motion in areas of the wrist not included in the arthrodesis. Although this compensatory change may be asymptomatic in some cases, a few patients have developed mild pain in the area of increased motion. In our series of patients with midcarpal instability undergoing triquetrohamate arthrodesis, one individual developed radial wrist pain and a popping sensation approximately seven months postoperatively. Cineradiography revealed increased motion at the scapholunate joint associated with the "pop." This suggests that abnormal stress is created elsewhere in the wrist by triquetrohamate arthrodesis. This alteration of stress forces on the wrist may, perhaps, be extrapolated to other limited carpal arthrodeses involving articulations where significant motion normally occurs. The long-term results of limited carpal arthrodesis are still uncertain. Arthrodesis of the capitolunate joint or perhaps of both the capitolunate and the triquetrohamate joints ("four-corner fusion"), rather than of the triquetrohamate joint alone, may eliminate the development of a postoperative click in patients surgically treated for midcarpal instability and may improve the long-term results. For a detailed discussion of the technique of limited arthrodesis, refer to Chapter 30.

In our experience, the results of triquetrolunate arthrodesis for triquetrolunate instability are better than those of triquetrohamate arthrodesis for midcarpal instability. There is less alteration of pre-operative motion with triquetrolunate arthrodesis. This is to be expected, since there is less physiologic motion at the triquetrolunate articulation than at the triquetrohamate joint.

Extrinsic Midcarpal Instability

There are numerous complications of distal radial fractures.[3, 4, 9, 21, 33, 42] Several types of carpal instabilities are associated with distal radial fractures, including perilunar instability, dorsal and volar proximal carpal subluxation, and extrinsic midcarpal instability described recently by Taleisnik.[42] Perilunar instability, scapholunate dissociation, or rotatory subluxation of the scaphoid occurs with some intra-articular radial fractures as a continuation of the injury disrupting the radiocapitate ligament and possibly the interosseous scapholunate ligaments.[25, 33] Mayfield[25] noted in experimental studies on the pathomechanics of progressive perilunar instability that the radiocapitate ligament was avulsed with the radial styloid when a radial fracture occurred. Dorsal or palmar proximal carpal instability can occur with malunion of the distal radius; however, with this entity, intercarpal alignment remains normal (Figs. 20–11 and 20–12).

In 1972, Linscheid and colleagues[21] described a type of dorsiflexion wrist instability that could result from malunion of distal radial fractures. They felt that this alteration of intercarpal alignment was compensatory

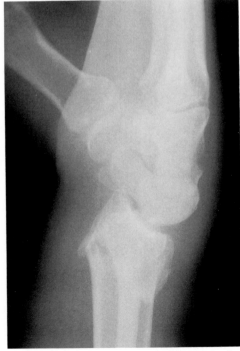

Figure 20–11. Dorsal carpal subluxation secondary to angulated distal radius fracture. Note that the intercarpal alignment is normal.

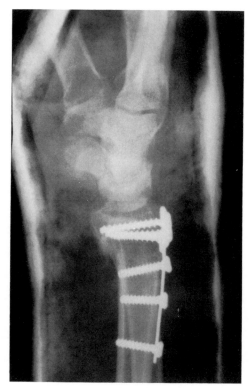

Figure 20–12. Postoperative lateral x-ray of the distal radius shown in Figure 20–11. The dorsal carpal subluxation has been corrected by anatomic reduction of the distal radius fracture.

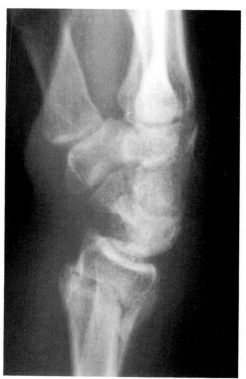

Figure 20–13. Extrinsic carpal instability with malalignment of the distal radius.

rather than true instability and could be corrected by radial osteotomy if the deformity was not "fixed." The patients presented by Taleisnik all had malunions of distal radial fractures not involving the articular surface, with an average palmar tilt of −23° (one exception had a minimal intra-articular component). In these cases, symptoms of subluxation or pain or both over the triquetrohamate joint developed several months after immobilization was discontinued. Subluxation was associated with a pop occurring with ulnar deviation when the hand was pronated, a symptom similar to that in patients with midcarpal instability. Routine lateral roentgenograms show normal lunate and capitate alignment in neutral deviation. Lateral x-rays in ulnar deviation reveal dorsiflexion of the lunate as expected, but the longitudinal axis of the capitate is parallel but dorsal to the longitudinal axis of the radius (Figs. 20–13 and 20–14). This change in the radiocapitate axis is probably secondary to the inability of the lunate to move palmarly with ulnar deviation because of the abnormal tilt of the radial articular surface. Radial osteotomy eliminated the abnor-

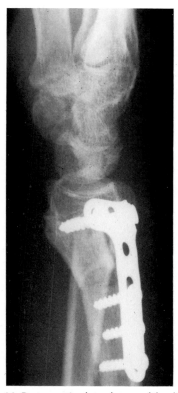

Figure 20–14. Postoperative lateral x-ray of the distal radius shown in Figure 20–13. After correction of the dorsal tilt of the distal radial articular surface, the intercarpal alignment is normal.

mal motion and symptoms in the majority of patients. In Fernandez's[5] series of cases of malunions treated with osteotomy, half of the patients presented with radiocarpal pain that was relieved postoperatively. It is possible that some of these patients might have had extrinsic midcarpal instability.

SUMMARY

Instabilities located on the ulnar aspect of the wrist and at the midcarpal joint appear to be much more common than previously suspected. In addition to a thorough clinical examination, the evaluation of patients with ulnar wrist pain should include a carpal instability series, an arthrogram, and cineradiography, when indicated. In the near future, wrist arthroscopy will be readily available. Further laboratory analysis is needed to better understand the pathomechanics of triquetrolunate instability and, particularly, midcarpal instability. The results of treatment of ulnar carpal instabilities have improved, in our experience, with the use of limited carpal arthrodesis rather than ligament reconstruction. Direct capsular reefing and advancement procedures are under investigation because the long-term effect of limited carpal fusions is still uncertain.

References

1. Arkless R: A detailed study of movement of the wrist joint. Am J Roentgenol 96:839–844, 1966.
2. Brumfield RH, and Champoux JA: A biomechanical study of normal functional wrist motion. Clin Orthop 187:23–25, 1984.
3. Chapman DR, Bennett JB, Bryan WJ, et al: Complications of distal radial fractures: pins and plaster treatment. J Hand Surg 7:509, 1982.
4. Cooney WP, Dobyns JH, and Linscheid RL: Complications of Colles' fractures. J Bone Joint Surg 62A:613–619, 1980.
4a. Dobyns JH, Linscheid RL, Wadih SM, et al: Carpal instability, non-dissociative (CIND). Presented at the Annual Meeting of the American Academy of Orthopaedic Surgeons, San Francisco, California, February, 1987.
5. Fernandez DL: Correction of post-traumatic wrist deformity in adults by osteotomy, bone-grafting, and internal fixation. J Bone Joint Surg 64A: 1164–1178, 1982.
6. Fisk G: Carpal instability and the fractured scaphoid. Ann R Col Surg Engl 46:63–76, 1970.
7. Fisk G: An overview of injuries of the wrist. Clin Orthop 149:137–144, 1980.
8. Fisk G: The wrist. J Bone Joint Surg 66B:396–407, 1984.
9. Frykman G: Fracture of the distal radius including sequelae—shoulder-hand-finger syndrome, disturbance in the distal radio-ulnar joint and impairment of nerve function. A clinical and experimental study. Acta Orthop Scand (Suppl 108), 1967.
10. Gilford W, Bolton R, and Lambrinudi C: The mechanism of the wrist joint. Guy's Hosp Rep 92:52–59, 1943.
11. Gilula LA, Totty WG, and Weeks PM: Wrist arthrography. Radiology 146:555–556, 1983.
12. Gilula LA, and Weeks PM: Post-traumatic ligamentous instabilities of the wrist. Radiology 129: 641–651, 1978.
13. Gilula LA: Carpal injuries: analytic approach and case exercises. Am J Roentgenol 133:503–517, 1979.
14. Glickel SZ, and Millender LH: Ligamentous reconstruction for chronic intercarpal instability. J Hand Surg 9:514–524, 1984.
15. Goldner JL: Treatment of carpal instability without joint fusion—current assessment. J Hand Surg 7:325–326, 1982.
16. Graner O, Lopes EI, Carvalho BC, et al: Arthrodesis of the carpal bones in the treatment of Kienböck's disease, painful ununited fractures of the navicular and lunate bones with avascular necrosis, and old fracture-dislocations of carpal bones. J Bone Joint Surg 48A:767–774, 1966.
16a. Johnson RP, and Carrera GF: Chronic capitolunate instability. J Bone Joint Surg 68A:1164–1176, 1980.
17. Kauer JMG: Functional anatomy of the wrist. Clin Orthop 149:9–20, 1980.
18. Levinsohn EM, and Palmer AK: Arthrography of the traumatized wrist. Radiology 146:647–651, 1983.
19. Lichtman DM, Schneider JR, Swafford AR, et al: Ulnar midcarpal instability. Clinical and laboratory analysis. J Hand Surg 6:515–523, 1981.
20. Lichtman DM, Noble WH, and Alexander CE: Dynamic triquetrolunate instability: case report. J Hand Surg 9:185–187, 1984.
21. Linscheid RL, Dobyns JH, Beabout JW, et al: Traumatic instability of the wrist. Diagnosis, classification, and pathomechanics. J Bone Joint Surg 54A:1612–1632, 1972.
22. Linscheid RL, Dobyns JH, Beckenbaugh RD, et al: Instability patterns of the wrist. J Hand Surg 8:682–686, 1983.
23. MacConaill MA: The mechanical anatomy of the carpus and its bearings on some surgical problems. J Anat 75:166–175, 1941.
24. Mayfield JK, Johnson RP, and Kilcoyne RF: The ligaments of the human wrist and their functional significance. Anat Rec 186:417–428, 1976.
25. Mayfield JK, Johnson RP, and Kilcoyne RF: Carpal dislocations: pathomechanics and progressive perilunar instability. J Hand Surg 5:226–241, 1980.
26. Mayfield JK: Patterns of injury to carpal ligaments. Clin Orthop 187:36–42, 1984.
27. McMurtry RY, Youm Y, Flatt AE, et al: Kinematics of the wrist. Clinical applications. J Bone Joint Surg 60A:955–961, 1978.
28. Mouchet A, and Belot J: Poignet à ressaut. (Subluxation médiocarpienne en avant). Bull Mem Soc Nat Chir 60:1243, 1934.
29. Palmer AK, Levinsohn EM, and Kuzma GR: Arthrography of the wrist. J Hand Surg 8:15–23, 1983.
30. Palmer AK, Dobyns JH, and Linscheid RL: Management of post-traumatic instability of the wrist secondary to ligament rupture. J Hand Surg 3:507–532, 1978.
31. Protas JM, and Jackson WT: Evaluating carpal instabilities with fluoroscopy. Am J Roentgenol 135:137–140, 1980.
32. Reagan DS, Linscheid RL, and Dobyns JH: Lunotriquetral sprains. J Hand Surg 9:502–513, 1984.
33. Rosenthal DI, Schwartz MC, Phillips WC, et al:

Fracture of the radius with instability of the wrist. Am J Radiol 141:113–116, 1983.

34. Sarrafian S, Melamed J, and Goshgarian G: Study of wrist motion of flexion and extension. Clin Orthop 126:153–159, 1977.

35. Sebald JR, Dobyns JH, and Linscheid RL: The natural history of collapse deformities of the wrist. Clin Orthop 104:140–148, 1974.

36. Sutro CJ: Treatment of nonunion of the carpal navicular bone. Surg 20:536, 1946.

37. Sutro CJ: Bilateral intercarpal subluxation. Am J Surg 72:110, 1946.

38. Taleisnik J: The ligaments of the wrist. J Hand Surg 1:110–118, 1976.

39. Taleisnik J: Post-traumatic carpal instability. Clin Orthop 149:73–82, 1980.

40. Taleisnik J, Malerich M, and Prietto M: Palmar carpal instability secondary to dislocation of the scaphoid and lunate: report of case and review of the literature. J Hand Surg 7:606–612, 1982.

41. Taleisnik J: Subtotal arthrodesis of the wrist joint. Clin Orthop 187:81–88, 1984.

42. Taleisnik J, and Watson HK: Midcarpal instability caused by malunited fractures of the distal radius. J Hand Surg 9:350–357, 1984.

43. Uematsu A: Intercarpal fusion for treatment of carpal instability. Clin Orthop 144:159–165, 1979.

44. Watson HK: Limited wrist arthrodesis. Clin Orthop 149:126–136, 1980.

45. Watson HK, and Hempton RF: Limited wrist arthrodeses. The triscaphoid joint. J Hand Surg 5:320–327, 1980.

46. Watson HK, Goodman ML, and Johnson TR: Limited wrist arthrodesis. Part II: Intercarpal and radiocarpal combinations. J Hand Surg 6:223–233, 1981.

47. Wright R: A detailed study of movement of the wrist joint. J Anat 70:137–143, 1933.

48. Youm Y, McMurtry RY, Flatt AE, et al: Kinematics of the wrist. 1. An experimental study of radial-ulnar deviation and flexion-extension. J Bone Joint Surg 60A:423–431, 1978.

PART IV

Developmental and Degenerative Conditions

CHAPTER 21

Degenerative Disorders of the Carpus

H. KIRK WATSON, M.D.,
and LAURENCE H. BRENNER, M.D.

INTRODUCTION

Degenerative arthritis of the wrist follows specific patterns. In examining over 4000 radiographs of wrists, 210 demonstrated some form of degenerative arthritis. The joints were evaluated for joint space narrowing, degree of loss of cartilage, cyst formation, sclerosis, and progression of degeneration. Specific patterns of degeneration allowed a categorization of degenerative arthritis of the human wrist. Over 90 percent of the observed changes involve the scaphoid and occur in three distinct patterns.

We have termed the most frequent form of degeneration the SLAC (scapholunate advanced collapse) wrist. The name implies the gradual collapse and loss of ligamentous support that accompanies the degeneration and also indicates the responsible bones. SLAC wrist accounts for 55 per cent of cases of unselected degenerative arthritis occurring in the human wrist. This pattern develops primarily because of malalignment of the scaphoid. Initially, changes then progress to the proximal scaphoradial articulation and then shift to the capitolunate articulation. The radiolunate joint is almost never involved.

Triscaphe arthritis, occurring in 20 percent of cases of degenerative arthritis of the

wrist, is the second most common form of degenerative arthritis. This disease pattern involves the articulation of the scaphoid, the trapezium, and the trapezoid. In a random cadaveric study of the triscaphe joint, 15 percent of the specimens, with an average age of 74.9, showed degenerative changes, although scaphotrapezial involvement alone (19 percent) was more than twice as great as scaphotrapezoidal involvement alone (9 percent). In only one instance was the trapeziotrapezoidal joint involved, and this involvement was considered to be mild.

The third most common form of degenerative arthritis occurs as a combination of the two previously described patterns and is seen in approximately 10 percent of degenerative wrist disorders. The remaining 15 percent is composed of cases of degeneration between the distal ulna and the lunate, the radiolunate and the lunotriquetral joints, and occasionally other areas, usually following a specific fracture or external force destruction of a joint. Recently, it has been demonstrated that congenitally incomplete carpal separation can lead to a painful arthrosis resembling degenerative arthritis. This is seen most commonly at the triquetrolunate joint. Prescribed treatment has been a limited wrist arthrodesis across the involved joint. Other common causes of

SLAC degeneration that result from carpal collapse include nonunion of the scaphoid and Kienböck's disease.

DEGENERATIVE PATTERNS

SLAC Wrist

A normal wrist will not usually develop arthritis. However, wrists with disruption or attenuation of the normal ligamentous carpal support are at risk for degeneration. This may result from trauma, may be occupationally related, or may be secondary to calcium pyrophosphate dihydrate deposition (CPPD) disease. The abnormal articulations can destroy the cartilaginous surfaces. This usually occurs when cartilage is subjected to shearing forces, especially high shear loading over very small contact surfaces.

The distal radius is composed of two fossae: an ovoid one for articulation of the scaphoid and a more spheroidal one for articulation of the lunate (Fig. 21–1). No matter which way the lunate is positioned, the proximal cartilage loading tends to remain perpendicular to the articular surface. The ovoid or elliptical shape of the scaphoid fossa does not allow for motion in certain planes. Envision two stacked spoons with their handles aligned and their bowls nested one within the other. If you rotate the handles away from one another in their flat plane even slightly, the upper spoon bowl rises out of the lower bowl, and what was

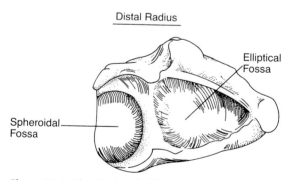

Figure 21–1. The distal end of the radius is made up of an elliptical and a spheroidal fossa. The lunate articulates in the spheroidal fossa and the scaphoid in the elliptical fossa. With rotary subluxation of the scaphoid, it spins out of place and articulates only with the edge of the spheroidal fossa, and rapid degeneration results. The radiolunate articulation, being spheroidal in shape, is not affected by malpositioning of the lunate, no matter which way it spins. Thus, shearing forces do not develop, and degenerative arthritis almost never occurs between the radius and the lunate.

total contact between the bowls becomes small surface edge contact (Fig. 21–2). This is essentially what happens in rotary subluxation of the scaphoid, which is far more prevalent than was previously thought. There are many wrists that have sustained ligamentous damage sufficient to allow the scaphoid to spin but only under significant loading. These wrists appear normal on radiographs but are symptomatic and can be diagnosed clinically. This disorder is termed dynamic rotary subluxation of the scaphoid, as opposed to the static rotary subluxation with radiographic changes.

Changes that occur with nonunion of the scaphoid support this hypothesis. Standard SLAC degeneration is seen at the distal radioscaphoid joint, then at the proximal radioscaphoid joint, and then at the capitolunate joint with preservation of the radiolunate joint (Fig. 21–3). In scaphoid nonunion, the degeneration begins in the same radiostyloscaphoid area but progresses proximally only as far as the nonunion site. The proximal fragment of the scaphoid is now acting as a sphere in the more spherical ulnar portion of the elliptical radial fossa. The radius proximal fragment cartilage is now like that of the radiolunate joint and is always preserved, even with severe late destruction of the radius distal fragment joint (Fig. 21–4). This supports the theory of scaphoid rotation as the basic cause of SLAC degeneration. We therefore recommend grafting of scaphoid nonunions, even in less symptomatic cases.

SLAC degeneration initially involves only the radioscaphoid joint. As the radioscaphoid cartilage disappears, further shift and collapse of the scaphoid occur, along with increasing load at the capitolunate joint. The loaded capitate is driven off the radial side of the lunate and between the lunate and the scaphoid with shear loading of the capitolunate cartilage. This joint degenerates rapidly once the radioscaphoid cartilage has narrowed significantly. This same phenomenon occurs with a Silastic scaphoid implant in place, except in a limited number of wrists in which the ligamentous support is strong and tight enough to maintain the capitate directly on the distal lunate without a concomitant limited wrist arthrodesis.

TREATMENT OF THE SLAC WRIST

Silastic material provides an adequate spacing mechanism for light loading. Medium to

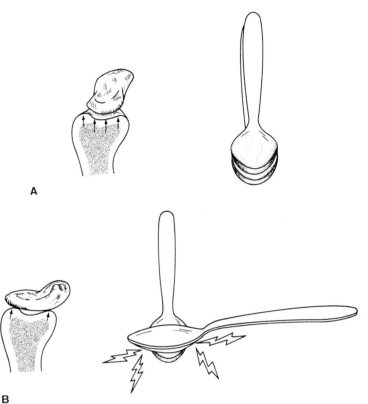

Figure 21–2. *A, B,* The articular shape of the radioscaphoid joint is not unlike that of two stacked spoons. With even the slightest amount of volar rotation, as in rotary subluxation of the scaphoid, the congruous joint surface contact is lost, with all the load now transferred along the edges, as demonstrated by the perpendicular, stacked spoons. This results in rapid degeneration of the joint.

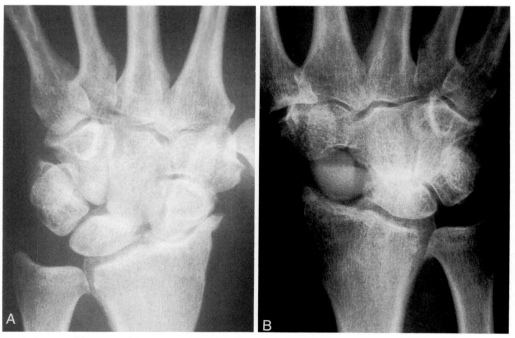

Figure 21–3. Rotary subluxation of the scaphoid results in SLAC wrist. *A,* Degenerative change occurs at the radioscaphoid joint and at the capitolunate joint. The radiolunate joint is spared, even in advanced disease. *B,* Anteroposterior x-ray film demonstrates the same wrist with long-term result of SLAC wrist deformity treated with limited wrist arthrodesis and Silastic scaphoid implant.

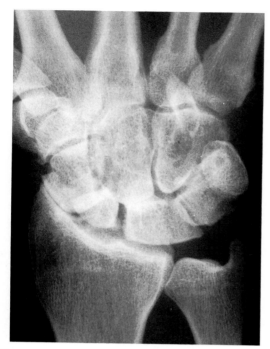

Figure 21–4. Degenerative changes occurring with non-union of the scaphoid tend to support the hypothesis of SLAC wrist. Degenerative changes occur at the radial styloid but progress only as far as the nonunion site. The proximal pole, having been detached from the elongated scaphoid, acts within the wrist as if it were a second lunate. This proximal ununited pole has become a spheroidal shape in a spheroidal cup, and degenerative arthritis does not occur at the proximal pole, just as it does not occur between the radius and the lunate.

heavy loading requires the provision of a stable load-bearing path through bone or Silastic synovitis will occur; that is, a Silastic lunate is in the load path between the capitate and the radius and can never stand alone, except in debilitated patients. The addition of a triscaphe arthrodesis provides an adequate load-carrying mechanism from the hand to the radius.

The technique of reconstruction of the SLAC wrist is based on the fact that the radiolunate joint is highly resistant to degenerative change, even in the most severe late cases. By fusion of the capitolunate joint, all of the wrist load can be taken on by this preserved joint. A proximal row carpectomy, as advocated for nonunited fractures of the scaphoid and rotary subluxation of the scaphoid, would waste the proximal lunate articular surface and replace it with the less congruous shape and the often eburnated surface of the proximal capitate. Adding the hamate and the triquestrum to the capitolunate fusion does not seem to change the

eventual range of motion and definitely enhances the healing of the arthrodesis. The principle of the surgery, however, is capitolunate arthrodesis with a Silastic scaphoid prosthesis. In cases in which this prosthesis has been left out, the resting wrist tends toward a radial deviation position.

This reconstruction is indicated for the symptomatic, degenerated wrist having the SLAC pattern that does not respond to a program of conservative management. SLAC reconstruction is not designed for systemic arthritis or inflammatory conditions.

OPERATIVE TECHNIQUE

A dorsal transverse incision is made at a level ¼ inch distal to the radial styloid tip. Wound spread technique is used, and the branches of the superficial radial nerve and dorsal veins are identified and retracted. The extensor pollicis longus and the extensor carpi radialis longus and brevis are identified and retracted. A transverse incision is made in the capsule at the level of the capitolunate joint. With a dental rongeur, the cartilage is removed entirely from the adjacent surfaces of the lunate, capitate, hamate, and triquetral articulations. High-speed burs are not recommended, because thermal necrosis can interfere with healing. The scaphoid is removed, protecting primarily the radial and the volar ligaments. Ordinarily, in limited wrist arthrodesis, the space between the joints must be maintained by packing with cancellous bone. However, some collapse of the capitate and the hamate onto the lunate and the triquetrum can be allowed in this particular operation because no other joints will be affected by the slight degree of collapse.

A Silastic scaphoid prosthesis is chosen to fill the scaphoid deficit. Dow Corning now makes a stemless, amorphously shaped scaphoid for SLAC wrist reconstruction.

A short 3-cm transverse incision is made approximately 1 inch proximal to the first incision, running from the line of Lister's tubercle dorsally to just volar to the first dorsal tendinous compartment. Spread technique will quickly identify the branches of the superficial radial nerve and the dorsal veins, and they should be protected from injury. A tiny longitudinally aligned periosteal artery is always present and lies between the first and second dorsal compartments. A periosteal incision along this artery and subperiosteal dissection between the first and second dorsal compartments reveal a cortical area that can average 2 cm in length and 1.5 cm in width. An oval window of nearly this size is cut with an osteotome, and a number 2 curette is used to obtain sufficient cancellous bone for grafting. One-half to 1 cm of trabecular bone is left to support the distal radial articular surface. There have been no complications in 256 consecutive bone grafts obtained by us in this manner.

Pins (0.045-in) are then preset to run from the capitate to the lunate, from the triquetrum to the lunate, from the hamate to the lunate, and from the triquetrum to the hamate. Initial cancellous bone graft is packed into the volar joint spaces and tamped into place with a dental tamp. The pins are driven across the assigned joints, but never into the radius or the ulna. The remaining bone graft is packed in place. The Silastic scaphoid implant is put in place.

Note: The capitate angle must be corrected by moving the capitate volarly and dorsiflexing it in relation to the lunate. If the abnorml DISI alignment of the lunate is not corrected, then painful, limited wrist dorsiflexion results.

In our original series of 20 wrists previously reported, there were only two complications. The first complication, a nonunion, was treated successfully by a second bone graft. The second complication was an infection related to the prosthesis, which was removed; the infection cleared, and the prosthesis was replaced seven months later.

There were no other complications in the 20 wrists studied or in the remaining patients. No patients found it necessary to change vocation postoperatively because of problems in the wrist. They retained an average of 60 percent of both flexion-extension and radioulnar deviation in the repaired wrist as compared with contralateral non-operated wrists.

In no instance did follow-up radiographs demonstrate degenerative changes in the radiolunate joint or other unfused joints.

Triscaphe Degenerative Arthritis

Focal degenerative arthritis of the triscaphe joint (the articulation between the trapezoid, trapezium, and scaphoid) is the second most common form of noninflammatory arthritis of the wrist and is usually attributed to osteoarthritis. This pattern was seen alone in 20 percent of affected wrists.

Patients commonly complain of aching at the thumb base and weakness. The onset of symptoms is slow and may be precipitated by trauma, especially a dorsiflexion injury. Occasionally, these individuals will complain of symptoms relating to carpal tunnel syndrome.

Physical examination reveals swelling and tenderness over the triscaphe joint dorsally and a loss of motion in both the flexion-extension and radioulnar deviation planes. Weakness of pinch or grasp has been documented as well as the presence of radiovolar ganglia. As with degenerative joint disease of other joints of the hand, if the symptoms are mild and localized to this joint, initial treatment is splinting, or the injection of steroids into the triscaphe joint, or both.

Early degenerative change is seen here during operations treating severe rotary subluxation of the scaphoid. The collapse of the radial column brings the trapezium and the trapezoid onto the dorsum of the neck of the scaphoid just proximal to the scaphoid distal articular cartilage. Treatment of isolated triscaphe disease is achieved with fusion of the joints between the trapezium, the trapezoid, and the scaphoid (triscaphe arthrodesis).

Operative Technique

The operative technique in triscaphe arthrodesis is very similar to that of the SLAC procedure, except that different bones are fused, and there is no Silastic prosthesis implanted. A slide program, with sound, on triscaphe surgical technique is available from the American Academy of Orthopaedic Surgeons—Program Number 791. The distal radial bone graft technique is exactly the same as that used in the SLAC procedure, and the skin incision is very similar. One has to remember to inspect the proximal scaphoid cartilage and to reduce the scaphoid until it is in proper position before pin fixation. This is best accomplished by excising ½ cm of the styloid process of the radius. If left in place, the styloid is occasionally symptomatic years later. One frequent mistake in this reduction is to overcorrect the scaphoid to the extreme "inline" position of the forearm. The fused scaphoid should lie approximately 45° to 50° to the long axis of the forearm, when viewed from a lateral position. Pin fixation in triscaphe arthrodesis is usually accomplished by two pins from the trapezoid to the scaphoid and one from the trapezium to the trapezoid.

Occasionally, a pin from the scaphoid to the capitate helps in reducing significant rotary subluxation of the scaphoid.

Postoperative care is exactly the same as that after the SLAC procedure.

An acceptable surgical technique is described in detail in Chapter 30.

POSTOPERATIVE RESULTS

Sixty-one triscaphe arthrodeses are currently being followed. At an average follow-up of 36 months, with a range of 13 months to 13 years, the patients retain an average of 80 percent of flexion-extension and 66 percent of radioulnar deviation, as compared with the contralateral nonoperated wrists. No further degenerative changes in unfused carpal joints have been noted. Short-term results of triscaphe arthrodesis for rotary subluxation of the scaphoid have been published.

Combination of SLAC Wrist and Triscaphe Degenerative Arthritis

Combination of the SLAC wrist and triscaphe degenerative arthritis is usually treated as if it were purely SLAC wrist. There are cases in which the triscaphe disease is severe, and the changes of the radioscaphoid and capitolunate joints are not as extensive. Triscaphe arthrodesis is the procedure of choice in these cases. Sclerosis is usually the hallmark of the significant pain source. This radiographic finding, combined with the clinical picture, helps in determining the area of surgery. If there is only narrowing without sclerosis, there is probably enough cartilage remaining in that particular joint for continued function. The scaphoid replacement procedure done in SLAC reconstruction is used to treat the triscaphe joint when the SLAC wrist joints are more severely degenerated.

CONCLUSION

There are very specific patterns of progression in degenerative arthritis of the wrist. About 90 percent of cases occur as the result of problems involving the scaphoid. The most likely pathogenic mechanism of SLAC wrist involves the specialized movement of the scaphoid in its elliptical articulation with the radius. This joint poorly tolerates certain positional scaphoid changes and, unfortunately, the scaphoid ligamentous support is easily disrupted. Degeneration occurs

between the radius and the scaphoid and then between the lunate and the capitate. Treatment consists of limited wrist arthrodesis of the capitate, lunate, hamate, and triquetrum combined with Silastic scaphoid arthroplasty. Painless, full-power, tolerant wrists result.

References

1. Bertheussen K: Partial carpal arthrodesis as treatment of local degenerative changes in the wrist joints. Acta Orthop Scand 52:629–631, 1981.
2. Brenner LH, Watson HK, Strickland JW, et al: Triquetral-lunate arthritis secondary to congenitally incomplete carpal separation. In preparation.
3. Campbell CJ, and Koekarn T: Total and subtotal arthrodesis of the wrist. J Bone Joint Surg (Am) 46:1520–1533, 1964.
4. Carstam N, Eiken O, and Andren L: Osteoarthritis of the trapezioscaphoid joint. Acta Orthop Scand 39:354–358, 1968.
5. Chernin MM, and Pitt MJ: Radiographic disease patterns at the carpus. Clin Orthop 187:72–80, 1984.
6. Cockshott WP: Pisiform hamate fusion. J Bone Joint Surg (Am) 51:778–780, 1969.
7. Crosby EB, Linscheid RL, and Dobyns JH: Scapho-trapezial trapezoid arthrosis. J Hand Surg 3:223–234, 1978.
8. Inglis AE, and Jones EC: Proximal-row carpectomy for diseases of the proximal row. J Bone Joint Surg (Am) 59:460–463, 1977.
9. Kempf L, Copin B, and Forster JP: Wrist arthrodesis, critical study, apropos of 28 cases. Ann Chir 23:81–88, 1969.
10. Kleinman WB, Steichen JB, and Strickland JW: Management of chronic rotary subluxation of the scaphoid by scaphotrapezio-trapezoid arthrodesis. J Hand Surg 7(2):125–136, 1982.
11. Mack GR, Bosse MJ, Gelberman RH, et al: The natural history of scaphoid non-union. J Bone Joint Surg (Am) 66:504–509, 1984.
12. North ER, and Eaton RG: Degenerative joint disease of the trapezium: a comparative radiographic and anatomic study. J Hand Surgery 8(2):160–166, 1983.
13. Patterson AC: Osteoarthritis of the trapezioscaphoid joint. Arthritis Rheum 18:375–379, 1975.
14. Peterson HA, and Lipscomb PR: Intercarpal arthrodesis. Arch Surg 95:127–134, 1967.
15. Rechnasel K: Arthrodesis of wrist. Acta Orthop Scand 42:441, 1971
16. Resnik CS, Miller BW, Gelberman RH, et al: Hand and wrist involvement in calcium pyrophosphate deposition disease. J Hand Surg 8:856–863, 1983.
17. Ricklin P: L'arthrodèse radiocarpienne partielle. Ann Chir 30:909–911, 1976.
18. Schwartz S: Localized fusion at the wrist joint. J Bone Joint Surg (Am) 49:1591–1596, 1967.
19. Simmons BP, and McKenzie WD: Symptomatic carpal coalition. J Hand Surg 10:190–193, 1985.
20. Smith RJ, Atkinson RE, and Jupiter JB: Silicone synovitis of the wrist. J Hand Surg 1:47–60, 1985.
21. Swanson AB: Silicone rubber implants for the replacement of the carpal scaphoid and lunate bones. Orthop Clin North Am 1:299–309, 1970.

22. Watson HK, Hempton RF: Limited wrist arthrodesis. Part I: The triscaphoid joint. J Hand Surg 5:320–327, 1980.

23. Watson HK, Goodman ML, and Johnson TR: Limited wrist arthrodesis. Part II: Intercarpal and radial carpal combinations. J Hand Surg 6:223–233, 1981.

24. Watson HK, and DiBella A: Triscaphe Arthrodesis—Operative Technique. Sound Slide Program #791. Anaheim, California, American Academy of Orthopaedic Surgeons, 1983.

25. Watson HK, and Ryu J: Degenerative disorders of the carpus. Orthop Clin North Am 15:337–353, 1984.

26. Watson HK, Ryu J, and Akelman E: Limited triscaphjoid intercarpal arthrodesis for rotary subluxation of the scaphoid. J Bone Joint Surg 68A(3):345–349, 1986.

27. Watson HK, Ryu J, and DiBella A: An approach to Kienböck's disease: triscaphe arthrodesis. J Hand Surg 10:179–187, 1985.

28. Zielinski CJ, and Gunther SF: Congenital fusion of the scaphoid and trapezium—case report. J Hand Surg 6:220–222, 1981.

CHAPTER 22

Scaphoid Nonunion

GREGORY R. MACK, M.D.
and DAVID M. LICHTMAN, M.D.

Scaphoid nonunion frequently challenges the physician who treats the wrist. Management is difficult because (1) treatment does not assure union, (2) the time required to obtain union may be long, (3) union alone does not always assure a good result, and (4) problem nonunions most commonly occur in young men in their second or third decade, for whom prolonged treatment may create significant economic hardship.[23, 32, 68, 88, 100] To treat scaphoid nonunion, it is therefore important to have a clear understanding of its etiology, natural history, clinical presentation, classification, and prognosis.

ETIOLOGY

Many factors are believed to contribute to the development of scaphoid nonunion: severity of the initial injury, fracture pattern and location, displacement of fracture fragments, associated ligamentous injury, dorsal intercalated segment instability (DISI) between the proximal and distal carpal rows, loss of blood supply to the proximal fragment, delayed diagnosis, ineffective immobilization, and premature removal of the cast. Clearly, both extrinsic factors relating to treatment and intrinsic factors peculiar to the individual injury are involved.

Extrinsic Factors

The factors that most commonly cause scaphoid nonunion are extrinsic. Most fractures are undisplaced and heal well if promptly immobilized. Most nonunions are seen in patients who failed to seek medical attention at the time of their initial injuries

and in those whose diagnoses were initially missed or whose immobilization was discontinued too soon or both. These observations were clearly stated by London[52] and have been confirmed by both retrospective and prospective reviews of our own patients. Many nonunions can thus be prevented by early recognition and treatment. Early diagnosis of scaphoid fracture requires a high index of suspicion, proper positioning of the wrist for roentgenograms, and timely follow-up roentgenograms after cast removal for all wrist injuries with localized snuffbox tenderness. Roentgenographic techniques are discussed in Chapters 7 and 8. Primary health care providers for susceptible populations, including athletic trainers, team physicians, and emergency room physicians, need to be aware of the relative ease of treating acute scaphoid fractures versus the difficulty of managing neglected nonunions. The majority of our previously reported scaphoid nonunions of five to ten years' duration, all of which were symptomatic, were due to injuries sustained in organized athletic programs.

Occasionally, nonunion occurs because immobilization is discontinued prematurely, before trabeculation is clearly demonstrated across the fracture site. Care must be taken not to mistake overlap of the fragments for healing (Fig. 22–1). When doubt exists about the healing of an adequately immobilized fracture, we routinely obtain additional roentgenograms. The most useful views are oblique views with the forearm positioned in 45° pronation and 45° supination and an anteroposterior view in maximum voluntary ulnar deviation.[8] We do not recommend traction views for fractures that are healing. The most definitive assessment will be obtained from plain tomography in two planes with 2 mm cuts. The need to

---

The illustrations in this chapter were redrawn from Gregory R. Mack's original renderings.

293

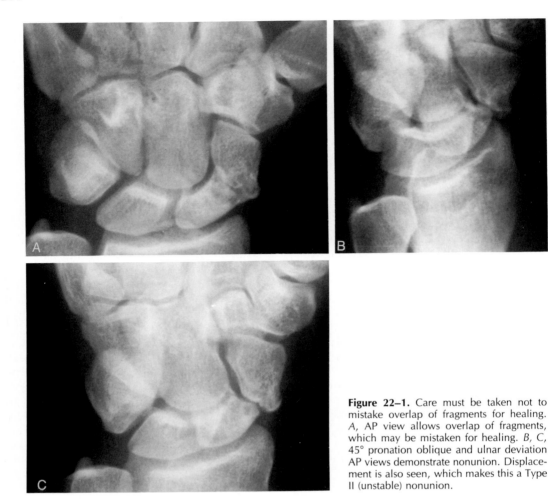

Figure 22–1. Care must be taken not to mistake overlap of fragments for healing. *A,* AP view allows overlap of fragments, which may be mistaken for healing. *B, C,* 45° pronation oblique and ulnar deviation AP views demonstrate nonunion. Displacement is also seen, which makes this a Type II (unstable) nonunion.

clearly document union before releasing the patient cannot be overemphasized. We have not seen a case of so-called reversal of trabecular healing, but we have had patients come to us with established nonunions, who had previously been told by physicians that their treated scaphoid fractures were healed.

Intrinsic Factors

In order to heal, a scaphoid fracture requires coaptation of the fracture fragments, adequate blood supply, and immobilization from the time of injury until union is established. Factors that interfere with these three requirements will delay or prevent union. These may include displacement, carpal instability, avascular necrosis, and fracture location.

Displacement. Significant displacement is defined as cortical offset of the fracture surfaces from their anatomically opposed position by 1 mm or more as seen in roentgeno-grams taken in any plane (Fig. 22–2).[23, 24, 28, 54] Leslie[47] observed that fractures that displaced under treatment had a lower rate of union. Displacement alone, however, does not preclude union. When performing delayed open reduction and internal fixation of displaced fractures, we have found some fractures of the middle or distal thirds to be already healing as early as three weeks after injury. We have not seen this with fractures of the proximal third, fractures with DISI deformity, or fractures with true cystic change. In our opinion, displacement is most significant as a cause of nonunion, when associated either with loss of blood supply to the proximal pole or with motion at the fracture site. We reduce and fix *all* displaced scaphoid fractures, however, to prevent both nonunion and late degenerative change.

Instability. Instability between the proximal and distal carpal rows, characterized by an abnormally increased scapholunate angle (SLA) or radiolunate angle (RLA) or both

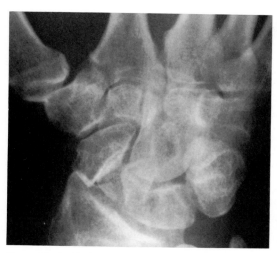

Figure 22–2. Displacement is present if cortical offset of 1 mm or more is demonstrated in any roentgenographic view.

(see Fig. 22–10), is perhaps the most significant cause of scaphoid nonunion. It may be associated with notable displacement at the fracture site, fracture angulation, loss of fragment apposition, ligamentous damage, and/or significant bone resorption at the fracture site. The pathomechanics of carpal instability have been well described by Linscheid.[51] Normally, the intact scaphoid serves as a link between the proximal and distal carpal rows, allowing dorsiflexion and palmar flexion to occur synchronously through two centers of rotation.[35] If the scaphoid is broken, disruption of the link allows a collapse deformity to occur. The proximal row, no longer restrained by the scaphoid, slides volarly into a position of lowest potential energy, resulting in the characteristic DISI deformity, with dorsiflexion of the lunate and proximal fragment of the scaphoid. In stable, undisplaced fractures, the axis of the scaphoid remains unbroken, collapse deformity is not present, and the fracture surfaces are still in contact with each other. Resorption associated with a DISI pattern is probably due to motion and chronic microshearing of trabeculae. This may result in a cystic appearance on the anteroposterior roentgenogram, as the wedge-shaped volar defect allows the scaphoid to angulate (Fig. 22–3A and B). This should be distinguished, however, from true cyst formation at the fracture site, which may heal with prolonged immobilization and does not preclude union (Fig. 22–3C).[60]

Avascular Necrosis. In the context of scaphoid fractures, avascular necrosis (AVN) is commonly understood as the phenomena that result when the blood supply to the proximal pole is interrupted by fracture. Obletz[73] demonstrated that 13 percent of 297 cadaver specimens had no arterial foramina proximal to the waist of the scaphoid and that an additional 20 percent had only one foramen proximal to the waist. Gelberman[34] also found that in 14 percent of specimens, the proximal pole of the scaphoid was dependent on blood supply from vessels entering the distal half of the bone. This anatomic finding is believed to account for the increased radiographic density of the proximal pole that is seen in some scaphoid fractures.[60] Radiographically defined avascularity may represent a relative increase in the density of the proximal pole of the scaphoid as compared with the remainder of the carpus, which may become somewhat porotic due to immobilization and hyperemia. In promptly treated fractures, this is a potentially reversible phenomenon[78] that may be a useful indicator of fracture healing (Fig. 22–4). Green,[38] however, has reported that increased density seen on the roentgenograms of scaphoid nonunions may not necessarily correlate with the true vascularity of the proximal pole. He observed and recorded the number and quality of punctate bleeding points in the cancellous portion of the bone when performing Russe's volar inlay bone grafting, and found vascularity to be a reliable prognostic indicator for the success of bone grafting. He concluded that pre-operative roentgenograms did not accurately predict avascularity found at surgery. So-called necrosis of the proximal pole represents its fragmentation or collapse or both following loss of blood supply. It is unusual, however, to see secondary collapse of the proximal pole in fractures less than 20 years old. Collapse is more commonly a late phenomenon due primarily to the mechanical changes that eventually cause carpal collapse in old scaphoid nonunions rather than the direct results of loss of blood supply alone (Figs. 22–5 and 22–3C).

Fracture Pattern and Location. The pattern and location of scaphoid fracture (Fig. 22–6) may affect its ability to heal. In a prospective study of 100 consecutive fractures, Morgan[66] concluded that fractures of the proximal third and vertical oblique fractures in the middle third had a greater risk of nonunion. Injuries involving the proximal third take longer to heal, both when treated as acute

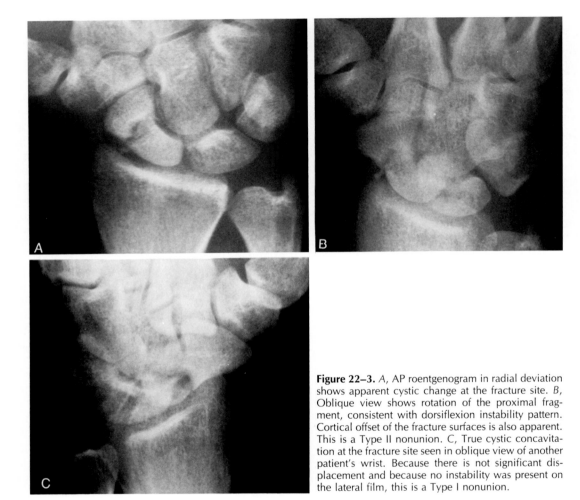

Figure 22–3. *A,* AP roentgenogram in radial deviation shows apparent cystic change at the fracture site. *B,* Oblique view shows rotation of the proximal fragment, consistent with dorsiflexion instability pattern. Cortical offset of the fracture surfaces is also apparent. This is a Type II nonunion. *C,* True cystic concavitation at the fracture site seen in oblique view of another patient's wrist. Because there is not significant displacement and because no instability was present on the lateral film, this is a Type I nonunion.

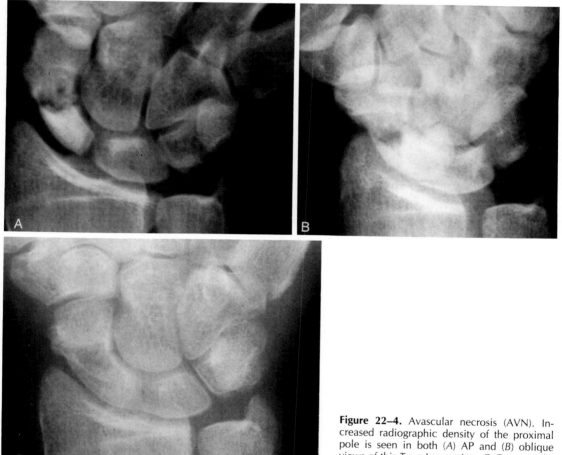

Figure 22–4. Avascular necrosis (AVN). Increased radiographic density of the proximal pole is seen in both (*A*) AP and (*B*) oblique views of this Type I nonunion. *C*, Two months later, AVN has resolved with fracture healing.

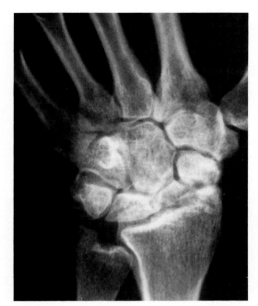

Figure 22–5. Old scaphoid nonunion shows a relative "collapse" of the proximal pole. Note arthritic change between capitate and proximal scaphoid fragment and cystic degenerative changes in the capitate and lunate, consistent with a Type IVa nonunion. This nonunion is 27 years old.

fractures[26, 43] and when grafted as nonunions.[23, 99] This may be related to the smaller diameter of the proximal pole or to interruption of its blood supply, or both.

NATURAL HISTORY

Fracture of the scaphoid characteristically results in bone resorption at the fracture site within three weeks.[59, 87] With prompt diagnosis and adequate immobilization, new bone will slowly bridge the fracture site and healing will occur in most cases in approximately seven to 12 weeks.[3, 14, 28, 52, 66] If the fracture is not immobilized, however, or if

it is so unstable that displacement occurs and apposition of the fragments is lost, no trabeculation will develop across the fracture site, and the fracture will become roentgenographically more obvious with time.

Changes with Time

Once a fracture becomes a nonunion, a specific sequence of degenerative changes occurs. Cyst formation, radioscaphoid arthritis, and extensive arthritis of the wrist develop progressively during the first three decades after injury. Apparent cyst formation is first seen at the fracture site as early as six weeks after injury.[59] Soto-Hall[85] believed that early cystic degeneration is not true cyst formation and suggested that this phenomenon was simply cavitary resorption at the fracture site. True cystic degenerative changes may not appear until much later in the first decade. During this time, additional resorptive change and sclerosis tend to be confined to the scaphoid (Fig. 22–7). Radioscaphoid arthritis, characterized by joint space narrowing, subchondral sclerosis, and pointing of the radial styloid, usually begins before ten years and becomes most prominent during the second decade (Fig. 22–8). After 20 years, extensive arthritis of the wrist develops, with sclerosis and narrowing of the capitolunate and scaphocapitate joints and eventual degenerative changes throughout the carpus (Fig. 22–9). By 30 years, advanced arthritis is invariably present. Involvement of the radiolunate joint is unlikely.[77, 101]

Relation of Displacement and Instability to Arthritis

The pathogenesis of arthritis in patients with scaphoid nonunion is best understood by

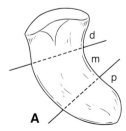 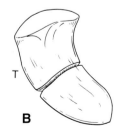 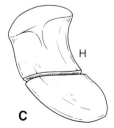 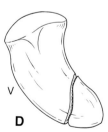

Figure 22–6. Fracture pattern and location as described by Russe: *A,* Nonunion may be located in the proximal, middle, or distal third of the scaphoid. *B,* Transverse fracture pattern. Line of nonunion is perpendicular to the longitudinal axis of the scaphoid. *C,* Horizontal oblique pattern. Line of nonunion is oblique with respect to the scaphoid axis but horizontal with respect to the long axis of the radius. *D,* Vertical oblique pattern. Line of nonunion is oblique with respect to the scaphoid axis but somewhat vertical when compared with the axis of the radius.

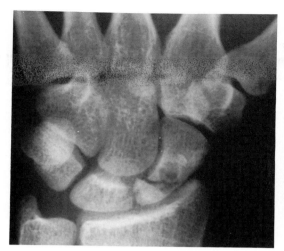

Figure 22–7. Scaphoid nonunion with changes confined to the scaphoid. This nonunion is 29 months old.

correlating the observed patterns of roentgenographic change with fracture displacement and carpal instability. In the natural history of scaphoid nonnion, these factors correlate strongly with degenerative change.[54] Fisk[30] has suggested that displacement occurs in acute fractures because of associated perilunar ligamentous damage,

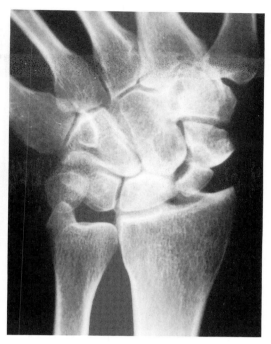

Figure 22–9. Scaphoid nonunion with degenerative arthritis. Note significant involvement of both the radioscaphoid and capitolunate joints. Involvement of the midcarpal joint is consistent with a Type IVa nonunion. Note relative sparing of the radiolunate joint. This nonunion is 20 years old.

which also predisposes the wrist to collapse into a dorsiflexion intercalated segment instability (DISI) pattern of deformity. Such instability may also be caused by a second injury to a previously undisplaced stable nonunion. Mayfield and Johnson[44, 61, 62] have shown that displaced fractures of the scaphoid occur in a similar fashion to that in Grade I perilunate dislocation (i.e., scapholunate dissociation) but that in the displaced fracture, the force takes a wider arc through the carpus. Watson[101] has stated that osteoarthritis of the wrist begins at the radioscaphoid joint, owing to abnormal "nesting" of the scaphoid in the lateral elliptical fossa of the distal radius, and then progresses to the capitolunate joint. Because a DISI pattern is usually present in advanced arthritis, he has coined the term "SLAC wrist" to characterize the "scapholunate advanced collapse."

Lunate Dorsiflexion

Lunate dorsiflexion is a characteristic part of the DISI deformity. Because the proximal scaphoid fragment is attached to the lunate by the intact interosseous portion of the

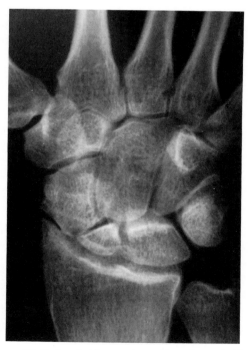

Figure 22–8. Scaphoid nonunion with radioscaphoid arthritis. The radial styloid is pointed, and there is a relative loss of height of the joint space between the styloid and the distal fragment of the scaphoid. Displacement is also apparent. This Type III scaphoid nonunion is 11 years old.

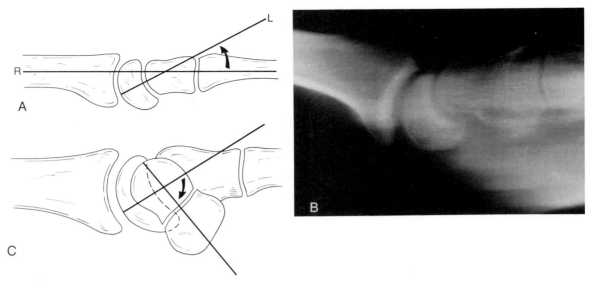

Figure 22–10. *A,* Lunate dorsiflexion is a characteristic finding with the DISI deformity and may be determined by measuring the radiolunate angle. Normally the angle formed by the axes of the radius and the lunate should be less than 10°.[79] Note that the third metacarpal is parallel to the radius. *B,* Lateral tomogram of Figure 22–3A, B demonstrates abnormal lunate dorsiflexion consistent with the rotated proximal scaphoid fragment and indicative of collapse deformity at the midcarpal joint. *C,* Scapholunate angle. The scapholunate relationship should be less than 70°.[51] For scaphoid nonunion, we measure this as the angle formed by the axis of the lunate and the axis of the distal scaphoid fragment.

scapholunate ligament, lunate dorsiflexion causes it to rotate upward, changing not only its angulation with respect to the distal fragment but also its orientation within the elliptical fossa of the radius (Fig. 22–10). When this occurs in acute fractures, contact is lost between the fracture surfaces. In old nonunions, however, the proximal and distal fragments often remain in contact, but the scaphoid is shortened; chronic resorption and wear appear to erode bone at the fracture site, especially from the volar cortices, causing the nonunion to angulate (Fig. 22–11).

Late Displacement

Displacement may develop as a late phenomenon in previously undisplaced fractures. In our experience, reinjury is not necessary for this to occur. We believe that it is possible for the wrist to settle into the DISI position as chronic resorption creates a wedge-shaped volar scaphoid defect. Although some asymptomatic nonunions may not undergo these changes, we expect the majority of all scaphoid nonunions to develop arthritis with time; those that are displaced or unstable are likely to do so at a faster rate.

Advanced Changes

Additional changes in the carpal architecture may occur after the appearance of capitolunate and scaphocapitate arthritis. These changes include radial migration of the distal carpal row, collapse of the proximal pole, and loss of carpal height. They occur to a significant degree in slightly less than half of nonunions of more than 20 years' duration. As degenerative changes continue, the distal radius may take on a triple-scalloped appearance in the anteroposterior roentgenogram. The styloid remodels and may appear to develop a third articular fossa in response to chronic abutment of the distal pole of the scaphoid (Fig. 22–12).

Symptoms

The symptoms of scaphoid nonunion are pain, weakness, and loss of motion. Symptoms may occur any time after a scaphoid fracture has become a nonunion. Many nonunions are continuously symptomatic from the time of the initial injury; others remain asymptomatic for an indefinite period[52, 53] and then become symptomatic either when degenerative changes begin to appear or when the wrist is reinjured.[46, 52, 81] Occasionally, a nonunion is discovered as an inciden-

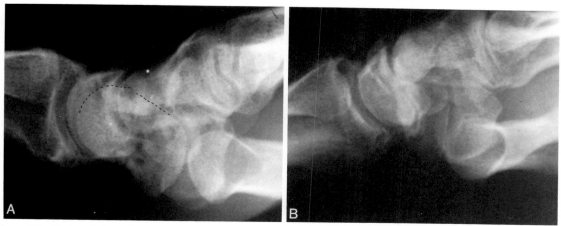

Figure 22–11. Angulation of scaphoid nonunion. Chronic resorption appears with time to selectively erode more bone from the volar cortices than from the dorsal aspect of the bone. *A*, Angulated scaphoid nonunion, eight months old. *B*, Angulated nonunion, 25 years old.

tal radiographic finding in a patient who presents with another problem in the hand. When a nonunion that is asymptomatic comes to medical attention, it may be diffi-

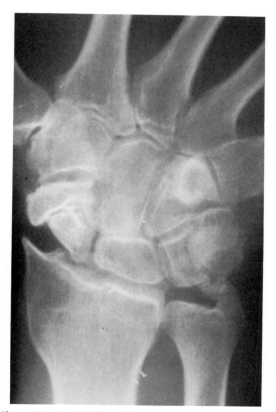

Figure 22–12. "Triple-scallop" appearance of the distal radial articular surface, owing to remodeling of the styloid as a result of chronic degenerative change, seeming to form a third articular fossa for the distal fragment in this Type IVa scaphoid nonunion. This nonunion is 35 years old.

cult to predict when symptoms will occur and how severe they will become. We advise the patient that all scaphoid nonunions are expected to develop degenerative changes with time, and that the onset and severity of eventual symptoms cannot be accurately predicted. Generally speaking, however, displaced or unstable nonunions are likely to undergo degenerative change more rapidly than undisplaced nonunions. Displaced nonunions, in our experience, are also likely to have more severe symptoms than undisplaced nonunions. Regardless of the displacement factor, symptoms of any scaphoid nonunion are likely to be aggravated by reinjury. It is not uncommon for symptoms to be aggravated by minor trauma or exertional stress of a repetitive nature. The intensity of symptoms varies with the patient's use of the wrist, occupation, hand dominance, age, ability to tolerate symptoms, and with predisposition to arthritis.

CLASSIFICATION

There are four types of scaphoid nonunion; they are identified by the presence or absence of displacement and carpal instability and the extent of degenerative change (Table 22–1).

Type I: Simple Nonunion

There is no significant displacement, carpal instability, or degenerative change in any plain roentgenogram, nor is any separation or shift of the fragments seen in ulnar deviation or traction views (Fig. 22–13). Displace-

Table 22–1. **CLASSIFICATION OF SCAPHOID NONUNION**

Classification	Characteristics
Type I: Simple nonunion	Undisplaced Stable No degenerative change
Type II: Unstable nonunion	Displaced > 1 mm or SLA* > 70° or RLA† > 10°
Type III: Nonunion with Early Degenerative Change	Radioscaphoid arthritis
Type IV: Nonunion with Late Degenerative Change	Capitolunate arthritis Generalized arthritis

*SLA = scapholunate angle
†RLA = radiolunate angle

ment, if present at all, is less than one millimeter. The relationship of the lunate to the radius and the distal carpal row is normal. The criterion for this relationship is the absence of significant lunate dorsiflexion in the lateral roentgenogram. For this roentgenogram, the third metacarpal must be parallel

to the radius; the scapholunate angle is less than 70°, and the radiolunate angle is less than 10°.

Type II: Unstable Nonunion

There is significant displacement or instability but no degenerative change. The displaced nonunion is potentially unstable[23, 24] (Fig. 22–14). Displacement is present if there is offset of the fracture fragments by one millimeter or more[23, 24, 28, 54] (see Fig. 22–2). If there is no displacement in standard views, yet the fragments can be separated or shifted by stress or traction views, the nonunion should be considered unstable. If the scapholunate angle[51] is greater than 70° or the radiolunate angle is greater than or equal to 10°, or both,[54] the nonunion is unstable and stress views are unnecessary.

Type III: Nonunion with Early Degenerative Change

Radioscaphoid arthritis is present, with joint space narrowing, subchondral sclerosis, or

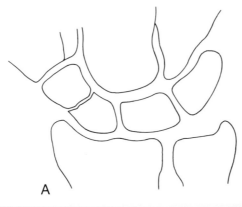

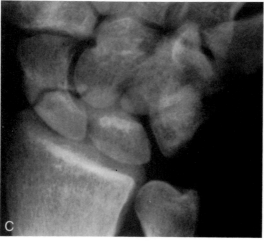

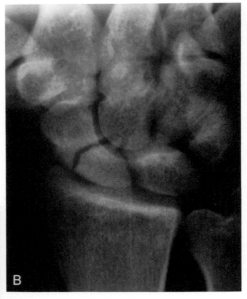

Figure 22–13. *A*, Type I nonunion. There is no displacement, carpal instability, or degenerative change. *B*, Standard AP roentgenogram. *C*, Ulnar deviation (AP view) fails to displace the nonunion.

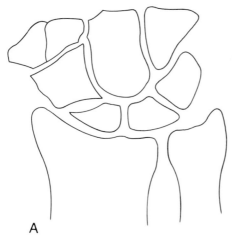

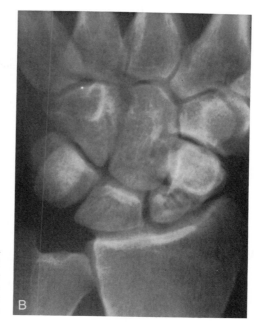

Figure 22–14. *A,* Type II nonunion. If displacement of the nonunion is present, the midcarpal joint is potentially unstable. Traction views are unnecessary. *B,* AP roentgenogram demonstrates displacement. Cortical displacement need not be present, however, if a DISI deformity is seen in the lateral roentgenogram.

pointing of the radial styloid, or both (Fig. 22–15). Displacement or carpal instability or both may or may not be present.

Type IV: Nonunion with Late Degenerative Change

Arthritis is present not only in the radioscaphoid joint but in other joints as well. Watson has observed that radioscaphoid arthritis is invariably followed by capitolunate arthritis.[101] This is the key radiographic find-

ing that distinguishes Type III from Type IV nonunion: In Type IV nonunion the midcarpal joint is affected. Type IV nonunions may be subdivided into (a) those with capitolunate or scaphocapitate arthritis or both, and (b) those with generalized arthritis (Fig. 22–16).

CLINICAL EVALUATION

Evaluation of scaphoid nonunion will be as successful as it is organized. The essential

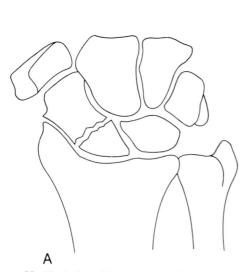

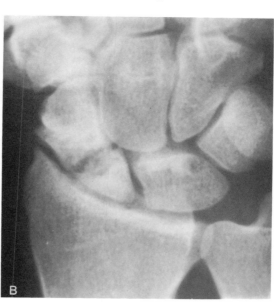

Figure 22–15. *A,* Type III nonunion. Arthritis is confined to the radioscaphoid joint. *B,* AP roentgenogram. Note absence of arthritis in the capitolunate joint.

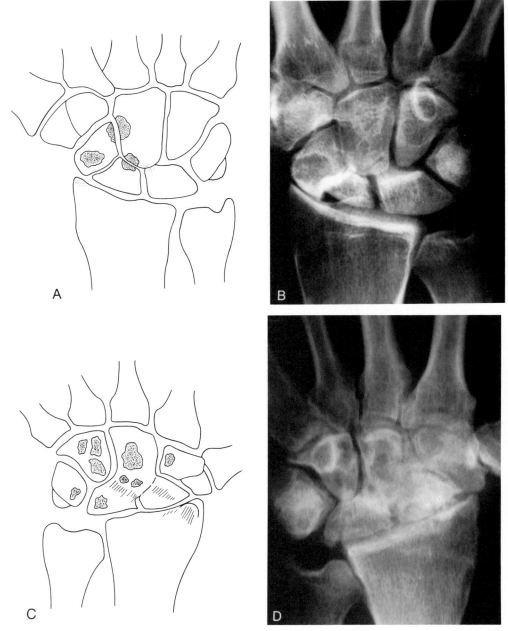

Figure 22–16. Type IV nonunion. *A,* Type IVa demonstrates radioscaphoid and midcarpal arthritis. *B,* Scaphoid nonunion with periscaphoid arthritis. There is midcarpal arthritis with involvement of articulation of the capitate with the proximal scaphoid fragment. *C, D,* In Type IVb, arthritis is generalized.

elements of a complete evaluation are an accurate history, an appropriate but thorough physical examination, a detailed analysis of roentgenograms, and a determination of the character and prognosis of nonunion.

History

Accurately document the chronologic events leading to nonunion, including all prior in-

juries to the wrist and their treatment. The most common and most significant historical error is failure to identify a prior injury, which leads to the misdiagnosis of a new fracture that is actually a reinjured nonunion. A good history and careful scrutiny of roentgenograms will prevent this error. We question all patients with nonunions about prior injury and specifically inquire about wrist "sprains," participation in organized athletics, any history of wrist soreness, and "normal" roentgenograms from emergency rooms. This issue must be addressed not only to apportion causality of any disability to the original and recent injuries, but also to determine the prognosis. If a nonunion was previously treated as a fracture, it is important to inquire about the type and duration of the treatment in order to determine if it was adequate. This is helpful to know because certain Type I nonunions may heal if immobilized long enough. Generally, however, the likelihood of successfully treating a nonunion by prolonged immobilization decreases progressively after it is six months old.

Complaints must be listed to evaluate both the functional and the objective needs of the patient. Most patients will describe some pain, weakness, or loss of motion. Record the patient's hand dominance, occupation, and work status since injury. Note the relation of symptoms to the patient's work. Because most symptomatic scaphoid nonunions occur in young adult males, facts elicited from the history should constructively address two issues: whether the patient's present symptoms impair his ability to work and, if so, whether treatment will help return him to a full-duty status. In older patients whose symptoms are readily controlled by nonsteroidal anti-inflammatory agents, aggressive therapy is rarely indicated.

Physical Examination

Thorough examination will help substantiate subjective complaints with objective findings, assess the severity of impairment, and provide baseline data to document improvement following treatment. Key elements to be recorded include grip strength, range of motion, crepitus, swelling, and localized tenderness. Scars, neuromata, arthritic findings in other joints, and motion of the shoulder, elbow, and forearm are also noted. All measurements are compared with those of the opposite, normal limb. Wrist motion is recorded in four directions: dorsiflexion, palmar flexion, radial deviation, and ulnar deviation. Attempts are made to specifically elicit tenderness in the anatomic snuffbox, over the scaphoid tuberosity, on the radial styloid, over the radiocarpal joint dorsally, and along the course of the first dorsal compartment. Swelling is identified

both by direct palpation and by visual and palpable comparison with the opposite, normal wrist. Ganglia must be sought, especially in the arthritic wrist, since these may be the basis of symptom exacerbations. We have identified these on the volar, dorsal, and radial sides of wrists with well-established scaphoid nonunions. The wrist is then carefully stressed in each of the four standard directions of motion to identify maneuvers that cause pain or reproduce symptoms. Pain elicited only on radial deviation may correlate with radioscaphoid arthritis. Pain at the extremes of dorsiflexion and palmar flexion is less specific but not uncommon and may be related by the examiner to occupational aggravation of symptoms.

Radiographic Analysis

Our preferred views for roentgenographic evaluation of scaphoid nonunion include anteroposterior (AP) view, AP view of the wrist in ulnar deviation, lateral view with the third metacarpal parallel to the radius, and oblique view of the wrist with the forearm in 45° pronation. These views are assessed for fracture pattern and location (see Fig. 22–6), displacement (see Fig. 22–2), carpal instability (see Fig. 22–10), and arthritic change. The criteria for displacement, instability, and degenerative change have been described in the previous discussion of the etiology and classification of scaphoid nonunion. If a nonunion is asymptomatic and undisplaced on these standard views, traction views may be helpful to rule out any latent instability that would predispose to early degenerative change. The ulnar deviation AP view may demonstrate separation of the fragments, which would indicate that the nonunion is unstable.[4] Plain tomograms are useful for evaluating healing and defining displacement. We most commonly use them for evaluation of (1) fractures that have been adequately immobilized, usually for longer than three months, but show no signs of union; (2) acute fractures with minimal fragment separation, to rule out displacement; (3) treated nonunions, to document the course of healing or bone graft incorporation, or both, as early as six weeks after surgery and at four- to six-week intervals thereafter; and (4) neglected fractures and nonunions of the proximal third of the scaphoid to clearly assess fragment size and possible displacement because standard views are not always reliable for this purpose.

TREATMENT

When faced with the decision of how to treat a scaphoid nonunion, the surgeon has a variety of procedures to choose from. No single procedure, however, is appropriate for all nonunions. It is therefore important to understand the general principles of treating scaphoid nonunion, to identify which procedures are appropriate for each type of nonunion, and to know the prognosis, pitfalls, and techniques of each procedure considered for and recommended to the patient.

Principles of Treatment

Undisplaced Fractures Less Than Six Months Old May Be Treated by Prolonged Immobilization. In our experience, the majority of fractures less than six months old will heal if immobilization is adequate and continued until healing is clearly demonstrated roentgenographically. It is important to clearly establish the date of injury, however, to rule out the possibility that the presumed fracture may be a reinjury of an old nonunion, and to be certain that neither displacement nor carpal instability is present. If there is any doubt about the position of the fracture, we obtain stress views and traction views or tomograms or both before embarking on a long period of closed treatment. The time may be prolonged for union of a neglected fracture that is between six weeks and six months old. For fractures more than six months old, the efficacy of closed treatment alone decreases with the age of the nonunion.

Simple (Type I) Nonunion May Be Treated by Bone Graft Alone or by Electrical Stimulation. Pins have been shown to improve the probability of union with bone grafting in selected nonunions.[23] In our experience, however, nondisplaced, stable nonunions treated by volar inlay bone grafting are just as likely to heal without them. It is imperative, however, for the surgeon to be absolutely certain that the nonunion is undisplaced. Careful scrutiny of all roentgenograms is mandatory, and additional studies, including stress views, traction views, and tomograms, may be necessary. Electrical stimulation of scaphoid nonunions has been

shown to achieve union rates of 67 percent to 95 percent.* This may be a reasonable alternative for the patient with an undisplaced stable nonunion who does not want surgery.

If a Nonunion Is Displaced or Unstable or Both (Type II), Open Reduction and Internal Fixation Are Necessary. Because the goals of treatment are not only to obtain union but also to prevent degenerative change, it is necessary to restore the proper length, position, and alignment of the scaphoid in order to make it "nest" properly in the scaphoid fossa of the radius.[101] If chronic resorption has shortened the scaphoid, interposition bone grafting is necessary to restore its length. Interposition bone graft will also help to correct associated DISI deformity and may improve wrist dorsiflexion. Secure internal fixation of both fragments and the interposed bone graft is *always* mandatory in these cases. If a DISI deformity was present pre-operatively and is not corrected by interposition bone grafting, the bone graft may be too small. In some cases it is necessary to first reduce and pin the lunate to the radius to facilitate graft placement.

Osteosyntheses of Proximal Third Nonunions Take Longer to Heal and May Be Technically Difficult to Perform. It is well established that grafted nonunions of the proximal third of the scaphoid take longer to heal than grafted nonunions of the middle or distal thirds.[23, 100] This is probably due to the fact that a small proximal fragment is more likely to be avascular and is more difficult to stabilize. If the length of the proximal pole is less than 4 mm after the nonunion is resected or less than 20 percent of the scaphoid on the pre-operative roentgenogram, fixation and grafting will be difficult, and alternative treatment should be considered. Alternatives include simple excision, excision and replacement with a carved Silastic spacer, replacement of the entire scaphoid with a silicone prosthesis, and proximal row carpectomy.

If Degenerative Change Is Present, Alternative Treatment Should Be Considered. Scaphoid nonunion with arthritis limited to the radioscaphoid joint (Type III) may be treated by bone grafting, internal fixation, and radial styloidectomy if the arthritis is not severe and if the patient is less than 35 years old.

---

*References 5, 9, 10, 14, 15, 17, 31, 65.

Table 22–2. **GUIDELINES FOR TREATMENT OF SCAPHOID NONUNION**

Classification of Nonunion	Treatment	Alternative Treatment
Type I: Simple Nonunion	Bone graft: Volar inlay (Russe) Dorsal inlay (Matti)	Electrical stimulation: Direct (semi-invasive) Indirect (noninvasive) Inductive (PEMFs*) Capacitive coupling
Type II: Unstable Nonunion	Bone graft plus internal fixation: Block graft + screw Wedge graft + screw or pins	If proximal fragment small (<20 percent), avascular: Proximal row carpectomy Excision of proximal pole +/− silicone spacer Intercarpal arthrodesis
Type III: Nonunion with Early Degenerative Change	Patient age <35: Bone graft, internal fixation, and radial styloidectomy	Patient age >35: Proximal row carpectomy Silicone replacement arthroplasty if DISI† not present Radial styloidectomy
Type IV: Nonunion with Late Degenerative Change		
Midcarpal Arthritis (IVA)	Silicone replacement arthroplasy plus midcarpal arthrodesis (SLAC wrist procedure)	Conservative treatment
Generalized Arthritis (IVB)	Wrist arthrodesis	Conservative treatment

*PEMFs = pulsing electromagnetic fields
†DISI = dorsal intercalated segment instability

Prolonged immobilization of the arthritic wrist after surgery may cause stiffness and loss of motion. Loss of wrist dorsiflexion may decrease grip strength. If the patient with a Type III nonunion has a history of arthritis or is over 35, an alternative form of treatment should be considered. Alternative procedures include proximal row carpectomy[25, 42, 45, 72, 89–91] and silicone replacement arthroplasty.[93] If a DISI deformity is also present, implant arthroplasty should not be performed without a limited wrist arthrodesis (SLAC wrist procedure)[101, 102] to stabilize the midcarpal joint. Radial styloidectomy alone may be considered for the older patient whose symptoms can be clearly localized to the radioscaphoid joint. Relief will be only temporary, however, if the distal carpal row shifts further radially without the styloid to abut it and if degenerative change continues.

If degenerative change involves the midcarpal joint in addition to the radioscaphoid joint (Type IVa), treatment alternatives include scaphoid implant arthroplasty with limited wrist arthrodesis (SLAC wrist procedure) between the capitate and the lunate, and wrist arthrodesis. We do not recommend proximal row carpectomy if the head of the capitate is affected by arthritic change.

If degenerative change is extensive (Type IVb), wrist arthrodesis is the surgical treatment of choice.

These guidelines for treatment of scaphoid nonunion are summarized in Table 22–2.

THERAPEUTIC TECHNIQUES

Surgical Anatomy

The scaphoid receives its Greek name from its unique "boat-like" shape. Its major convexity articulates with the distal radius, and its major concavity contains and helps stabilize the head of the capitate. Volarly, the proximal two thirds form a minor concavity, and the distal third a minor convexity that is palpable as the tuberosity. Except for the tuberosity, the dorsal ridge, and the area of its proximal ligamentous attachments to the radius and the lunate, most of the scaphoid's surface is articular. The scaphoid is connected proximally to the lunate by the interosseous and dorsal scapholunate ligaments, and also to the radius by the deep radioscapholunate ligament. Distally, it is tightly secured to the trapezium and the trapezoid, chiefly by palmar ligaments. The distal scaphoid is also connected to the radius— by the radial collateral ligament—and to the capitate.[96] The scaphoid is nested obliquely in a position that allows its radial convexity to conform with the lateral articular facet of the distal radius, with the longitudinal axis tilted approximately 45° toward the palm.[101]

The scaphoid receives its blood supply chiefly from the radial artery by means of vessels that enter dorsally and volarly. The dorsal vessels enter foramina located on the dorsal ridge between the scaphoid's radial and trapezial articular surfaces. The volar vessels enter the scaphoid in the area of the tuberosity.[34] Immediately proximal to the tuberosity, on the palmar surface, is a small, rough triangular area in which vascular perforations may be identified.[95] Small vessels entering here are reflected when the tuberosity is exposed through the extended volar approach to the scaphoid. A denser network of small vessels perforates the lateral cortex of the distal end of the scaphoid and may be identified surgically as small punctate bleeding points when the tuberosity is exposed through an extended volar approach. The vascularity of the proximal 70 to 80 percent of the bone is supplied by the dorsal vessels. The distal 20 to 30 percent of the bone is supplied by the volar vessels. In approximately 14 percent of scaphoids, the dorsal vessels enter just distal to the waist.[34] The reader is referred to Chapter 3 for details.

Volarly, the scaphoid is crossed by the flexor carpi radialis. The first dorsal compartment is radial to the scaphoid and volar to its proximal two thirds. Dorsally, it is crossed by the tendons of the second compartment, the extensor carpi radialis longus and brevis (see Fig. 22–18B).

The scaphoid is palpable at the base of the palm, where the tuberosity lies just beyond the volar wrist flexion crease in line with the flexor carpi radialis. The midportion of the scaphoid is palpable in the anatomic snuffbox.

Surgical Approaches

The scaphoid may be approached volarly, through the sheath of the flexor carpi radialis (FCR); dorsally, beneath the extensor carpi radialis brevis (ECRB) and extensor carpi radialis longus (ECRL); and radially, through the anatomic snuffbox, between the extensor pollicis longus (EPL) and the extensor pollicis brevis (EPB).

Volar Approach. This is the simplest and safest approach because it is least likely to

disrupt the scaphoid blood supply or cause injury to the superficial sensory branch of the radial nerve (SBRN).[34, 78] It is the preferred approach to inlay bone grafting. With extended distal dissection, it may be used for placement of a Herbert screw. Its chief disadvantage is that it requires division and repair of the strong, inelastic volar wrist capsule, including the radiocapitate ligament, which may result in excessive scarring and may decrease wrist dorsiflexion.

Begin the incision directly over the center of the scaphoid tuberosity in the palm and continue proximally 1½-in directly over the FCR (Fig. 22–17A). The scaphoid is exposed proximal to the tuberosity by longitudinally dividing both the roof and floor of the sheath of the FCR; this keeps the plane of dissection away from the radial artery and out of the carpal tunnel. Retract the tendon ulnarly. Expose and open the volar wrist capsule in line with the skin incision. Create continuous capsuloperiosteal flaps radially and ulnarly by sharply dissecting Sharpey's fibers off the distal radius with an end-cutting knife blade. This relaxes the interval for better exposure. Division of the distal fibers of the pronator quadratus may be necessary. The scaphoid and its nonunion can be easily manipulated in the fossa of the distal radius with a curved blunt instrument such as a narrow Langenbeck elevator.

If distal exposure is required, extend the skin incision distally from the tuberosity to the middle of the trapezium in a line that parallels the axis of the thumb. Divide the superficial fascia of the thenar muscles and reflect the muscle ulnarly. At this point the superficial branch of the radial artery is likely to cross the distal portion of the operative field and should be retracted radially. Continue the capsule incision distally onto the tuberosity and trapezium. Take care not to damage the cartilage on either side of the scaphotrapezial joint. Reflect capsuloperiosteal flaps radially and ulnarly sufficiently to expose this joint (Fig. 22–17B and C) but avoid excessive lateral reflection of the capsuloligamentous attachments so as not to interfere with vascularity. Radial styloidectomy can be performed through this approach by slight extension of the proximal incision, exposing the styloid subperiosteally.

Dorsal Approach. This approach is slightly more difficult than the volar approach because care must be taken not to injure the

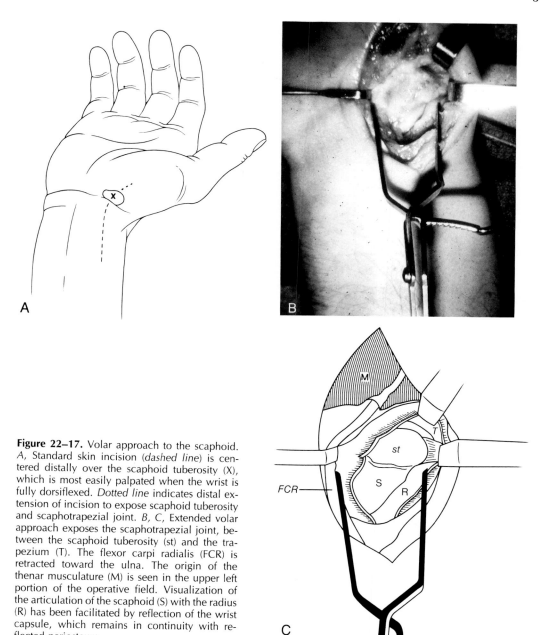

Figure 22–17. Volar approach to the scaphoid. *A,* Standard skin incision *(dashed line)* is centered distally over the scaphoid tuberosity (X), which is most easily palpated when the wrist is fully dorsiflexed. *Dotted line* indicates distal extension of incision to expose scaphoid tuberosity and scaphotrapezial joint. *B, C,* Extended volar approach exposes the scaphotrapezial joint, between the scaphoid tuberosity (st) and the trapezium (T). The flexor carpi radialis (FCR) is retracted toward the ulna. The origin of the thenar musculature (M) is seen in the upper left portion of the operative field. Visualization of the articulation of the scaphoid (S) with the radius (R) has been facilitated by reflection of the wrist capsule, which remains in continuity with reflected periosteum.

vessels that enter the dorsal ridge, because the superficial sensory branch of the radial nerve and accompanying dorsal vein cross the field (Fig. 22–18A), and because the tendons of the second and third dorsal compartments must be mobilized and retracted for exposure (Fig. 22–18B). The advantage of this approach is that it does not disrupt the strong volar wrist capsule. It is the preferred approach for excision of the proximal pole and for silicone replacement arthroplasty. It can also be extended ulnarly to

permit proximal row carpectomy or for exploration in cases of an acute naviculocapitate syndrome.

Locate Lister's tubercule, the radiocarpal joint, and the EPL. Begin the skin incision distally in line with the EPL, and curve it toward the ulna proximally at the level of the radiocarpal joint, just distal to Lister's tubercle (Fig. 22–19A). The ulnar limb of the skin incision may be extended if more exposure is needed. The sensory branch of the radial nerve and the accompanying vein

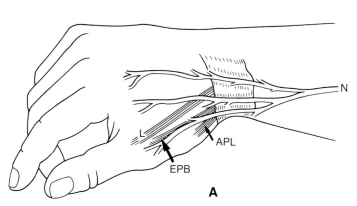

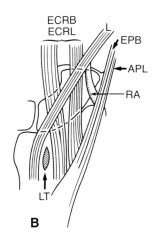

Figure 22–18. Anatomic structures that overlie the dorsal and radial aspects of the scaphoid include the superficial branch of the radial nerve (N), extensor pollicis longus (L), extensor carpi radialis brevis (ECRB), extensor carpi radialis longus (ECRL), radial artery (RA), extensor pollicis brevis (EPB), and abductor pollicis longus (APL). *A,* The terminal sensory branches of the radial nerve cross the tendons of the first three extensor compartments. The radial wrist extensors, which are crossed by the EPL, are not shown. *B,* Location of the scaphoid, as seen from its dorsal aspect, with respect to the tendons of the first three extensor compartments, Lister's tubercle (LT), and the radial artery.

will cross the radial half of the operative field and can be first recognized by their surrounding fat. Protect the nerve by first mobilizing it proximally and distally and then by retracting it gently to either side of the operative field. Identify the EPL, the ECRL, and the ECRB, and free each from investing fascia and synovial tissue until each can be gently retracted to either side of the wound (Fig. 22–19B and C). Division of

the extensor retracululm proximal to Lister's tubercle is not necessary.

Move the wrist, and identify the radioscaphoid joint with a blunt instrument. Incise the wrist capsule transversely over the proximal third of the scaphoid. The capsular incision may be extended distally along the axis of the scaphoid, provided that the dorsal ridge vessels are directly visualized and protected from injury. To expose the distal third

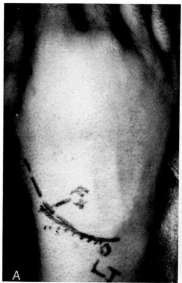
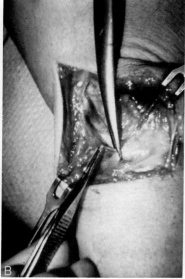
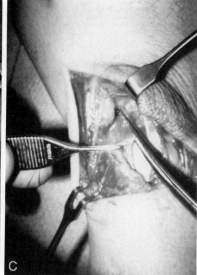

Figure 22–19. *A,* Skin incision (*dashed line*) for dorsal approach to the scaphoid. *Solid line* indicates distal margin of the radius. Lister's tubercle (LT) and the level of the nonunion (Fx) are also indicated on this patient's wrist. *B,* Tendovaginotomy of the extensor pollicis longus (EPL). Branches of the superficial branch of the radial nerve have been mobilized and retracted along with their fat. The tendon is mobilized by clearly identifying its surrounding tissue and carefully dividing the extensor retinaculum to the level of Lister's tubercle. Extra care is necessary to avoid damage to the tendon itself where it "turns the corner" around the tubercle. *C,* In similar fashion, each of the two radial wrist extensor tendons is mobilized, from the radiocarpal joint to its metacarpal insertion. The EPL is retracted ulnarly.

of the scaphoid, a second capsular incision is sometimes necessary. For removal of the scaphoid, care must be taken distally when soft tissue is dissected superficial to the capsule so as not to injure the deep branch of the radial artery, which lies dorsoradial to the scaphotrapezial joint. For proximal row carpectomy, continue the skin and capsular incisions over the lunate and triquetrum toward the ulnar styloid.

Radial Approach

The radial approach exposes the scaphoid directly through the anatomic snuffbox in the interval between the EPL and the EPB (Fig. 22–20). It is the preferred approach for simple radial styloidectomy[7] and may also be used for dorsoradial inlay bone grafting[23] or for wrist arthrodesis.[39] It has also been preferred by some surgeons for fixing the scaphoid dorsally from distal to proximal, using either pins or a simple navicular lag screw. Its advantage over the dorsal approach is protection of the sensory branch of the radial nerve under its dorsal flap. Because the radial artery crosses the operative field when the distal pole of the scaphoid or the scaphotrapezial joint is approached, it is important that the artery be identified and carefully retracted. Retraction of the artery facilitates the procedure, whereas failure to identify it risks a serious vascular injury.

The incision is curvilinear and begins distally over the proximal quarter of the thumb metacarpal; it courses through the snuffbox and curves toward the ulna over the radiocarpal joint to the EPL[33] (Fig. 22–21A). Branches of the SBRN are retracted within the dorsal flap. The capsule is exposed between the EPL and the EPB. The radial artery lies distally in the wound beneath the EPB and must be protected. A transverse capsular

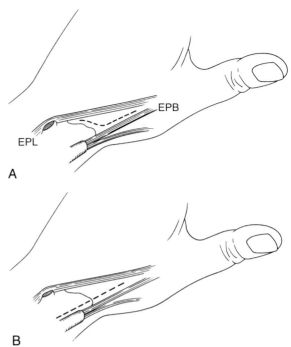

A

B

Figure 22–21. Radial approach to the scaphoid. *A,* Skin incision for exposure of the scaphoid in the anatomic snuffbox. The incision is centered distally between the EPL and EPB and parallels the EPB before curving dorsally and ulnarly at the radiocarpal joint. Dorsally, incision may extend to the EPL. *B,* Skin incision for radial styloidectomy is centered over the styloid and parallels the EPB. This incision is also appropriate for the Dobyns-Lipscomb technique of dorsoradial inlay bone grafting.

incision is made with the wrist in ulnar deviation and may be continued proximally and ulnarly for more exposure.

If radial styloidectomy is to be performed through this approach, the skin incision is made longitudinally, directly over the radial styloid[7] (Fig. 22–21B).

TREATMENT OF TYPE I NONUNION

Appropriate techniques for treating Type I scaphoid nonunion include bone grafting alone and electrical stimulation. We prefer bone grafting to electrical stimulation because our results in undisplaced nonunions have been favorable, and the required period of immobilization (12 to 20 weeks) is predictable in most cases.

Bone Grafting

Bone grafting a scaphoid nonunion is most likely to be successful when the following conditions are met: (1) pseudarthrotic tissue is resected; (2) the nonunion is well bridged

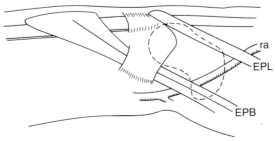

Figure 22–20. Location of the scaphoid and radial styloid relative to the radial artery (ra) and the extensor pollicis longus (EPL) and extensor pollicis brevis (EPB) tendons.

by autogenous, preferably cancellous, bone; (3) the blood supply and viability of the fragments are not disturbed, either by surgical dissection or by the use of power instruments; (4) the bone fragments are stable at the conclusion of the procedure.

Three bone grafting techniques have been described for treating scaphoid nonunion: volar inlay bone grafting (Russe),[78] dorsal inlay bone grafting,[56] and dorsal peg grafting with cortical bone.[69-71] Of these three, we prefer the Russe procedure because favorable results have been obtained by different authors* and because it is the simplest procedure to perform without jeopardizing scaphoid vascularity. Cooney,[23] however, reported comparable results with dorsoradial inlay grafting combined with radial styloidectomy. Murray reported that 96 of 100 nonunions he treated by dorsal peg grafting healed in an average time of 3.3 months. Comparable results with his technique were obtained by Palmer[74] but have not been reported by other authors.[23, 32, 97]

Volar Inlay Bone Grafting Technique. Russe[78] modified the technique that he published in 1960 and described it to Green,[38] who reported his own experience with the modified technique.

Carefully expose the scaphoid through a volar approach. Expose the nonunion, but do not disturb its dorsal or lateral surfaces. Resect pseudarthrotic tissue with a fine curette and an end-cutting knife blade to expose the opposing bone surfaces of the proximal and distal fragments. Cut a 3 × 12 mm cortical window in the volar aspect of the scaphoid with small, sharp osteotomes. Curette the fragments by hand, until bleeding bone is seen on either side of the nonunion and a trough is created to accept the bone graft. If the bone is viable, small punctate bleeding points may be observed even with the tourniquet inflated.[38] It may be necessary to thoroughly excavate all cancellous bone from the proximal fragment. Obtain two corticocancellous bone grafts from the ilium or the distal radius. These should measure slightly more than 2 mm in width. Bone graft from the distal radius may be preferable because its cortex is thinner.[38] Insert the strut grafts into the cavity, with the cortical sides outward (Fig. 22–22). Fill the remainder of the cavity with small chips of cancellous bone graft. The wrist should be immobilized

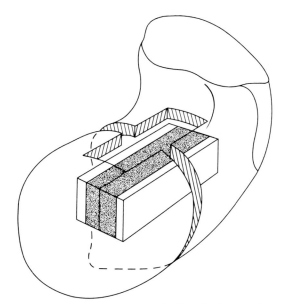

Figure 22–22. Russe technique of volar inlay bone grafting, as described by Green. Two struts of corticocancellous graft are countersunk within the bone, cortical sides outward. Multiple 1 to 2 mm "chips" of cancellous graft (not shown) fill the remainder of the cavity prepared for the strut grafts. Green prefers graft obtained from the distal radius because its cortex is thinner than the cortex of graft obtained from the ilium.

by a well-fitting long-arm thumb spica cast in slight flexion and slight radial deviation. Change the cast every six to eight weeks until healing occurs. After the first six weeks, we use a short-arm thumb spica cast. All fingers should be freely mobile throughout the postoperative period.

Dorsoradial Inlay Bone Grafting Technique. Matti[56] introduced the excavation concept for bone grafting of the scaphoid in 1936. He performed his procedure through a dorsal approach. We do not recommend inlay grafting through the dorsal approach because of the possibility of disrupting the dorsal ridge vessels. Barnard and Stubbins[7] and Dobyns and Lipscomb[23] modified the Matti technique by using a radial approach between the tendons of the first and second extensor compartments. Whereas Matti bridged the curetted defect with cancellous bone from the ilium, Dobyns and Lipscomb resected the radial styloid, used it to make a corticocancellous bone graft, and inlayed it on the dorsoradial aspect of the scaphoid (Fig. 22–23). The styloid is resected proximal to the level of the nonunion, and a 5 × 20 mm graft is used. Cooney[23] compared the results of dorsal inlay grafting through the radial approach with the results of volar inlay grafting and reported union in 91 percent

---

*References 23, 27, 29, 36, 41, 63, 67, 68, 80, 86, 98, 99.

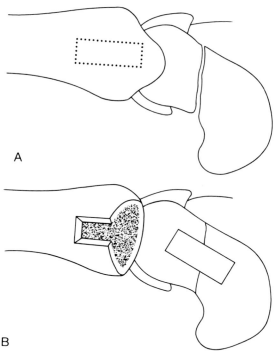

A

B

Figure 22–23. Dobyns-Lipscomb modification of dorsoradial inlay bone grafting. *A,* A 5 × 20 mm corticocancellous graft is obtained from the radial styloid, which is then resected. *B,* The graft is mortised into a corresponding slot in the dorsoradial aspect of the scaphoid.

and 87 percent of the cases, respectively; his series included both stable and unstable nonunions treated both with and without internal fixation.

Dorsal Bone Peg Technique (Murray). Murray[69] published the first description of his procedure in 1934. He used a radial approach and inserted a cortical bone graft from the tibia into a 5/16-in drill hole made through the dorsal distal aspect of the scaphoid. Murray himself emphasized that this technique might fail, however, if the surgeon was inexperienced, had not seen the operation performed correctly, and was doing it himself for the first time. To achieve best results with his technique, he emphasized that the graft must be large enough, that it must cross the fracture line well into the proximal fragment, that the drill hole must not violate articular cartilage, that the graft must be firmly impacted into the proximal fragment, that the wrist and first metacarpal must be completely immobilized after surgery, and that immobilization must be continued until healing is demonstrated roentgenographically.[71]

Electrical Stimulation

An alternative to bone grafting an undisplaced scaphoid nonunion is to stimulate it electrically while it is immobilized in a cast. Electricity may be delivered to the site of nonunion either directly or indirectly. Clinical experience with scaphoid nonunion supports *direct treatment with percutaneous electrodes*[5, 14, 15, 17, 65] and *indirect treatment with pulsating electromagnetic fields (PEMFs)*.[9, 10, 31] *Capacitive coupling* is an additional noninvasive technique that uses direct current to induce electromagnetic fields in the bone. Only preliminary results of its use have been reported, however.

Direct Method, or Semi-Invasive Techniques. This method delivers a constant 20-microampere (μA) current from an external battery pack to each of three or four stainless steel pins that act as cathodes. The pins are drilled through the scaphoid tuberosity into the nonunion, under regional anesthesia with fluoroscopic control. A remote anode pad is attached to the skin under the cast. The pins are Teflon-coated, except for their tips; maximum electrical activity occurs at the junction of the bare metal and the insulation. Treatment is continued for 12 weeks; Bora[14, 15] recommends that a long-arm cast that allows slight elbow flexion-extension but prevents forearm pronation-supination be used for the first six weeks of immobilization. After the semi-invasive technique was used, 71 to 95 percent (84 percent overall) of scaphoid nonunions healed, as reported by different authors[5, 14, 17, 65]

Indirect Method. The PEMF or inductive technique uses a pair of external coils supplied by a pulse generator to produce time-varying magnetic fields that induce weak electric currents in bone.[9] The coils are centered over the nonunion and may be incorporated into the cast. Beckenbaugh[10] reported that union was more likely to be achieved with a long-arm cast than with a short-arm cast and that treatment may be needed for four to six months. After use of PEMFs, 67 to 85 percent (79 percent overall) of scaphoid nonunions healed, as reported by different authors.[9, 10, 31] The results of electrical stimulation compare favorably with those of bone grafting, considering the lower risk of the noninvasive and semi-invasive techniques. The volume of published material is much larger for bone grafting than for electrical stimulation, however, and the rates of union are slightly higher for the grafting techniques. No series directly compares bone grafting with electrical stimulation in a prospective fashion.

Internal Fixation

Internal fixation without bone graft has been used for scaphoid nonunion, but reported union rates vary from 0 to 80 percent.[33, 36, 48, 57, 64] McLaughlin[64] advocated internal fixation of scaphoid fractures, delayed unions, and nonunions in order to preserve motion and permit use of the wrist throughout the period of healing. None of the five nonunions he reported treating by this method healed. Maudsley[51] and Cooney[23] also reported low union rates with internal fixation alone. Gasser[33] immobilized some of the nonunions he treated and reported union in 11 of 20 cases. Glass[36] used Gasser's method and reported union in seven of nine nonunions; he compared results of internal fixation with those of the Russe procedure and concluded that the latter was simpler, safer, and more effective. Leyshon[48] reported that eight of ten nonunions healed following internal fixation with an A–O scaphoid lag screw. He emphasized that the nonunion must not be disturbed and reported union, as demonstrated radiologically, to occur at an average of seven months.

We do not advocate internal fixation alone, because volar inlay grafting is likely to produce union in a higher percentage of cases with no greater morbidity.

TREATMENT OF TYPE II NONUNION

The goals of treatment of Type II nonunion are to reduce and stabilize the fracture fragments and to establish union. Because the Type II nonunion is inherently unstable, internal fixation is required, in addition to resection of pseudarthrotic tissue and bone grafting.

Choice of Bone Graft

The size and shape of bone graft are determined chiefly by the size of the bone defect at the nonunion. This is determined by resecting the nonunion through a volar approach, reducing the fragments, and observing the size of the volar defect. The graft should fill the cavity left by resection of the

nonunion, conforming to the approximate shape of the defect left by resection of pseudarthrotic tissue and, prior to instrumentation, should distract the fragments slightly beyond the desired final position. The fracture fragments and bone graft are then reduced and compressed with a Herbert jig and secured with a bone screw of the same size as that indicated on the jig. As compression is applied, the graft will collapse slightly, making intimate contact with the fracture surfaces on either side. If the graft is fragmented, of poor quality, or too small, no correction of alignment will be obtained. This is a useful technique because rigid internal compressive fixation may allow a shorter period of external immobilization. This technique is contraindicated if the proximal pole is avascular or too small to accept the narrow threads of the Herbert screw. Herbert has demonstrated that a small proximal fragment can be secured with his screw through a dorsal approach. Curettage and iliac cancellous graft are still required. Dorsal screw insertion is more difficult, however, because instrumentation is performed freehand, without the jig. It requires thorough understanding of the shape and position of the scaphoid. A shorter screw is used to avoid cortical penetration by the leading threads of the screw.

An alternative graft for a Type II nonunion with a small volar defect is a volar inlay graft as described above for Type I nonunion, stabilized by two or three 0.035-in stainless steel pins. If the volar scaphoid defect is greater than 2 mm, an interposition graft should be used to restore the length of the scaphoid and to correct the carpal instability pattern. This graft may be wedge- or block-shaped and must be stabilized, either with Kirschner wires or a Herbert screw.

Block Interposition Technique

Approach the scaphoid volarly and extend the incision distally to expose the scaphotrapezial joint (Fig. 22–17B and C). Reflect capsuloperiosteal flaps off the proximal ridge of the trapezium, the scaphoid tuberosity, and the distal radius. Using a 5/16-in small osteotome, resect the nonunion. The osteotomy cuts should be made through trabecular bone to remove the sclerotic faces of the nonunion, which would impair healing. The cuts should be perpendicular to the long axis of the scaphoid (Fig. 22–24). If carpal instability is present, reduce it by applying

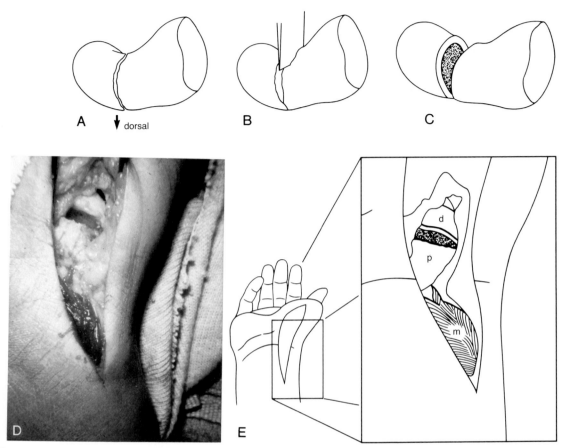

Figure 22–24. Osteotomy of the scaphoid for block or wedge bone grafting. *A,* Nonunion of right scaphoid viewed from radial aspect. *B,* Resection of nonunion with sharp ⁵⁄₁₆-in small osteotome. *C,* A volar wedge-shaped defect is usually demonstrated by realignment of the nonunion fragments to their proper anatomic position. *D, E,* Dorsiflexion of the wrist will also demonstrate the size of the volar defect between the proximal (p) and distal (d) fragments to be bridged and/or filled by interposition grafting. Proximal muscle (m) is a portion of the flexor carpi radialis. If the bone defect is substantial and is not restored, loss of wrist dorsiflexion may result.

pressure on the palmar pole of the lunate with a blunt instrument such as a narrow Langenbeck periosteal elevator. This will help demonstrate the size and configuration of the scaphoid defect and the correct orientation of the proximal carpal row; gentle dorsiflexion of the wrist over a bump will achieve the same result (Fig. 22–24D and E). Soft tissue adherent to the dorsal aspect of the nonunion should not be disturbed. Measure the scaphoid defect to determine the size of corticocancellous bone graft required. The cancellous portion of the graft should be slightly longer than the defect before compression is applied.

Expose the most lateral aspect of the iliac crest. Make two parallel cuts in the periosteum on the top of the crest, 3 cm apart, and connect these cuts with a third periosteal incision along the lateral margin of the crest (Fig. 22–25A). Do not elevate the periosteum. Through the periosteal incisions, os-

teotomize the cortex of the crest to create a 3.0 × 1.5-cm "lid," which is hinged medially (Fig. 22–25B). Now reflect periosteum and muscle inferiorly to expose the outer cortex. From the exposed area, obtain a corticocancellous block of bone slightly larger than the measured scaphoid defect (Fig. 22–25C). Bone cuts should be made precisely, with sharp hand instruments. Do not use power tools, which may burn and devitalize the periphery of the graft. Trim and fit the graft to the defect. The cancellous part of the graft should be slightly longer than its cortex. The cortical surface of the graft should face outward on the volar side of the scaphoid and should be firmly seated with a bone tamp to abut the cortices on either side of the nonunion (Fig. 22–26). Apply the jig for the Herbert screw.[40] This is perhaps the most critical and most difficult part of this procedure. The screw must pass through both fracture fragments and the graft from distal

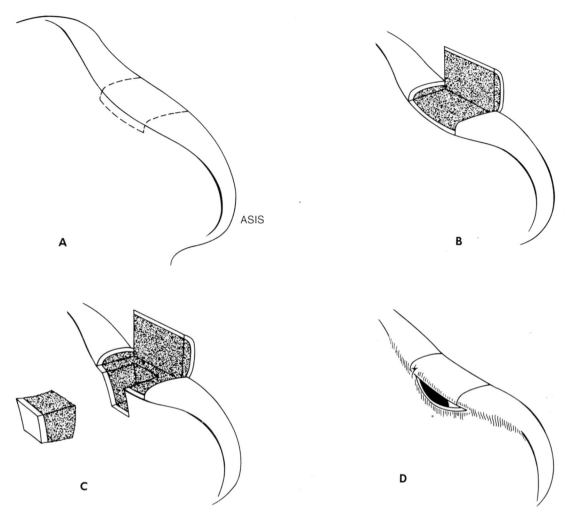

Figure 22–25. *A*, Periosteal incision on the superolateral aspect of iliac crest. Palpable landmarks are the superolateral margin of the crest itself and the anterior superior iliac spine (ASIS). *B*, Periosteal cuts are deepened with very sharp osteotomes to create a medially-hinged cortical lid. *C*, Corticocancellous block is removed by sharp cuts on all sides using osteotomes. The medial vertical cut is made along the medullary face of the inner table of the ilium. *D*, Closure of the cortical "lid" and its attached periosteum.

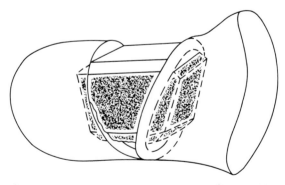

Figure 22–26. Diagrammatic representation of interposition block graft bridging volar scaphoid defect, with its cortical side abutting the volar cortices of the proximal and distal fragments. The cancellous edges of the graft extend beyond its cortex and are tapered to achieve a "lozenge" shape.

to proximal. If the hook of the jig is too far in the ulnar direction, the screw will miss the proximal pole; if too radial, it will slip and score the cartilage; if too volar, the screw will tend to "bowstring" volar to the graft; and if the hook is too dorsal, placement of the barrel distally will be difficult. For accurate barrel placement, it will be necessary to lever the distal pole of the scaphoid palmarly and to position the barrel against the distal articular surface. Resection of a small portion of the trapezial ridge may facilitate placement of the barrel but is usually not necessary if scaphoid angulation is adequately corrected. Compress the fragments

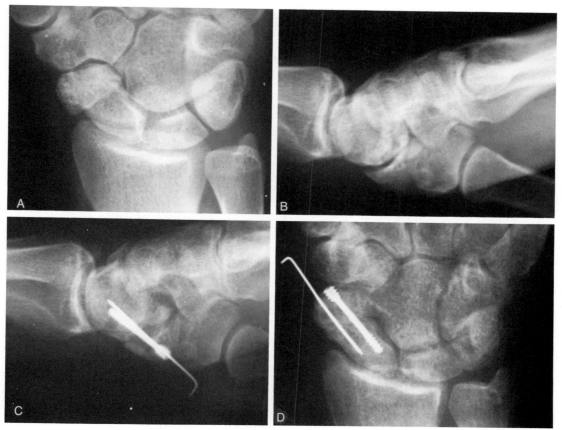

Figure 22–27. Type II scaphoid nonunion treated by interposition bone block technique. *A,* Preoperative AP view demonstrates displacement. *B,* Preoperative lateral view suggests dorsiflexion of lunate and proximal scaphoid fragment. *C,* Postoperative lateral view demonstrates Herbert's screw and a 0.035-in pin transfixing both the scaphoid fragments and the interposition graft. The pin is removed after the fracture has healed. *D,* At six weeks, the graft appears to be incorporated. Tissue at the wide end of the screw is somewhat proud but not symptomatic.

and the graft together by tightening the jig. If the osteotomy cuts are not parallel, the graft may tend to extrude; if it does so, re-reduce it and stabilize the fragments with a single 0.035-in wire, which is inserted parallel to the path for screw placement (Fig. 22–27). If the wire is inserted first, it may also provide a small amount of leverage for manipulating the scaphoid while applying the jig. At this point, the surgeon who is not experienced with the Herbert system should confirm jig placement radiographically. A single 0.028-in wire may be driven through the barrel of the jig and down the intended screw path to help visualize the position of the jig radiographically. Confirm final screw placement with roentgenograms. Trim the periphery of the graft flush with the margins of the proximal and distal fragments with fine-tipped rongeurs.

Wedge Graft

The technique of interposition wedge grafting is similar to the block technique described earlier (Figs. 22–28 and 22–29). Pins may be used in lieu of a compression screw.

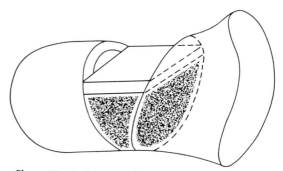

Figure 22–28. Diagram of wedge graft prior to fixation.

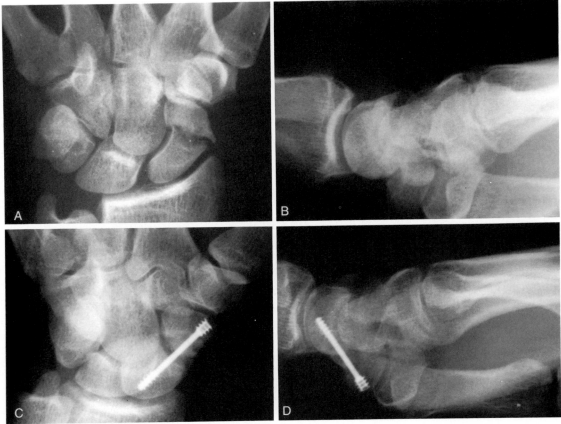

Figure 22–29. Type II scaphoid nonunion treated by interposition wedge graft technique. A, Preoperative AP roentgenogram. B, Preoperative lateral view. Note angulation of scaphoid. C, Postoperative oblique view. D, Lateral view eight weeks after surgery shows incorporation of wedge graft.

OSTEOSYNTHESIS OF TYPE III SCAPHOID NONUNION

Bone grafting and internal fixation of the Type III scaphoid nonunion are similar to the techniques described for the Type II nonunion. We prefer the volar approach, interposition grafting, and compressive fixation with the Herbert screw. Pin fixation is more likely to require prolonged immobilization, which may cause wrist stiffness. Radial styloidectomy should be performed as part of the procedure. This is done through the same incision, by subperiosteally exposing the volar and radial cortices of the styloid with an end-cutting knife blade, retracting the tendons of the first dorsal compartment, and resecting the styloid with a 5/16-in osteotome. The osteotome must be sharp to make an accurate cut, and adjacent soft tissues must be protected while the cut is being made. A second alternative is to perform dorsoradial inlay bone grafting as modified by Dobyns and Lipscomb.[23] Their

technique resects the radial styloid as part of the approach (see Fig. 22–23). Pins to stabilize the fragments can be introduced through the distal fragment, but care must be taken to protect the radial artery, its intercarpal branch, and the dorsal ridge vessels.

ARTHROPLASTY FOR SCAPHOID NONUNION

Arthroplasty may be indicated for the symptomatic patient with scaphoid nonunion if the proximal fragment is small, or collapsed, or both, if previous bone grafting has failed, and for the treatment of symptoms due to degenerative arthritis. Four procedures recommended by different authors are appropriate for some or all of these indications: excision of the proximal pole, with[103] or without insertion of a carved silicone spacer; silicone replacement of the scaphoid;[92] proximal row carpectomy;[25, 42, 45, 72, 89–91] and radial styloidectomy[7, 18, 32, 49, 58, 88] (Fig. 22–30). We

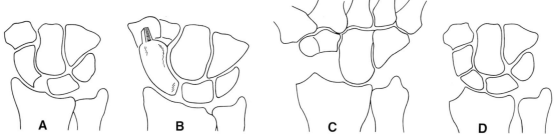

Figure 22–30. Four types of arthroplasty for scaphoid nonunion: *A,* Excision of the proximal fragment. *B,* Silicone replacement arthroplasty. *C,* Proximal row carpectomy. *D,* Radial styloidectomy.

do not advocate soft tissue interposition arthroplasty, as described by Bentzon,[11] because it does nothing to correct or prevent the pathomechanics of carpal collapse and will not, in our opinion, prevent the late degenerative changes characteristic of scaphoid nonunion.

Proximal Pole Excision

Proximal pole excision is indicated for the symptomatic nonunion if the proximal pole is less than 20 percent of the length of the scaphoid. This may relieve symptoms due to nonunion. If a DISI deformity is also present, proximal pole excision is less likely to be effective. The procedure should therefore be limited to undisplaced nonunions with proximal poles that are too small or that are unsuitable for grafting. Nonunions with small proximal poles and carpal collapse may be more suitably treated by proximal row carpectomy or by capitolunate fusion and silicone replacement of the scaphoid. Watson[102] has cautioned that excision of the proximal pole may led to capitolunate arthritis.

Proximal pole excision is easily performed through a dorsal approach between the second and third extensor compartments if the proximal pole is small. Care must be taken not to disrupt the radial or lunate attachments of the deep radioscapholunate ligament.

Zemel[103] reported on the use of a spacer carved from medical grade silicone rubber combined with proximal fragment excision. His procedures were performed through a volar approach. He found that results were clinically satisfactory in 20 of 21 patients, although measurable carpal displacement occurred in 17 wrists followed for two years after surgery. We do not use this technique because we believe that carved silicone implants are more susceptible to tear propaga-

tion, and their use thus predisposes the area to late foreign-body synovitis.

Silicone Replacement Arthroplasty

Replacement of the scaphoid with a molded silicone (or Swanson's) prosthesis is a useful procedure for the scaphoid nonunion that is unsuitable for grafting or has associated degenerative arthritis, or both. Abnormal loading of the implant, including shear stresses and compressive loading, will cause microfibrillation of its surface and possibly a late foreign-body synovitis of the wrist.[21, 75, 83] Swanson[94] reported severe degenerative or cystic changes in four of 55 scaphoid implant arthroplasties. If a pin is used to stabilize an implant and synovitis occurs, cystic changes may develop in the vicinity of the pin tract. Because a pre-operative DISI pattern is likely to abnormally load the implant, we do not recommend silicone arthroplasty as an isolated procedure if a nonunion is displaced or unstable, or both. This, unfortunately, limits the indications for use of this implant because most nonunions with degenerative changes are displaced and unstable,[54] and most nonunions without degenerative changes may be more reliably treated by reduction, bone grafting, and osteosynthesis. Because premature wear of the prosthesis may be prevented by stress-shielding silicone replacement arthroplasty may be combined with midcarpal arthrodesis to relieve radioscaphoid arthritis and to preserve some wrist motion, with theoretically less risk of late synovitis than treatment by arthroplasty alone would afford. Until the advantage of stress-shielding is proved, however, the combination of implant arthroplasty and midcarpal arthrodesis should be reserved for nonunions with arthritis limited to the radioscaphoid, the scaphocapitate, and the capitolunate joints (Type IVa).

The technique of silicone replacement arthroplasty has been described by Swanson (see Chapter 28).[93] A dorsal approach is used. The scaphoid is exposed through the interval between the second and third extensor compartments, with care taken to avoid injury to the branches of the radial artery and nerve. We use an oblique capsular incison that begins proximally at Lister's tubercle, parallels the radiocarpal joint, and follows the thumb axis distally as far as the scaphotrapezial joint. It is necessary to preserve the capsule. Intraoperative roentgenograms may be required to correctly identify both fragments and the nonunion. The bone is completely excised, preserving all capsular attachments. A hole is then fashioned, using curettes, in the center of the articular surface of the trapezium to accept the stem of the scaphoid implant. The size of the implant is determined by insertion of trial implants. After implant insertion, the capsule is carefully repaired with nonresorbable sutures. A short-arm cast is worn for four to six weeks, and full use of the wrist is allowed at 12 weeks.[93] We do not pin the implant because we do not believe that pins prevent late subluxation of carpal implants, because pins may cause tear propagation in the implant, and because their use may be associated with late foreign-body synovitis.

The principles of intercarpal arthrodesis are described in Chapter 30. When performing midcarpal arthrodesis, it is essential to restore the correct alignment of the proximal row, in this case the lunate. If lunate dorsiflexion is not corrected, dorsal subluxation of the scaphoid implant will occur.

Proximal Row Carpectomy

Proximal row carpectomy has been successfully used for scaphoid nonunion,[25, 72] and favorable results as long as 20 years after surgery have been reported.[25, 42] Because resection of the proximal row repositions the dome of the capitate in the lunate fossa of the distal radius, intact, healthy articular cartilage on these two surfaces favors a better long-term result. This procedure may be performed if radioscaphoid arthritis is present (Type III), but a good result is less likely if capitolunate arthritis is present (Type IVa). It is indicated for Type II nonunions not suitable for bone grafting. It is also a good procedure for the older patient with a displaced Type III nonunion as an alternative to implant arthroplasty and midcarpal ar-

throdesis. It is unnecessary for Type I nonunions with viable proximal poles and is contraindicated in Type IV nonunions. Its advantages are a shorter period of immobilization than that following bone grafting and the fact that it avoids the risk of implant failure. It preserves an arc of wrist motion that is functional but, of course, not normal. After proximal row carpectomy, the wrist appears broader than normal, and grip is usually slightly weaker than normal, probably owing to the effect that shortening of the wrist has on the length-tension (Blix) curve of the long flexors. If proximal row carpectomy fails to relieve pain, it may be converted to a wrist arthrodesis.

Proximal row carpectomy is performed as follows: Make a transverse skin incision over the radiocarpal joint. The incision is made along a line drawn from the ulnar styloid to the radial styloid. We recommend curving the radial third of the incision slightly distally to facilitate exposure and removal of the scaphoid. The dorsal cutaneous branches of the radial and ulnar nerves should be identified and protected. The distal half of the extensor retinaculum is divided and will later be repaired. Mobilize and retract the tendons of the second, third, and fourth dorsal compartments. The direction of retraction is determined by the area to be exposed. Incise the wrist capsule transversely over the proximal row; "T" it centrally and distally if necessary.[72] The proximal row can also be exposed by making two capsular incisions on either side of the fourth compartment, but correct positioning of the capitate on the radius after excising the proximal row is easier to visualize when a single transverse incision is used. Separate the dorsal capsule from the bones of the proximal row. Take care not to damage the radial artery when exposing the scaphoid. Do not disturb the volar capsule.

It is easiest to remove the triquetrum first. Portions of the proximal row may be removed piecemeal with rongeurs to facilitate their dissection from the palmar capsule. The scaphoid is the most difficult to remove because of its distal and volar ligamentous attachments and is removed last; it is sometimes helpful to insert a 0.062-in pin into the distal fragment to manipulate and to help expose it.

After the proximal row is removed, release the tourniquet and obtain hemostasis. Position the capitate in the lunate fossa of the distal radius. If the radial styloid abuts the trapezium in either the neutral position or in radial deviation, resect the styloid. Repair the dorsal capsule and close the wound.

Apply a sterile dressing and splints to immobilize the wrist in a neutral position. Remove the sutures and apply a well-molded short-arm cast at 10 to 12 days. Continue immobilization for approximately four weeks. Apply a removable volar wrist splint, carefully molded to the new contour of the wrist (prefabricated devices may not fit properly) for an additional month and prescribe a nonresistive exercise program for that period to gradually mobilize the wrist. Maximum strength may not be regained for six or more months postoperatively.

Radial Styloidectomy

Radial styloidectomy is a useful procedure for the symptomatic management of old scaphoid nonunions. It may be indicated for a Type III or IV nonunion in an older patient with symptoms localized to the radioscaphoid joint, in lieu of a more extensive procedure such as proximal row carpectomy or wrist arthrodesis. Bone scan may be used to identify the site of inflammation prior to making this decision.

Styloidectomy works by relieving painful impingement of the distal scaphoid fragment on the radial styloid. It is a simple procedure with minimal risk and does not require prolonged postoperative immobilization. Its chief disadvantage is that the relief it affords may be only temporary because it does not prevent further radial migration of the distal carpal row[18] (Fig. 22–31).

The technique of radial styloidectomy has been described by Barnard[7] and Smith.[82] The skin incision may be longitudinal or transverse. The transverse incision is more cosmetic, but the longitudinal incision is safer because injury to the fine terminal sensory branches of the radial nerve is less likely.

Make a 4-cm incision directly over the

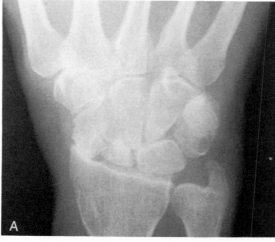
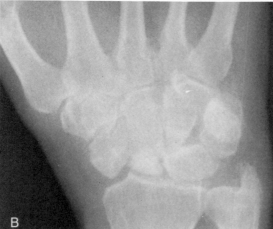
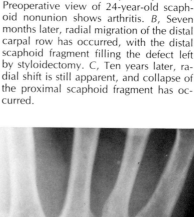
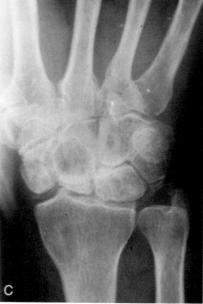

Figure 22–31. Scaphoid nonunion treated by radial styloidectomy for symptoms localized to the radioscaphoid joint. *A,* Preoperative view of 24-year-old scaphoid nonunion shows arthritis. *B,* Seven months later, radial migration of the distal carpal row has occurred, with the distal scaphoid fragment filling the defect left by styloidectomy. *C,* Ten years later, radial shift is still apparent, and collapse of the proximal scaphoid fragment has occurred.

radial styloid (see Fig. 22–24). Retract the cephalic vein dorsally. Carefully free up the sensory nerves with their fat from the deep structures, and gently retract them with the skin flaps. Open the first dorsal compartment and retract its tendons dorsally. Incise and reflect the periosteum over the styloid and continue the incision longitudinally in the mid-portion of the radial collateral ligament. The radial styloid and distal fragment of the scaphoid should be well exposed. No more than 1.5-cm of the articular surface should be excised or the carpus may become unstable radially; therefore, this procedure may be contraindicated in proximal pole fractures. Resect the styloid just proximal to the level that corresponds with the nonunion, when the wrist is in radial deviation. Repair the radial collateral ligament and the periosteum. For patient comfort, splint the wrist for seven to 10 days. Progressive wrist motion may then be encouraged.

Soft Tissue Interposition Arthroplasty

Bentzon[11] described soft tissue interposition arthroplasty for painful pseudarthrosis of the scaphoid. This procedure interposes a fat-fascia flap between the proximal and the distal scaphoid fragments. Bentzon did not recommend this procedure in cases with a small proximal fragment. Perey[76] and Agner[2] reported favorably on this procedure. Boeckstyns[12] combined radial styloidectomy with Bentzon's technique and reported satisfactory clinical results. We do not use either technique, however, because soft tissue procedures for nonunion will not stabilize the carpus or prevent degenerative change.

INTERCARPAL ARTHRODESIS FOR SCAPHOID NONUNION

A limited wrist arthrodesis may be appropriate for a scaphoid nonunion that is not suitable for grafting. A Type III nonunion with a small proximal fragment, for example, is unlikely to unite after bone grafting if the proximal pole is truly avascular[38] and may still be symptomatic if the proximal fragment is simply excised. Gordon and King[37] reported favorable results with adequate follow-up in five scaphoid nonunions treated by partial wrist arthrodesis, including four with arthrodesis of the radius to the scaphoid and the lunate. The types and techniques of intercarpal arthrodeses and their indications are discussed in Chapter 30.

WRIST ARTHRODESIS

Wrist arthrodesis is the treatment of choice for advanced degenerative arthritis due to scaphoid nonunion. Because the symptoms of arthritis may be controlled by rest, short periods of splinting, and nonsteroidal anti-inflammatory medication, we reserve arthrodesis for older patients with severe symptoms and for manual laborers with Type IV nonunions. The advantage of arthrodesis is that it is the most effective means of controlling wrist pain. Its disadvantage is permanent loss of motion in the midcarpal and radiocarpal joints.

There are two basic techniques of wrist arthrodesis, which differ chiefly in the surgical approach to the carpus. The two standard approaches are dorsal and radial. A third approach through the distal radioulnar joint was described by Smith-Peterson[84] and modified by Seddon,[55] but wrist arthrodesis through the medial approach is not appropriate when the distal radioulnar joint is not also affected by the arthritic process. Techniques for both the radial and dorsal approaches include resection of articular cartilage, autogenous bone grafting, and postoperative immobilization in a long-arm cast for eight to 12 weeks or until union occurs. With both techniques, it is best to extend the fusion to the base of the index and long metacarpals, in order to prevent the occurrence of late symptoms at the second and third carpometacarpal joints. The radial approach is more difficult because its exposure of the carpus is limited, but one of us (Mack) prefers it because it does not add bulk to the wrist or significantly disturb the extensor retinaculum.

Wrist Arthrodesis Through a Radial Approach (Haddad and Riordan)[39]

Begin the skin incision on the lateral side of the distal forearm, 1½-in proximal to the radial styloid. Follow the radius distally to the radial styloid and then curve the incision gently upward to the base of the index metacarpal (Fig. 22–32). Identify the superficial sensory branch of the radial nerve, mobilize it from the deep structures, and gently reflect and retract it with the volar skin flap; by so doing, the extensor tendons of the first, sec-

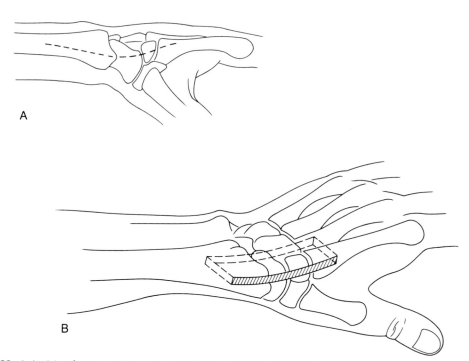

Figure 22–32. *A,* Incision for wrist arthrodesis through radial approach. *B,* Radial slot extending from distal radius to base of index and long metacarpals.

ond, and third compartments are easily exposed.

Incise the dorsocarpal ligament and the periosteum of the distal radius between the first and second dorsal compartments. Elevate periosteal flaps dorsally and volarly, and reflect the tendons of the first compartment with the volar periosteal flap. If the interval between the first and second compartments has been clearly identified and cleanly incised, it is not necessary to open the first compartment. Identify the insertion of the extensor carpi radialis longus on the base of the index metacarpal, and transect it 1 cm proximal to its insertion; it is helpful to first secure the proximal end of the tendon with a 2–0 suture for later retrieval and repair. Expose the dorsal and radial aspects of the carpus by reflecting the capsular flaps in continuity with the periosteal flaps reflected off the radius. The dorsal and radial aspects of the scaphoid, the lesser multangular, the capitate, and the lunate, and the base of the index and long metacarpals should be exposed.

Throughout the dissection, great care must be taken to avoid injury to the radial artery in the anatomic snuffbox (see Fig. 22–20). The intercarpal branch of this artery may be ligated and divided, but the radial artery itself should be gently retracted palmarly with the volar flap.

Denude the articular surfaces of the radius, scaphoid, lunate, capitate, lesser multangular, and proximal ends of the index and long metacarpals with rongeurs. Do not disturb the hamate, the triquetrum, the ulnar two metacarpals, or the triangular fibrocartilage. Position the wrist in 5° to 10° ulnar deviation and approximately 15° dorsiflexion. These angles are formed by the axes of the radius and the long metacarpal; in this position a line extended from the axis of the radial shaft should roughly bisect the web between the opposed thumb and digits.[16]

Cut a slot in the lateral cortex of the distal radius, and extend it distally through the carpus to the base of the index and long metacarpals. This is done by using a sharp oscillating saw with a 1-in blade, while one assistant secures the position of the wrist and a second assistant retracts the soft tissue flaps. The slot should be large enough to accept a corticocancellous graft approximately 2.5 cm wide, 5 cm long, and 5 mm thick (Fig. 22–32B). The graft is obtained from the inner table of the ilium, near the iliac crest. The inner table is recommended because its cortical surface is concave and its cancellous surface is convex.[39] We also

use cancellous bone chips for the arthrodesis. Key the bone graft into the rectangular
slot, and fill the spaces of the denuded joints
with the cancellous chips.

With the graft in place, the wrist should
be stable with slight upward pressure on the
palm, an important point to keep in mind
when applying the postoperative dressing
and subsequent casts. Because the inner table of the ilium is thin, the graft may break
when the wrist is dorsiflexed. If this occurs
or if the wrist is unstable, or both, a nonthreaded Kirschner wire should be passed
obliquely across the arthrodesis to maintain
position. Close the capsuloperiosteal flaps,
repair the extensor carpi radialis longus, and
close the skin.

Apply a sterile dressing and long-arm
splints to maintain rigid immobilization of
the elbow at 90°, the forearm in neutral
rotation, and the wrist in slight dorsiflexion
and ulnar deviation. At 10 days, remove the
sutures and apply a long-arm cast in the
same position. We routinely change the cast
and obtain roentgenograms at the sixth and
twelfth weeks after surgery, but more frequent cast changes and repairs are sometimes necessary in active patients.

Wrist Arthrodesis Through a Dorsal Approach

The basic technique for wrist arthrodesis has
been well described by Abbott.[1] Variations
of the dorsal technique differ chiefly in the
source and shape of the bone graft and in
the extent of the fusion.[20, 22, 50, 92] The following technique is based on our own experience and incorporates what we believe are
the key principles of dorsal arthrodesis of
the wrist.

Use a longitudinal incision and center it
over Lister's tubercle for optimal exposure
(Fig. 22–33). Making the incision slightly
curvilinear may facilitate exposure but will
not improve the appearance of the postoperative scar, which is likely to widen with
time. The incision should extend from 1½-
in above the radiocarpal joint to the base of
the index and long metacarpals.

Incise the dorsocarpal ligament between
the third and fourth extensor compartments.
It is safest to do so by incising over the jaws
of a slightly opened hemostat, which is positioned radially within the fourth compartment. Repair of the dorsocarpal ligament
will prevent bowstringing of the extensor

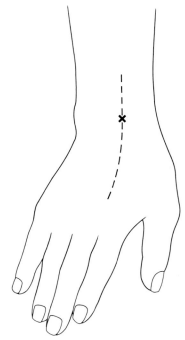

Figure 22–33. Incision for wrist arthrodesis through dorsal approach is centered over Lister's tubercle (X).

tendons, but this may be difficult because
the ligament is inelastic and its fibers are
transversely oriented. If the ligament is thin,
it may be opened with a step-cut to facilitate
closure. Complete the incision between the
third and fourth compartments to the bone
and elevate the second, third, and fourth
compartments subperiosteally.

The extent of fusion should include all
the affected joints but should exclude the
distal radioulnar joint and the fourth and
fifth carpometacarpal joints (Fig. 22–34). Incise the capsule to its distal insertion on the
base of the second and third metacarpals.
The capsule may be "T'd" if necessary at
the radiocarpal joint to increase exposure.
Proliferative synovium, if present, should be
excised, but the margins of the incised dorsal
capsule should be preserved to present a
smooth gliding surface to the underside of
the extensor and to help contain the bone
graft.

Denude the cartilage and resect subchondral bone from all joints to be fused,
and resect any fibrous tissue from the nonunion. Do not disturb the attachment of the
palmar capsule to any of the carpal bones,
and take care not to injure the triangular
fibrocartilage.

Inlay a corticocancellous iliac bone graft
from the radius to the base of the index and

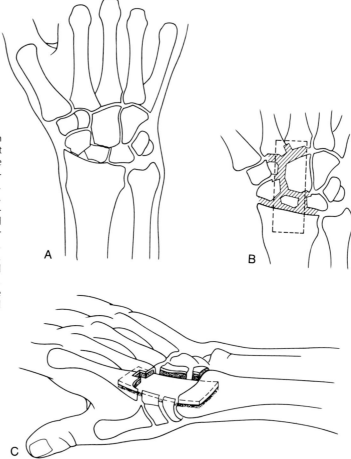

Figure 22–34. A, Diagrammatic representation of a Type IVa scaphoid nonunion prior to wrist arthrodesis. B, Cartilage and subchondral bone resected from radiocarpal, midcarpal, and carpometacarpal joints, denoted by shaded area. Note that the articulations of the trapezium, hamate, triquetrum, fourth and fifth metacarpals, and distal ulna are not disturbed. Dashed line denotes rectangular bed to be prepared for corticocancellous iliac bone graft (see text). C, Corticocancellous iliac bone graft in place, extending from medullary cavity of the distal radius into base of index and long metacarpals. In this illustration, the ends of the graft are countersunk beneath the cortices of the distal radius and the index and long metacarpals.

the long metacarpals. The graft should be long enough to bridge the fusion area, approximately 2 cm wide, 6.5 cm long, and 0.5 cm thick. The graft should be carefully countersunk into slots in the distal radius and in the base of the index and the long metacarpals. Use an oscillating saw to make the slots, and resect the dorsal aspect of the carpal bones to accept the graft and make good contact with its undersurface (Fig. 22–34C).

Fill the interstices of the denuded intercarpal, radiocarpal, and second and third carpometacarpal joints with small cancellous chips of iliac bone graft.

Countersink the graft into the distal radius and the second and third metacarpals by dorsiflexing the wrist approximately 15°. If stability is not achieved with the graft in place and the wrist slightly dorsiflexed, insert a nonthreaded pin through the distal radius and across the carpus into the base of the third metacarpal.

Postoperative care is the same as that described for arthrodesis through the radial approach.

References

1. Abbott LC, Saunders JB, and Bost FC: Arthrodesis of the wrist with the use of grafts of cancellous bone. J Bone Joint Surg 24:883–898, 1942.
2. Agner O: Treatment of ununited fractures of the carpal scaphoid by Bentzon's operation. Acta Orthop Scand 33:56–65, 1962.
3. Alho A, and Kankaanpaa U: Management of fractured scaphoid bone. A prospective study of 100 fractures. Acta Orthop Scand 46:737–743, 1975.
4. Arkless, R.: Cineradiography in Normal and Abnormal Wrists. Am J Radiol 96:837–844, 1966.
5. Aversa JM: Electrical treatment of scaphoid nonunions. Fiftieth Annual Meeting of the American Academy of Orthopaedic Surgeons, Anaheim, 1983.
6. Bannerman MM: Fractures of the carpal scaphoid bone. An analysis of sixty-six cases. Arch Surg 53:164–168, 1946.
7. Barnard L, and Stubbins SG: Styloidectomy of the radius in the surgical treatment of non-union of

the carpal navicular. J Bone Joint Surg 30A:98–102, 1948.

8. Barr JS, Elliston WA, Musnick H, et al: Fracture of the carpal navicular (scaphoid) bone. An end-result study in military personnel. J Bone Joint Surg 35A:609–625, 1953.

9. Bassett CAL, Mitchell SN, and Gaston SR: Pulsing electromagnetic field treatment in ununited fractures and failed arthrodeses. JAMA 247:623–628, 1982.

10. Beckenbaugh RD: Noninvasive pulsed electromagnetic stimulation in the treatment of scaphoid nonunion. 52nd Annual Meeting of the American Academy of Orthopaedic Surgeons, Las Vegas, 1985.

11. Bentzon PGK, and Randlov-Madsen A: On fracture of the carpal scaphoid. A method for operative treatment of inveterate fractures. Acta Orthop Scand 16:30–39, 1946.

12. Boeckstyns MEH, and Busch P: Surgical treatment of scaphoid pseudarthrosis: evaluation of the results after soft tissue arthroplasty and inlay bone grafting. J Hand Surg 9A:378–382, 1984.

13. Bongers KJ, and Ponsen RJG: Operative and nonoperative management of fractures of the carpal scaphoid: five years' experience. Neth J Surg 32:142–145, 1980.

14. Bora FW, Osterman AL, and Brighton CT: The electrical treatment of scaphoid nonunion. Clin Orthop 161:33–38, 1981.

15. Bora FW, Osterman AL, Woodbury DF, et al: Treatment of nonunion of the scaphoid by direct current. Orthop Clin North Am 15:107–112, 1984.

16. Boyes JW: Surgical Repair of Joints. In Bunnell S: Bunnell's Surgery of the Hand. 5th ed, Philadelphia, JB Lippincott Co, 1970, p 297.

17. Brighton CT, Black J, Friedenberg ZB, et al: A multicenter study of the treatment of non-union with constant direct current. J Bone Joint Surg 63A:2–13, 1981.

18. Brown PE, and Dameron TB: Surgical treatment for nonunion of the scaphoid. South Med J 68:415–421, 1975.

19. Burnett JH: Further observations on treatment of fracture of the carpal scaphoid (navicular). J Bone Joint Surg 19:1099–1109, 1937.

20. Butler AA: Arthrodesis of the wrist joint. Graft from inner table of the ilium. Am J Surg 78:625–630, 1949.

21. Carter PR, and Benton LJ: Late osseous complications of carpal Silastic implants. 40th Annual Meeting of the American Society for Surgery of the Hand, Las Vegas, 1985.

22. Colonna PC: A method for fusion of the wrist. South Med J 37:195–199, 1944.

23. Cooney WP, Dobyns JH, and Linscheid RL: Nonunion of the scaphoid: analysis of the results from bone grafting. J Hand Surg 5:343–354, 1980.

24. Cooney WP, Linscheid RL, and Dobyns JH: Scaphoid fractures. Problems associated with nonunion and avascular necrosis. Orthop Clin North Am 15:381–391, 1984.

25. Crabbe WA: Excision of the proximal row of the carpus. J Bone Joint Surg 46B:708–711, 1964.

26. Dickison JC, and Shannon JG: Fractures of the carpal scaphoid in the Canadian Army. A review and commentary. Surg Gynecol Obstet 79:225–239, 1944.

27. Dooley BJ: Inlay bone-grafting for non-union of

the scaphoid bone by the anterior approach. J Bone Joint Surg 50B:102–109, 1968.

28. Eddeland AE, Eiken O, Hellgren E, et al: Fractures of the scaphoid. Scand J Plast Reconstr Surg 9:234–239, 1975.

29. Eitenmuller JP, and Haas HG: Behandlungsergebnisse bei 258 Kahnbeinverletzungen an der Hand. Arch Orthop Trauma Surg 91:45–51, 1978.

30. Fisk GR: Carpal instability and the fractured scaphoid. Ann R Coll Surg Engl 46:63–76, 1970.

31. Frykman GK, Helal B, Kaufman R, et al: Pulsing electromagnetic field treatment of nonunions of the scaphoid. 37th Annual Meeting of the American Society for Surgery of the Hand, New Orleans, 1982.

32. Gartland JJ: Evaluation of Treatment for Non-Union of the Carpal Navicular. J Bone Joint Surg 44A:169–174, 1962.

33. Gasser H: Delayed union and pseudarthrosis of the carpal navicular: treatment by compression-screw osteosynthesis. J Bone Joint Surg 47A: 249–266, 1965.

34. Gelberman RH, and Menon J: The vascularity of the scaphoid bone. J Hand Surg 5:508–514, 1980.

35. Gilford WW, Bolton BM, and Lambrinudi C: The mechanism of the wrist joint. With special reference to fractures of the scaphoid. Guy's Hosp Rep 92:52–59, 1943.

36. Glass KS, and Hochberg F: Nonunion of carpal navicular bone: comparison of two methods of treatment. Bull NY Acad Med 54:865–868, 1978.

37. Gordon LH, and King D: Partial wrist arthrodesis for old ununited fractures of the carpal navicular. Am J Surg 102:460–464, 1961.

38. Green DP: The effect of avascular necrosis on Russe bone grafting for scaphoid nonunion. J Hand Surg 10A:597–605, 1985.

39. Haddad RJ, and Riordan DC: Arthrodesis of the wrist. A surgical technique. J Bone Joint Surg 49A:950–954, 1967.

40. Herbert TJ, and Fisher WE: Management of the fractured scaphoid using a new bone screw. J Bone Joint Surg 66B:114–123, 1984.

41. Hull WJ, House JH, Gustillo RB, et al: The surgical approach and source of bone graft for symptomatic nonunion of the scaphoid. Clin Orthop 115:241–247, 1976.

42. Inglis AE, and Jones EC: Proximal-row carpectomy for diseases of the proximal row. J Bone Joint Surg 59A:460–463, 1977.

43. Jahna H: Die konservative Behandlung des veralteten Kahnbeinbruchs der Hand. Verh Dtsch Ges Orthop 43:156–160, 1955.

44. Johnson RP: The acutely injured wrist and its residuals. Clin Orthop 149:33–44, 1980.

45. Jorgensen EC: Proximal-row carpectomy. An end-result study of twenty-two cases. J Bone Joint Surg 51A:1104–1111, 1969.

46. Kessler I, Heller J, Silberman Z, et al: Some aspects in nonunion of fractures of the carpal scaphoid. J Trauma 3:442–452, 1963.

47. Leslie IJ, and Dickson RA: The fractured carpal scaphoid. Natural history and factors influencing outcome. J Bone Joint Surg 63B:225–230, 1981.

48. Leyshon A, Ireland J, and Trickey EL: The treatment of delayed union and non-union of the carpal scaphoid by screw fixation. J Bone Joint Surg 66B:124–127, 1984.

49. Lichtman DM, and Alexander CE: Decision-mak-

ing in scaphoid nonunion. Orthop Rev 11:55–67, 1982.

50. Liebolt FL: Surgical fusion of the wrist. Surg Gynecol Obstet 66:1008–1023, 1938.

51. Linscheid RL, Dobyns JH, Beabout JW, et al: Traumatic instability of the wrist. J Bone Joint Surg 54A:1612–1632, 1972.

52. London PS: The broken scaphoid bone. The case against pessimism. J Bone Joint Surg 43B:237–243, 1961.

53. Louis DS, Calhoun TP, Garn SM et al: Congenital bipartite scaphoid—fact or fiction? J Bone Joint Surg 58A:1108–1112, 1976.

54. Mack GR, Bosse MJ, Gelberman RH, et al: The natural history of scaphoid non-union. J Bone Joint Surg 66A:504–509, 1984.

55. MacKenzie IG: Arthrodesis of the wrist in reconstructive surgery. J Bone Joint Surg 42B:60–64, 1960.

56. Matti H: Technik und Resultate meiner Pseudarthrosenoperation. Zentralblatt Chir. 63:1442–1453, 1936.

57. Maudsley RH, and Chen SC: Screw fixation in the management of the fractured carpal scaphoid. J Bone Joint Surg 54B:432–441, 1972.

58. Mazet R, and Hohl M: Radial styloidectomy and styloidectomy plus bone graft in the treatment of old ununited carpal scaphoid fractures. Ann Surg 152:296–302, 1960.

59. Mazet R, and Hohl M: Conservative treatment of old fractures of the carpal scaphoid. J Trauma 1:115–127, 1961.

60. Mazet R, and Hohl M: Fractures of the carpal navicular. J Bone Joint Surg 45A:82–111, 1963.

61. Mayfield JK: Mechanism of carpal injuries. Clin Orthop 149:45–54, 1980.

62. Mayfield JK, Johnson RP, and Kilcoyne RK: Carpal dislocations: pathomechanics and progressive perilunar instability. J Hand Surg 5:226–241, 1980.

63. McDonald G, and Petrie D: Un-united fracture of the scaphoid. Clin Orthop 108:110–114, 1975.

64. McLaughlin HL: Fracture of the carpal navicular (scaphoid) bone. Some observations based on treatment by open reduction and internal fixation. J Bone Joint Surg 36A:765–774, 1954.

65. Meyer RD, Sherill J, and Daniel W: Electrical stimulation for treatment of non-union of navicular fractures. 50th Annual Meeting of the American Academy of Orthopaedic Surgeons, Anaheim, 1983.

66. Morgan DAF, and Walters JW: A prospective study of 100 consecutive carpal scaphoid fractures. Aust NZ J Surg 54:233–241, 1984.

67. Mulder JD: Pseudarthrosis of the scaphoid bone. J Bone Joint Surg 45B:621, 1963.

68. Mulder JD: The results of 100 cases of pseudarthrosis in the scaphoid bone treated by the Matti-Russe operation. J Bone Joint Surg 50B:110–115, 1968.

69. Murray G: Bone-graft for non-union of the carpal scaphoid. Br J Surg 22:63–68, 1934.

70. Murray G: Bone graft for non-union of the carpal scaphoid. Surg Gynecol Obstet 60:540–541, 1935.

71. Murray G: End results of bone-grafting for non-union of the carpal navicular. J Bone Joint Surg 28:749–756, 1946.

72. Neviaser RJ: Proximal row carpectomy for post-traumatic disorders of the carpus. J Hand Surg 8:301–305, 1983.

73. Obletz BE, and Halbstein BM: Non-union of fractures of the carpal navicular. J Bone Joint Surg 20:424–428, 1938.

74. Palmer I, and Widen A: Treatment of fractures and pseudarthrosis of the scaphoid with central grafting (autogenous bone-peg). Acta Chir Scand 110:206–212, 1955.

75. Peimer CA, Medige J, Eckert BS, et al: Invasive silicone synovitis of the wrist. 40th Annual Meeting of the American Society for Surgery of the Hand, Las Vegas, 1985.

76. Perey O: A re-examination of cases of pseudarthrosis of the navicular bone operated on according to Bentzon's technique. Acta Orthop Scand 23:26–33, 1952.

77. Ruby LK, Stinson J, and Belsky MR: The natural history of non-union of the scaphoid. A review of fifty-five cases. J Bone Joint Surg 67A:428–432, 1985.

78. Russe O: Fracture of the carpal navicular. Diagnosis, non-operative treatment, and operative treatment. J Bone Joint Surg 42A:759–768, 1960.

79. Sarrafian SK, Melamed JL, and Goshgarian GM: Study of wrist motion in flexion and extension. Clin Orthop 126:153–159, 1977.

80. Schneider LH, and Aulicino P: Nonunion of the carpal scaphoid: the Russe procedure. J Trauma 22:315–319, 1982.

81. Scott JHS: Assessment of ununited fractures of the carpal scaphoid. Proc R Soc Med 49:961–962, 1961.

82. Smith L, and Friedman B: Treatment of ununited fracture of the carpal navicular by styloidectomy of the radius. J Bone Joint Surg 38A:368–375, 1956.

83. Smith RJ, Atkinson RE, and Jupiter JB: Silicone synovitis of the wrist. J Hand Surg 10A:47–60, 1985.

84. Smith-Petersen MN: A new approach to the wrist joint. J Bone Joint Surg 22:122–124, 1940.

85. Soto-Hall R, and Haldeman KO: The conservative and operative treatment of fractures of the carpal scaphoid (navicular). J Bone Joint Surg 23:841–850, 1941.

86. Southcott R, and Rosman MA: Non-union of carpal scaphoid fractures in children. J Bone Joint Surg 59B:20–23, 1977.

87. Speed K: The fate of the fractured navicular. Ann Surg 80:532–535, 1924.

88. Sprague B, and Justis EJ: Nonunion of the carpal navicular. Arch Surg 108:692–697, 1974.

89. Stack JK: End results of excision of the carpal bones. Arch Surg 57:245–252, 1948.

90. Stamm TT: Excision of the proximal row of the carpus. Proc R Soc Med 38:74–75, 1944.

91. Stamm TT: Developments in orthopaedic operative procedures. Guy's Hosp Rep 112:1–14, 1963.

92. Stein I: Gill turnabout radial graft for wrist arthrodesis. Surg Gynecol Obstet 106:231–232, 1958.

93. Swanson AB: Silicone rubber implants for the replacement of the carpal scaphoid and lunate bones. Orthop Clin North Am 1:299–309, 1970.

94. Swanson AB, Wilson KM, Mayhew DE, et al: Long-term bone response around carpal bone implants. 40th Annual Meeting of the American Society for Surgery of the Hand, Las Vegas, 1985.

95. Taleisnik J, and Kelly PJ: The extraosseous and intraosseous blood supply of the scaphoid bone. J Bone Joint Surg 48A:1125–1137, 1966.

96. Taleisnik J: The ligaments· of the wrist. J Hand Surg 1:110–118, 1976.

97. Torngren S, and Sandqvist S: Pseudarthrosis in the scaphoid bone treated by grafting with autogeneous bone-peg. Acta Orthop Scand 45:82–88, 1974.

98. Trojan E: Grafting of ununited fractures of the scaphoid. Proc R Soc Med 67:1078–1080, 1974.

99. Unger HS, and Stryker WC: Nonunion of the carpal navicular: analysis of 42 cases treated by the Russe procedure. South Med J 62:620–622, 1969.

100. Verdan C, and Narakas A: Fractures and pseudarthrosis of the scaphoid. Surg Clin North Am 48:1083–1095, 1968.

101. Watson HK, Goodman ML, and Johnson TR: Limited wrist arthrodesis. Part II: Intercarpal and radiocarpal combinations. J Hand Surg 6:223–233, 1981.

102. Watson HK, and Ballet FL: The SLAC wrist: scapholunate advanced collapse pattern of degenerative arthritis. J Hand Surg 9:358–365, 1984.

103. Zemel NP, Stark HH, Ashworth CR, et al: Treatment of selected patients with an ununited fracture of the proximal part of the scaphoid by excision of the fragment and insertion of a carved silicone-rubber spacer. J Bone Joint Surg 66A:510–517, 1984.

CHAPTER 23

Kienböck's Disease

A. HERBERT ALEXANDER, M.D., F.A.C.S.
and DAVID M. LICHTMAN, M.D., F.A.C.S.

Kienböck's disease (avascular necrosis of the lunate) should be considered in any patient presenting with wrist pain of uncertain origin. Often, the early stages of the disease are clinically and roentgenographically indistinguishable from other causes of wrist pain. The patient is usually young, 20 to 40 years old, and may complain of pain and stiffness in the wrist. The male to female ratio is two to one.[49, 50] The lesion, though not rare, is uncommon, and the average orthopedist can expect to see a case once every year or two. The incidence of bilateral Kienböck's disease is extremely low, and there are few reports of this occurrence.[51, 55]

Clinically, the patient notes tenderness dorsally about the lunate, which is sometimes associated with synovial swelling consistent with localized synovitis. Early on, however, the patient may appear to simply have a wrist sprain. With progression, symptoms of synovitis predominate, and in the late stage arthritis is the predominant pathologic condition.

Invariably, the grip strength is significantly decreased compared with that of the normal hand,[49, 50] and the range of motion of the wrist may be somewhat reduced. The diagnosis is established through radiographs, particularly in the later stages of the disease, when the sclerotic appearance of the lunate is so characteristic. Early in the course of Kienböck's disease, the radiographs may actually be normal. Because of the varying appearance of the radiographs of a patient with Kienböck's disease, at least two classifications have been devised.[49, 50, 72] Figures 23–1 through 23–4 represent a simple classification that is useful for determining the degree of involvement and for choosing appropriate treatment based upon the extent of involvement.

ETIOLOGY

The various names (lunatomalacia, aseptic necrosis, osteochondritis, traumatic osteoporosis, osteitis) used synonymously for Kienböck's disease are an indication that its exact etiology remains in dispute. Peste,[64] in 1843, first described collapse of the carpal lunate. His discovery, before the advent of the roentgenogram, was based on studies of anatomic specimens. He believed the lesion to be a fracture with a traumatic etiology. Kienböck, in 1910, also thought this lesion to be the result of trauma. He believed that repeated sprains, contusions, or subluxations lead to ligamentous and vascular injury, resulting in loss of blood supply to the lunate.[43, 44] Since then, numerous authors

Acute

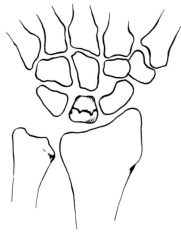

Figure 23–1. Schematic representation of the roentgenographic appearance of Stage I Kienböck's disease. (From Lichtman DM, Alexander AH, Mack GR, et al: J Hand Surg 7:343–347, 1982.)

Density Changes

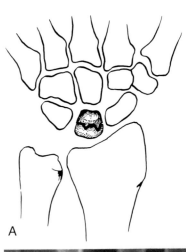

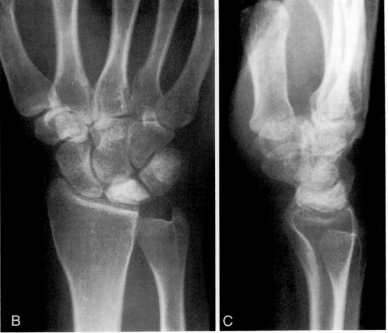

Figure 23–2. *A*, Schematic representation of the roentgenographic appearance of Stage II Kienböck's disease. *B, C*, Anteroposterior and lateral views of a patient with Stage II Kienböck's disease. Note the obvious density change and slight amount of collapse of the lunate on the radial border. The overall shape of the lunate, however, remains intact, and there is no proximal migration of the capitate. This patient also has negative ulnar variance. (From Lichtman DM, Alexander AH, Mack GR, et al: J Hand Surg 7:343–347, 1982.)

Collapse of Lunate

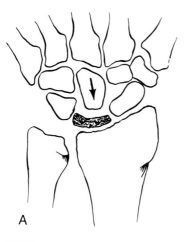

Figure 23–3. *A,* Schematic representation of the roentgenographic appearance of Stage III Kienböck's disease. *B, C,* Anteroposterior and lateral views of a patient with Stage III Kienböck's disease. The lunate is collapsed, the capitate displaced proximally, the scaphoid is rotated, and there is negative ulnar variance. (From Lichtman DM, Alexander AH, Mack GR, et al: J Hand Surg 7:343–347, 1982.)

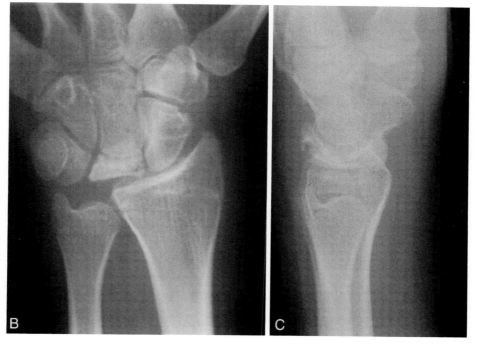

Pan Carpal Arthrosis

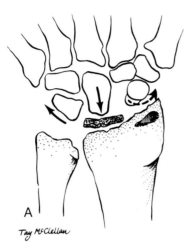

A

Tay McClellan

Figure 23–4. A, Schematic representation of the roentgenographic appearance of Stage IV Kienböck's disease. B, C, Anteroposterior and lateral views of a patient with early Stage IV Kienböck's disease. Note that in addition to severe collapse of the lunate, there is sclerosis and osteophyte formation in the remaining carpus. (From Lichtman DM, Alexander AH, Mack GR, et al: J Hand Surg 7:343–347, 1982.)

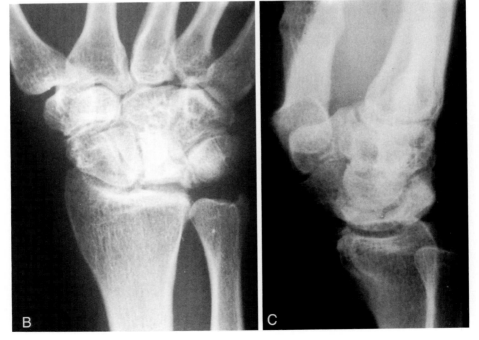

have described the pathologic changes as avascular necrosis.*

In 1928, Húlten[37] noted that a short ulna was present in 78 percent of his patients with Kienböck's disease, whereas only 23 percent of normal patients had a short ulna. He called this condition *ulna minus variant* (Fig. 23–5). Since the condition was first discovered, many other authors have confirmed negative ulnar variance in their patients with Kienböck's disease.† Theoretically, a short ulna, relative to the distal articular surface of the radius, causes increased shear forces on the ulnar side of the wrist and particularly on the lunate. This is thought to be a contributing factor in the development of avascular necrosis.

Gelberman and associates[29] described a method for establishing the degree of ulnar variance (Fig. 23–6). This is done by extending the line from the distal radial articular surface toward the ulna and measuring the distance between this line and the carpal surface of the ulna.

Palmer and coworkers[59] further standardized the method for determining ulnar variance. They found that the position of the distal ulna, in relation to the distal radial

---

*References 1, 2, 5, 7, 27, 28, 49–51, 57, 78.
†References 5, 28, 29, 47, 49, 50, 55, 74, 81.

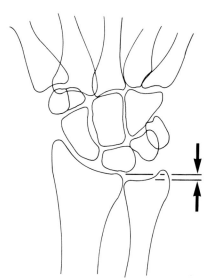

Figure 23–6. Measurement of ulnar variance. Ulnar variance may be determined by extending a line from the articular surface of the radius to the ulna and measuring in millimeters the distance between this line and the carpal surface of the ulna. (After Gelberman RH, Salamon PB, Jurist JM, et al: J Bone Joint Surg 57A:674–676, 1975.)

surface, changes with varying degrees of forearm rotation and that the change in variance was least with the elbow flexed 90°. The standard view recommended is a posteroanterior wrist radiograph obtained with the patient's shoulder abducted 90°, the elbow flexed 90°, and the forearm in neutral rotation. They then utilized a template of concentric circles (similar to the one used in establishing sphericity in Legg-Calvé-Perthes disease).[56] The concentric circle that best approximates the distal radial surface is selected as a reference and compared in millimeters to the carpal surface of the ulna. The importance of accurate measurement of ulnar variance is highlighted by the recent gain in popularity of ulnar lengthening and radial shortening techniques to treat Kienböck's disease.

Acute fracture or trauma as an etiology has been implicated in many series,[5, 41, 48–50, 72] as the majority of patients report a history of injury predating the exacerbation of symptoms. Beckenbaugh and coworkers[5] found lines suggestive of fracture on radiographs of 82 percent of their patients. More and more investigators are documenting the presence of these fractures in Kienböck's disease, particularly with tomographic techniques; however, it remains unclear whether these fractures are the cause or the result of the avascular necrosis.

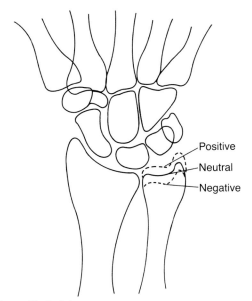

Figure 23–5. Schematic representation of the roentgenographic appearance of ulnar variance. Neutral variance occurs when the carpal surfaces of the radius and ulna are equal. If the ulna is shorter relative to the radius, negative ulnar variance exists; if the ulna is longer than the radius, the relationship is described as positive variance.

Stahl[72] believed that in a lunate with an already tenuous blood supply, traumatic compression fracture leads to avascular necrosis. Lee[48] found three vascular patterns in lunates from cadavers: (1) a single vessel, either volar or dorsal, supplying the entire bone; (2) several vessels at both volar and dorsal surfaces of the lunate without central anastomosis; and (3) several vessels at both volar and dorsal surfaces of the lunate with central anastomosis. Therefore, according to Lee, patients with the former two patterns are at greater risk for developing Kienböck's disease. Injection studies by Panagis and coworkers[60] support this contention, since they found a single palmar nutrient vessel in 20 percent of fresh lunate specimens.

In fresh specimens, Gelberman and associates[28, 30] also studied the extraosseous and intraosseous blood supply of the lunate. They found the extraosseous supply to be extensive, with branches of the radial and anterior interosseous arteries forming a dorsal lunate plexus. Branches of the radial, ulnar, and anterior interosseous arteries and recurrent deep palmar arch arteries form a volar plexus. In most specimens, vascularity reached the lunate through one or two foramina from the volar plexus and through one or two foramina from the dorsal plexus; in only 7 percent of specimens was there only a volar contribution. These lunates with a single volar contribution theoretically would be at greatest risk for a single traumatic event (e.g., fracture or dislocation of the carpus) resulting in avascular necrosis. However, seldom is this history present in a patient with Kienböck's disease. Gelberman and associates found that the intraosseous blood supply consisted of three patterns: Y in 59 percent, I in 31 percent, and X in 10 percent, with the dorsal and volar anastomosis just distal to the center of the lunate (Fig. 23–7).

Evaluation of the terminal vessels in the lunate allowed Gelberman and associates to conclude that the proximal subchrondral bone, adjacent to the radial articular surface, was least vascular. Because of the rich extraosseous blood supply, they discounted the theory held by some that interruption of vessels entering a single pole of the lunate caused avascularity. Based on this work, Gelberman and coworkers suggested that it is intraosseous disruption of vascularity, owing to repeated trauma with compression fracture, that causes Kienböck's disease.

To summarize current thinking on the

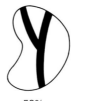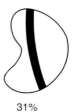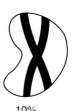

59%   31%   10%

Figure 23–7. Three patterns of the lunate's intraosseous blood supply. (After Gelberman RH, Salamon PB, Jurist JM, et al: J Hand Surg 5:272–278, 1980.)

etiology of Kienböck's disease, trauma or repeated minor trauma due to excessive shear force leads to interruption of the blood supply to the susceptible or "at risk" lunate: Avascular necrosis results. The susceptible lunate is one that has a single nutrient vessel supplying the entire bone or a limited intraosseous blood supply.

DIAGNOSIS

Kienböck's disease is an isolated disorder of the lunate diagnosed from characteristic roentgenographic density changes, often accompanied by fracture lines, fragmentation, and progressive collapse. It should be distinguished from other causes of wrist pain and swelling, particularly in the early stages, when the roentgenograms may be negative. Disorders to be ruled out include rheumatoid arthritis, post-traumatic arthritis, synovial-based inflammatory disease, acute fracture, carpal instability, and ulnar abutment syndromes. The radiographic hallmark of increased density typically seen in Kienböck's disease should be distinguished from transient vascular compromise. White and Omer[82] recently described this radiographic condition seen following fracture-dislocation or dislocation of the carpus. In three of 24 patients sustaining this injury, there was a postinjury transient increase in lunate radiodensity that could have been confused with Kienböck's disease. This radiodensity lasted from five to 32 months. Patients with this finding should be treated expectantly.

In more severe Kienböck's disease, as the lunate collapses, there is proximal migration of the capitate, widening of the proximal carpal row, and, frequently, rotation of the scaphoid, causing it to appear foreshortened on anteroposterior radiographs. This foreshortening has been referred to as the "ring" sign (Fig. 23–8A and B). Tomograms may be helpful to identify linear fractures or local-

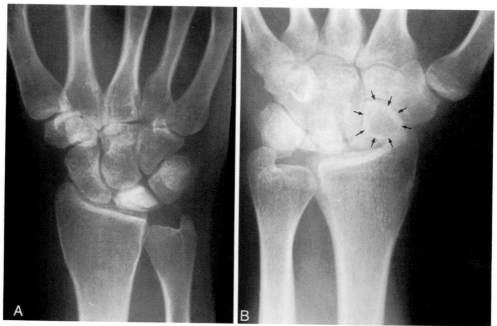

Figure 23–8. *A* is an anteroposterior view of an early stage of Kienböck's disease, demonstrating a normal relationship of the scaphoid to the remaining carpus. *B* is a late stage, in which scaphoid rotation has led to a characteristic appearance referred to as the "ring" sign, as seen on an anteroposterior view.

ized area of sclerosis not readily apparent on plain radiographs. Scintigraphic imaging may be of benefit in patients who have otherwise negative radiographs.[20]

Rarely has Kienböck's disease been reported in association with other conditions. There are case reports of Kienböck's disease in sickle cell disease,[47] carpal coalition,[52] and gout.[14] One article identified streptococcal infection in several cases and attempted to cite this as the causative organism.[65] Rooker and Goodfellow[68] found five cases of Kienböck's disease in a group of 53 adults with cerebral palsy. An abnormally flexed wrist posture was the common feature in all five cases. This suggested to them that this extreme posture compromised the blood supply to the lunate. The authors have seen one case of bilateral Kienböck's disease and one case associated with Madelung's deformity.

Once the diagnosis of Kienböck's disease is established, determination of the degree of involvement should be made in order to assist in guiding one through the maze of treatment options. Plaster immobilization for two to three weeks in uncertain cases will usually bring out the diagnosis by relative disuse osteoporosis of the adjacent carpal bones.

STAGING

Stahl's[72] original classification has been modified by Lichtman and coworkers[49, 50] and consists of four stages of Kienböck's disease.

Stage I. Roentgenograms are normal except for the possibility of either a linear or a compression fracture (Fig. 23–1). Unless a compression fracture is visible, this stage is clinically indistinguishable from a wrist sprain. Scintigraphic and magnetic resonance imaging may be helpful.

Stage II. There are definite density changes apparent in the lunate relative to the other carpal bones; however, the size, shape, and anatomic relationship of the bones are not significantly altered. Fracture lines may be noted. Later in this stage, anteroposterior roentgenograms show loss of height on the radial side of the lunate (Fig. 23–2). The patient exhibits symptoms of recurrent pain, swelling, and tenderness in the wrist.

Stage III. The entire lunate has collapsed in the frontal plane and is elongated in the sagittal plane (Fig. 23–3). The capitate migrates proximally. Scapholunate dissociation, rotation of the scaphoid (the ring sign), and ulnar deviation of the triquetrum may be seen on the anteroposterior roentgeno-

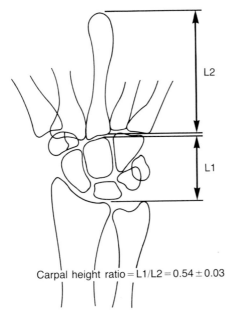

Carpal height ratio = L1/L2 = 0.54 ± 0.03

Figure 23–9. Carpal height ratio is defined as the carpal height (L1) divided by the length of the third metacarpal (L2). In normal individuals, this is 0.54 ± 0.03. (After Youm Y, McMurty RY, Flatt AE, et al: J Bone Joint Surg 60A:423–431, 1978.)

grams. To better assess the degree of collapse in Stage III, it is helpful to establish the *carpal height ratio*:[84] Carpal height is the distance between the base of the third metacarpal and the distal radial articular surface (Fig. 23–9), as determined on a posteroanterior roentgenogram of the wrist; the carpal height ratio is defined as the carpal height divided by the length of the third metacarpal. In normal persons, this ratio is 0.54 ± 0.03. Knowledge of carpal height ratio is becoming more important, since the factors determining results of treatment in Stage III appear to be tied to the degree of collapse. We now divide Stage III into Stage IIIA (lunate collapse without fixed scaphoid rotation) and Stage IIIB (lunate collapse with fixed scaphoid rotation and other secondary derangements). Clinically, patients in these stages have the same symptoms as those in Stage II but with an increased level of wrist stiffness.

Stage IV. All findings characteristic of Stage III are present as well as generalized degenerative changes in the carpus (Fig. 23–4).

TREATMENT

Kienböck's disease may be treated by immobilization, revascularization, ulnar lengthening or radial shortening, simple excision, silicone replacement arthroplasty (SRA), soft tissue replacement arthroplasty, limited intercarpal fusion, or salvage procedures. Table 23–1 lists the various treatment modalities for Kienböck's disease, along with the stage for which the procedure is recommended by the authors.

Immobilization. Prolonged immobilization of the wrist has been tried in all stages of Kienböck's disease. Stahl[72] advocated immobilization, yet in some series it has been shown to lead to continued collapse of the lunate or to otherwise unsatisfactory results, owing to the need for prolonged treatment.[50, 69, 80] Lichtman and colleagues[50] reported on 22 unstaged patients treated with cast or splint immobilization, of which 17 had progressive collapse while immobilized and 19 had unsatisfactory results. For Stage I, however, immobilization may be indicated in hopes that the vascular insult be kept to a minimum and to give the lunate a chance to heal. Immobilization by external fixator may be a more efficient method to unload the lunate and prevent collapse. Because diagnosis in this stage often is difficult, a trial period of immobilization may result in the characteristic radiographic changes that establish the diagnosis.

Revascularization. In Stage II Kienböck's disease, before there has been collapse of the lunate, it is theoretically possible for the lunate to regain blood supply without significant alteration of wrist anatomy. Braun[8, 9] has described a method by which a small piece of volar radial bone, still attached to the pronator quadratus muscle, is grafted to the avascular lunate (Fig. 23–10). This procedure is done through a volar approach with division of the palmar and transverse carpal ligaments, in order to mobilize the median nerve. After the volar wrist is entered, the lunate is burred with a high-speed drill in preparation for receiving a 1 to 1.5 cm piece of radial bone, still attached to the

Table 23–1. **TREATMENT MODALITIES RECOMMENDED FOR STAGES OF KIENBÖCK'S DISEASE**

Treatment	Stage
Immobilization	I
Revascularization	II, IIIA
Ulnar lengthening or radial shortening	II, IIIA
Silicone replacement arthroplasty (SRA)	IIIA
Excision + autogenous tendon graft	IIIA
Capitohamate fusion ± SRA	IIIA, B
Triscaphe fusion ± SRA	IIIB
Limited intercarpal fusion	IIIB, IV
Salvage (proximal row carpectomy, wrist arthrodesis)	IV

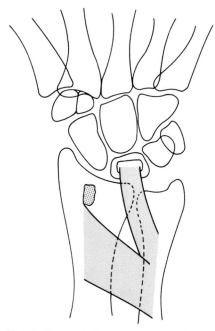

Figure 23–10. Revascularization procedure for pronator quadratus muscle pedicle.

pronator quadratus muscle. This is secured with pull-out wires and the fixation augmented with transarticular Kirshner wires. Braun[10] has found this procedure to be successful in seven to eight patients with the longest follow-up period (seven years). He recommends that the procedure be done only in those cases without significant collapse. Chacha[16] has also reported on this technique in three patients.

A similar revascularization procedure uses the pisiform. Pisiform transfer on its vascular pedicle was reported by Erbs and Böhm[24] in 32 patients. They found uniformly good results at five years' follow-up. Presumably, most of these patients were in Stage II of the disease. Of 14 with advanced Kienböck's disease, however, 50 percent became symptom-free or had pain only under stressful conditions. Eckardt[21] reported the same technique with good results in two patients with four-year follow-up for Stage I.

Direct transplantation of a vascular bundle into the avascular lunate was described by Hori and coworkers.[36] They had successful results in eight out of nine patients.

It must be remembered, however, that none of the revascularization procedures is likely to work in the face of severe collapse (Stage III), because even if there is success in re-establishing blood supply, lunate height and normal carpal kinematics will not be restored.

Ulnar Lengthening or Radial Shortening. Based on the theory that ulnar minus variance is a significant causative factor in Kienböck's disease, some have advocated equalization of the distal articular surfaces either by ulnar lengthening[2, 4, 34, 62, 63, 74] or by radial shortening.* Good results have been reported in both of these procedures; however, they cannot restore an already collapsed lunate; therefore, these procedures remain questionable in the treatment of advanced Stage III disease.

Both radial shortening and ulnar lengthening require osteotomy. A segment of bone is removed when radial shortening is done and a segment of bone graft inserted when ulnar lengthening is done. After either procedure, fixation is usually accomplished with a compression plate. It is generally recommended that the ulnar variance be changed to 1 or 2 mm positive variance by placing an appropriate-sized interpositional graft when performing ulnar lengthening. Sundberg and Linscheid[74] found this to be successful in all but one of 19 patients followed for an average of 8.2 months. They reported no nonunions. Ulnar lengthening per se "burns no bridges," and therefore further treatment in the event of failure is not precluded.

Radial shortening may be preferable to some because it does not require a second surgical incision to harvest bone graft. As with ulnar lengthening, options for further treatment are available. Almquist and Burns[1] obtained good results in 11 out of 12 patients (minimum follow-up five years) and noted that the literature reported good results in an additional 58 of 67 patients (87 percent) treated with radial shortening.

Excision of the Lunate. Lunate excision was one of the first surgical procedures devised for the treatment of Kienböck's disease. The rationale of this procedure is the removal of sequestered bone that is provoking painful synovitis. Some have reported good results from simple excision,[15, 19, 32, 53] whereas others criticize the operation,[6, 54, 72] predicting late proximal migration of the capitate. There is at least one report of the same results from either excision or immobilization.[78] Nahigian and associates[57] combined

*References 1, 12, 23, 34, 44–46, 51, 69, 80.

simple excision with dorsal capsular flap arthroplasty to prevent migration of the capitate and reported good results in four patients. Schmitt and coworkers[71] reported a similar technique of capsuloplasty using "epitendinous" tissue from the flexor tendons to fill the gap. They reported 80 percent satisfactory results in 42 cases. Another similar technique is excisional arthroplasty and replacement with a rolled tendon (palmaris longus) graft. This is performed much like the procedure of metacarpotrapezial joint arthroplasty described by Froimson.[26] Ishiguro[39] also reported on the use of autogenous tendon graft (generally the palmaris longus, the plantaris, or a portion of flexor carpi radialis) placed in the bed of the excised lunate. Twenty-four of 26 patients with an average follow-up of 2.5 years were satisfied with their result. Using the criteria of Lichtman and colleagues,[50] he further noted that six out of 10 patients with Stage III disease and 11 out of 16 patients with Stage IV disease had satisfactory results. More recently, Kato and associates[42] treated patients with either silicone replacement arthroplasty or a coiled palmaris longus tendon and concluded that the latter is preferable once carpal collapse has occurred. Because in Stages I and II of Kienböck's disease there still exists a chance for lunate revascularization, soft tissue (palmaris longus) replacement arthroplasty is best reserved for those patients with Stage III disease.

Silicone Replacement Arthroplasty (SRA). SRA is simply another way to prevent carpal migration following lunate excision. There are many advocates of this procedure.* After excision, the lunate may be replaced by a hand-carved Silastic wafer[35, 73] or, more commonly, by a Swanson design carpal lunate (Fig. 23–11) manufactured from high-performance silicone elastomer (Dow-Corning, Midland, Michigan). SRA is not indicated in Stage IV disease, once pancarpal arthrosis is present. In Stages II and III, however, SRA has been shown to be successful in many series, although, prior to the development of the most recently designed implant, dislocation of the prosthesis made SRA contraindicated in Stage III disease.[50] Subsequently, the deeper concavity for capitate articulation and the more anatomic design of the newer implant have reduced the risk of its dislocation.

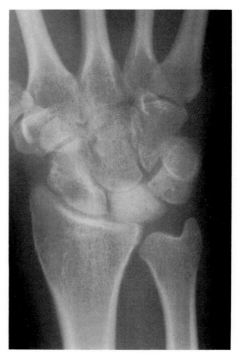

Figure 23–11. Silicone replacement arthroplasty (SRA); postoperative roentgenogram of the same patient shown in Figure 23–3B.

The advantages of SRA include rapid rehabilitation and return to work. It is also technically an easy operation to perform, and it does not require a second operation. However, recent reports of silicone synovitis are disturbing. Atkinson and associates[3] described nine patients with this entity, who presented following carpal or radiocarpal silicone replacement arthroplasty. Four of the nine had lunate replacements. In all cases in which the synovium was studied, silicone debris was noted, surrounded by multinuclear foreign body giant cell reaction. Similarly, Peimer and colleagues[61] reported four lunate and six scaphoid SRAs that were followed by silicone synovitis. They documented progressive bone destruction and cyst formation in patients followed sequentially. Carter and Benton[13] followed 33 of 49 patients with carpal Silastic implants (10 lunates), of which 17 (51 percent) had cyst formation adjacent to the implant. The largest series, by Swanson and coworkers,[77] had 260 Silastic carpal implants (followed for 12 to 207 months), of which 14 of 42 patients with lunate replacements (33 percent) developed minimal to moderate cystic changes. Most of the changes were noted to occur within the first three years

---

*References 5, 22, 35, 49–51, 66, 67, 73, 75, 76.

following surgery, and only six of the 260 required additional surgery.

The preceding reports have led the manufacturer to issue a warning that "wear particles from silicone elastomer implants... may participate in, or exacerbate synovitis or bone cyst complications in contiguous bone."[25]

It is our impression that most of the cases of silicone synovitis are seen in young, active patients; in patients with preoperative cysts or degenerative changes, or both; in patients who had temporary Kirschner wire or suture fixation of the implant or in those who had post-operative implant instability, or both. Therefore, SRA should not be done in the young patient with extreme functional demands, unless it is combined with a procedure (e.g., radial shortening, ulnar lengthening, or limited carpal arthrodesis) that reduces the bearing and shear stress and concomitant microfragmentation of the implant surface. Furthermore, the surgeon must avoid Kirschner wire or suture fixation and must achieve intraoperative stability of the lunate implant (see Chapter 28).

Lunate SRA is performed through a small transverse incision directly over the lunate. A distally based rectangular flap of wrist capsule is developed, and the lunate is removed piecemeal with a small rongeur, curette, or osteotome. One must be certain to maintain a thin cortical shell of palmar lunate along with its soft tissue attachment, in order to avoid volar dislocation into the carpal canal. A small hole is then made in the triquetrum to receive the stem of the prosthesis. A set of trial prostheses is used to aid in the selection of the appropriate-sized implant. Too large an implant will tend to be squeezed out, whereas too small an implant may subluxate radially, allowing the stem to disengage from the triquestrum. Full range of wrist motion should be possible without subluxation of the implant. The dorsal capsular flap may be manually held closed to prevent dorsal subluxation while stability is being tested. Careful suturing of the dorsal capsular flap is then done to prevent dorsal subluxation. Temporary Kirschner wire or suture fixation of the implant is no longer recommended, as previously mentioned, nor is it usually necessary. If intraoperative stability cannot be achieved, then a tendon soft tissue interposition arthroplasty should be done instead. Postoperatively, patients are immobilized for six weeks in a plaster cast.

Limited Intercarpal Fusion. Graner and coworkers[33] described arthrodesis of the lunate to adjacent carpal bones for advanced Kienböck's disease—presumably Stage III or Stage IV. They considered it as appropriate treatment only if conventional methods failed to provide relief of symptoms. Its most important advantage is that radiocarpal motion is maintained, unlike results after complete wrist arthrodesis. In this series, 18 patients with an average of 22 months' follow-up underwent limited intercarpal arthrodesis; all had satisfactory results. Patients with severe fragmentation of the lunate undergo resection of the necrotic bone, osteotomy of the capitate in its midportion, and proximal displacement of the proximal capitate fragment (Fig. 23–12), which is secured to the scaphoid and the triquetrum with bone pegs. Essentially, the space vacated by excision of the lunate is filled by the proximal half of the capitate, and the space left by osteotomy of the capitate is filled by autogenous bone graft. The procedure is then completed by arthrodesing contiguous surfaces of the hamate, capitate, scaphoid, and triquetrum by first denuding articular surfaces and securing the bones with small cortical bone pegs. When the lunate remains suitably intact, osteotomy of the capitate is omitted, as is lunate excision, and the contiguous surfaces of the lunate, scaphoid, triquetum, hamate, and capitate are arthrodesed (Fig. 23–13).

Capitohamate Fusion. Chuinard and Zeman[17] advocated capitohamate fusion as a method of preventing proximal capitate migration in the face of a collapsed lunate. Depending on the degree of collapse of the lunate in patients in their series, SRA may or may not be performed in conjunction with capitohamate fusion. Capitohamate fusion alone is not a method currently recommended by the authors because the hamate is already bound to the capitate by strong ligaments; furthermore, collapse of the capitate is accompanied by proximal migration of the entire distal carpal row (including the hamate) and widening of the proximal carpal row. Thus, it seems unlikely that capitohamate fusion alone can prevent proximal migration of the distal carpal row.

Triscaphe Fusion. Watson and colleagues[81] described triscaphe arthrodesis with and without SRA. Patients underwent fusion of the scaphoid, trapezium, and trapezoid, and half of them underwent concomitant SRA. In their article, Watson and colleagues

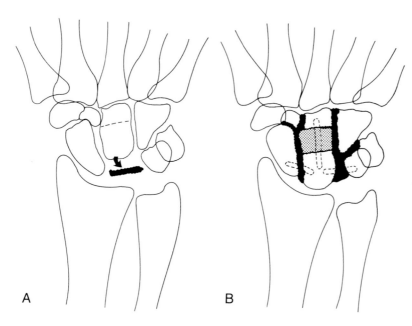

Figure 23–12. *A, B,* Limited intercarpal fusion in the face of severe collapse and fragmentation of the lunate. Excision of the fragmented lunate is performed as well as an osteotomy of the capitate in its midportion. The proximal pole of the capitate is displaced proximally, the gap in the capitate is filled with bone graft, and arthrodesis is carried out on the contiguous surfaces of the capitate, scaphoid, triquetrum, and hamate. (After Graner O, Lopes EI, Carvalho BC, et al: J Bone Joint Surg 48:767–774, 1966.)

graphically demonstrate roentgenograms of the clenched fist of a patient with SRA, showing a 22 percent reduction (compression of the implant) in capitoradial space, when compared with views of the wrist in the relaxed position. They suggest that triscaphe arthrodesis is capable of supporting the remaining carpus in the case of either a collapsed lunate or when performing SRA. Ten of 16 patients (average follow-up, 20 months) had complete relief of symptoms, with six reporting aching in the affected wrist only after activity.

Salvage Procedures. For severe Kienböck's disease (Stage IV), good results have been reported from proximal row carpectomy[18, 38, 40] and wrist arthrodesis.[49, 50, 78] As noted above, limited intercarpal arthrodesis in the method of Graner[33] is another option. Denervation of the wrist joint has been described by several authors to be successful in relieving pain without impairing function or mobility.[11, 31, 70, 83]

PITFALLS AND COMPLICATIONS

Because of the varied treatments advocated for Kienböck's disease, it is apparent that no single treatment stands out as the best. Choice of treatment must be predicated on the experience of the surgeon, on the desires, activity level, and goals of the patient, and on the stage of the disease. Finally, consideration of the risks involved with each treatment, including pitfalls and complications,

may help one to select the optimal treatment for an individual patient.

SRA has consistently yielded good results in both Stage II and III disease, but growing concern over silicone synovitis and progressive cystic degeneration in contiguous bones makes this treatment inadvisable in the young patient or in the patient who will have great functional demands. The other significant risk with SRA is the complication of implant dislocation. This is best avoided by proper selection of implant size, by preservation of the lunate volar shell of bone along with its soft tissue attachments, and by careful suture of the dorsal capsule. Results of the 20- and 30-year follow-up studies of SRA are yet to be determined, as is the fate of the silicone implants over long periods of time in relatively young patients. In some of our patients, we have noted a slight amount of scapholunate dissociation accompanied by mild scaphoid rotation, detectable on postoperative radiographs. To date, this seems not to have affected results of SRA, but these patients, too, will have to be followed to determine if the rotation progresses or becomes symptomatic.

The pronator muscle pedicle flap procedure is tedious and requires fastidious attention to detail. It is important to release the pronator fascia sufficiently, in order to ensure adequate length of the muscle and to prevent its vascular compromise. Dislodgement of the graft has also been reported and, if pull-out wires are used, it is possible to

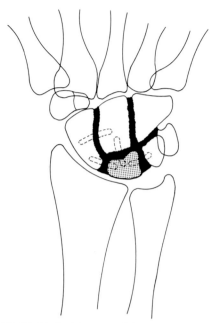

Figure 23–13. Limited intercarpal fusion in the face of a relatively intact lunate. Arthrodesis of the contiguous surfaces of the lunate, scaphoid, capitate, hamate, and triquetrum is performed. When the lunate is intact, capitate osteotomy and excision of the lunate are omitted. (After Graner O, Lopes EI, Carvalho BC, et al: J Bone Joint Surg 48:767–774, 1966.)

is lengthened, the anatomy at the distal radioulnar joint is affected and may be a source of postoperative discomfort. Care must be taken not to overlengthen the ulna. For the same reason, ulnar deviation may also be restricted by this procedure.

Following limited intercarpal arthrodesis, there may be moderate to marked limitation of the range of motion of the wrist. Loss of intercarpal motion may also lead to arthrosis of the radiocarpal joint.

In triscaphe arthrodesis, overcorrection of the scaphoid rotation can result in decreased range of motion and incongruity at the scaphoradial joint; furthermore, if it is performed alone, SRA may be required as a second procedure. Overall, Watson and coworkers reported two out of eight patients requiring delayed SRA after triscaphe arthrodesis. Also, the long-term results of triscaphe arthrodesis must be evaluated, especially since wrist kinematics are significantly altered.

In summary, Kienböck's disease is an isolated disorder of the lunate, resulting from vascular compromise to the bone. The symptoms include wrist pain, limited range of motion, and decreased grip strength. The diagnosis is made from characteristic changes seen in the lunate on radiographs of the wrist. The severity of the disease can be categorized by staging the degree of involvement. This is helpful in guiding the practitioner through the maze of treatment options. The treatment of Kienböck's disease begins with conservative measures that include immobilization and analgesics or anti-inflammatory medication or both. If symptoms are not relieved, then, based on the degree of involvement, several surgical options exist that will provide a successful result. These include autogenous tendon replacement arthroplasty, revascularization, radial shortening, ulnar lengthening, limited intercarpal arthrodesis, and silicone replacement arthroplasty. Salvage procedures for Kienböck's disease include wrist denervation, wrist arthrodesis, and proximal row carpectomy.

Currently, we prefer immobilization for treatment of Stage I Kienböck's disease. For Stage II, a revascularization procedure may be attempted or ulnar lengthening/radial shortening may be done, particularly if there is significant negative ulnar variance. Ulnar lengthening/radial shortening is also successful in early Stage III disease. In later

entrap the extensor tendons. This procedure, even if successful in re-establishing blood supply of the lunate, cannot be expected to restore lunate height and normal kinematics and therefore is not recommended for advanced Stage III disease.

Radial shortening and ulnar lengthening are relatively simple procedures and have yielded consistently good results in Stage II and early Stage III disease. There are a few drawbacks, though. With radial shortening, nonunion of the radius is possible. Furthermore, a second operation may be required for plate removal. This operation as well as ulnar lengthening should not be done in the presence of significant collapse of the lunate, as these procedures are unlikely to restore height and normal carpal kinematics. Their application in patients with neutral and positive ulnar variance is questionable, though Grassi and associates[34] noted good results, even in these patients.

Ulnar lengthening, like radial shortening, may result in nonunion of the ulna or delayed incorporation of the bone graft, requiring prolonged immobilization. In this procedure, too, a second operation may be required for plate removal. Because the ulna

Stage III, replacement arthroplasty and triscaphe intercarpal arthrodesis are our treatments of choice; for Stage IV, one of the salvage procedures is indicated.

References

1. Almquist EE, and Burns JF: Radial shortening for the treatment of Kienböck's disease—a 5- to 10-year follow-up. J Hand Surg 7:348–352, 1982.

2. Armistead RB, Linscheid RL, Dobyns JH, et al: Ulnar lengthening in the treatment of Kienböck's disease. J Bone Joint Surg 64A:170–178, 1982.

3. Atkinson RE, Smith RJ, and Jupiter JB: Silicone synovitis of the wrist. Presented at the 40th Annual Meeting of the American Society for Surgery of the Hand, January, 1985.

4. Axelsson R: Niveauoperationen bei mondbeinnekrose. Handchirurgie 5:187–196, 1973.

5. Beckenbaugh RD, Shives TC, Dobyns JH, et al: Kienböck's disease: the natural history of Kienböck's disease and consideration of lunate fractures. Clin Orthop 149:98–106, 1980.

6. Blaine ES: Lunate osteomalacia. JAMA 96:492, 1931.

7. Bolhofner B, and Belsole RJ: Kienböck's disease: current concepts in diagnosis and management. Contemp Orthop 3:713–720, 1981.

8. Braun R: The pronator pedicle bone grafting in the forearm and proximal carpal row. Presented at the 38th Annual Meeting of the American Society for Surgery of the Hand, March, 1983.

9. Braun RM: Viable pedicle bone grafts. What's New and What's True Orthopaedic Symposium (abst), UC Davis, March, 1985, pp 28–29.

10. Braun RM: Personal communication, July, 1985.

11. Buck-Gramcko D: Denervation of the wrist joint. J Hand Surg 2:54–61, 1977.

12. Calandriello B, and Palandri C: Die behandlung der lunatum malazie durch speichenverkurzung. Zh Orthop 101:531–534, 1966.

13. Carter PR, and Benton LJ: Late osseous complications of carpal Silastic implants. Presented at the 40th Annual Meeting of the American Society for Surgery of the Hand, January, 1985.

14. Castagnoli M, Giacomello A, Argentina RS, et al.: Kienböck's disease in gout. Arthritis Rheum 24:974–975, 1981.

15. Cave EF: Kienböck's disease of the lunate. J Bone Joint Surg 21:858–866, 1939.

16. Chacha PB: Vascularized pedicular bone grafts. Int Orthop 8:117–138, 1984.

17. Chuinard RG, and Zeman SC: Kienböck's disease: an analysis and rationale for treatment by capitate-hamate fusion. Orthop Trans 4:18, 1980.

18. Crabbe WA: Excision of the proximal row of the carpus. J Bone Joint Surg 46B:708–711, 1964.

19. Dornan A: The results of treatment in Kienböck's disease. J Bone Joint Surg 31B:518–520, 1949.

20. Duong RB, Nishiyama H, Mantil JC, et al: Kienböck's disease: scintigraphic demonstration in correlation with clinical, radiographic, and pathologic findings. Clin Nucl Med 7:418–420, 1982.

21. Eckardt K: Spätergebnisse nach Pissiforme-Verpflanzung bei Lunatum-Malazie. Handchir Mikrochir Plast Chir 16:90–92, 1984.

22. Eiken O, and Necking LE: Lunate implant arthroplasty, evaluation of 19 patients. Scand J Plast Reconstr Surg 18:247–252, 1984.

23. Eiken O, and Niechajev I: Radius shortening in malacia of the lunate. Scand J Plast Reconstr Surg 14:191–196, 1980.

24. Erbs G, and Böhm E: Langzeitergebnisse der Os Pisiforme-verlagerung bei Mondbeinnekrose. Handchir Mikrochir Plast Chir 16:85–89, 1984.

25. Frisch EE: Possible complications—carpal bone implants. Dow Corning Wright (letter), December 28, 1984.

26. Froimson AI: Tendon arthroplasty of the trapezio-metacarpal joint. Clin Orthop 70:191–199, 1970.

27. Fu FH, and Imbriglia JF: An anatomical study of the lunate bone in Kienböck's disease. Orthopedics 8:483–487, 1985.

28. Gelberman RH, Bauman TD, Menon J, et al: The vascularity of the lunate bone and Kienböck's disease. J Hand Surg 5:272–278, 1980.

29. Gelberman RH, Salamon PB, Jurist JM, et al: Ulnar variance in Kienböck's disease. J Bone Joint Surg 57A:674–676, 1975.

30. Gelberman RH, and Szabo RM: Kienböck's disease. Orthop Clin North Am 15:355–367, 1984.

31. Geldmacher J, Legal HR, and Brug E: Results of denervation of the wrist and wrist joint by Wilhelm method. Hand 4:57, 1972.

32. Gillespie HS: Excision of the lunate bone in Kienböck's disease. J Bone Joint Surg 43B:245–249, 1961.

33. Graner O, Lopes EI, Carvalho BC, et al: Arthrodesis of the carpal bones in the treatment of Kienböck's disease, painful ununited fractures of the navicular and lunate bones with avascular necrosis, and old fracture-dislocations of carpal bones. J Bone Joint Surg 48:767–774, 1966.

34. Grassi G, Santoro D, Coli G, et al: The surgical treatment of Kienböck's disease. Ital J Orthop Traumatol 4:149–154, 1978.

35. Hedeboe J: Individually fashioned prostheses in the treatment of Kienböck's disease. Scand J Plast Reconstr Surg 16:87–89, 1982.

36. Hori Y, Tamai S, Okuda H, et al: Blood vessel transplantation to bone. J Hand Surg 4:23–33, 1979.

37. Húlten O: Uber anatomische variationen der handgelenkknochen. Acta Radiol Scand 9:155, 1928.

38. Inglis AE, and Jones EC: Proximal-row carpectomy for diseases of the proximal row. J Bone Joint Surg 59A:460–463, 1977.

39. Ishiguro T: Experimental and clinical studies of Kienböck's disease—excision of the lunate followed by packing of the free tendon. J Jpn Orthop Assoc 58:509–522, 1984.

40. Jorgensen EC: Proximal-row carpectomy: an end result study of 22 cases. J Bone Joint Surg 51A:1104–1111, 1969.

41. Kashiwagi D, Fukiwara A, Inoue T, et al: An experimental and clinical study of lunatomalacia. Orthop Trans 1:7, 1977.

42. Kato H, Usui M, and Minami A: The long-term results of Kienböck's disease treated by excisional arthroplasty using a silicone implant and a coiled palmaris longus tendon. Presented at the 40th Annual Meeting of the American Society for Surgery of the Hand, January, 1985.

43. Kienböck R: Concerning traumatic malacia of the lunate and its consequences: degeneration and compression fractures. Clin Orthop 149:4–8, 1980.

44. Kienböck R: Uber traumatische Malazie des

Mondbeins und ihre Folgezustande: Entartungsformen und Kompressionsfrakturen. Fortschritte auf dem Gebiete der Roentgenstrahlen 16:78–103, 1910.

45. Kinnard P, Tricoire JL, and Basora J: Radial shortening for Kienböck's disease. Can J Surg 3:261–262, 1983.

46. Kleven H: The treatment of lunatomalacia. Tidsskr Nor Laegeforen 91:1944–1946, 1971.

47. Lanzer W, Szabo R, and Gelberman R: Avascular necrosis of the lunate and sickle cell anemia. Clin Orthop 187:168–171, 1984.

48. Lee M: The intraosseous arterial pattern of the carpal lunate bone and its relation to avascular necrosis. Acta Orthop Scand 33:43–55, 1963.

49. Lichtman DM, Alexander AH, Mack GR, et al: Kienböck's disease—update on silicone replacement arthroplasty. J Hand Surg 7:343–347, 1982.

50. Lichtman DM, Mack GR, MacDonald RI, et al: Kienböck's disease: the role of silicone replacement arthroplasty. J Bone Joint Surg 59A:899–908, 1977.

51. Lin E, Engel J, and Marganitt B: Surgery in Kienböck's disease. Orthop Rev 12:51–57, 1983.

52. Macnicol MF: Kienböck's disease in association with carpal coalition. Hand 14:185–187, 1982.

53. Marek RM: Avascular necrosis of the carpal lunate. Clin Orthop 10:96–107, 1957.

54. McMurtry RY, Youm Y, Flatt AE, et al: Kinematics of the wrist. II. Clinical applications. J Bone Joint Surg 60A:955–961, 1978.

55. Morgan RF, and McCue FC III: Bilateral Kienböck's disease. J Hand Surg 8:928–932, 1983.

56. Mose K: Methods of measuring in Legg-Calvé-Perthes disease with special regard to prognosis. Clin Orthop 150:103–109, 1980.

57. Nahigian SH, Li CS, Richey DG, et al: The dorsal flap arthroplasty in the treatment of Kienböck's disease. J Bone Joint Surg 52A:245–251, 1970.

58. Ovesen J: Shortening of the radius in the treatment of lunatomalacia. J Bone Joint Surg 63B:231–235, 1981.

59. Palmer AK, Glisson RR, and Werner FW: Ulnar variance determination. J Hand Surg 7:376–379, 1982.

60. Panagis JS, Gelberman RH, Taleisnik J, et al: The arterial anatomy of the human carpus. Part II: the intraosseous vascularity. J Hand Surg 8:375–382, 1983.

61. Peimer CA, Medige J, Ecker BS, et al. Invasive silicone synovitis of the wrist. Presented at the 40th Annual Meeting of the American Society for Surgery of the Hand, January, 1985.

62. Persson M: Causal treatment of lunatomalacia. Further experiences of operative ulna lengthening. Acta Chir Scand 100:531–544, 1950.

63. Persson M: Pathogenese und Behandlung der Kienböckschen Lunatummalazie; der Frakturtheorie im Lichte der Erfolge operativer Radiusverkürzung (Hultén) und einer neuen Operationsmethode—Ulnaverlängerung. Acta Chir Scand (Suppl 98) 92:1–58, 1945.

64. Peste: Discussion. Paris, Bull Soc Anat, 18:169–170, 1843.

65. Phemister DB, Day L: Streptococcal infections of the epiphyses and short bones, their relation to Kohler's disease of the tarsal navicular, Legg-Perthes disease and Kienböck's disease of the os lunatum. JAMA 95:995–1002, 1930.

66. Ramakrishna B, D'Netto DC, Sethu AU: Long-term results of silicone rubber implants for Kienböck's disease. J Bone Joint Surg 64B:361–363, 1982.

67. Roca J, Beltran JE, Fairen MF, et al: Treatment of Kienböck's disease using a silicone rubber implant. J Bone Joint Surg 58A:373–376, 1976.

68. Rooker GD, and Goodfellow JW: Kienböck's disease in cerebral palsy. J Bone Joint Surg 59B:363–365, 1977.

69. Rosemeyer B, Artmann M, and Viernstein K: Lunatummlacie nachuntersuchungsergebnisse und therapeutische erwagungne. Arch Orthop Unfallichir 85:119–127, 1976.

70. Rostlund T, Somnier F, and Axelsson R: Denervation of the wrist joint—an alternative in conditions of chronic pain. Orthop Scand 51:609–616, 1980.

71. Schmitt E, Hassinger M, and Mittelmeier: Die Lunatummalazie und ihre behandlung mit lunatumexstirpation. Zh Orthop 122:643–650, 1984.

72. Stahl F: On lunatomalacia (Kienböck's disease), a clinical and roentgenological study, especially on its pathogenesis and the late results of immobilization treatment. Acta Chir Scand [Suppl] 126:1–133, 1947.

73. Stark HH, Zemel NP, and Ashworth CR: Use of a hand-carved silicone-rubber spacer for advanced Kienböck's disease. J Bone Joint Surg 63A:1359–1370, 1981.

74. Sundberg SB, and Linscheid RL: Kienböcks' disease—results of treatment with ulnar lengthening. Clin Orthop 187:43–51, 1984.

75. Swanson AB: Flexible Implant Resection Arthroplasty in the Hand and Extremities. St Louis, CV Mosby Co, 1973.

76. Swanson AB: Silicone rubber implants for the replacement of the carpal scaphoid and lunate bones. Orthop Clin North Am 1:299–309, 1970.

77. Swanson AB, Wilson KM, Mayhew DE, et al: Long-term bone response around carpal bone implants. Presented at the 40th Annual Meeting of the American Society for Surgery of the Hand, January, 1985.

78. Tajima T: An investigation of the treatment of Kienböck's disease. J Bone Joint Surg 48A:1649–1655, 1966.

79. Taleisnik J: Fractures of the carpal bones. In Green DP (ed): Operative Hand Surgery. New York, Churchill Livingstone Inc, 1982, pp 669–702.

80. Viernstein K, and Weigert M: Die radiusverkurzungsosteotomie bei der lunatummalzie. Munch Med Wochenschr 109:1992, 1967.

81. Watson HK, Ryu J, and DiBella A: An approach to Kienböck's disease: triscaphe arthrodesis. J Hand Surg 10A:179–187, 1985.

82. White RE, and Omer GE: Transient vascular compromise of the lunate after fracture-dislocation or dislocation of the carpus. J Hand Surg 9A:181–184, 1984.

83. Wilhelm A: Die gelenkdenervation und ihre anatomischen grundlagen. Ein neues behandlungsprinzip in der handchirurgie. Hefte Unfallheilkd 86:1–109, 1966.

84. Youm Y, McMurtry RY, Flatt AE, et al: Kinematics of the wrist, Part I—an experimental study of radial-ulnar deviation and flexion-extension. J Bone Joint Surg 60A:423–431, 1978.

CHAPTER 24

Inflammatory and Rheumatoid Arthritis

DONALD C. FERLIC, M. D.

DIFFERENTIAL DIAGNOSIS

There are over 100 types of arthritic and rheumatic disorders, but rheumatoid arthritis is second only to degenerative joint disease in frequency of occurrence. Knowledge of patterns of joint involvement is helpful in the diagnosis of arthritis. Clinically, the disease is polyarticular and symmetric. Typically, the small joints of the hands and feet swell initially, but wrist disease is almost invariably noted.[62] Active synovitis can be observed on the dorsum of the wrist as a boggy, soft tissue swelling. Median nerve compression may develop, owing to volar tenosynovitis. Later, in the diseased wrist, immobility results from fibrous or bone ankylosis. Commonly, forearm rotation is painful or limited, owing to distal radioulnar joint involvement.

A patient with systemic lupus erythematosus (SLE) can present with wrist and hand deformities that appear similar to those caused by rheumatoid arthritis. Joint involvement is the most common manifestation of SLE.[63] Joint pain or swelling may precede the onset of this multisystem disease by many years. Arthritis, evidenced objectively by painful motion, tenderness, or effusion, is present in 75 percent of SLE patients at the time of diagnosis. The joints most commonly involved are the proximal interphalangeal joints, the knees, the wrists, and the metacarpophalangeal joints. Joint involvement is remarkably symmetric.[62] Generally, the deformities are passively correctible, but over time they can also become fixed.[39] The articular cartilage is usually well preserved until late in the disease, with joint spaces roentgenographically normal. Because there can be severe deformities despite normal results of x-ray studies, the problems

in planning reconstructive surgery may be puzzling. Oftentimes, soft tissue reconstruction of the wrist affected by painful carpal collapse and volar subluxation is inadequate. In these cases, wrist arthroplasty should be considered.[24]

Progressive systemic sclerosis incorporates scleroderma as one of its components. Hand involvement is almost universal with this condition, as 98 percent of the patients have Raynaud's phenomenon.[62] Polyarthralgias and joint stiffness affecting both small and large peripheral joints are common. Many patients develop severe deformities of the fingers and wrists, owing to intense fibrosis of the synovium. X-ray studies reveal subcutaneous calcinosis as well as absorption of the tufts of the terminal phalanges. Other areas of bone absorption include the distal portions of the radius and the ulna as well as the ribs and the mandible.[62]

Psoriatic arthritis classically affects the distal interphalangeal joints but can affect any of the joints, including the wrists. It has a pattern of symmetric polyarthritis clinically indistinguishable from that of rheumatoid arthritis. Arthritis mutilans may be a component, and, except for this condition, psoriatic arthritis tends to cause less pain and disability than rheumatoid arthritis.

Belsky and coworkers[5] found patterns of hand and wrist involvement in psoriatic arthritis to differ from those typically seen in rheumatoid disease. Their patients had multiple joint involvement in the hands, with joint destruction and stiffness as characteristic findings rather than the typical instability seen in rheumatoid arthritis. Palmar subluxation of the carpus, common in the rheumatoid patient, was not found, but spontaneous wrist fusion was common.

Osteoarthritis is the most common joint

344

disease. This condition can be divided into primary and secondary, depending on the presence of some pre-existing condition. While primary osteoarthritis commonly involves the thumb basal joints and the digits with Heberden's and Bouchard's nodes in the distal and proximal interphalangeal joints, wrist joint involvement is less common. Secondary degenerative arthritis of the wrist is very common and is due to old trauma.

Gouty arthritis is caused by sodium urate crystals in the synovium as a result of chronic hyperuremia. In the majority of patients, recurrent bouts of acute joint inflammation constitute the first manifestation of the disease, but in 10 to 15 percent of patients, it is preceded by nephrolithiasis.[62] A family history is common. It is a disease of middle-aged and older men, but women can also be affected. The initial attacks are typically monarticular and most often affect the great toe or other foot joints, ankles, and knees. The acute episode can be confused with sepsis because of the presence of local swelling, redness, and heat. The patient may also have a low-grade fever and leukocytosis. Initially, the attacks are separated by long periods of time, but as the disease progresses, they become more frequent and affect fingers, wrists, and elbows. Primarily, the joints return to normal during the remissions, but later, permanent, chronic arthritis persists. Before effective control of hyperuremia was available, up to 60 percent of gout patients developed tophi. Medical treatment with uricosuric agents is usually all that is necessary to control or shrink gouty tophi, but it may be necessary to débride and decompress tendons and nerves involved with gouty tenosynovitis in the wrist.[55, 72]

Pseudogout caused by a deposition of calcium pyrophosphate crystals is marked by inflammation in one or more joints, lasting for several days or longer. These episodes are usually self-limited and are less painful than gout.[62] This disease can be similar to rheumatoid arthritis, with multiple symmetric joint involvement lasting for weeks or months. The wrists are the second most commonly affected joints, after the knees. Metacarpophalangeal joints, hips, shoulders, elbows, and ankles follow in that order in frequency of occurrence. Flexion deformities develop. X-ray studies demonstrate crystal deposition in articular cartilage in the menisci of the knees, the intervertebral discs, the

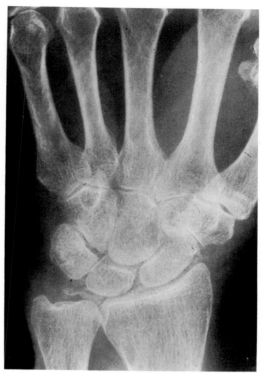

Figure 24–1. Pseudogout with opacification in the triangular fibrocartilage of the wrist.

symphysis pubis, and the articular fibrocartilage of the wrist (Fig. 24–1).

Some of the other conditions that result in wrist deformities similar to those caused by rheumatoid arthritis are juvenile rheumatoid arthritis, mixed connective tissue disease, ankylosing spondylitis, Reiter's syndrome, rheumatoid fever with Jacod's syndrome, infectious arthritis, sarcoidosis, and hemachromatosis.

MEDICAL CONSIDERATIONS AND MANAGEMENT

Rheumatoid arthritis is a generalized medical disease, and surgeons are called upon only when the disease process cannot be controlled medically. At this time, there is no cure for rheumatoid arthritis, although there are many claims of cures. The Arthritis Foundation states that frauds and rackets robbed arthritis victims of more than 400 million dollars last year, and for every dollar spent this year by responsible organizations in legitimate research into the cause of and cure for arthritis, many more will be spent on useless quack cures and remedies.

One reason that charlatans can claim to

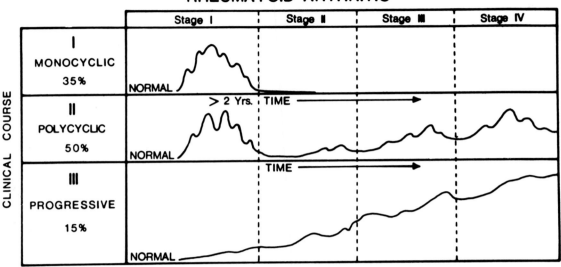

Figure 24–2. Various clinical courses of rheumatoid arthritis.[26, 69]

have a cure for rheumatoid arthritis is the unpredictable course of this disease. Rheumatoid arthritis can present three hypothetical courses: monocyclic, polycyclic, and progressive[26, 69] (Fig. 24–2). According to the best available estimates, rheumatoid arthritis might be expected to follow a monocyclic course with complete spontaneous recovery in 35 percent of patients, a polycyclic course with periods of unpredictable swings in disease activity in 50 percent of cases, and a progressive, unremitting course in 15 percent of patients. Because of the variable potential courses that this illness may follow without any therapy, it is exceedingly difficult to judge the degree of response to any of the modes of therapy, whether drug, physical, or surgical. One must, therefore, be constantly aware that what appears to be a favorable change may be due to a natural remission and may not be a beneficial response to therapy.[1] Conversely, an unfavorable change may reflect a spontaneous relapse rather than an adverse effect of an agent or procedure being used.[2] It is for this reason that early surgical treatment is avoided in the beginning stages of the disease.

Therapeutic Pyramid

It is useful to consider a stepwise approach to the treatment of rheumatoid arthritis[26, 70] (Fig. 24–3). This therapeutic pyramid offers a realistic approach to the treatment of patients in various stages of the disease.

LEVEL I

The basic therapeutic program is the foundation of the pyramid; it consists of patient and family education, rest, pain relief with salicylates, measures to combat anemia, controlled exercise, and a well-balanced diet. Psychological support is extremely important, since patients in whom the diagnosis of rheumatoid arthritis is made may present with relatively few symptoms and no joint destruction, but they will see in their physician's waiting room other patients with severe destruction and disability.

For many patients with low-grade disease and little disability, this basic program (Level I) may provide adequate control for long periods, and no additional measures will be necessary.

LEVEL II

In cases of moderately severe rheumatoid arthritis with multiple joint involvement and considerable constitutional disturbance and disability, when the basic medical treatment proves inadequate after several weeks of trial, additional measures are needed. These include the use of nonsteroidal anti-inflammatory drugs, antimalarials, and anthranilic acid derivatives. Also included in this second level of therapy are intra-articular injections of corticosteroids.

LEVEL III

The drugs that make up the third level of the treatment pyramid include gold, D-penicillamine, and corticosteroids.

Gold. Of all the anti-inflammatory agents commonly used in treatment of rheumatoid arthritis, only gold salts may alter the clinical course or stop the progression of the disease.

Toxic reactions to gold are of the utmost seriousness and may even be fatal. The most common toxic manifestation is dermatitis, and gold therapy should be stopped when itching appears.

D-Penicillamine. D-Penicillamine (D-3-mercaptovaline) is used in the treatment of patients with rheumatoid arthritis who have not responded to nonsteroidal anti-inflammatory drugs. Its use is limited by side effects that are similar to those encountered with gold therapy and that may be equally hazardous. Nausea, vomiting, and diminution of the sense of taste can be annoying, but thrombocytopenia and proteinuria are far more hazardous to the patient.

Oral Corticosteroids. The corticosteroids are the most powerful anti-inflammatory compounds available. There is no convincing evidence to show that corticosteroids can stop or significantly alter the natural course of the underlying disease. They are used for their palliative effect in suppressing symptoms and in alleviating general fatigue.

Candidates for oral corticosteroid therapy are those patients who have severe unremitting disease with fever, anemia, weight loss, effusion, neuropathy, vasculitis, and deformities, in spite of an adequate trial of conservative treatment. Few people can take therapeutic amounts of corticosteroids without some unwanted side effects.

LEVEL IV

This level of rheumatoid arthritis requires hospitalization either for reconstructive surgery or because of lack of response to the measures already mentioned.

There is a growing recognition of the value of four to six weeks of intensive hospitalization, in which the team approach is used for meeting the patient's needs. The cooperative efforts of professional personnel trained in rheumatology, orthopedic surgery, hand surgery, and rehabilitation medicine have proved to be of great value in providing a truly comprehensive and maximally effective approach to the care of the patient with rheumatoid arthritis.

In addition to hospitalization and surgery, the immunosuppressive drugs are indicated in Level IV; these are used only in those patients who have progressive rheumatoid arthritis that is unresponsive to all of the other usual forms of therapy or in those who require high doses of steroids for adequate control of synovitis. The side-effects of bone

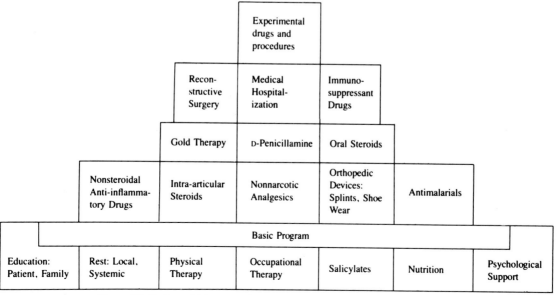

Figure 24–3. Pyramidal approach to the treatment of rheumatoid arthritis.[26, 70]

marrow suppression, loss of hair, hematuria, sterility, and liver inflammation are not to be taken lightly. A major unanswered question is the possibility of the risk of induction of malignant changes with use of these drugs.

LEVEL V

Treatment at this level is investigational in nature. It includes orthopedic procedures and devices as well as drugs and such treatment as irradiation of lymphoid tissue and "cryopheresis." It is hoped that, in the future, drugs for immunization against the very agent that causes rheumatoid arthritis will be available.

CONSERVATIVE TREATMENT

The wrist is the most commonly involved upper extremity joint in the rheumatoid patient. It is the one part of the hand that can be splinted for long time periods with some success. Resting the wrist with a simple splint may provide relief of pain and some subsidence of inflammation; however, a complex, burdensome device will be abandoned by the patient.[13] A single steroid injection may be useful, but local steroid injections have been implicated in tendon rupture, so they are used sparingly for dorsal tenosynovitis. We also teach proper joint positioning and other education techniques and call upon the hand therapists to instruct patients in these areas.

INDICATIONS FOR SURGERY

Indications for surgery are progressive pain and deformity in the joints or progression of the synovial disease in tendon sheaths despite adequate general medical treatment. Ideally, any patient with rheumatoid arthritis who is selected for surgery should be properly motivated and be willing to cooperate in the pre-operative and postoperative regimen. Surgery of the wrist, however, may be indicated even in the lackadaisical patient because of the known disastrous natural course of tendon rupture that occurs if surgery is withheld, and because a good result may be obtained without a formal postoperative exercise program.

Synovitis

Synovitis may involve the distal radioulnar joint, the ulnar styloid process, and the ra-diocarpal, intercarpal, and metacarpocarpal joints as well as the tendon sheaths, both volar and dorsal.

Radioulnar synovitis. Occasionally, rheumatoid disease in the wrist will involve only the distal radioulnar joint and the prestyloid recess, which is the cause of ulnar head and styloid process erosion.[81] The patient presents with swelling and pain localized to the ulnar side of the wrist. Treatment consisting of synovectomy with partial or complete ulnar head resection may be indicated.

Radiocarpal synovitis. Taleisnik[81] has described the mechanism of the deformities seen in the rheumatoid wrist. This consists of malrotation of the scaphoid, loss of carpal height and radial rotation, and supination of the metacarpals. The carpus is normally "suspended" from the radius by a ligamentous sling that originates predominantly from the volar-radial and dorsal-ulnar corners of the distal radius. Loss of the ulnar component of the radiocarpal sling allows the medial "column" to subluxate volarly with an increased metacarpal descent angle.[80]

On the radial side of the carpus, alteration or destruction of the deep radioscapholunate and radiocapitate ligaments effectively results in loss of stability of the proximal pole of the scaphoid, which gradually assumes a volar flexed position perpendicular to the radius. Further destruction of the volar radiocarpal support leads to dissociation of the scapholunate joint, rapidly accelerating wrist collapse.[81]

Dorsal Tenosynovitis

Rheumatoid tenosynovitis on the dorsum of the wrist begins beneath the dorsal carpal ligament and extends distally, causing swelling below this rigid ligament. Occasionally, this is misdiagnosed as a ganglion. Ligamentous involvement and instability of the distal radioulnar joint are often present, producing the so-called caput ulnae syndrome.[3] The clinical manifestations of this syndrome are[76, 77]

1. increasing weakness of the wrist, crepitation on movement, especially on rotation, and pain, which may be sudden, sharp, severe, and may momentarily prevent use of the hand;

2. loss of rotation and dorsiflexion of the wrist;

3. dorsal prominence and instability of the head of the ulna;

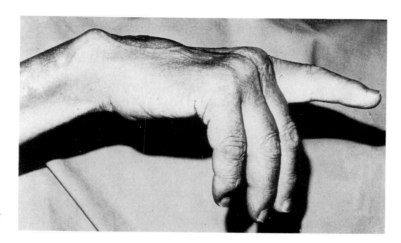

Figure 24–4. Rupture of the extensor tendons of the ulnar three digits.

4. soft tissue swelling over the ulnar dorsal surface of the wrist caused by synovial proliferation;

5. descent of the fourth and fifth metacarpals;

6. occasional rupture of the extensor tendons to the digits;

7. loss of normal action of the extensor carpi ulnaris, which produces some of the deformities seen in the rheumatoid hand, including radial rotation of the wrist.

If dorsal tenosynovitis persists despite splinting, rest, and adequate medication, surgical treatment is indicated to prevent tendon damage.

Rupture of the extensor tendons at the wrist level has been blamed solely on the erosive effect of the distal end of the ulna, but tendon rupture has also occurred after distal ulnar resection when no other wrist surgery has been performed. Our experience[14] indicates that extensor tendon rupture results from a combination of factors such as (1) erosion caused by bone irregularity, (2) compressive effect of the dorsal carpal ligament, and (3) direct rheumatoid invasion of the tendons. Other causes of rupture, demonstrated at least in flexor tendons, are local steroid injections and occlusion by hypertrophic rheumatoid tissue around vincular vessels, causing localized infarcts in the tendon.[47]

The diagnosis of rupture of the extensor tendons at the wrist usually poses no problem (Fig. 24–4), but three other conditions must be considered in the differential diagnosis in the rheumatoid patient. The first is the result of metacarpophalangeal synovitis, in which the extensor tendons have slipped off the metacarpal heads into the intermetacarpal areas, so that these tendons are below

the axis of rotation, which impedes their mechanical advantage. The second is that of posterior interosseous nerve palsy, resulting from rheumatoid involvement at the elbow[49, 51] (Fig. 24–5). The third is rupture of the extensor tendons over the metacarpal heads.[18]

Tendon rupture of the extensor tendons at the wrist in rheumatoid arthritis is not just an academic issue. There have been many articles* in the literature dealing with spontaneous tendon rupture in the arthritic wrist, beginning with Vaughan-Jackson,[85] who reported two cases in 1948.

Early dorsal wrist surgery, consisting of tenosynovectomy, synovectomy, resection of the distal end of the ulna, and transposition of the dorsal carpal ligament beneath the extensor tendons, will, indeed, prevent ten-

---

*References 14, 42, 52, 54, 58, 61, 71, 77.

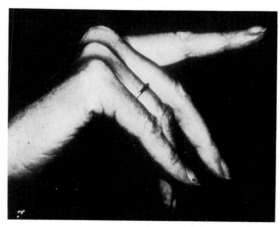

Figure 24–5. Hand with posterior interosseous nerve palsy, which appears similar to a hand with tendon rupture or one unable to extend the fingers, owing to metacarpophalangeal destruction.

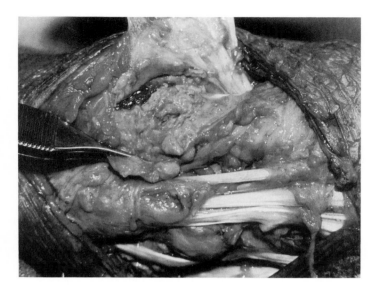

Figure 24–6. Marked dorsal tenosynovitis. The dorsal retinaculum is reflected, exposing each extensor compartment.

don rupture, although Abernathy and Bennyson[1] do not feel that tenosynovectomy is even necessary, since they found that dorsal tenosynovitis resolved in 81.5 percent of their 54 cases after the dorsal carpal ligament was simply transposed.

SURGICAL TECHNIQUE

A straight-line longitudinal dorsal incision is made. This may be diagonal or placed more to the radial or ulnar side, depending on where the tenosynovitis is more prominent. The incision is long enough so that retraction is gentle. The skin is not undermined, and the subcutaneous fat is left attached, in order to minimize the chance of skin necrosis. Dorsal veins should be preserved as much as possible. Dorsal sensory nerves are protected. The dorsal carpal ligament is reflected from the ulnar side, leaving it attached radially (Fig. 24–6). All extensor compartments are opened, and each extensor tendon is isolated. A tenosynovectomy is performed. Bony spicules are removed from the carpus and the distal radius. The capsule of the distal ulna is opened longitudinally, and if the triangular fibrocartilage is absent, the distal 1 to 2 cm of the ulna are resected. If the triangular fibrocartilage is intact and will give some support to the carpus, the entire ulnar head is not resected, but instead, the radial portion of the head is excised, as described by Bowers[8] and Watson.[90] This will preserve the triangular ligament, thus maintaining support on the ulnar side.

Other methods of treating the distal ulna have been described, including the Lauenstein procedure, in which the distal ulna is fused to the radius and a pseudarthrosis is created just proximal to the arthrodesis by removing a section of ulna. In the Baldwin procedure, the distal radioulnar joint is already fused or stiff, and a proximal pseudarthrosis is created again by removing a portion of the ulna.[32] We have not had experience with these two procedures in the rheumatoid wrist, but they may occasionally be useful.

The radioulnar disk is often destroyed, but if it is not, an incision is made into the radiocarpal joint longitudinally, taking care to avoid any intact radiocarpal ligaments. The wrist is distracted, and a ronguer is placed in the radiocarpal joint, where a synovectomy is carried out. The wrist ligaments are then reconstructed. The key point of the reconstruction consists of passing the ulnar retinaculum beneath the extensor carpi ulnaris and suturing the retinaculum and ulnar volar capsule to the dorsum of the distal radius. This reconstructs the radioulnocarpal complex and helps prevent later ulnar sliding and supination deformities (Fig. 24–7). The dorsal carpal ligament is then passed beneath the extensor tendons and is sutured to its cut edge on the ulnar side, leaving a small strip to be passed around the extensor carpi ulnaris to keep it dorsalized and to help stabilize the distal ulna (Fig. 24–8). Silicone capping of the distal ulna is not done by us; however, indications and techniques for the procedure can be found in Chapter 28. The tourniquet is lowered

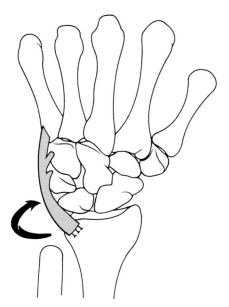

Figure 24–7. Reconstruction of the ulnar side of the wrist.[82] (From Thirupathi RG, Ferlic DC, and Clayton ML: J Hand Surg 8:848–856, 1983.)

before wound closure, and drains are inserted. Protective splinting is carried out for two to four weeks postoperatively.

Using this operative technique before tendons rupture usually prevents this complication in the rheumatoid wrist.[17, 82]

Wound breakdown is another complication encountered with dorsal wrist surgery. We have seen this in about 5 percent of our cases; most often it involves a very small area and heals without any problem. There will rarely be a significant area of wound

breakdown that necessitates débridement or even grafting. This complication can be minimized by making an almost straight, longitudinal, ample incision; by not undermining the skin; by leaving all the fat on the skin flaps, preserving all possible dorsal veins; by avoiding strong retraction; by lowering the tourniquet and obtaining hemostasis; by wound drainage; by dressing the wrist up to the finger tips with much padding; and by using only light compression and splinting.

One potential complication in moving the entire retinaculum is bowstringing of the extensor tendons (Fig. 24–9). This problem may be avoided by leaving the dorsal fascia in the forearm proximal to the dorsal carpal ligament. If it is necessary to release this fascia, then it may be necessary to make a checkrein ligament with a thin strip of dorsal carpal ligament. To prevent the carpus from sliding off the radius, the key suture is made to join the ulnar volar wrist capsule and the retinaculum to the dorsal radius.

The use of a silicone ulnar cap also remains controversial. Swanson[76] states that the advantages of the implant over simple resection are (1) less bone needs to be removed; (2) the physiologic length of the ulna is maintained, thus helping to prevent ulnar carpal shift and to provide greater wrist stability; (3) there is a smooth articular surface in contact with the radius and carpus that provides freer movements of the distal radioulnar and carpoulnar joints; (4) there is a smooth surface on which the overlying extensor tendons can glide; (5) the incidence

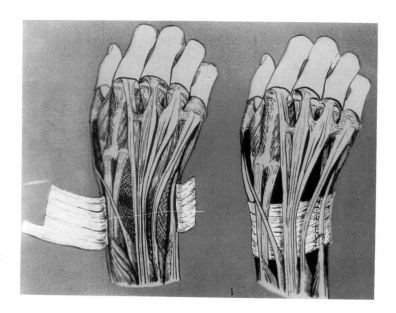

Figure 24–8. The dorsal carpal ligament is passed beneath the extensor tendons, and a flap is used to dorsalize the extensor carpi ulnaris.

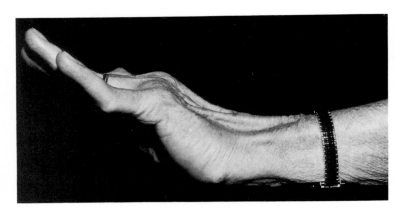

Figure 24–9. Bowstringing of extensor tendons after dorsal tenosynovectomy.

of bone overgrowth is decreased; (6) ligament reconstruction is possible; (7) the important extensor carpi ulnaris tendon may be rerouted over the dorsum of the ulna; (8) the cosmetic appearance is improved. We do not feel that the use of this implant prevents the complications it is supposed to avoid; intead, we feel that stabilizing the ulnar side of the wrist and the distal ulna by soft tissue reconstruction is the preventative measure one should take.

The last point of emphasis in the surgical technique is the reconstruction of a flap of retinaculum around the extensor carpi ulnaris, which keeps this tendon on the dorsum of the wrist. This helps to stabilize the distal ulna and prevents the bases of the fourth and fifth metacarpals from descending and adding to the supination deformity of the hand. Other techniques for stabilization of the ulnocarpal complex can be found in Chapter 17.

We are confident that dorsal wrist surgery will minimize extensor tendon rupture, but what happens to the wrist joint itself after synovectomy? Does the reconstruction on the dorsal side prevent further destruction of the wrist with collapse of the carpus and ulnar translocation? In order to answer these questions, we reviewed our patients after a minimum five-year follow-up study and found that 95 percent of the patients had excellent relief of pain.[82] Motion increased somewhat. Seventy percent of the patients' wrists maintained good carpal height. Carpal collapse of more than 5 mm occurred progressively over two years, not just suddenly. Ulnar translocation of more than 5 mm also occurred in a linear fashion. Progressive carpal collapse was associated with an increase in ulnar deviation of the fingers. An attempt was made to predict which wrists would

deteriorate with time, and this long-term study showed that once collapse and ulnar translocation progressed beyond 5 mm, the wrist was likely to continue to change further. Synovectomy does not cure the disease, but it is an effective procedure in the wrist to minimize the destructive effects of the arthritis.

The results of our long-term follow-up study can also be compared with those of Kulick and colleagues,[41] who had similarly satisfactory results, but synovitis recurred in 20 percent of their patients.

There are other methods to prevent ulnar translocation and to preserve motion. Ryu, Watson, and Burgess[64] have described an operation in which an apparent fusion of the radiocarpal joint is carried out, but the fixation pins are left in for a short period of time, creating a stable pseudarthrosis with some painless motion. Another procedure is a lunate radial fusion, which will maintain some motion but will also prevent ulnar translocation. These methods may be particularly useful when the wrist has already started slipping off to the ulnar side even before surgery.

Extensor Tendon Rupture

Many patients with dorsal tenosynovitis experience ruptured tendons, and repair of these structures needs to be considered at the time of wrist reconstruction. Rarely, if ever, can a ruptured extensor tendon in the rheumatoid patient be repaired primarily. In order to reconstruct these tendons, it is necessary to resect a considerable amount of frayed tendon, leaving them too short for end-to-end suture. An acute tendon rupture in the wrist should, however, be treated with some urgency,[52, 53] the reason being that a single rupture is often followed by a second one, and prompt surgery may prevent this. The result of surgery for ruptured tendons is directly proportional to the number of tendons ruptured. Surgical repair in a hand with a triple rupture (extensor tendons to the little, ring, and long fingers) cannot be expected to turn out as well as surgery in the hand in which only the tendons to the little finger were separated.

Extensor pollicis longus rupture is common. It is often overlooked because of minimal functional deficit due to the action of the intrinsic thumb muscles. In the isolated case, a number of alternatives are available. Arthrodesis of the interphalangeal joint of the thumb may be all that is warranted if the joint is already destroyed or does not have satisfactory passive motion. In cases in which thumb motion needs to be preserved, our preferred treatment for this rupture is to transfer the indicis proprius. We have also successfully used a free graft in thumbs in which the tissue bed is relatively unaffected. Goldner[31] has suggested that the brachioradialis or the extensor carpi radialis longus be used as a motor.

For treatment of the rupture of the finger extensors, individual transfers work better than mass transfer of one tendon into all that are ruptured. If the extensor tendons to the little finger are gone, transfer of the communis into the adjacent intact ring finger extensor works well. The same principle applies if any single finger extensor tendon is ruptured. If the extensors to the little and ring fingers have ruptured, the ring finger extensor is sutured into the long finger tendon and the indicis proprius is used as the motor in the little finger. The proximal muscles of the ruptured tendon are sutured into the transferred tendon motor. If the adjacent tendon is frayed, it may not be suitable for transfer and should be bypassed, using the next tendon. In such a case, a tendon graft is used to reinforce the weakened area.

In the case of triple rupture, several options are available, but goals will be limited. The extensor carpi radialis longus can be transferred into all three ruptured tendons. This is often the best method, considering the extensive pathologic condition involved. Normal finger motion cannot be expected because of the limited excursion of this muscle. If the wrist is supple, a tenodesis effect will help with the motion, but usually the wrist has limited motion in such a case. Another alternative is to transfer the ruptured long finger tendon into the intact index extensor, then to transfer the extensor indicis proprius to the little finger, and to use a superficialis into the ring finger. One may consider the possibility of using the extensor pollicis longus for transfer if arthrodesis of the metacarpophalangeal or interphalangeal joints of the thumb is to be performed at the same time.

Many other possibilities of tendon transfer have been advocated[30, 37, 52, 65, 83, 86] and alternatives often need to be considered, owing to the specific conditions found at the time of surgery. In cases in which the wrist as well as the finger extensors are ruptured, reconstruction is not possible unless the wrist is fused. The wrist tendons can then be used for transfers.[15] Surgery to these hands certainly has limited goals, and the patient needs to be aware of this before reconstructive attempts are carried out.

The hand with ruptured wrist extensors and fixed volar subluxated metacarpophalangeal joints presents a special problem in reconstruction. The metacarpophalangeal joints must be mobilized and the tendon transfers need to be immobilized; however, doing both of these procedures together is not advisable. In these cases, the metacarpophalangeal joints should be replaced first and held in extension with dynamic rubber band traction. Motion is started as usual. Wrist surgery and tendon transfers are then performed at a second operation.

Ulnar Drift

The hypothesis that radial rotation and deviation of the carpus initiate ulnar drift of the fingers has been presented.[12, 29, 44, 57, 66, 67] Ulnar drift with a proliferative synovitis of the metacarpophalangeal joints causes loss of dorsal, radial, and volar support. Thus, the fingers may progressively drift toward the ulnar side owing to dynamic influences within the hand,[13, 25, 73, 92] the normal anatomy of the hand,[25, 30, 35] and external forces acting upon the hand.[4, 28, 29]

Although radial rotation of the metacarpals may not be the sole initiating factor, it is an important one (Fig. 24–10). If radial rotation of the wrist is not corrected, ulnar drift is more prone to occur or recur after ulnar deviation has been corrected. In addi-

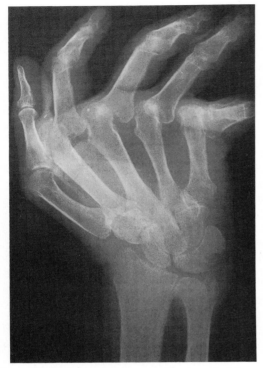

Figure 24–10. Rheumatoid hand with ulnar deviation of the fingers and radial rotation of the wrist.[16]

tion to tenosynovectomy, synovectomy of the wrist, resection of the distal ulna, and transposition of the dorsal carpal ligament, it has been our practice to transfer the extensor carpi radialis longus to the extensor carpi ulnaris in patients who do not have the ability to actively ulnar deviate the wrist or in those in whom the extensor carpi ulnaris is attenuated or ruptured[16] (Fig. 24–11). This transfer may also help prevent "metacarpal descent," which Zancolli[92] feels is a major cause of ulnar deviation of the fingers and of progressive ulnar dislocation of the long extensor tendons.

The extensor carpi radialis longus inserts on the radial side of the second metacarpal, making this tendon a strong radial deviator. Therefore, using this muscle for a transfer not only provides active ulnar deviation of the metacarpals but also removes a strong deforming force.

Others have disputed the concept that radial rotation of the wrist affects ulnar deviation of the fingers.[9, 38] In spite of these conflicting reports, we continue to perform the transfer and believe we have shown that it favorably affects ulnar deviation of the fingers.

Flexor Tenosynovitis

In many patients, hand pain may be interpreted as arthritic pain but is, in fact, pain from carpal tunnel syndrome caused by rheumatoid tenosynovitis.[40] This may also be the initial symptom of rheumatoid arthritis.[11, 56] There may actually be locking or triggering of tendons at the level of the transverse carpal ligament[14] (Fig. 24–12). Initial treatment consists of splinting and perhaps a local injection of a steroid into the carpal canal. Failure to respond to this treatment after a single injection is an indication for surgery.

Flexor tenosynovectomy is carried out when hypertrophic synovium is found when the volar carpal ligament is incised to decompress the nerve. It is also necessary to inspect the floor of the carpal canal, since we have seen bone spicules from the carpus as well as synovium ruptured through the volar capsule, resulting in a space-occupying lesion in the carpal tunnel.

The ulnar nerve may also be entrapped at the wrist when it passes through Guyon's canal. Surgical decompression of the nerve in Guyon's canal is the preferred treatment for ulnar nerve compression at the wrist. More common than with the median nerve, the so-called double crush[56] phenomenon may compress the ulnar nerve in more than one place, and in the rheumatoid patient,

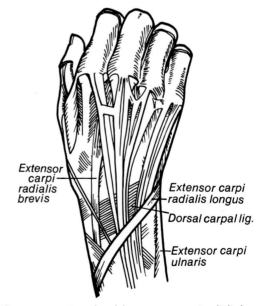

Extensor carpi radialis brevis

Extensor carpi radialis longus

Dorsal carpal lig.

Extensor carpi ulnaris

Figure 24–11. Transfer of the extensor carpi radialis longus to the extensor carpi ulnaris.[16]

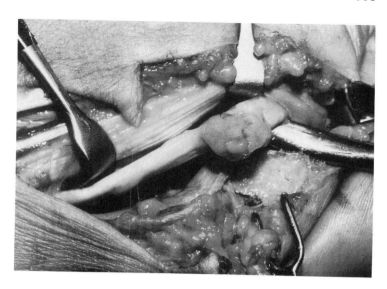

Figure 24–12. Rheumatoid granuloma of a flexor tendon, causing triggering beneath the volar carpal ligament.

involvement at the elbow or cervical radiculopathy may also be present.

Rupture of the flexor tendons is not nearly as common as rupture of the extensor tendons in the rheumatoid patient, but the flexor tendons are more difficult to reconstruct satisfactorily. The most common flexor tendon to rupture is that of the flexor pollicis longus, followed by that of the profundus to the index finger (Fig. 24–13).

With regard to reconstruction of the ruptured flexor tendons, one must keep in mind that it is necessary to start motion early after volar tenosynovectomy or motion may be lost forever. It may be more advisable to perform arthrodesis or tenodesis in the distal joint of a finger if only the profundus is ruptured. If only a superficialis is ruptured, no reconstruction is indicated. To reconstruct a ruptured flexor pollicis longus, the ring superficialis may be transferred, but a free tendon graft can be used if there is minimal tenosynovitis. Arthrodesis of the interphalangeal (IP) joint of the thumb is the treatment of choice if the joint is destroyed or if there is little chance of mobilizing the thumb. Reconstruction of the finger when both flexor tendons are ruptured at the wrist can usually be carried out by transferring one of the remaining superficialis tendons to the ruptured profundus. The anastomosis site must be secure enough for motion to be started immediately.

Probably the most important treatment for flexor tendon rupture at the wrist is to prevent additional tendons from rupturing by performing a flexor tenosynovectomy, de-

compressing the volar carpal ligament, exploring the carpal canal, and removing bone spicules that could cause further tendon damage.

WRIST ARTHROPLASTY

A stable, balanced, and painless wrist is necessary for optimal hand function. A wrist arthrodesed in the neutral position with preserved forearm pronation and supination is compatible with useful hand function, but elimination of wrist motion may be nonessential or even objectionable in the patient with progressive disease in adjacent joints. To be acceptable, an arthroplasty must relieve pain, be stable, correct deformity, provide motion, and leave a reasonable alternative for salvage in case of failure.

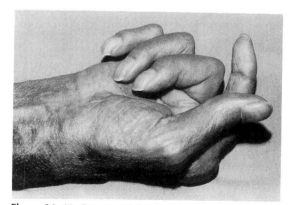

Figure 24–13. Rupture of the flexor tendons to the index finger and the flexor pollicis longus.

Arthroplasties without implants have been used. Synovectomy and limited arthroplasty or radiocarpal fusion, or both, have been previously discussed. Proximal row carpectomy has been useful in treating wrist trauma. We have performed this procedure in a few patients with rheumatoid arthritis in whom the articular surface of the capitate and the lunate fossa of the radius have been preserved, but long-term results were unsatisfactory because of progressive deterioration.

The second type of arthroplasty for the rheumatoid wrist without implant is palmar shelf arthroplasty.[2] Instead of removing bone from the carpus, the distal end of the radius is shaped, and a volar lip of bone is preserved, giving the wrist stability.

Our experience with this procedure is limited. We have encountered one case of persistent lateral deviation that could possibly have been prevented by a longer period of splinting. We do not use this procedure at the present time.

Silicone Wrist Arthroplasty

Joint replacement at the wrist level has taken two forms: silicone interpositional arthroplasty and total joint replacement. The radiocarpal flexible-hinge implant was designed as an adjunct to resection arthroplasty to maintain alignment and adequate joint space, while supporting the capsuloligamentous system (Fig. 24–14). The proximal stem of the implant fits the intramedullary canal of the radius, and the distal stem passes through the capitate and fits the intramedullary canal of the third metacarpal. Swanson[78] lists the advantages of his prosthesis as (1) providing reasonable wrist mobility, stability, and pain relief for finger function; (2) maintaining joint space; (3) supporting and orienting joint incapsulation; (4) allowing reconstruction and balancing of musculotendinous systems; (5) being well tolerated by bone and soft tissues; (6) providing high flexural durability and early postoperative motion. Indications for use are rheumatoid disabilities of the radiocarpal joint with (1) instability of the wrist due to subluxation or dislocation of the radiocarpal joint; (2) wrist deviation causing digital imbalance; (3) stiffness where movement is required for hand function. Swanson and coworkers[78, 79] reported excellent results with this prosthesis, with 90 percent of the

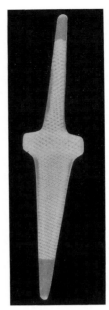

Figure 24–14. Silicone wrist prosthesis.

rheumatoid patients having excellent pain relief and a reasonable amount of motion. Fracture of the prosthesis was the most common reason for failure.

In 1982, Swanson[79] introduced metal grommets around the implants to prevent cutting of the implant in cases where the bones are sharp or thin. He has not recorded any fractured implants since he has started using these devices.

Our experience suggests that further collapse of the carpus over the implant with more loss of motion and a high rate of implant breakage occurs with time. We have used the silicone prosthesis in the rheumatoid wrist and have obtained results similar to those previously reported.[21, 33, 78, 79] Silicone arthroplasty is especially useful in treating the juvenile rheumatoid wrist with very small bones, in which other available total wrist components are too large to be inserted.

Problems with the silicone wrist prosthesis have been breakage (Fig. 24–15), silicone synovitis, and collapse of the carpus over the prosthesis, which results in decreased motion over a period of time.

OPERATIVE TECHNIQUE

The silicone prostheses are flexible hinges. They do not and are not supposed to provide stability. Maintenance of the correction is dependent on adequate soft tissue release and bone resection to repair the deformity

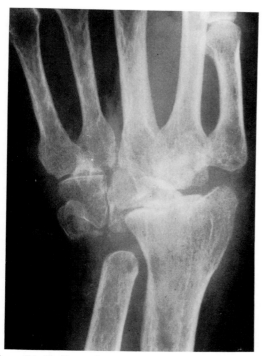

Figure 24–15. X-ray of a wrist with a silicone arthroplasty. The prosthesis has fractured, resulting in pain and recurrence of the deformity.

and to restore alignment. The external mechanical forces must also be balanced to prevent angular deformity.

A dorsal midline straight incision is made. The cutaneous veins and nerves are preserved. The skin is not undermined. Retraction must be gentle in order to minimize the possibility of skin necrosis. The dorsal retinaculum is reflected from the ulnar side of the wrist, opening each of the extensor compartments, except the first. The tenosynovium is removed from the involved tendons. The distal end of the ulna is excised. An ulnar prosthesis is not used. The dorsal capsule is detached from the radius and reflected distally. The carpus is hyperflexed to expose the wrist joint. A partial carpectomy is carried out, removing enough bone to get a flat surface for prosthetic seating. This may entail half the scaphoid, lunate, and triquetrum, but the entire scaphoid and half the capitate may need to be removed to correct a deformity.

The distal 1 cm of radius is excised at right angles to the shaft of the bone. Enough bone must be resected in order to correct any deformity. An opening is then made into the capitate and extended into the third metacarpal. A trial reduction is made. The size of the bones distal to the wrist is the limiting factor for determining the size of the prosthesis, so the distal hole is made before the opening into the radius in order to avoid excess bone resection from the radius.

It is necessary to trim any sharp bone edges. The prosthesis should sit squarely against the carpus and the radius and should not buckle when motion is attempted. The volar capsule can be stripped, if necessary, to avoid excessive bone resection.

The prosthesis is inserted. The dorsal capsule is reattached to the distal radius through drill holes. The radial and ulnar ligaments are tightened, if necessary, and the ulnovolar capsule is pulled up and sutured to the dorsal capsule, reconstructing the ulnar side of the wrist.

As in wrist synovectomy, the extensor retinaculum is passed beneath the extensor tendons and sutured to the ulnar side of the wrist, leaving a strip of retinaculum placed around the extensor carpi ulnaris to keep it on the dorsum of the wrist, thus stabilizing the distal ulna as well as preventing volar migration of the ulnar metacarpals. Tendon transfers for ruptured finger extensors can now be carried out. The tourniquet is lowered, hemostasis is achieved, a suction drain is inserted, and the subcutaneous tissue and skin are closed.

In the loose type of rheumatoid joint, the wrist is splinted for four to six weeks before motion is begun. Motion may be started earlier in the stiff type.

The reader is referred to Chapter 28 for additional details concerning the silicone wrist prosthesis.

Total Wrist Arthroplasty

Total wrist arthroplasty has gained popularity as total replacement in other joints has progressed. Two types of artificial wrist joints, the Meuli (Fig. 24–16) and the Volz (Fig. 24–17), have gained the widest acceptance, although others, such as the Hamas[36] and the spherical-triaxial wrist prostheses,[59, 60] have been developed.

The Meuli Prosthesis. Meuli[48, 49] has used his prosthesis since 1971. In a 1980 report[48] on 41 wrist arthroplasties, he listed two infections, five reactions to polyester, seven technical errors, two dislocations, and one breakage. Fifteen wrists mandated re-operation, of which six required a change of pros-

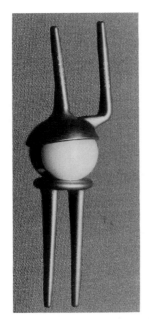

Figure 24–16. Meuli total wrist.[27]

thesis, and five needed arthrodesis. The problem in centering this prosthesis can be overcome by bending the fixation stems. This is not possible with other designs.

In 1977[6] and 1984,[20] the Mayo Clinic results with the Meuli prosthesis were reported, with a high rate of revision and re-operation found to be necessary. They discovered that the probability of revision increases with time for major complications requiring re-operation.

Volz Prosthesis. Volz[87, 88] reviewed the first 100 wrist arthroplasties performed using his prosthesis by 15 collaborating surgeons; 83 cases had rheumatoid arthritis. The overall results were good or excellent in 86 percent, and 6 percent resulted in failure. The most frequent postoperative problem was wrist motor imbalance. In addition, 6 percent demonstrated wound healing problems, all of which occurred in rheumatoid patients. Four patients experienced a single episode of subluxation, three of these in the immediate postoperative period. Two patients developed a wound infection requiring removal of the prosthesis. One patient demonstrated loosening of the distal component. Of the six failures, five required removal of the prosthesis, resulting in solid ankylosis in three and fibrous ankylosis in two.

Since this first report, Volz[89] has changed the design of his prosthesis to a single-prong distal component. This more accurately duplicates the instant center of motion determined by Youm and associates[91] to be at the base of the capitate. In 25 wrist arthroplasties with the single-stemmed prosthesis in 22 patients, 19 of whom were rheumatoid, there were no cases of radioulnar imbalance, nor were there any cases of dislocation, infection, or loosening. Pain relief was excellent. In addition, the Volz prosthesis press-fits the distal component without cement in cases where a secure fit is possible.

SURGICAL TECHNIQUE

A straight-line dorsal skin incision is made. The skin and subcutaneous tissue are divided in one layer. The extensor retinaculum is reflected radially from between the fifth and sixth compartments to the first. The distal ulna is resected and a tenosynovectomy carried out. The integrity of the extensor carpi radialis brevis is checked carefully, because if it is ruptured, a wrist arthrodesis should be done. The dorsal capsule is elevated subperiosteally from the radius. Synovectomy is performed as necessary. The volar radiocarpal ligament is then released subperiosteally from the radius.

Prepare the carpals, metacarpals, and distal radius to accept the two components by cutting the distal radius at a right angle to the longitudinal axis and removing the lunate, proximal half of the scaphoid and triquetrum, and by cutting the distal row off straight. An appropriate amount of bone must be resected to allow insertion of the 2 cm prosthesis. The distal articulating end should be exactly in line with the third metacarpal, corresponding to the resected end of the capitate. Trial reduction is per-

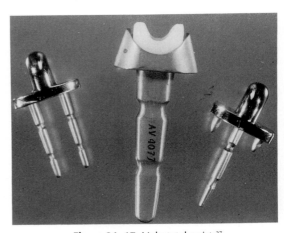

Figure 24–17. Volz total wrist.[27]

formed, and range of motion is checked. There should be no bone or soft tissue projections to interfere with the full range of motion permitted by the design of the prosthesis.

Balance is then determined: On the hand table, the wrist should lie in the neutral position in the radioulnar plane. If the wrist has a pre-operative contracture in ulnar deviation, an extensive amount of rebalancing may be necessary. This consists of positioning the radial component further to the ulnar side, tenotomizing the flexor carpi ulnaris and the palmaris longus, and performing a more extensive capsular release on the ulnar side.

The components are then cemented in place with methylmethacrylate. The canals should be plugged and, if feasible, cement injected under pressurization. If a tight press-fit can be obtained, the distal component may be secured without bone cement. The dorsal radiocarpal ligament is sutured into the radius to further preserve balance, to keep the wrist from subluxating volarly, and to prevent supination of the ulnar metacarpals.

The entire dorsal retinaculum is reattached beneath the extensor tendons. The ulnar aspect of the retinaculum and capsule is secured to the radius, so that any wrist supination deformity is decreased. The extensor carpi ulnaris is positioned dorsally, with a strip of extensor retinaculum utilized as a sling. Ruptured finger extensor tendons are repaired. The subcutaneous tissue is loosely closed over a drain, and the skin is closed. The wrist and forearm are immobilized in a bulky dressing with a volar plaster splint to hold the wrist in neutral position. The splint is removed for active exercises, which are started after two weeks. At four weeks, the patient may perform light activities without the splint, which is completely discarded at three months. Active flexion as well as extension is emphasized.

RESULTS

We have now performed over 50 total wrist replacements in rheumatoid patients using the Volz prosthesis and have reported on the first 20 cases that were done in patients with rheumatoid arthritis.[43] These patients were followed for an average of 18 months. In this early report, we found 90 percent to have no significant pain. There was an increase in grip strength in all patients except one. Three wrists remained unbalanced after surgery. Good or excellent motion was obtained in 75 percent. The overall rating showed 70 percent with good or excellent results (Fig. 24–18). No patient was made worse, but there were two (10 percent) with poor results.

Our complications were similar to Volz's, with balance being the greatest problem. In the original 20, there were two cases of carpal tunnel syndrome after surgery. One postoperative hematoma resolved without surgery. In two patients, the prosthesis dislocated immediately after surgery but was reduced without subsequent problems. One patient dislocated both of her total wrist replacements following a fall seven years after bilateral arthroplasty was performed. These dislocations were reduced completely without sequelae.[22] One patient had inadequate wrist extensors and was re-operated on in an attempt to balance these motors but without success.

We were encouraged by these results and have continued to perform this procedure and to follow up the earliest cases. Those cases with a three-year minimum and a nine-year maximum follow-up study (average, 70

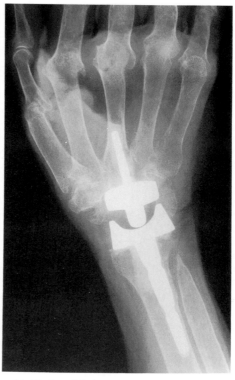

Figure 24–18. A well-balanced wrist after a Volz total wrist arthroplasty.[27]

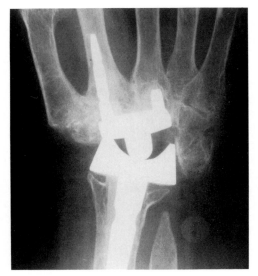

Figure 24–19. Bone resorption beneath the radial component seven years after a Volz wrist implant.[27]

months) have recently been reviewed.[23, 27] Eighty-six percent had no pain or only mild pain and felt that the wrist was improved after arthroplasty, but our critical review with the same criteria used in the 1980

preliminary study showed 60 percent with good and excellent results and 13 percent with poor results.

In addition to clinical follow-up, we reviewed the x-ray studies of these long-term patients and found a significant number with bone resorption beneath the collar of the radial component (Fig. 24–19) and some with loosening and settling of the carpus proximally onto the distal component (Figs. 24–20A and B). Although proximal component loosening did not present a problem, there were a number of prostheses that developed a radiolucent line, a finding that may become more significant with the passage of time, along with the possibility of loosening in additional cases.

Balancing has been the major problem after total wrist arthroplasty. Postoperative imbalance was discovered most often in patients who had pre-operative x-ray evidence of an ulnarly translocated, subluxated, or dislocated carpus; a resting posture of flexion or supination of the hand; a grasp pattern of finger flexion and wrist flexion rather than finger flexion and wrist extension; or a loss of voluntary active wrist extension.[43] The

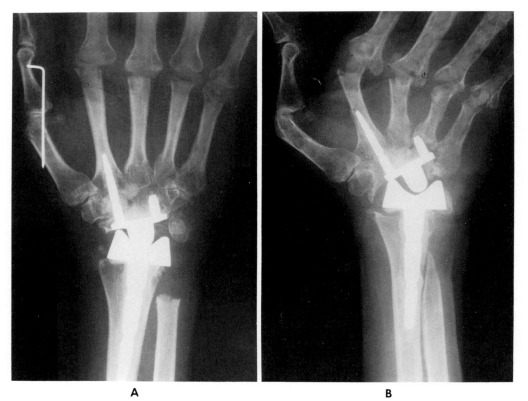

A   **B**

Figure 24–20. *A,* Immediate postoperative x-ray of the wrist.[27] *B,* Seven years later, x-ray showing loosening and proximal migration of the carpus onto the prosthesis.[27]

redesign of the distal component to only one prong has helped alleviate this problem, but we still have had balancing problems. Some contracted wrists still need release of the flexor carpi ulnaris. The functional integrity of the extensor carpi radialis brevis and the degree of volar and ulnar contracture are the most important factors influencing the ultimate result.

Component size is another problem. Even though the radial portion of the prosthesis is available in a small size, this component is still very large. We have had to change the procedure in adults with juvenile rheumatoid arthritis in whom we had planned to insert the prosthesis, because the radial canal could not be sufficiently reamed.

The question of when to use a silicone implant as opposed to a total wrist replacement is frequently asked. We have had considerable experience with both options in rheumatoid patients. We use the total wrist in those patients in whom destruction and deformity have been the greatest and when the bone structure is not small. We continue to use the silicone prosthesis when the wrist has an intermediate amount of destruction or deformity, or in a patient with small bone structure, or when 2 cm of bone should not be sacrificed.

Beckenbaugh[7] uses the total wrist replacement for advanced destructive changes of rheumatoid arthritis in patients over 50 years of age. Meuli[49] feels that patients who engage in heavy manual work or rely on walking aids such as canes or crutches are not suitable candidates. Volz's[87-89] indications are (1) a functionally or potentially restorable hand, (2) diffuse Stage III or IV disease of the carpus, (3) a functional elbow, (4) intact dorsiflexion of the wrist, (5) healthy skin over the dorsal aspect of the wrist, and (6) a highly motivated outlook on the part of the patient.

In an attempt to compare the results of total wrist arthroplasty with those of silicone replacement, Summers and Hubbard[75] studied six Meuli total wrist arthroplasties and six silicone replacements. They found that both gave a pain-free stable joint with some degree of useful motion, with the Meuli giving a greater range of motion. They concluded that both prostheses were satisfactory, but their present practice is to use the Swanson Silastic prosthesis because it eliminates the use of cement, making revision easier.

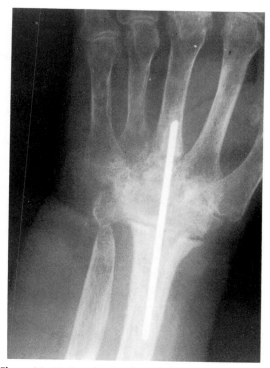

Figure 24–21. Fused wrist after a failed Volz arthroplasty. An interpositional bone graft was used.[27]

Any arthroplasty may fail completely, so a reasonable salvage procedure must be available. Four options are (1) reimplantation and revision of the prosthesis, (2) resectional arthroplasty, (3) arthrodesis, and (4) soft tissue reconstruction. The components can be reinserted or removed and a flexible hinge used.[20] A poorly balanced wrist may be salvaged by tendon transfers or by reinserting the prosthesis in another position. This, however, is difficult.

Arthrodesis must be considered for a failed wrist implant (Fig. 24–21). This procedure has a reasonable chance of success, using internal fixation and bone grafting.

For further details on total wrist arthroplasty in rheumatoid patients, the reader is referred to Chapter 29.

ARTHRODESIS

There is still a place for arthrodesis of the wrist in selected patients with rheumatoid arthritis. Wrist fusion is sometimes desirable and, occasionally, bilateral wrist fusion may be necessary. Sometimes patients retain better function in the distal joints after wrist arthrodesis.[68] Indications for wrist fusion are (1) ankylosis in marked flexion, (2) marked instability as the result of carpal destruction, (3) rupture of the extensor carpi radialis longus and brevis, and (4) moderate changes in the wrist but marked pain in those patients using crutches.

The general recommendation has been fusion in 10° of dorsiflexion (Hadad and Riordan[34]); Boyes[10] has recommended 20° to 30.° For bilateral wrist fusions, it has sometimes been recommended that one wrist be fused in dorsiflexion and the other in palmar flexion. We recommended fusion in the neutral position for uni- or bilateral cases.[19] By placing the wrist at neutral, the arc of motion for pronation and supination substitutes for palmar and dorsiflexion without shoulder or elbow substitution.

TECHNIQUE

A method of fusion was devised in about 1962 that utilized an intramedullary pin with a local or iliac bone graft. This method has continued to be used successfully with minor variations.[14, 15, 19, 46, 50, 84]

The general principles for wrist arthrodesis are (1) neutral position, (2) internal fixation, (3) bone contact (bone graft), (4) compression, and (5) rotation of forearm obtained or maintained.

The dorsal approach is used with a long, straight incision extending distally between the second and third metacarpals. As many dorsal veins as possible are preserved. The fat and subcutaneous tissues are carefully reflected with the skin. The sensory nerves are protected.

The dorsal carpal ligament is incised directly over the ulna and reflected radially. The distal 1.5 to 2 cm of the ulna is resected subperiosteally. A longitudinal incision is made in the capsule of the wrist, exposing the bases of the second and third metacarpals and the distal radius. The dorsal surface of the carpal bones is removed. The cartilage and cortical bone are removed from all joint surfaces to be fused. In some cases, local bone graft from the ulnar head or a sliding radial graft will suffice, but if necessary, an iliac graft is used. A slot is sawed sagittally in the carpus from the base of the second and third metacarpals to the radius, at a depth of 1.0 to 1.2 cm and at a width of 2.5 cm. An opening is undercut into the radius and the bones of the second and third metacarpals. A unicortical inner table iliac graft or the sliding distal radial graft is removed, shaped to fit the prepared bed, and tightly

wedged proximally and distally. Fixation is obtained with a 1/8-in Rush pin, introduced at the distal end of the third metacarpal from the radial side into the radius for about 15 to 20 cm. If a bone graft has been utilized, it is shaped and placed either through or volar to the Rush pin, so that the pin holds it in position. Manual compression is then applied, and a staple or a Kirschner wire can be driven into the second metacarpal and the radius to maintain contact and compression and to prevent rotation. Special length staples can be made from small pins and used for compression.

With this technique, the position of the wrist is automatically set at neutral. If a few degrees' alteration is desired, the intramedullary pin can be bent manually after insertion. The dorsal wrist capsule is closed and the dorsal carpal ligament passed beneath the long thumb and finger extensors, and the dorsal carpal ligament is repaired snugly to stabilize the distal end of the resected ulna.

The tourniquet is released, hemostasis obtained, a drain inserted, and the wound closed. After two weeks, a short-arm cast or a simple volar splint is utilized for protection if the internal fixation is rigid, but if a large graft was necessary or if there is no cross-fixation, a long-arm cast is mandated for about six weeks. Union is obtained between two and three months.

The fusion should extend to the metacarpals in the rheumatoid patient. We have seen patients in whom this was not done; the results were instability and the development of destructive changes or flexion deformity in the metacarpocarpal joints.

Additional details are given for arthrodesis of the rheumatoid wrist in Chapter 25.

References

1. Abernathy PJ, and Bennyson WG: Decompression of the extensor tendons at the wrist in rheumatoid arthritis. J Bone Joint Surg 61B:64, 1979.
2. Albright JA, and Chase RA: Palmar-shelf arthroplasty of the wrist in rheumatoid arthritis. J Bone Joint Surg 52A:896, 1970.
3. Backdahl M: The caput ulnae syndrome in rheumatoid arthritis. Acta Rheum Scand (Suppl) 5:1, 1963.
4. Backhouse KM: The mechanics of normal digital control in the hand and an analysis of the ulnar drift of rheumatoid arthritis. Ann Col Surg Engl 43:154, 1968.
5. Belsky MR, Feldon P, Millender LH, et al: Hand involvement in psoriatic arthritis. J Hand Surg 7:203, 1982.
6. Beckenbaugh RD, and Linscheid RL: Total wrist

arthroplasty: a preliminary report. J Hand Surg 2:339, 1977.

7. Beckenbaugh RD: Implant arthroplasty in the rheumatoid hand and wrist: current state of the art in the United States. J Hand Surg 8:675, 1983.

8. Bowers WH: Distal radioulnar joint arthroplasty: the hemiresection-interposition technique. J Hand Surg 10A:169, 1985.

9. Boyce T, Youm Y, Sprague BL, et al: Clinical and experimental studies on the effect of extensor carpi radialis longus transfer in the rheumatoid hand. J Hand Surg 3(4):390, 1978.

10. Boyes JH: Bunnell's Surgery of the Hand. Philadelphia, JB Lippincott Co, 1970, p. 296.

11. Chamberlain MA, and Corbett M: Carpal tunnel syndrome in early rheumatoid arthritis. Ann Rheum Dis 29:149, 1970.

12. Chaplin D, Pulkki T, Saarimaa A, et al: Wrist and finger deformities in juvenile rheumatoid arthritis. Acta Rheum Scand 15:206, 1969.

13. Clayton ML: Surgery of the rheumatoid hand. Clin Orthop 36:47, 1964.

14. Clayton ML: Surgical treatment at the wrist in rheumatoid arthritis. J Bone Joint Surg 47A:741, 1965.

15. Clayton ML: Wrist arthrodesis and tendon reconstruction in rheumatoid arthritis. (Movie) Am Acad Ortho Surg Film Lib, 1966.

16. Clayton ML, and Ferlic DC: Tendon transfer for radial rotation of the wrist in rheumatoid arthritis. Clin Orthop 100:176, 1974.

17. Clayton ML, and Ferlic DC: The wrist in rheumatoid arthritis. Clin Orthop 106:182, 1975.

18. Clayton ML, Thirupathi R, Ferlic DC, et al.: Extensor tendon rupture over the metacarpal heads. Hand 15:149, 1983.

19. Clayton ML, and Ferlic DC: Arthrodesis of the arthritic wrist. Clin Orthop 187:89, 1984.

20. Cooney WP, Beckenbaugh RD, and Linscheid RL: Total wrist arthroplasty. Problems with implant failures. Clin Orthop 187:121, 1984.

21. David RF, Weiland AJ, and Dawling SV: Swanson implant arthroplasty of the wrist in rheumatoid patients. Clin Orthop 166:132, 1982.

22. Dennis DA, Clayton ML, Ferlic DC, et al: Bilateral traumatic dislocations of Volz total wrist arthroplasties: a case report. J Hand Surg 10A:503, 1985.

23. Dennis DA, Ferlic DC, and Clayton ML: Long-term results of Volz total wrist arthroplasty. Submitted to J Hand Surg, 11A:483, 1986.

24. Dray GJ, Millender LH, Nalebuff EA, et al.: The surgical treatment of hand deformities in systemic lupus erythematosis. J Hand Surg 6:339, 1981.

25. Ellison M, Flatt AE, and Kelly KJ: Ulnar drift of the fingers in rheumatoid disease. J Bone Joint Surg 53A:1061, 1971.

26. Ferlic DC, Smyth CJ, and Clayton ML: Medical considerations and management of rheumatoid arthritis. J Hand Surg 8:662, 1983.

27. Ferlic DC: Implant arthroplasty of the rheumatoid wrist. Hand Clin North Am 3:169, 1987.

28. Flatt AE: Some pathomechanics of ulnar drift. Plast Reconstr Surg 37:295, 1966.

29. Flatt AE: The pathomechanics of ulnar drift. Final Report, Social and Rehabilitation Services. Grant Number RD 2226M, 1971.

30. Flatt AE: The Care of the Arthritic Hand. 4th ed. St Louis, CV Mosby Co, 1983.

31. Goldner JL: Tendon transfers in rheumatoid arthritis. Orthop Clin North Am 5:425, 1974.

32. Goncalves D: Correction of disorders of the distal radioulnar joint by artificial pseudarthrosis of the ulna. J Bone Joint Surg 56B:462, 1974.

33. Goodman MJ, Millender LH, Nalebuff EA, et al: Arthroplasty of the rheumatoid wrist and silicone rubber: an early evaluation. J Hand Surg 5:114, 1980.

34. Haddad RJ Jr, and Riordan DC: Arthrodesis of the wrist. J Bone Joint Surg 49A:950, 1967.

35. Hakstian RW, and Butiana R: Ulnar deviation of the fingers. In Proceedings of the American Society for Surgery of the Hand. J Bone Joint Surg 48A:608, 1966.

36. Hamas RS: A quantitative approach to total wrist arthroplasty: development of a precentered total wrist prosthesis. Orthopedics 2(3):245, 1979.

37. Harrison S, Swannell AJ, and Ansell BM: Repair of extensor pollicis longus using extensor pollicis brevis in rheumatoid arthritis. Ann Rheum Dis 31:490, 1972.

38. Hastings DE, and Evans JA: Rheumatoid wrist deformities and their relation to ulnar drift. J Bone Joint Surg 57A:930, 1975.

39. Hastings DE, and Evans JA: The lupus hand: a new surgical approach. J Hand Surg 3(2):1979, 1978.

40. Henderson ED, and Lipscomb P: Surgical treatment of the rheumatoid hand. JAMA 175:431, 1961.

41. Kulick RG, DeFiore JC, Straub LR, et al: Long-term results of dorsal stabilization in the rheumatoid wrist. J Hand Surg 6:272, 1981.

42. Laine VAI, and Vainio KJ: Spontaneous rupture of tendons in rheumatoid arthritis. Acta Orthop Scand 24:250, 1955.

43. Lamberta FJ, Ferlic DC, and Clayton ML: Volz total wrist arthroplasty in rheumatoid arthritis. A preliminary report. J Hand Surg 5:245, 1980.

44. Landsmeer JMF: Studies in the anatomy of articulation. II. Patterns of movement of bimuscular biarticular systems. Acta Morphol Neerl Scand 3:304, 1960.

45. Mannerfeldt L, and Norman O: Attrition ruptures of flexor tendons in rheumatoid arthritis caused by bone spurs in the carpal tunnel. J Bone Joint Surg 51B:270, 1969.

46. Mannerfeldt L, and Malmsten M: Arthrodesis of the wrist in rheumatoid arthritis. A technique without external fixation. Scand J Plast Reconstr Surg 5:124, 1971.

47. Marmor L, Lawrence JF, and Duboid EL: Posterior interosseous nerve palsy due to rheumatoid arthritis. J Bone Joint Surg 49A:381, 1967.

48. Meuli HC: Arthroplasty of the wrist. Clin Orthop 149:118, 1980.

49. Meuli HC: Meuli total wrist arthroplasty. Clin Orthop 187:107, 1984.

50. Millender LH, and Nalebuff EA: Arthrodesis of the rheumatoid wrist. J Bone Joint Surg 55A:1026, 1973.

51. Millender LH, Nalebuff EA, and Holdsworth DE: Posterior interosseous nerve syndrome secondary to rheumatoid arthritis. J Bone Joint Surg 55A:753, 1973.

52. Millender LH, Nalebuff EA, Albin R et al: Dorsal tenosynovitis and tendon ruptures in the rheumatoid hand. J Bone Joint Surg 56A:601, 1974.

53. Millender LH, and Nalebuff EA: Preventive surgery: tenosynovectomy and synovectomy. Ortho Clin North Am 6:765, 1975.

54. Moberg E: Tendon grafting and tendon suture in rheumatoid arthritis. Am J Surg 109:375, 1965.

55. Moore JR, and Weiland AJ: Gouty tenosynovitis in the hand. J Hand Surg 10A:291, 1985.

56. Nakaro KK: The entrapment neuropathy of rheumatoid arthritis. Ortho Clin North Am 6:837, 1975.

57. Pahle I, and Raunio P: The influence of wrist position in finger deviation in the rheumatoid hand. J Bone Joint Surg 51B:664, 1969.

58. Rana NA, and Taylor AR: Excision of the distal end of the ulna in rheumatoid arthritis. J Bone Joint Surg 55B:96, 1973.

59. Ranawat CS: Anatomical considerations and design features of total wrist joint. ONA J 6:61, 1979.

60. Ranawat CS, Green NA, Inglis, AE, et al: Spherical-triaxial total wrist replacement. Inglis AE (ed): Symposium on Total Joint Replacement of the Upper Extremity. St Louis, CV Mosby Co, 1982.

61. Rasmussen KB, and Sneppen O: Operativ behandlung of polyarthritis. Nord Med 77:433, 1967.

62. Rodman GP, and Schumacher R (eds): Primer on the Rheumatic Diseases. 8th ed, Atlanta, Arthritis Foundation, 1983.

63. Rothfield NF: Systemic lupus erythematosis: clinical and laboratory aspects. In McCarty DJ (ed): Arthritis and Allied Conditions: A Textbook of Rheumatology. 9th ed, Philadelphia, Lea & Febiger, 1979, p 691.

64. Ryu J, Watson HK, and Burgess RC: Rheumatoid wrist reconstruction utilizing a fibrous nonunion and radiocarpal arthrodesis. J Hand Surg 10A:830, 1985.

65. Shannon FT, and Barton NJ: Surgery for rupture of extensor tendons in rheumatoid arthritis. Hand 8(3):279, 1976.

66. Shapiro JS: The etiology of ulnar drift. In Proceedings of the American Society for Surgery of the Hand. J Bone Joint Surg 48:634, 1968.

67. Shapiro JS: A new factor in the etiology of ulnar drift. Clin Orthop 68:32, 1970.

68. Smith-Petersen MM, Aufranc OE, and Larson CB: Useful surgical procedures for rheumatoid arthritis involving joints of the upper extremity. Arch Surg 36:764, 1943.

69. Smyth CJ: Optimum therapeutic program in seropositive nodular rheumatoid arthritis. Med Clin North Am 52:687, 1968.

70. Smyth CJ: Therapy of rheumatoid arthritis. A pyramidal plan. Postgrad Med J, Monograph Issue 51:31, 1972.

71. Straub LR, and Wilson EH: Spontaneous rupture of extensor tendons in the hand associated with rheumatoid arthritis. J Bone Joint Surg 38A:1208, 1956.

72. Straub LR, Smith JW, Carpenter GK Jr, et al: The surgery of gout in the upper extremity. J Bone Joint Surg 43A:731, 1961.

73. Straub LR: Surgical rehabilitation of the hand and upper extremity in rheumatoid arthritis. Bull Rheum Dis 12:265, 1962.

74. Straub LR, and Ranawat CS: The wrist in rheumatoid arthritis. J Bone Joint Surg 51A:1, 1969.

75. Summers B, and Hubbard MJ: Wrist joint arthroplasty in rheumatoid arthritis: a comparison between the Meuli and Swanson prostheses. J Hand Surg 9B:171, 1984.

76. Swanson AB: The ulnar head syndrome and its treatment by implant resection arthroplasty. Proceedings of the American Society for Surgery of the Hand. J Bone Joint Surg 54A:906, 1972.

77. Swanson AB, and Swanson G de G: Pathogenesis and pathomechanics of rheumatoid deformities in the hand and wrist. Orthop Clin North Am 4:1039, 1973.

78. Swanson AB, and Swanson G de G: Flexible implant resection arthroplasty: a method for reconstruction of small joints in the extremities. AAOS Instr Course Lect 27:27, 1978.

79. Swanson AB, Swanson G de G, and Maupin BK: Flexible implant arthroplasty of the radiocarpal joint. Surgical technique and long-term study. Clin Orthop 187:94, 1984.

80. Taleisnik J: The ligaments of the wrist. J Hand Surg 1:110, 1976.

81. Taleisnik J: Rheumatoid synovitis of the volar compartment of the wrist joint: its radiological signs and its contribution to wrist and hand deformity. J Hand Surg 4:526, 1979.

82. Thirupathi R, Ferlic DC, and Clayton ML: Dorsal wrist synovectomy in rheumatoid arthritis. A long-term study. J Hand Surg 8:848, 1983.

83. Vainio KJ: Hand. In Milch RA (ed): Surgery of Arthritis. Williams & Wilkins, 1964, p 130.

84. Vakvanen V, and Talbroth K: Arthrodesis of the wrist by external fixation in rheumatoid arthritis: a follow-up study of forty-five consecutive cases. J Hand Surg 9A:531, 1984.

85. Vaughan-Jackson OJ: Rupture of extensor tendons by attrition at the inferior radioulnar joint. J Bone Joint Surg 30B:528, 1948.

86. Vaughan-Jackson OJ: Tendon ruptures in the hand. Hand 1:122, 1969.

87. Volz RG: Total wrist arthroplasty. Clin Orthop 128:180, 1978.

88. Volz RG: Total wrist arthroplasty. A review of 100 patients. Orthop Trans 3:268, 1979.

89. Volz RG: Total wrist arthroplasty. A clinical review. Clin Orthop 187:112, 1984.

90. Watson HK: Personal communication, 1984.

91. Youm Y, McCurtry RY, Flatt AE, et al: Kinematics of the wrist. I. J Bone Joint Surg 60A:423, 1978.

92. Zancolli E: Structural and Dynamic Basis of Hand Surgery. Philadelphia, JB Lippincott Co, 1972.

CHAPTER 25

Arthrodesis of the Rheumatoid Wrist: Indications and Surgical Technique

EDWARD A. NALEBUFF, M.D., JOHN F. FATTI, M.D., and CRAIG E. WEIL, M.D.

INTRODUCTION

A stable, pain-free wrist is a necessary pre-requisite for normal hand function. It is commonly agreed that if the wrist joint has been destroyed by arthritic processes, a "salvage" procedure such as arthroplasty or arthrodesis is indicated. In patients with moderate wrist deformity, good bone stock, adequate wrist motors, and a spontaneous or surgical fusion on the opposite side, a Swanson flexible implant arthroplasty is a good alternative to wrist arthrodesis. Alternatively, in those wrists with severe deformity, poor bone stock, or poor soft tissue support, arthrodesis is our choice of treatment. Because of the propensity of rheumatoid disease for affecting mainly the radiocarpal joints and for selectively sparing the midcarpal area, reconstructive procedures may only be necessary on a limited portion of the wrist joint.

Therefore, when wrist arthrodesis has been chosen as the treatment procedure, we perform either a limited (radiocarpal) wrist arthrodesis or a total wrist arthrodesis. We use Steinmann pin fixation to stabilize a total wrist fusion. Either an intermetacarpal or an intrametacarpal technique is utilized. The choice of fixation technique is dictated by certain pre-operative and intra-operative criteria that are described along with the indications and surgical details for the three types of wrist fusion procedures.

PARTIAL WRIST FUSION
(Radiocarpal)

Indications

This operation is warranted in patients whose wrist x-rays show sparing of the midcarpal joints, with destruction limited to the radiocarpal area (Fig. 25–1A). Clinically, these wrists are painful, minimally deformed, and usually retain a significant amount of mobility. Radiographs often reveal ulnar translocation of the carpus, since the main target of the rheumatoid disease is the volar supporting ligaments. The extent of ulnar translocation is best determined by checking the relationship of the lunate to the ulnar border of the distal radius.

Contraindications to this procedure include a rapidly progressive destructive rheumatoid process, nonfunctioning or ruptured wrist extensor tendons, or intra-operative discovery of significant arthritic involvement of the midcarpal joints.

Surgical Technique

The technique for achieving a limited (radiocarpal) wrist fusion begins with a longitudinal oblique dorsal skin incision, which is done more toward the radius distally and more toward the ulna proximally (Fig. 25–6A). The dorsal veins and cutaneous nerves are meticulously preserved in the subcutaneous flaps. These flaps are kept as

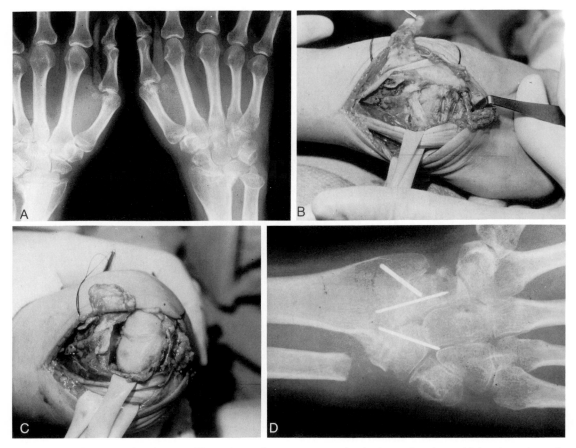

Figure 25–1. Indication and technique of limited wrist fusion. A, Patient has had an arthroplasty of left wrist and now has a painful right wrist. Note preservation of midcarpal joints and ulnar translocation. B, Dorsal radiocarpal ligament. Note preserved cartilage of the midcarpal area. C, With dorsal radiocarpal ligament divided, the proximal carpal row is exposed. Note the loss of articular cartilage. D, X-ray demonstrates improved alignment of the proximal carpal row with K-wire fixation.

thick as possible by taking the dissection directly down to the extensor retinaculum after the skin and subcutaneous tissues are incised. Dissection directly on top of the retinaculum both ulnarly and radially serves to preserve the integrity of these flaps, while minimizing the risk of injury to the cutaneous nerves. The dorsal retinaculum is next reflected as an ulnarly based flap. The extensor compartments (two through six) are opened and the tendons retracted, exposing the dorsal wrist capsule (Fig. 25–1B). The terminal portion of the posterior interosseous nerve, located at the radial side of the fourth dorsal extensor compartment, is routinely divided 3 cm proximal to the wrist joint. The dorsal wrist capsule, including the dorsal radiocarpal ligament, is transversely divided and left as a distally based flap, as the radiocarpal and midcarpal joints are exposed. To increase exposure, the distal

ulna is resected if it is unstable or if it is a source of pain, as determined pre-operatively. Care is taken to preserve the ulnocarpal ligaments for later reconstruction.

With the radiocarpal joint exposed, the remaining articular cartilage and subchondral bone are removed from the distal radius, proximal scaphoid, and proximal lunate (Fig. 25–1C); this procedure is facilitated by acute wrist flexion. The ulnarly translocated radiocarpal joint is shifted radially into a more anatomic position. Multiple Kirschner wires are passed from the radius into the scaphoid and lunate, with care taken not to enter into the distal carpal row (Fig. 25–1D). Bone chips obtained from the distal ulnar resection or from a window in the distal radius adjacent to Lister's tubercle are added to the fusion site. If preservation of the articular surface of the scaphoid is discovered intra-operatively, only a solitary radi-

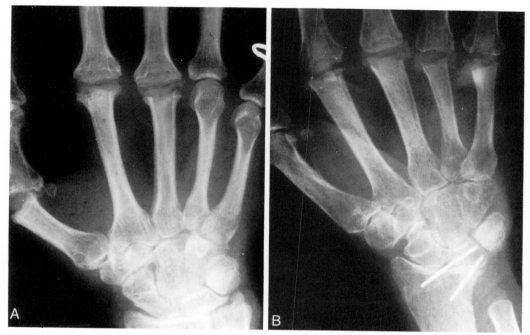

Figure 25–2. An example of radiolunate fusion. *A,* Note narrowing of the radiolunate joint with ulnar translocation. *B,* Ulnar translocation is corrected. Note preservation of the articular cartilage between the scaphoid and the radius.

olunate arthrodesis is performed (Fig. 25–2). This halts continued ulnar translocation of the wrist, while preserving more motion than a total radiocarpal arthrodesis. This approach has recently been advocated by Chamay and associates[4] and by Linscheid and Dobyns.[3]

Postoperatively, a volar plaster splint with the wrist in neutral position is used until suture removal. A short-arm plaster cast is then applied for six weeks. The status of the fusion is radiographically evaluated, and the Kirschner wires are removed if healing is progressing as anticipated. Gentle range-of-motion exercises for the wrist are then instituted, but a volar wrist splint is worn between exercise periods until the fusion is shown radiographically to be complete (Fig. 25–3).

TOTAL WRIST ARTHRODESIS

Indications

Total wrist arthrodesis is indicated in the significantly deformed rheumatoid wrist with poor quality bone stock and limited soft tissue support. When wrist extensor tendons are ruptured or nonfunctioning, an increasing deformity can be anticipated. A patient with this amount of wrist disease is not a candidate for a reconstructive procedure that preserves motion.[5, 6] In addition, when radiographic evaluation discloses destruction of both the radiocarpal and midcarpal joints, the wrist is no longer considered suitable for a limited carpal fusion. In our opinion, a history of a previous wrist joint infection or the permanent need for crutch support also precludes wrist arthroplasty as a reconstructive procedure, making total wrist arthrodesis our choice in this situation.[7]

Once this decision is made, there are several methods to choose from to accomplish this goal. Since 1965, the method used almost exclusively by one of the authors (Nalebuff) has involved Steinmann pin internal fixation.[7] This method's advantage is its relative simplicity, allowing other procedures to be performed concomitantly. This fusion technique also allows for a briefer period of postoperative immobilization (approximately three weeks in a short-arm splint). Other techniques that require longer periods in an arm cast postoperatively increase morbidity, may lead to joint stiffness and muscle weakness, and prevent patients who need crutches from walking until the cast is removed.

We use two different methods for Steinmann pin fixation in our total wrist arthro-

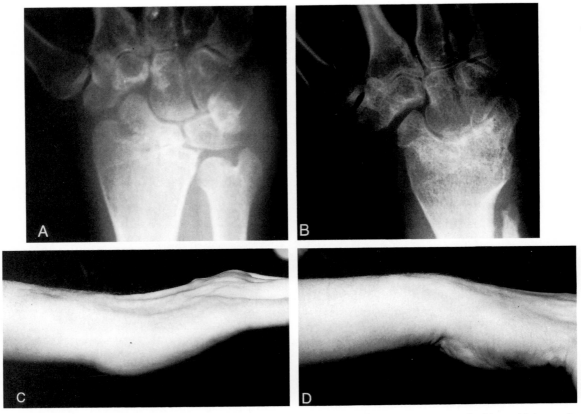

Figure 25–3. Another example of limited wrist fusion. *A,* Pre-operative x-ray demonstrates preserved midcarpal joints and ulnar translocation of the carpus. *B,* Postoperative x-ray demonstrates solid fusion with improved carpal alignment. *C,* Early postoperative wrist extension. *D,* Postoperative wrist flexion.

desis. One calls for placement of the distal aspect of the Steinmann pin between the second and third metacarpal (intermetacarpal arthrodesis), whereas the other method calls for placement of the pin within the medullary canal of the third metacarpal (intrametacarpal arthrodesis)[8] (Fig. 25–4). When a substantial amount of carpus remains for bone fixation distally, the *intermetacarpal technique of total wrist fusion* is employed. This is also the method chosen if the third metacarpophalangeal joint is functioning well and not deemed expendable. This technique is our choice if the medullary canals of the metacarpals are particularly narrow, as is commonly seen in former juvenile arthritis patients. In this situation, the small-diameter Steinmann pin that is needed to enter the medullary canal of the metacarpal would fit loosely in the radius, and solid fixation would not be obtained.

However, in wrists with severe bone loss, distal stability must be gained by inserting the Steinmann pin within the shaft of the third metacarpal (Fig. 25–5). This is known as the *intrametacarpal wrist fusion technique.* The added bone fixation with the pin in this intramedullary position is mandatory in patients with the "arthritis mutilans" variant, because the carpus may be completely destroyed, and the attempted fusion is essentially between the radius and the bases of the metacarpals.

Surgical Technique—Intermetacarpal

The operation is performed through the same dorsal incision described earlier in this chapter. Once the retinaculum is prepared for relocation, the distal ulna is excised and the radiocarpal joints exposed; traction and moderate flexion of the carpus facilitate removal of synovium, remaining cartilage, and subchondral bone. A flat surface over the distal end of the radius is fashioned to match a similar flat surface of the proximal aspect of the remaining carpus. A small oscillating saw is helpful in forming these surfaces.

The medullary canal of the radius is entered with a pointed awl, and the largest-

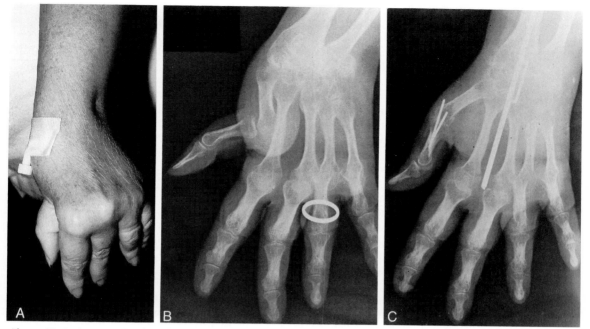

Figure 25–4. An example of total wrist fusion with intermetacarpal technique. *A*, pre-operative appearance of the wrist. Note ulnar shift of the carpus. *B*, X-ray demonstrates severe deformity. Midcarpal joints are severely involved. *C*, Postoperative x-ray shows improved wrist alignment, with Steinmann pin fixation between the second and third metacarpals.

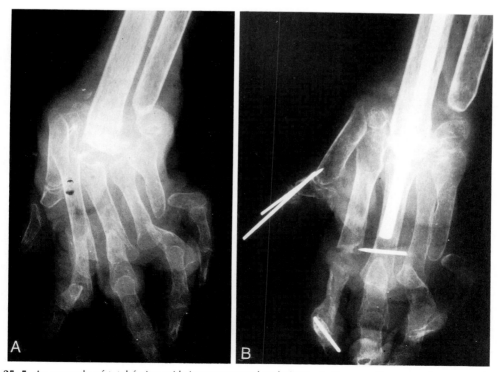

Figure 25–5. An example of total fusion with intrametacarpal technique. *A*, Pre-operative x-ray shows complete loss of the carpus. *B*, Postoperative fixation with a large Steinmann pin. Transverse K wire is used to prevent distal migration.

sized Steinmann pin that can be inserted by hand into the medullary canal of the radius is selected. The length of the pin (to be cut later) is also determined. The pin is then removed from the radius and placed on a power drill. With the wrist in flexion and the tool aimed toward the space between the second and third metacarpal heads, the pin is carefully drilled distally through the carpus. It is critical that the pin be parallel with the metacarpal shaft to avoid unwanted lateral deviation of the hand when the pin is finally reinserted into the radius. After emerging through the skin between the metacarpal heads, the pin is withdrawn until the tip is flush with the proximal aspect of the carpus. The pin is cut distally to the appropriate length so that it can be buried in the distal intermetacarpal space upon completion of the procedure.

After bone chips from the distal ulna or the resected radial styloid are added to the radiocarpal space, the pin is tapped into the radius and countersunk into the intermeta-

carpal space. Careful tapping, instead of drilling, of the rod into the radius will prevent its perforating the cortex of the radius. To provide additional fixation, a bone staple or obliquely placed Kirschner wire can be used but is seldom needed if a large enough pin is chosen. Correct alignment of the hand in relationship to the forearm should be confirmed before final tapping of the pin between the metacarpal heads.

Surgical Technique—Intramedullary

The same techniques as those described previously are used to gain exposure and to prepare the bone surfaces of the radiocarpal joint. Again, the Steinmann pin is hand-placed into the medullary canal of the radius in order to determine the length of the pin that it will accept (Fig. 25–6B). The total pin length is determined by whether or not a simultaneous metacarpophalangeal (MP) arthroplasty is to be performed; in that case, the distal end of the Steinmann pin must be

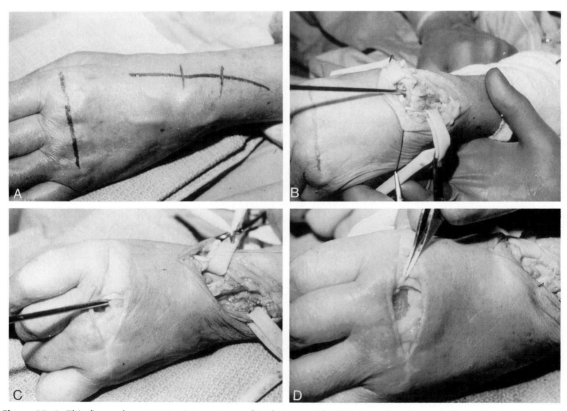

Figure 25–6. This figure demonstrates intrametacarpal technique with MP joint arthroplasty. *A,* Typical wrist incision for limited or total wrist fusion. *B,* Steinmann pin is inserted into the radius to predetermine length. *C,* Final insertion of Steinmann pin via the third metacarpal head, prepared for prosthesis insertion. *D,* Note Swanson prosthesis inserted after Steinmann pin wrist fixation.

finally countersunk sufficiently to allow the proximal stem of a prosthesis to be inserted, and this factor must be considered in the final determination of pin length. In contrast to the "retrograde" intermetacarpal technique, the Steinmann pin is directly inserted into the canal of the metacarpal through the resected head (Fig. 25–6C). It is then tapped into the prepared opening in the radius. When it is fully inserted, there should be just sufficient space to accommodate the proximal stem of a prosthesis (Fig. 25–6D). If the MP joint is not yet in need of replacement, the Steinmann pin can still be introduced through the distal articular surface of the metacarpal, which is opened with a small awl. The defect produced later becomes covered with fibrocartilage. If the MP joint is pristine, one can avoid its penetration by using the intramedullary Rush rod technique, as advocated by Mannerfelt and Malmsten.[9] This method allows more leeway in determining wrist position, since the flexible pin can be bent to provide wrist extension. However, it is more difficult to insert than a Steinmann pin and may not provide as rigid fixation. In addition, we have seen considerable erosion of the metacarpal shaft following its use.

Comparisons: Intermetacarpal and Intrametacarpal Methods

The intrametacarpal method is technically easier to perform than the intermetacarpal method, and good alignment is assured by lining up the medullary canals of the third metacarpal and the radius. With the latter technique, care must be used to avoid aligning the wrist in exaggerated ulnar deviation, which can occur if the pin is not inserted parallel to the third metacarpal shaft. In both methods, the ideal pin size is determined by the size of the medullary canal of the radius. In the intramedullary method, it may be necessary to use a smaller-diameter pin, thus reducing the fixation. Late removal of the pin is often necessary but easy to accomplish with the intermetacarpal method. The intramedullary pin is not ordinarily removed, but this can be done with difficulty, if required.

Both angular deformities and lateral shift of the carpus in relation to the radius can be corrected with these two methods of total wrist fusion. Because of the rigidity of the Steinmann pin, the wrist is automatically held in neutral flexion-extension. This has been found to be an excellent wrist position for most rheumatoid patients.[10] By adjustment of the osteotomy planes and the direction of the Steinmann pin as it is driven into the radius, the surgeon can vary the degree of flexion or extension of the wrist, but only by 5 to 10 degrees. However, most activities can be carried out by the patient with the wrist in a neutral or slightly flexed position.

Aftercare

Postoperatively, a bulky dressing and a volar plaster splint are applied. A solid plaster cast is not needed or advisable because of swelling of the wrist. We change the dressing and the splint the following day. The wrist is continuously splinted for two to three weeks, but finger and thumb motion are encouraged from the beginning. After two to three weeks, the patient is either weaned from the volar wrist splint, or it is simply discarded.

Patients who required crutches pre-operatively are instructed in the use of platform crutches, which are utilized for several months until the fusion has consolidated. Steinmann pin removal has not been routinely performed but can be done as early as four months after the procedure, if discomfort so dictates.

CONCLUSION

Pain relief, stability, and strength are important goals in any reconstructive procedure for the rheumatoid wrist. When the wrist demonstrates relative midcarpal sparing from rheumatoid arthritic destruction, partial wrist fusion can accomplish these goals, while preserving some motion. It is an excellent alternative to arthroplasty, if the condition of the wrist warrants it. Total wrist arthrodesis, accomplished by one of the two methods described that use the Steinmann pin, restores stability and strength to those rheumatoid wrists with more significant deformity and destruction.

References

1. Taleisnik J: Rheumatoid arthritis of the wrist. In Strickland JW, and Steichen JB (eds): Difficult Problems in Hand Surgery. St Louis, CV Mosby Co, 1982.

2. Nalebuff EA, and Garrod KJ: Present approach to the severely involved rheumatoid wrist. Orthop Clin North Am 15(2):369–380, 1984.

3. Linscheid RL, and Dobyns JH: Radiolunate Arthrodesis. Hand Surg 10A6:821–829, 1985.

4. Chamay A, Della Santa D, and Vilaseca A: Radiolunate arthrodesis, factor of stability for the rheumatoid wrist. Ann Chir Main 2:5–17, 1983.

5. Flatt AE: Care of the Arthritic Hand. 4th ed, St Louis, CV Mosby Co, 1983.

6. Carroll RE, and Dick HM: Arthrodesis of the wrist for rheumatoid arthritis. J Bone Joint Surg 53A:1365–1369, 1971.

7. Millender LH, and Nalebuff EA: Arthrodesis of the rheumatoid wrist. Bone Joint Surg 55A:1026–1034, 1973.

8. Millender LH, Nalebuff EA, and Feldon PG: Rheumatoid arthritis. In Green D (ed): Operative Hand Surgery. New York, Churchill Livingstone Inc, 1982, pp 1161–1262.

9. Mannerfelt L, and Malmsten M: Arthrodesis of the wrist in rheumatoid arthritis: a technique without external fixation. Scand Plast Reconstr Surg 5:124–130, 1971.

10. Linscheid RL, and Dobyns JH: Rheumatoid arthritis of the wrist. Orthop Clin North Am 2:649–665, 1971.

CHAPTER 26

Tumors of the Wrist

GEORGE P. BOGUMILL, Ph.D., M.D.

With the exception of the ubiquitous ganglion, tumors and tumorous conditions of the wrist are distinctly uncommon.[6] The true incidence of such lesions is almost impossible to ascertain, because most reports include them with lesions of the hand in general and do not restrict their description to those of the wrist alone. As is true of the hand, most lesions that occur in or about the wrist are benign, although malignancies do appear sporadically. Lesions may occur at any age, and size alone gives no specific clues as to whether they are benign or malignant. The majority of lesions arise in local tissues, although they may be associated with a generalized metabolic disorder, such as gout or xanthomatosis, or develop following trauma (e.g., a foreign-body granuloma).

Some of the smaller, more superficial lesions may be readily treated in outpatient surgery units; however, this presupposes that there is an adequate operating room with good lighting and good instruments as well as trained staff. Pre-operative evaluation of the lesion includes a carefully taken history, in which are recorded symptoms such as pain and numbness, duration of the lesion, history of trauma, and any other related factors. A careful general physical examination should include evaluation of the epitrochlear and axillary nodes. Laboratory studies and x-ray evaluations should be done prior to biopsy; these may rarely include CT scans, tomograms, arteriograms, and bone scans. A chest x-ray should be done if there is any suspicion that the lesion may be malignant.

Adequate anesthesia at the time of surgery is necessary. This may occasionally be local anesthesia, but the patient will frequently require axillary block or even general anesthesia. Use of the pneumatic tourniquet has been questioned because of the fear of aggre-

gates of cells being trapped at the level of the tourniquet and then freed as an embolus at the time of tourniquet release. Others argue that with no blood flow, the likelihood of individual cells or clusters of cells being washed the full length of the extremity to the tourniquet is unlikely, and that the benefits to be gained by operating in a bloodless field outweigh the theoretical risks of tumor aggregates.

A nerve stimulator is occasionally useful. One must remember that nerves stop conducting after the tourniquet has been in place for 15 or 20 minutes.

Standard extensile skin incisions and closures are used where possible but may need to be modified, depending on the location of the tumor or of a previous biopsy.

A full catalogue of the lesions that might possibly appear in the wrist would be impractical and would serve no useful purpose. Therefore, the discussion here will be limited to some of the more common entities.

BENIGN SOFT TISSUE LESIONS

Lesions of Synovial Tissues

The dorsal wrist ganglion (Fig. 26–1A) arising from the capsule over the scapholunate joint is the most common tumor in the hand in all reported series.[1, 2, 4, 6, 10, 18, 21] It can appear in patients of almost any age, but tends to predominate during the third to fifth decades. It is rare in old age and infancy. Two thirds to three fourths occur in women. Although it may disappear spontaneously, particularly in children, it usually persists for prolonged periods. The main symptom or presenting complaint is usually a painless mass. There is a history of trauma in approximately one third of these patients. Weakness of grip, occasional pain when the

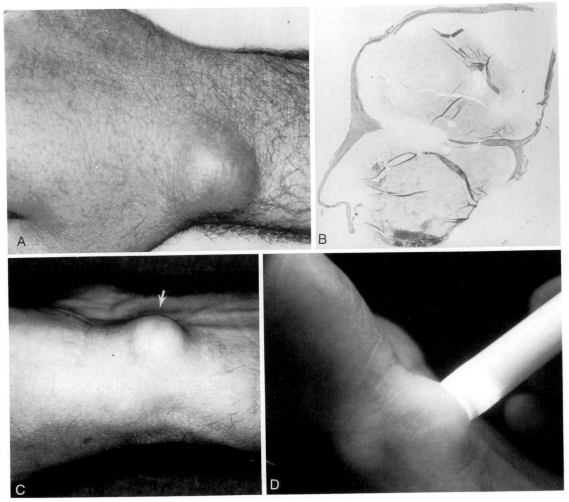

Figure 26–1. Ganglion. *A,* Typical dorsal wrist ganglion in the classic location. *B,* Microscopic section of the ganglion. The apparent trabeculation and multiloculation are deceiving; ganglia almost always have a single cavity. *C,* Volar wrist ganglion in the typical position. *Arrow* indicates a previous attempt at surgical excision. *D,* Transillumination of the ganglion confirms the diagnosis.

ganglion first appears, and, rarely, paresthesias or paralysis from nerve compression or irritation may bring the patient to see the doctor.

Most volar wrist ganglia also originate from the wrist joint capsule (Fig. 26–1B and C). Some originate from the trapezioscaphoid joint. They usually appear near the radial artery and may cause compression of it or distortion of its pathway. They may also be found in the carpal tunnel or in Guyon's canal, with compression of the deep branch of the ulnar nerve (Fig. 26–2A). A ganglion may dissect medially or laterally for a distance to reach the subcutaneous regions. Typically there is a single ganglion cavity, which is filled with a mucinous material. It may appear to be loculated but seldom has

true compartmentation (Fig. 26–1B). Early in its course, the wall of the ganglion is quite thin and easily ruptured; however, with the passage of time, the wall becomes thicker and more resilient. Even then, the wall is easily transilluminated with a penlight, the classic diagnostic test (Fig. 26–1D).

The etiology of ganglia is still being debated. The commonly accepted theory of causation involves remodeling of the fibrous capsular tissue of the joint.[2, 18, 23] Collagen fiber breakdown products and intercellular mucin collect in microscopic pools; as these collections of mucin coalesce and expand, dissecting toward the subcutaneous tissues, fibrous tissue around them is compacted, creating a pseudocapsule. Initially, the pseudocapsule is thin and easily ruptured, but with time it thickens, and then aspiration or rupture of the ganglion is usually not successful in preventing recurrence. Likewise resection of the ganglion may not be curative if the capsule adjacent to the stalk attachment is not also removed. This capsular tissue, which is also remodelling, could be the source of a new, not a truly recurrent, ganglion.

There have been many attempts to inject ganglia with radiopaque or colored dyes, in an effort to see if the dye will pass from the ganglion into the adjacent joint. This has been quite uniformly unsuccessful. However, Andren and Eiken[1] injected the wrist on the aspect opposite the ganglion until the joint space became distended. A significant percentage of the ganglia filled with dye from the joint, suggesting a one-way valve effect.

Treatment of a ganglion is also controversial.[2, 4, 8, 10, 18, 23] Aspiration or rupture by striking with a heavy book, the so-called Bible treatment, is followed by recurrence in more than 50 per cent of cases. Injection of sclerosing agents or steroids is followed by recurrence in 40 to 50 per cent of patients. Surgical excision under adequate anesthesia and tourniquet control with removal of a portion of the joint capsule has reduced the recurrence rate to 15 per cent or lower. When removing a volar ganglion, the surgeon should be prepared to identify the stalk at its origin, which at times requires an extensive dissection. Many surgeons (and patients) question the need for treatment at all, since the risks associated with surgery may indeed be more undesirable than the mild cosmetic deformity and minimal symptoms associated with the presence of the lesion.

Giant cell tumors of the tendon sheath, known by a variety of names, are much more common in the fingers than about the wrist, but they may arise in association with any of the synovial tendon sheaths on either the flexor or the extensor side. These lesions are benign growths containing numerous histiocytes and foreign-body giant cells adjacent to hemosiderin deposits from minor bleeding episodes secondary to trauma. When tendon sheath tumors do appear about the wrist, like those appearing around the fingers, they usually have a long history by the time they are brought to the attention of a doctor because they are slow-growing, painless masses. They may be large enough or have enough active circulation to cause hyperemic removal of adjacent bones, but this is uncommon.

Simple excision is the treatment of choice.

Lesions of Fat

Lipomas are common in the hand and usually appear in areas where fat normally is found in relatively large quantities, such as the thenar or hypothenar eminences or the mid-palm.[6, 15] Ordinarily, there is not much fat around the wrist, but occasionally a lipoma may arise there or extend there from the hand or forearm. A lipoma may be a surprise finding during carpal tunnel release, and there are numerous reports of large lipomas in the median nerve.[9, 17]

Lipomas are usually soft, lobulated, and slow-growing. Radiographically, they have the typical density of fat and are shaped by the surrounding tissues, such as the thenar space. They have a thin capsule and are quite clearly defined from the surrounding tissues. Deeper masses tend to follow the tissue planes and may extend far proximal or distal into the palm or hand. When they are widely spread or arborized, excision is very difficult and requires great patience. On rare occasions, the basic fatty tissue undergoes metaplastic change and appears as a mixture of fat and myxoid material and, if traumatized, may actually undergo osseous metaplasia (Fig. 26–2B through D). Of course, when that happens, the change is usually visible on radiograph.

Lesions of Vessels

Cavernous and capillary hemangiomas are very common around the hand and are frequently seen about the wrist. They can vary considerably in size and in symptoms. Related to the complex development of the vascular tree, angiomas can be predominantly cavernous (Fig. 26–3A) or capillary. Marginal excision of small, well-defined lesions is usually simple, and there is usually no recurrence. Larger lesions may extend widely into surrounding tissues, such as muscle, and be very difficult to eradicate without significant functional loss. Serious consideration and extensive experience are advised if one is contemplating surgical treatment of cavernous angiomas.

Arteriovenous shunts are common and are characterized by large dilated veins caused by the prompt shunting of the blood from

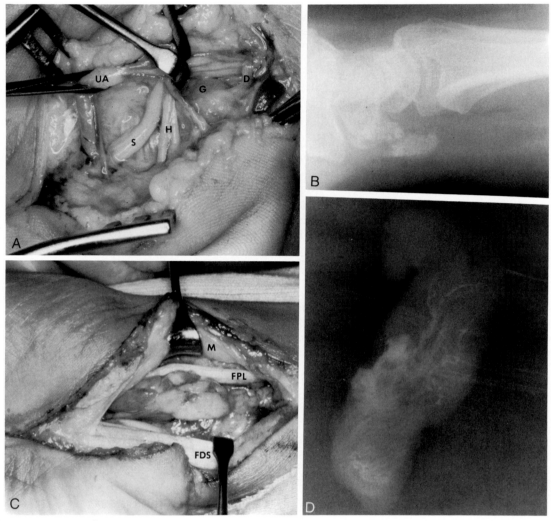

Figure 26–2. *A,* Ganglion compressing the deep branch of the motor nerve in Guyon's canal. *B,C,D,* Myxolipoma in the carpal canal. Lateral x-ray of ossifying myxolipoma illustrates its tenuous connection to the volar surface of the capitate (*B*); Myxolipoma presenting between flexor pollicis longus and flexor digitorum superficialis, after division of the flexor retinaculum (*C*); Lacy mineralization throughout the lesion proved to be bone on H & E preparation (*D*). D-deep motor branch of ulnar nerve; FDS-flexor digitorum superficialis; FPL-flexor pollicis longus; G = ganglion arising from hamate metacarpal joint; H-branch of ulnar nerve to hypothenar eminence; M-median nerve; S-sensory branch of ulnar nerve; U-ulnar artery.

artery to vein. These anomalous shunts can be either congenital or acquired. When the shunt is congenital, the vessels have histologic characteristics of both artery and vein in the same vessel.[5] The true nature of the vascular lesion is often best demonstrated by an arteriogram. The concern of major importance in arteriovenous fistulas is to recognize them as such and to avoid ligating the feeder vessels. The arterial head of pressure may be essential for perfusion of distal tissues; ligation of the feeder vessel often results in tissue infarction. Partial rather than thorough limb exsanguination prior to

inflation of the tourniquet facilitates dissection and ligation of associated feeder and drainage vessels.

Thromboses of vessels are frequently of concern to the patient; they manifest as firm, nontender masses. They are most common following intravenous infusions but may occur spontaneously following trauma. Aneurysms also tend to appear following trauma; the most common site for this to occur is the hypothenar area, owing to repeated use of this region when applying blows with the hand (Fig. 26–3B).

Glomus tumors have been described in

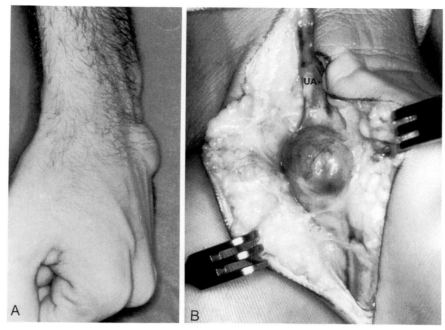

Figure 26–3. *A*, Cavernous hemangioma. This lesion consisted primarily of a large sacular dilatation that filled with blood when the hand was dependent and emptied readily when the hand was elevated. *B*, Aneurysm in the ulnar artery. This aneurysm appeared following repeated trauma to the heel of the hand while the patient was playing pinball machines for prolonged periods. UA-ulnar artery.

the carpal area.[12] As in the fingers, diagnosis is difficult and delayed because the lesion is small and seldom palpable. Also, it is seldom considered in the differential diagnosis of wrist and hand pain. Simple excision is curative, although multiple lesions do occur.

Lesions of Nerves

The most common lesion at the wrist, as elsewhere, is a traumatic neuroma following section of the nerve, with or without repair. They can be quite large but are usually diagnosed by history and by a positive percussion test result.

Any of the nerves crossing the wrist can give rise to either a neurofibroma or a neurilemoma[11, 19, 26, 27] (Fig. 26–4). The latter lesion is often associated with pain, tenderness, and paresthesias. It is usually readily shelled from the nerve without significant damage. It arises from Schwann's cells and is usually composed of two distinct types of tissue: The Antoni A cells compose the more solid portions of the tumor; they are well defined, orderly groups of cells and fibers. The Antoni B cells are in areas of myxomatous degeneration, leading to looser texture and haphazard fiber and cell arrangement, with sparse cellularity. These areas actually break down and form cystic areas that may coalesce into one large cyst with loss of the typical structure of the neurilemoma. This may be the origin of case reports of intraneural ganglia.

The neurofibroma originates from the fibrous tissue of the epineurium or endoneurium and tends to infiltrate more thoroughly between the nerve bundles. It is less clearly defined and, therefore, impossible to remove without causing significant damage to the nerve in which it arises.

Lipofibroma of nerve,[16, 20] of which Déjérine-Sottas disease may be a manifestation, is a hamartomatous enlargement of the median nerve, often accompanied by macrodactyly of fingers or of portions of the hand. It is fortunately a very rare condition, but causes great problems in treatment. Attempts have been made to excise the involved portion of the nerve and to use a nerve graft to bridge the resulting defect. The recommended treatment at present, however, is merely carpal tunnel release, possibly combined with an epineurotomy of the median nerve. Excision of the lesion without removing the nerve is impossible.

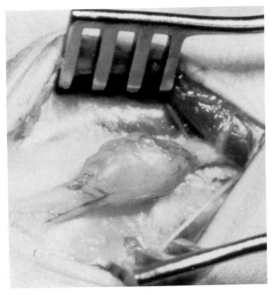

Figure 26–4. Neurilemoma in median nerve. This enlargement of the median nerve was a surprise finding at carpal tunnel release for median nerve compression. It was readily dissected from the nerve with no loss of nerve function.

Fibrous Lesions

This group includes a wide gamut of lesions, both benign and malignant. Stout, in 1954,[25] and Soule, in 1956,[24] tried to classify these lesions to bring order out of chaos, but there is still a great deal of difficulty in defining the borderline between the well differentiated fibrosarcoma and the benign but aggressive fibrous lesion.

Fibrous lesions can occur in the skin or the immediate subdermal tissues (Fig. 26–5A and B); these lesions are relatively common, may be single or multiple, and are usually self-limited and benign. Most fibrous lesions are poorly circumscribed because of the very nature of the tissue of which they are composed. They tend to infiltrate the adjacent fibrous planes, and it is almost impossible to identify this spread with the naked eye. Many of these lesions tend to be quite cellular and locally invasive; they may or may not have fine stippled calcifications, but this is usually not enough to be evident radiographically. They may be fixed to deeper structures, and unlike most of the other lesions, seldom have a pseudocapsule.

Lesions of the Skin

To my knowledge, there are no specific lesions that are more apt to occur in the region of the wrist than anywhere else. The whole range of benign to malignant lesions can be seen on either dorsal or palmar aspects of the wrist. The malignant lesions tend to create problems with treatment, because the wrist area is not usually considered a compartment; all of the structures from the forearm to the hand pass through the wrist area, and a localized resection is very difficult to accomplish. Malignancy that invades the deeper tissues usually requires amputation through the forearm rather than localized resection (Fig. 26–11B).

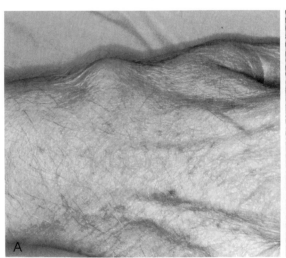
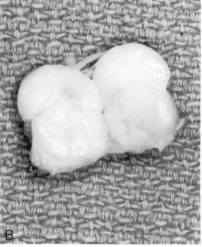

Figure 26–5. Fibroma. *A,* This mass appeared and grew rapidly over a period of three or four months in a 76-year-old man who had severe involvement of Dupuytren's disease in both hands. *B,* Cut section of the mass showed a glistening, white, shiny surface; it appeared to be well contained within a pseudocapsule.

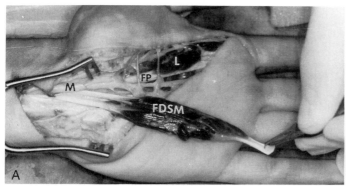
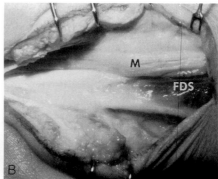

Figure 26–6. A, Anomalous muscle belly presented in the hand of an 18-year-old male who had symptoms consistent with carpal tunnel syndrome for three months. B, Prolongation of the flexor digitorum superficialis muscle belly into the carpal tunnel is a relatively frequent cause of carpal tunnel syndrome. FDS-flexor digitorum superficialis; FDSM-flexor digitorum superficialis manus; FP-flexor digitorum profundus; L-first lumbrical; M-median nerve.

Lesions of Muscle

The most common presenting mass of muscle tissue is usually normal muscle in an abnormal location (Fig. 26–6); for example, the extension of a flexor digitorum superficialis muscle belly into the carpal tunnel may present diagnostic problems or may cause carpal tunnel syndrome (Fig. 26–6B). Likewise, a muscle originating in the palm and extending proximally into the carpal tunnel can cause symptoms of median nerve compression (Fig. 26–6A). Tumors of muscle are decidedly rare.

BENIGN LESIONS OF THE WRIST SKELETON

Lesions of the Distal Radius and Ulna

A wide variety of lesions can be seen in either of these bones. The distal radius is one of the more common locations of the benign giant cell tumor of bone. Since it is not a weight-bearing bone, resection and grafting are the preferred treatments. The choice of source for graft tissue varies considerably among different surgeons, with fibula, tibia, iliac crest, and even allograft tissue being used. Curettage, with or without bone grafting, tends to be a less common operation, and is usually reserved for lesions that are quite small. Bone cysts, nonossifying fibromata, and a wide variety of other benign lesions can be found in either of these bones and are treated with conventional measures, usually curettage. Metastatic disease is relatively frequent, not as an isolated metastasis, but as part of a generalized metastatic disease, particularly from the breast.

Lesions of the Carpal Bones

A wide variety of accessory bones occurs in the carpal area; some of them are common enough to be named, such as the os epilunatum (Fig. 26–8A). Some can actually become large enough to be palpated as excrescences, the most common being the metacarpal boss at the base of the third or occasionally the second metacarpal.

Lytic (cystic) lesions are very common in the carpal bones. Radiographically, they usually present as rounded lucencies that are sharply demarcated by an endosteal reinforced trabecular margin (Fig. 26–7). They usually contain mucinous material and probably represent degenerative cysts. Occasionally, they are called intraosseous ganglia,[13] and since they originate in the same location as the routine ganglia (Fig. 26–7C and D), they may indeed be similar to such entities, in that they represent remodeling of the bone and capsular tissues.

Cartilaginous lesions, such as benign enchondromas, are relatively common and are frequently seen in conjunction with other enchondromas in the hand skeleton. Osteochondromas are quite unusual but can occur in the wrist as they do in the foot.

Osteoblastic lesions vary from the benign inactive bone island (Fig. 26–8C and D) or osteoma (Fig. 26–8B) to aggressive, fortunately rare, osteosarcoma. Bone islands are common, can occur in any carpal bone, are usually asymptomatic, and are picked up as incidental findings. Occasionally, one may be "hot" on bone scan, but more frequently, where there is increased radionuclide uptake, it represents a more active process such as an osteoid osteoma (Fig. 26–9). For some

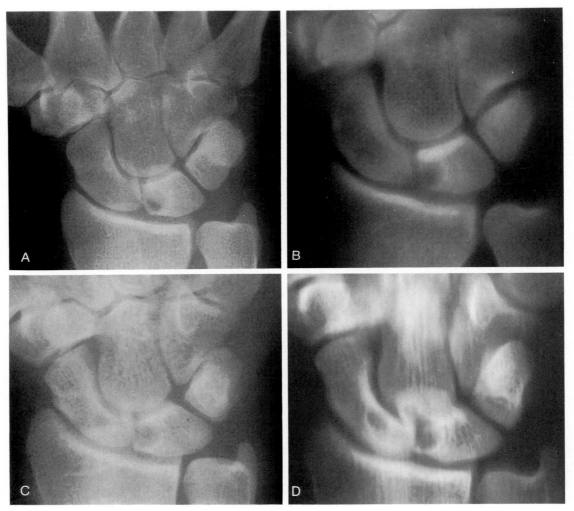

Figure 26–7. Examples of cystic lesions in bone. *A,C,* Plain films of two patients with well-defined cystic lesions. *B,D,* Tomograms through these areas. Note the rim of endosteal bone outlining the cysts.

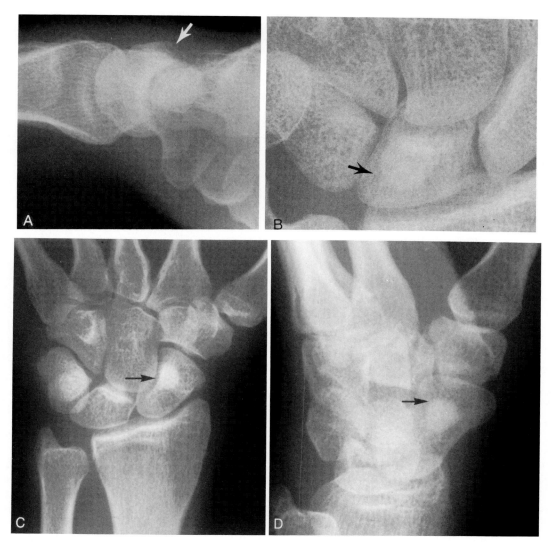

Figure 26–8. *A,* Os epilunatum. An example of an accessory ossicle occurring about the wrist. Such ossicles are quite common, and many have been given names. The arrow indicates the ossicle overlying the lunate bone dorsally. This patient also had a ganglion adjacent to this accessory bone. *B,* Osteoma, lunate bone. Histologic examination showed that this lesion consisted of portions of very dense reactive bone, without significant medullary space. Portions of this reactive bone showed avascular necrosis. *C,D,* Bone island. This lesion was present in a 16-year-old girl who had had symptoms in her wrist for three years. The lesion was "warm" on bone scan but did not change in appearance over a three-year period.

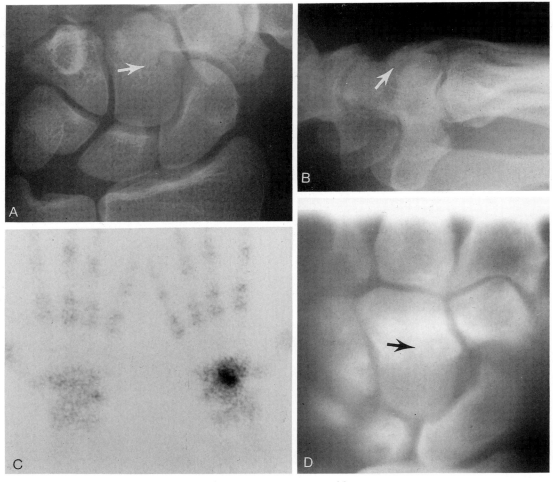

Figure 26–9. Osteoid osteoma of the capitate. *A,B,* AP and lateral radiographs of a relatively dense island of bone surrounded by a lucent zone and increased reactive sclerosis in the spongiosa of the capitate. *C,* Bone scan showed significant radionuclide uptake in the center of the wrist. *D,* Tomograms delineate the osteoid osteoma nidus clearly (*arrow*).

reason, osteoid osteoma is not an infrequent finding in the wrist area. It usually manifests with pain that is relieved more or less completely by salicylates. A tomogram or CT scan may be necessary to delineate the nidus. It is not unusual for symptoms to be present for a year or more before a diagnosis is made. Curettage of the nidus is curative.

Lesions of the Metacarpals

These short, tubular bones are prey to any of the lesions that one can find in the long tubular bones. Enchondromas are particularly common, but osteochondromas are not rare. Giant cell tumors are also quite common in the metacarpals, usually appearing in the metaphysis, which is located at the distal end of the bone. Simple curettage has

been condemned as leading to higher than 90 per cent recurrence;[3] however, that has not been my personal experience. A trial of thorough curettage, opening the cortex widely enough to see the entire endosteal cavity for excision of the full extent of the lesion, and cauterizing the remaining cavity with 89 percent phenol, has resulted in prolonged freedom from the disease for periods ranging from 18 months to four years in three patients. As most recurrences happen within the first year, I am encouraged that these results may last. The surgery is less disabling than attempts at resection, particularly of centrally placed metacarpals. Bone grafting these lesions has not been shown to be helpful, since the metacarpals are not weight-bearing bones. There is usually enough structural stability remaining after

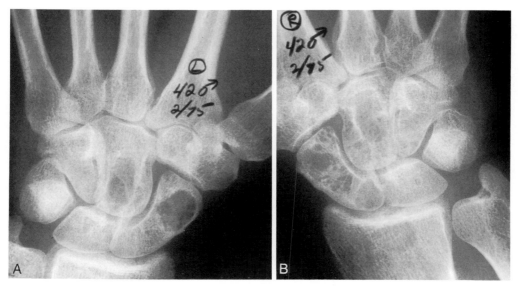

Figure 26–10. A, B, Amyloid deposits from widespread multiple myeloma. The erosions seen in the carpal bones were detected during work-up for carpal tunnel syndrome. Numerous amyloid deposits were also found in and around the flexor tendons passing through the carpal tunnel.

curettage to preserve length and shape until the body can refill the canal with normal bone, which it will do in a year or two.

MALIGNANT TUMORS OF THE WRIST

Such tumors are rare enough to cause problems in treatment for the surgeon who sees only an occasional malignant tumor of the extremities. Many of these tumors deserve a case report. They are usually seen early because of the superficial nature of the tissues and the fact that they cause a mass or pain; since they are found early, they have a good chance for cure. The question of incisional biopsy versus excisional biopsy continues to be debated.[21, 22] Certainly, if the lesion is large or is situated in an area in which wide resection would create considerable disability in the hand, an incisional biopsy would be appropriate. This is true for most aggressive malignant tumors but may actually be true for many benign ones as well, particularly the fibrous types of lesions. The nature of excisional biopsy in a malignant lesion usually results in a marginal resection that goes through the pseudocapsule of the tumor, thus leaving tumor cells behind. In many cases this result would make attempts at a limb-sparing procedure impossible. If the lesion is small and readily accessible in an area that can be easily removed, such as in the finger, excisional

biopsy may be acceptable; however, this is rarely the situation with regard to the wrist.

Metastatic Tumors

Although reports of metastatic tumors of the bones of the hand are quite rare,[7] a large number of malignant tumors of the wrist are metastatic.[14] There is no specific predilection of any given primary tumor to metastasize to the bones of the wrist. The incidence of any type tends to match the frequency of the tumors (breast, lung, kidney, and so forth) that metastasize to bone. When tumors do metastasize to the carpus, they tend to cause destruction in several bones simultaneously (Fig. 26–10), which is often a clue to the aggressive nature of the process. Generally, the tumor is treated systemically, although, occasionally, a local approach may be necessary for diagnostic reasons and for stabilization or pain relief.

Primary Malignant Tumors of the Wrist

Primary skeletal malignancies of the carpus are decidedly rare. Because of the central location of the wrist, in terms of structures passing through it from forearm to hand and in the reverse direction (Fig. 26–11A), a localized limb-sparing resection is seldom feasible. As in malignancies elsewhere, control of the primary tumor is usually surgical. Staging is essential to determine whether

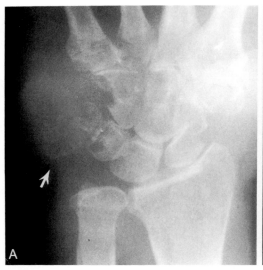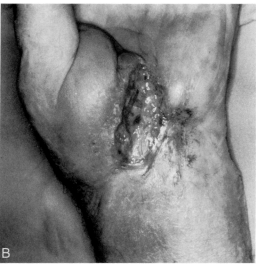

Figure 26–11. *A,* Malignant skeletal tumor with admixture of cartilage and fibrous elements. Note the aggressive nature of the lesion with erosion of multiple bones and a soft tissue mass that shows very little mineralization. Multiple bone destruction is characteristic of the more aggressive lesions, whether primary or metastatic. *B,* Squamous cell carcinoma. The central location of this lesion precludes attempts at limb-sparing procedures, because compromise in the form of resection in an effort to retain function leads to a high incidence of recurrence.

the tumor is indeed retained within a compartment, and it must also be biopsied to determine the grade. As mentioned previously, through-forearm amputation is usually required for malignancies in the region of the wrist, whether skeletal or soft tissue in origin.

References

1. Andren L, and Eiken O: Arthrographic studies of wrist ganglion. J Bone Joint Surg 53A:299–302, 1971.
2. Angelides AC, and Wallace PF: The dorsal ganglion of the wrist: its pathogenesis, gross and microscopic anatomy, and surgical treatment. J Hand Surg 1:228–235, 1976.
3. Averill RM, Smith RJ, and Campbell CC: Giant cell tumors of the bones of the hand. J Hand Surg 5:39–50, 1980.
4. Barnes WE, Larsen RD, and Posch JL: Review of ganglia of the hand and wrist with analysis of surgical treatment. Plast Reconstr Surg 34:570–578, 1964.
5. Bogumill GP: Clinico-pathological correlation in a case of congenital arterio-venous fistulae. Hand 9:60–64, 1977.
6. Bogumill GP, Sullivan DJ, and Baker GI: Tumors of the hand. Clin Orthop 108:214–222, 1975.
7. Chung TS: Metastatic malignancy to the bones of the hand. J Surg Oncol 24:99–102, 1983.
8. Crawford GP, and Taleisnik J: Rotatory subluxation of the scaphoid after excision of dorsal carpal ganglion and wrist manipulation. J Hand Surg 8:921–925, 1983.
9. Friedlander HL, Rosenberg NJ, and Graubard DJ: Intraneural lipoma of the median nerve. J Bone Joint Surg 51A:352–362, 1969.
10. Holm PCA, and Pandey SD: Treatment of ganglia of the hand and wrist with aspiration and injection of hydrocortisone. Hand 5:63–68, 1973.
11. Jenkins SA: Solitary tumors of peripheral nerve trunks. J Bone Joint Surg 34B:401–411, 1952.
12. Joseph FR, and Posner MA: Glomus tumors of the wrist. J Hand Surg 8:918–920, 1983.
13. Kambolis C, Bullough PG, and Jaffe HL: Ganglionic cystic defects of bone. J Bone Joint Surg 55A:496–505, 1973.
14. Kerin R: Metastatic tumors of the hand. A review of the literature. J Bone Joint Surg 65A:1331–1335, 1983.
15. Leffert RD: Lipomas of the upper extremity. J Bone Joint Surg 54A:1262–1266, 1972.
16. Louis DS, Dick HM: Ossifying lipofibroma of the median nerve. J Bone Joint Surg 55A:1082–1084, 1973.
17. Mikhail IK: Median nerve lipoma in the hand. J Bone Joint Surg 46B:726–730, 1964.
18. Nelson CL, Sawmiller C, and Phalen GS: Ganglions of the wrist and hand. J Bone Joint Surg 54A:1459–1464, 1972.
19. Rinaldi E: Neurilemomas and neurofibromas of the upper limb. J Hand Surg 8:590–593, 1983.
20. Rowland SA: Case report: ten year followup of lipofibroma of the median nerve in the palm. J Hand Surg 2:316–317, 1976.
21. Schultz RJ, and Kearns RJ: Tumors in the hand. J Hand Surg 8:803–806, 1983.
22. Smith RJ: Tumors of the hand. Who is best qualified to treat tumors of the hand? J Hand Surg 2:251–252, 1977.
23. Soren A: Pathogenesis and treatment of ganglion. Clin Orthop 48:173–179, 1966.
24. Soule EH: Tumors of fibrous tissues: a classification and problems in diagnosis and treatment. Am Acad Orthop Surg, Instr Course Lect XIII:265–274, 1956.
25. Stout AP: Juvenile fibromatoses. Cancer 7:953–978, 1954.
26. Strickland JW, and Steichen JB: Nerve tumors of the hand and forearm. J Hand Surg 2:285–291, 1976.
27. White NB: Neurilemomas of the extremities. J Bone Joint Surg 49A:1605–1610, 1967.

CHAPTER 27

Wrist Disorders in Children

PAUL W. ESPOSITO, M.D.
and ALVIN H. CRAWFORD, M.D.

INTRODUCTION

Fractures of the distal forearm compose an extremely high percentage of the total number of childhood upper extremity injuries. Conversely, carpal fractures and dislocations, especially with secondary chronic instability patterns, are uncommon. The treatment of distal forearm fractures and their complications is well covered in other texts. This chapter focuses on the development of the wrist, the relationship of the immature anatomy to specific injury patterns, as well as recommended treatment for specific childhood injuries. Because of the rarity of carpal fractures and of true ligamentous or carpal "sprains," this chapter emphasizes congenital, acquired, metabolic, developmental, and infectious disorders that may manifest with findings and complaints related to the wrist of a growing child.

Anatomy and Embryology

The child's wrist consists of the distal radial and ulnar metaphysis, physis, epiphysis, carpus, and metacarpal bases as well as the ligaments and the joint capsule. The carpus evolves by way of membranous ossification, with only the hamate and the capitate visible on radiographs at birth. The distal radial epiphysis ossifies at around 1 year of age. The triquetrum ossifies approximately at age 2 and a half. The lunate ossifies at age 4. The other carpal bones do not ossify until after age four. The scaphoid ossifies at approximately four and a half years of age in the female child, and at five and a half in the male, and the distal ulna at five in the female and at six in the male. There is a wide range in the time of onset of ossification with all of these centers. The pisiform does not ossify until about age 11 in males and nine in females. The variation in time of appearance of ossific centers makes interpretation of radiographs difficult and frequently mandates comparison x-ray studies of the opposite, presumed normal, side.[68]

The upper limb bud develops very early in gestation, with the structures of the wrist and hand being formed between the 20th and the 45th days. This is important for the clinician to understand, so that the frequently associated congenital defects that develop simultaneously can be recognized and treated. These wrist deformities and associated defects are discussed individually later in this chapter.

Pattern of Injury

The ligamentous attachments of the distal radius and ulna in the child attach to the epiphysis of the distal radius as well as to the carpal bones. The distal radial physis absorbs a great deal of energy during a fall on the outstretched hand prior to any bone or ligamentous injury to the carpus. This partially explains the relatively low incidence of carpal fractures in the young child, with an extremely high incidence of distal metaphyseal and physeal injuries instead. The other significant protective mechanism for the carpus is the resiliency of the carpal bones, provided by their thick, cartilaginous architecture. Conversely, a high-energy impact injury could conceivably occur prior to ossification of the carpal bones, and even with optimal evaluation and treatment, a significant long-term deformity could result. The lack of ossification can prevent diagnosis of significant ligamentous injury and instability or vascular compromise to the ossific centers of the carpus.

Other problems unique to the anatomy of the child's wrist include injuries to the radial or the ulnar physis or both. An injury to the radial physis can potentially lead to shortening or angular deformity of the distal radius, with potential for volar subluxation and proximal migration of the carpus, with overgrowth of the ulna (traumatic Madelung's deformity) (Fig. 27–1). Significant ulnar shortening from isolated traumatic growth arrest is extremely rare but has been reported. This injury in the younger child could lead to secondary bowing of the radius and to ulnar translocation of the distal radial epiphysis. In the older child, such a growth arrest may lead to an ulnar minus deformity[7, 19] (Fig. 27–2).

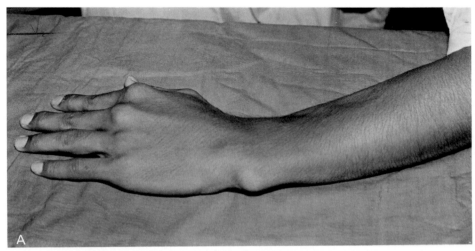

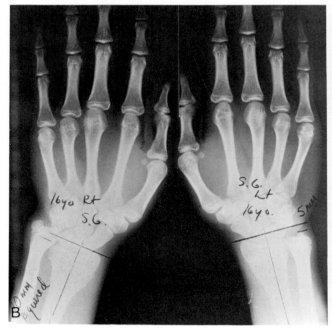

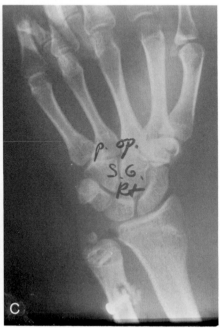

Figure 27–1. Post-traumatic Madelung's deformity. A, Clinical photo of the wrist of a 16-year-old male, three years following a distal radial physeal injury and subsequent growth arrest. There is overgrowth of the ulna relative to the radius, with radial and mild volar translocation of the wrist and hand. B, Radiographs of the same patient. There is obvious shortening of the radius and 10 mm of overgrowth of the ulna. The patient is now mature. C, Radiograph shortly following a Milch procedure, i.e., shortening of the ulnar diaphysis. In immature patients, typically under the age of 13, epiphyseal arrest of the distal ulna is also necessary to prevent recurrence.

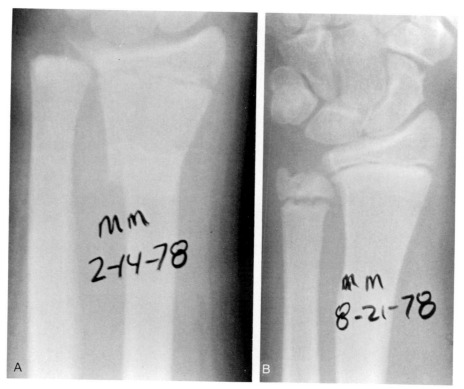

Figure 27–2. Distal ulnar growth arrest. *A,* Radiograph taken at the time of injury. Note the displaced distal radial metaphyseal fracture and a completely displaced distal ulnar physeal fracture. *B,* Radiograph taken six months after closed reduction and casting. There is widening and irregularity of the distal ulnar physis. This patient developed progressive ulnar shortening, with ulnar translocation of the carpus and mild radial bowing.

Radiologic Findings

There is a great variation in the appearance of the ossific centers in the carpus, with only the hamate and the capitate visible shortly after birth, as noted in the earlier anatomy and embryology discussion. The scaphoid and the lunate do not appear radiographically until, roughly, ages five and four, respectively. The scaphoid occasionally forms from several distinct ossification centers. The developmental cartilaginous rests can lead to the formation of osteochondromas of the scaphoid, i.e., dysplasia epiphysealis hemimelica.[18, 32, 35, 38] To complicate matters further, hematogenous septic arthritis, osteomyelitis, juvenile rheumatoid arthritis, and trauma may appear early with only soft tissue swelling. Radiographically demonstrable healing stages appear at a minimum of 10 days to two weeks after injury.

Carpal coalitions may cause difficulty in the radiographic differential diagnosis. These anomalies include hereditary symphalangism, fetal alcohol syndrome, Noonan's syndrome, and isolated variants[28, 33, 63] (Fig. 27–3). Other congenital wrist anoma-

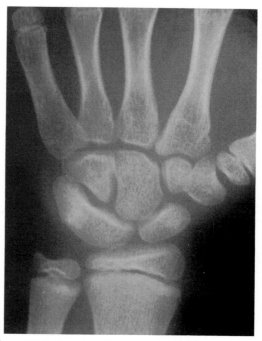

Figure 27–3. Carpal coalition. An asymptomatic 9-year-old male with bilateral triquetrolunate coalitions. These were noted as an incidental finding on radiographs of an acute distal ulnar physeal fracture.

lies are important to recognize because of the frequent association of other skeletal and nonskeletal anomalies.

Radial aplasia and hypoplasia are frequently part of the VATER syndrome (vertebral anomalies, anal atresia, tracheoesophageal fistula, renal and radial dysplasias)[39, 53, 62] (Fig. 27–4). Radial deficiencies may also be associated with cardiac defects (Holt-Oram syndrome), in association with pancytopenia (Fanconi's syndrome) or thrombocytopenia (TARR syndrome).[17, 22,] [39, 53] Ulnar hypoplasia typically is manifested by an absent distal ulna, absent fingers, frequently, and a dislocated or synostotic elbow. This syndrome is only associated with musculoskeletal anomalies[9] (Fig. 27–5).

Cleft or lobster claw hand is another embryologic defect that may accompany a wrist deformity. This disorder is associated with cleft feet, renal, cardiac, and anal anomalies, as well as cleft palate and cataracts, and other skeletal defects (Fig. 27–6).

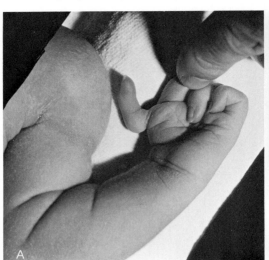

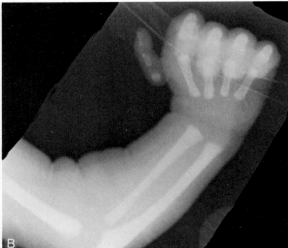

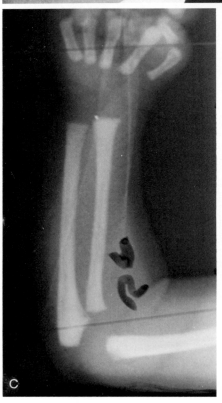

Figure 27–4. Radial hypoplasia. *A,* Clinical photograph of a floating thumb devoid of musculotendinous structures. The forearm, wrist, and hand otherwise appear grossly normal except for a mild radial tilt of the wrist. *B,* Radiograph of the same arm demonstrating mild radial hypoplasia. The distal ulnar physis is at the same level as the distal radial physis. *C,* The opposite, uninvolved forearm. Note that the radius is larger in general. In addition, the radial physis extends distally to the ulnar physis.

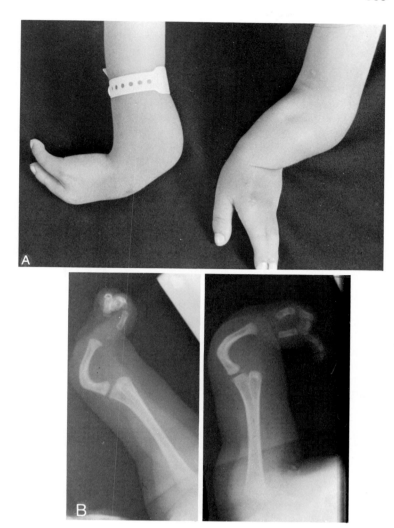

Figure 27–5. Radial meromelia (ulnar club hand). *A,* Clinical photograph demonstrating ectrodactyly of the ulnar border of the hand as well as relatively mild ulnar deviation of the wrist on the right despite aplasia of the ulna. Syndactyly, another frequent finding, is also present in this patient. *B,* Radiograph of this patient. These patients usually have reasonable wrist stability, but they frequently have unstable elbows.

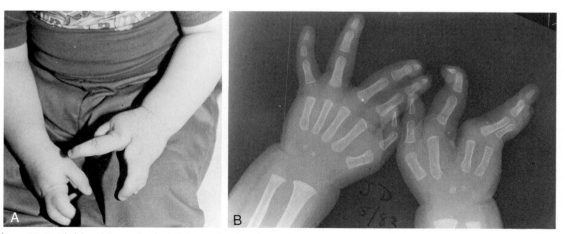

Figure 27–6. Cleft hand (central aplasia/lobster claw hand). *A,* Clinical photograph demonstrating bilateral but asymmetrical involvement. Aplasia most commonly involves the long finger. Involvement of the long and index or long and ring fingers also occurs. *B,* Radiographs of the same patient. There is ectrodactyly of the long finger and metacarpal in the right hand. There is minimal soft tissue involvement of the left hand.

METABOLIC DISORDERS

Rickets

Children occasionally present with wrist or forearm pain, or both, with x-ray studies revealing metabolic defects. Rickets is a condition that may be manifested by isolated wrist discomfort or swelling. The swelling is a clinical manifestation of disorganized endochondral growth of the distal radial physis (Fig. 27–7A and B). The swelling is occasionally painful and is noted at the ends of all long bones. Bachrach and coworkers[5] reported on vitamin D deficiency rickets secondary to nutritional, racial, cultural, and environmental factors. His patients presented with swollen wrists and other musculoskeletal symptoms, including refusal to use the extremity and developmental regression. Of his 24 cases, all the infants were breast-fed and all were black. Meat and dairy products were excluded from the diets of 21 of the 24 patients, and none were being given vitamin D supplementation. The importance of making the diagnosis early is demonstrated by the fact that although these pa-

tients show early response to vitamin D supplementation, few catch up on lost growth.[5, 49, 50] Others have also noted rickets on radiographs taken for dysmorphology evaluation and also as a diagnostic finding in neonates being given prolonged parenteral nutrition with chronic lung disease. The presence of rickets can also be indicated by wrist pain and swelling in patients with unrecognized renal disease, in those on prolonged anticonvulsant medications, in cases of delayed developmental milestones, and in patients with chronic liver disease.[42] Rickets may also simulate child abuse.[49]

Copper Deficiency in TPN

Chronic total parenteral nutrition (TPN), especially in neonates, can also lead to changes in the wrist, as a result of copper deficiency. The peak incidence occurs at seven to nine months of age, when the large hepatic reserves of copper are used up. The earliest changes are generalized demineralization with retardation or failure of epiphyseal ossification centers to appear. Late

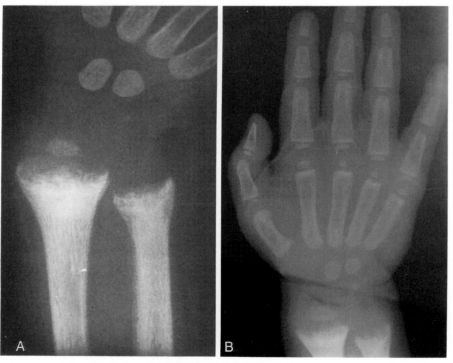

Figure 27–7. Rickets. *A*, An 18-month-old black male with dietary rickets. This child was fed breast milk only. Neither mother nor child had exposure to sunlight. The mother did not partake of milk products. Note the gross widening and irregularity of the physis, metaphyseal widening and cupping, and retarded radial epiphyseal ossification. *B*, Three and a half year old male with rickets secondary to renal osteodystrophy. The changes are similar to those seen in *A*, but are less severe because of the later onset of disease. Early diagnosis and treatment are vital in all cases of rickets to attempt to minimize long-term musculoskeletal problems and shortness of stature.

changes include metaphyseal widening and irregularity, extensive subperiosteal new bone formation, and ringlike or "bucket handle" deformities. There are striking similarities between this disorder and scurvy, both of which are caused by defects in collagen formation.[37, 74]

Hypervitaminosis A

Hypervitaminosis A may occur in the young child secondary to excessive ingestion of this substance. Our experience with this condition has been in adolescents who were prescribed vitamin A for their acne, who felt that the more vitamin tablets they took, the more quickly their pimples would go away. These patients present with hyperostosis of the ulna. This condition promptly resolves with cessation of vitamin A intake.[41] Caffey's disease, idiopathic cortical hyperostosis occurring in the young child, frequently appears with forearm and wrist pain and swelling because of involvement of the radius and the ulna.

CONGENITAL AND DEVELOPMENTAL DEFECTS OF THE FOREARM

Radial Hypoplasia

Radial hypoplasia may cause confusion in the differential diagnosis of wrist deformity and dysfunction in the neonate and in the young child (Fig. 27–4). However, these conditions are frequently associated with thumb hypoplasia and very commonly with defects in the muscles, tendons, and neurovascular structures on the radial aspect of the wrist and forearm. Thrombocytopenia and pancytopenia may also be associated with radial hypoplasia.[22, 39, 53]

Ulnar Hypoplasia

Ulnar hypoplasia, also known as radial meromelia, is not the mirror image of radial hypoplasia; it is typically a sporadic disorder. Unlike the case in radial club hand and hypoplasia, associated anomalies in ulnar hypoplasia usually involve only the musculoskeletal system. Both the preaxial and postaxial hand and wrist may be involved in ulnar hypoplasia, whereas in radial hypoplasia, there is typically involvement of the radial side only[9] (Fig. 27–5).

The carpus in the ulnar club hand is rarely normal. There is frequent ectrodactyly and syndactyly as well as thumb hypoplasia. With thumb and index aplasia, the trapezium and trapezoid are usually absent. With ectrodactyly of the ring and little fingers, the pisiform, the triquetrum, and the hamate are usually absent.

The wrist is typically in mild ulnar deviation, with restriction of radial motion. The involvement is rarely severe. Pollicization, metacarpal base derotation, and syndactyly release in the selected patient may allow improved function. However, wrist surgery is rarely indicated.[9]

Madelung's Deformity

Madelung's deformity is an idiopathic developmental arrest of the ulnar and volar aspects of the distal radius. There is usually secondary proximal and volar migration of the carpus and relative overgrowth of the ulna. This configuration presents a distal base triangulation or pyramidization of the proximal carpal row (Fig. 27–8). Both radius and ulna usually appear normal when this condition is seen early in childhood. The development of the classic radiographic findings of ulnar overgrowth, volar and proximal luxation of the carpus, and volar growth arrest of the distal radius is usually seen in early adolescence. Madelung's deformity is most frequently found in females. Even though the deformity is quite obvious, these patients typically have very minimal functional limitations.

Acquired Madelung's deformity may also be a result of distal radial physeal (posttraumatic) growth arrest (Fig. 27–1), dyschondrosteosis, diaphyseal aclasis, or genetic factors (Turner's syndrome).[16, 54]

Patients with mesomelic dysplasia (dyschondrosteosis) may have shortening of both bones of the forearm or only of the radius. If only the radius has significant shortening, then the typical Madelung's deformity will occur. This disorder is differentiated from idiopathic Madelung's deformity by demonstrating a significant reduction of the ratio of the tibial length to the femoral length, which, in Madelung's deformity, should be between 83 percent and 85 percent. Approximately 50 percent of those patients with mesomelic dysplasia will have significant tibiofibular deformity.[16, 54]

Osteochondromatosis

Multiple hereditary osteochondromatosis may lead to significant wrist deformity when

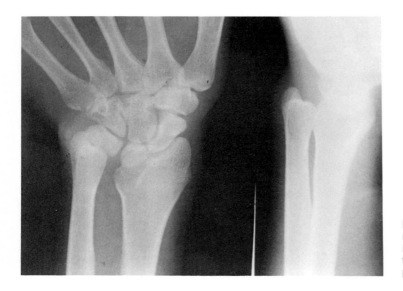

Figure 27–8. Madelung's deformity. Ulnar overgrowth with volar and proximal migration of the carpus. There is a distally based pyramidization of the carpus.

the distal radius and ulna are involved. Because the osteochondromas involve the physeal and metaphyseal regions of the growing long bones, significant growth-related deformities may occur. Up to 60 percent of patients with multiple osteochondromatosis have moderate to severe involvement of the forearm. Thirty-three percent of patients have moderate to severe limitation of pronation or supination but not usually both.[23, 61] Seventy-five percent of the growth of the radius and 85 percent of ulnar growth occur at the distal physis. Progressive and severe deformities occur in a significant number of cases. However, almost invariably, the involvement of the distal ulna is more severe.[23, 61]

The most commonly reported deformity consists of a relative shortening of the ulna, a bowing of one or both bones of the forearm, an ulnar drift of the carpus, and an ulnar tilt of the distal radius. This deformity differs from Madelung's, in which the ulna is excessively long and the carpus is subluxated volarly. In addition, with the progressive ulnar shortening seen in osteochondromatosis, the radial head frequently subluxates progressively and then dislocates. Early, aggressive treatment in an effort to correct the deformity, or at least to limit the eventual severity, is indicated. In the very immature child, excision of the osteochondroma may alter or prevent progressive deformity. However, there is a risk of further physeal injury. In the growing child who is developing ulnar shortening, with early ulnar tilt of the radius or subluxation of the radial head, or both, excision of the ulnar osteochondroma with

ulnar lengthening is indicated. In the child with distal radial tilt and growth remaining, osteotomy and distal radial epiphysiodesis should be combined with ulnar lengthening, as the discrepancy in length will otherwise recur.[23, 61]

If left untreated, these lesions may cause significant cosmetic deformity, wrist and elbow dysfunction, and potential neurologic and vascular compression. For these reasons, early, aggressive surgical treatment is indicated.[2]

Enchondromatosis

Multiple enchondromatosis (Ollier's disease) more typically causes angular and growth problems in the lower extremities than does osteochondromatosis; however, these patients may have very similar problems of wrist instability.[60] The condition is usually unilateral (Fig. 27–9).

Congenital Radioulnar Synostosis

Congenital radioulnar synostosis, which may severely restrict forearm motion, does not typically lead to wrist dysfunction. Patients demonstrate an amazing adaptability to the fixed forearm position. Cleary and Omer[10] reported on a group of 23 patients with 36 congenital synostoses. The average fixed pronation deformity was 30°, and the position of the forearm did not appear to be related to subjective functional limitations, employment status, or the results of objective hand function tests. Most of their patients were employed in jobs that demanded extensive use of the forearm. None of these patients had associated upper extremity anomalies or prior surgery. They concluded that operative treatment is rarely indicated, and that less emphasis should be placed on position and more on objective functional testing. Green and Mital,[29] on the other hand, reported a study of 15 patients, with an average pre-operative fixed pronation deformity of 76°. They recommended that one hand (preferably not the writing hand) in patients with bilateral deformity be shifted to 20° to 35° supination. With one hand in this position, the other can be left in considerable pronation. They recommended derotation of the second forearm to 30° to 45° pronation, only if function remains impaired after the initial derotation. They further suggested that maximal function could be obtained in unilateral cases if the arm is derotated to 10° to 20° supination. They recommended a transverse osteotomy through the conjoined mass of radius and ulna. One case of postoperative ischemic contracture occurred in 13 patients treated operatively. There is a significant neurovascular complication rate reported in all series, and the authors advise serious consideration of the benefits of potential functional improvement in light of potential complications, before recommending that osteotomy be performed.[3, 29]

Congenital and Acquired Dislocation of the Radial Head

Congenital dislocation of the radial head typically has little if any effect on wrist function.[3, 4] However, emphasis should be placed on the diagnosis of post-traumatic radial head dislocation, especially if it occurs in association with an ulnar fracture (Monteggia's fracture), since wrist function can be directly affected. Progressive contracture of the interosseous membrane with relative overgrowth of the ulna, restriction of forearm rotation, and secondary wrist pain may be the end result of a missed diagnosis. Traumatic or congenital dislocation of the radial head may occasionally lead to relative overgrowth of the ulna with wrist impingement but this is extremely uncommon. In

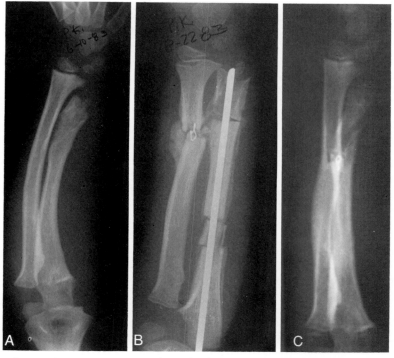

Figure 27–9. Enchondromatosis. *A,* Pre-operative radiograph of a 6-year-old male with shortening of the ulna secondary to osteochondromatosis. The radial head is subluxing as a result of this relative radial overgrowth. There is also ulnar tilt of the distal radial epiphysis and ulnar translocation of the carpus. *B,* Radiograph taken shortly after radial shortening and angulation osteotomy combined with ulnar lengthening. *C,* Radiograph at the time of osseous union. The distal radioulnar joint is reconstituted, and the radiohumeral articulation is normal. Continued distal radial growth may cause a recurrence of the deformity, but two years following this procedure this patient has a full, painless range of motion at the elbow, forearm, and wrist.

such an instance, shortening of the distal ulnar diaphysis as the patient approaches maturity may allow for relief of the impingement, while permitting the interosseous membrane to contract and resist further proximal migration of the radius. In addition, this may improve function of the distal radioulnar joint. Enchondromas or, more frequently, osteochondromas may likewise lead to progressive subluxation of the radial head or distal radioulnar joint. Early surgical resection of the lesion at the first signs of subluxation may prevent progressive wrist dysfunction.[23, 60, 61]

FRACTURES AND DISLOCATIONS

Fractures of the distal forearm and wrist are among the most frequent injuries sustained by the growing child. The great majority of these injuries require only straightforward nonoperative treatment.[1, 25, 55, 56] However, any injury in a child requires careful, diligent treatment to avoid potential lifelong problems. The following section is intended to highlight injuries that may affect wrist function. Treatment of the specific injuries is discussed, as is the treatment of complications arising from these injuries.

Diaphyseal Fractures

Diaphyseal fractures may lead to decreased wrist function, if significant malalignment or malrotation is permitted. Darnwalla[14] demonstrated that 52.8 percent of his patients had some limitation of supination or pronation secondary to healed diaphyseal fractures, all of which were compensated for at the glenohumeral joint. Angulatory deformity of the radius or the ulna was responsible for loss of rotation in 71 percent of those joints with limitation of rotation. Angulation of both bones with an apex toward the interosseous space limited motion, even with some opening of the interosseous space. Loss of pronation occurred because of disruption of the distal radioulnar joint in two of 53 patients. Several children in the study had loss of rotation without significant angulation or malrotation. Darnwalla further stated that angulation of 15° in healed metaphyseal fractures close to the radial physis would remodel in the patient under five years of age, but those of more than 10° were unlikely to remodel in the patient who is six to 10 years old.[14] No

malrotation should be accepted, as this will not remodel at any age. The interosseous space must be maintained at all times, and angulation of more than 10° in the distal radius and ulna should be corrected in patients older than 10 years. Bayonet apposition and mild angulation are well tolerated in the immature patient, as long as malrotation and closure of the interosseous space are avoided.* However, even with anatomic reduction and osseous healing, some loss of rotation is common although rarely symptomatic.

Physeal Injuries

Injuries to the distal radial and ulnar physis are quite common; these areas often absorb energy that would produce a carpal fracture or ligamentous injury in an adult. The fracture most frequently occurs through the physeal zone of provisional calcification. In view of the marked frequency of this injury, the incidence of growth arrest, malunion, and subsequent deformities is quite rare. However, these patients should all be evaluated serially for at least the first year after injury to detect an unlikely but potentially significant growth arrest. If a partial growth arrest occurs in an actively growing child, such as a bridging transphyseal bony "bar" involving less than 40 percent of the physeal line, the authors recommend resecting the bony bridge with Silastic interposition.[8, 40] Without treatment of the radial arrest, continued ulnar overgrowth may lead to a Madelung's type of deformity (Fig. 27–1). Opening wedge dorsal osteotomy or arrest of the distal ulnar physis, or both, may be necessary for optimal wrist function in those patients who sustain complete distal radial physeal arrest.[7] Ipsilateral fractures of the distal radial physis and carpal scaphoid have been reported but are rare.[30, 32]

Isolated, complete post-traumatic arrest of the distal ulnar epiphysis has also been reported, with variable long-term significance.[45, 48] Such an isolated ulnar growth arrest can lead to significant bowing of the radius as well as ulnar translocation of the carpus and ulnar tilt of the distal radial articular surface (Fig. 27–2). Isolated physeal injury without permanent growth arrest may also occur with repetitive axial loading and rotation.[27]

---

*References 14, 15, 25, 55, 56, 67, 71.

There have been several reports of "irreducible" fractures of the distal radius and ulna, with interposition of flexor tendons or neurovascular structures across and within the fracture sites.[19, 43] Significant neurovascular deficits that do not rapidly resolve with gentle reduction with traction or that worsen after manipulation require urgent exploration and reduction. However, most neurovascular compromise associated with closed physeal injuries resolves with closed anatomic reduction.[43, 55, 56, 66]

In the great majority of these fractures, residual dorsal angular displacement following a reduction maneuver usually remodels. Therefore, repetitive manipulations are unnecessary and may cause injury to the germinal layer of the physis.[1, 11, 55, 56, 68]

Epiphyseal Fractures

Intra-articular fractures of the distal radius in the child are extremely rare but mandate anatomic reduction with fixation, as necessary, to maintain a congruous articular surface and to avoid physeal bars secondary to bone overlap of the physis. However, a Type V injury to the physis may not manifest itself until six to 12 months after injury; therefore, prolonged radiographic follow-up is indicated. If an immature patient with significant growth remaining is noted to have a bony bridge, resection of the bony bridge with Silastic interposition is recommended.

Fractures of the Ulnar Styloid and Injury to the Triangular Fibrocartilage

The ulnar styloid does not ossify until late in the first decade and slowly assumes its adult configuration over several years. Fractures in this region frequently lead to nonunion, with the formation of a distinct ossicle. These injuries may well go undetected prior to the appearance of the ossification center or may be associated with disruption of the triangular fibrocartilage. Isolated tears or degenerative lesions involving the triangular fibrocartilage, often associated with athletic injuries, may also occur. These lesions may only be demonstrable by arthrography or by surgical exploration.[69] The authors, therefore, feel that a "sprain" in a child's wrist is a diagnosis of exclusion that frequently cannot be made at the time of injury. For this reason, any child with a tender or swollen wrist or both after trauma should be treated with aggressive immobilization.

Distal Radioulnar Joint Disruption

Disruption of the distal radioulnar joint, in association with fracture of the distal radius (Galeazzi's fracture) can usually be treated by closed means in the child.[46, 56] However, in the adolescent, this injury may well require operative fixation of the fracture to maintain reduction of the distal radioulnar joint. Isolated dislocation of the distal radioulnar joint without fracture may also occur, usually with a pulling, twisting mechanism of injury. Reduction can usually be obtained and maintained with closed manipulation in the child. Occasionally, temporary fixation by smooth Steinmann pins is necessary for stabilization. However, because of the intimate involvement of the triangular fibrocartilage in this joint, associated tears of this cartilage may lead to long-term discomfort. The key to diagnosis is a high index of suspicion in a patient presenting with a painful wrist without fracture. It is mandatory that a true lateral radiograph be obtained demonstrating superimposition of all four metacarpals.[4, 13, 64] In our experience, the CT scan is the most definitive study available if there is any question about the possibility of disruption of the distal radioulnar joint.

Carpal Fractures

Carpal fractures and ligamentous injuries of the wrist are extremely uncommon, especially prior to age 10. There is one report in the literature of a patient presenting at age seven with a chronic scapholunate dissociation, presumed to have been caused by an injury at age three months. This resulted in a chronic palmar flexion instability that was surgically corrected after two weeks of traction by ligamentous reconstruction.[26] Occasional fractures of the other carpal bones may also occur but are extremely rare, infrequently displace, and heal readily without long-term sequelae with casting, if the diagnosis is recognized.[22] However, reduction and fixation are occasionally necessary to ensure articular congruity and stability. These injuries appear more frequently in the older adolescent with a more adult type of anatomy.[75]

Fractures of the carpal scaphoid do occur in children, with the greatest number taking place between ages 10 and 14. In a series of 108 carpal scaphoid fractures in children under age 14 reported by Vahvanen and Westerlund,[72] 94 (87 percent) involved the distal one third of the scaphoid (Fig. 27–10). Forty-one of these were avulsion fractures from the dorsal radial aspect. This fracture pattern, with sparing of the proximal pole, has been verified in other series. Twelve percent were waist fractures, with only one avulsion fracture of the proximal pole (Fig. 27–11). None of these fractures progressed to avascular necrosis or nonunion, including three cases in which the diagnosis was made and treatment initiated three weeks after injury. There was marked resorption at the fracture site, but healing was not affected (Fig. 27–12). Seventy-two of these fractures occurred with falls on the outstretched hand, twenty-one in bicycling accidents, eight in falls from a height, and seven in twisting or direct-blow injuries incurred during a game or in a motor vehicle accident. Five of the 53 waist fractures were visible on the original radiographs, and five of the 108 had associated fractures in the same extremity. The average time in cast treatment in this series was four to eight weeks, with all patients reported to have complete bone healing, with full wrist motion and no symptoms at follow-up. Avascular necrosis of the scaphoid in the skeletally immature child is exceedingly rare.[72]

Nonunion of the carpal scaphoid has been reported but is extremely rare, and healing

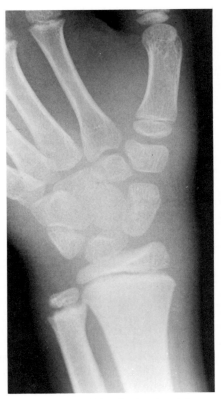

Figure 27–11. Fracture of the distal waist of the scaphoid. Fractures of the proximal pole of the scaphoid in immature patients are uncommon.

almost always occurs with prolonged casting or bone grafting, especially in the younger child[29, 42, 44, 62] (Fig. 27–13). Trans-scaphoid perilunate dislocation with post-traumatic instability in children has rarely been reported in the literature but deserves an aggressive reconstructive approach if encountered.[26, 51, 75]

Posterior dislocation of the trapezoid and trapezium in a young child has been described, but such an injury is exceedingly rare and only occurs as the result of major trauma.[22]

Thumb Metacarpal Fractures

Fractures at the base of the thumb metacarpal are quite common and typically involve angulation. There is rarely any malrotation. These metaphyseal fractures are frequently impacted, and significant angulation will remodel with remaining growth (Fig. 27–14).

Physeal injuries at the base of the thumb may be irreducible by closed means if significantly displaced. The displaced metaphyseal fragment may buttonhole through

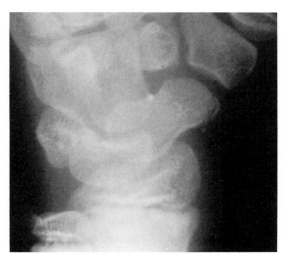

Figure 27–10. Avulsion fracture of the distal pole of the scaphoid in a 9-year-old child.

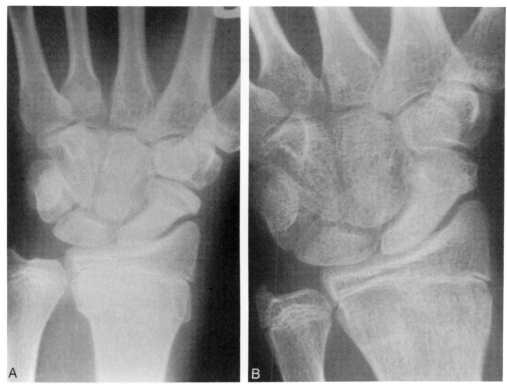

Figure 27–12. A, An acute Salter II fracture of the distal radius in a 13-year-old male, including an incidentally noted nonunion of a distal waist fracture of the scaphoid. The scaphoid fracture was presumably sustained in a fall nine months prior to diagnosis. B, Radiograph taken after 12 weeks of thumb spica cast immobilization, demonstrating complete union of both the radius and the scaphoid.

the thick periosteum and may require open reduction.

In the adolescent near the end of growth, the medial aspect of the physis remains

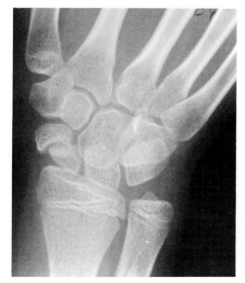

Figure 27–13. Nonunion of the scaphoid in an asymptomatic 12-year-old female one year after a fall.

open, whereas the lateral aspect is closed; this may fracture in a manner reminiscent of Tillaux's fracture. This is the adolescent equivalent of Bennett's fracture, with the thumb musculature displacing the metacarpal proximally. Anatomic reduction is mandatory, with percutaneous wire fixation frequently required to maintain the reduction. A thumb spica cast is the most effective means of immobilization in all three types of fractures. Great care must be exercised to avoid hyperextension of the thumb metacarpal to avoid further fracture displacement and hyperextension contracture of the thumb.

Carpometacarpal Joint Injuries

In our experience, these injuries occur more frequently than the literature describes. Reduction is usually straightforward with traction but, in the authors' experience, frequently requires percutaneous pin fixation, even in the younger child[34] (Fig. 27–15). Growth arrest of the metacarpals is obviously not a problem, because the physis is

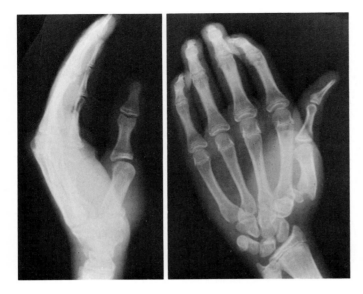

Figure 27–14. A physeal fracture through the base of the thumb metacarpal in an 8-year-old male.

in the distal metacarpal. However, there is a great potential for carpometacarpal incongruity and a dorsal prominence without anatomic reduction.

INFECTIONS

Since the advent of antibiotic treatment, hematogenous osteomyelitis of the carpal bones has been extremely uncommon. More often, the metaphyseal portions of the long bones are involved with hematogenous osteomyelitis (Figs. 27–16 and 27–17). Joint involvement typically occurs in those joints in which the metaphysis is intracapsular, such as the shoulder and the hip, and not in the distal radius or the ulna. Involvement of the carpal bones without direct contamination is extremely rare. One case involving the scaphoid in an 11-year-old male, secondary to a contralateral paronychia, has been reported.[59] *Mycobacterium fortuitum* synovitis and osteomyelitis have been reported in immunocompromised patients. In addition, osteomyelitis of the carpus, with infection due to *Brucella* and *Salmonella* as well as *Escherichia coli* and *Histoplasma*, has been reported.[58, 67] In the series of 258 chil-

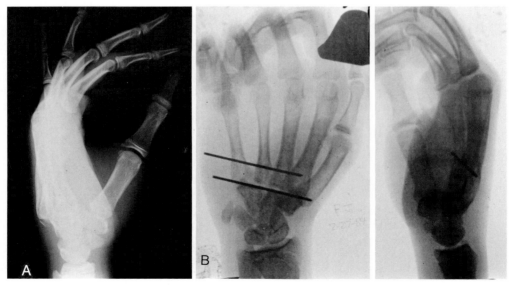

Figure 27–15. Fracture separation of the base of the fourth and fifth metacarpals. *A*, Lateral radiograph at the time of the injury. *B*, Intraoperative radiograph. These fractures are usually relatively easy to reduce but frequently require percutaneous pinning for stability.

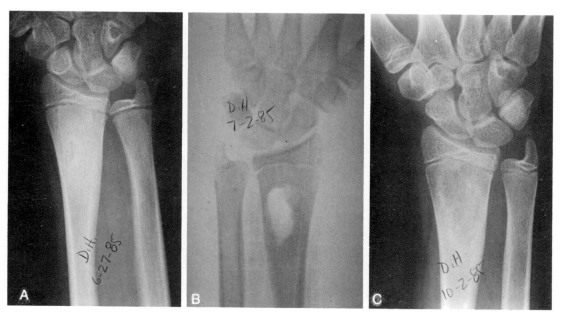

Figure 27–16. Osteomyelitis. *A,* A 14-year-old female who presented with a six-week history of wrist pain. Radiograph of the distal radius at the time of presentation. *B,* Intra-operative radiograph at the time of surgical débridement and saucerization. *C,* Radiograph four months after surgery. There is continued normal radial growth. Early aggressive surgical management, coupled with appropriate antibiotic treatment, is vital to preventing growth arrest and deformity. These patients must also be followed over a period of several years to detect the onset of late deformity.

dren with hematogenous osteomyelitis reported in 1982 by Jackson and Nelson,[36] only two had carpal bone involvement. The authors have seen a child with hematogenous *Mycobacterium* infection of the wrist, acquired in the Far East. The condition manifested as a cool, boggy synovitis, initially with few, if any, changes on radiographs,

that responded well to débridement and medical treatment. Even though such a presentation is extremely uncommon in the United States, tuberculosis should be included in the differential diagnosis of the swollen wrist. Infection with *Neisseria gonorrhoeae* should likewise be considered in the child with a swollen wrist, especially if

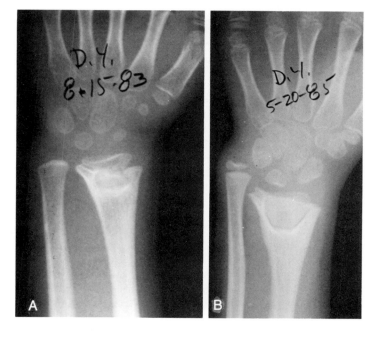

Figure 27–17. Osteomyelitis. *A,* Growth arrest of the distal radial physis following medical management of acute hematogenous osteomyelitis. *B,* Approximately two years following attempted resection of the bony physeal bar and silastic interposition. There is a persistent failure of distal radial growth and severe overgrowth of the ulna.

there is any suggestion of sexual abuse. Direct aspiration is indicated in any painful, swollen wrist without a clear-cut traumatic etiology, if there is no history of a bleeding disorder.

Growth arrest of the distal radius, secondary to osteomyelitis, may occur and can lead to significant shortening of the radius and disruption of the distal radioulnar joint. Radial lengthening has been described as a means of treating this uncommon problem[52] (Fig. 27–17).

SPORTS INJURIES

Among the most common injuries of the upper extremities sustained by the immature sports enthusiast are distal radial and ulnar fractures. However, the recent increase in popularity of certain sports activities necessitates mention of potential wrist problems peculiar to this era. As many as 50 percent of the children's fractures reported are sports-related.[6]

Gymnastics can lead to stress fractures and a unique wrist synovitis similar to those that have long been found in the lower extremities in runners.[70] Involvement of the scaphoid and the lunate with stress fractures because of the repetitive loading of the radial aspect of the wrist is a distinct example. Degenerative lesions involving the triangular fibrocartilage after such repetitive trauma have also been reported.[69] The physician's most important role in caring for such patients is probably educational, not only to instruct the young patient but also the parents and the coaches. These individuals, although well-meaning, may push children beyond their physiologic capabilities in an effort to have them excel. Restricted activities followed by resumption of the offending activities in a graduated fashion is the treatment of choice. These patients and their parents are typically highly motivated to do whatever is necessary to promote healing but will cooperate better with restricted participation (i.e., avoidance of repetitive use of the wrist) than with complete cessation of gymnastics. This is also true in other sports.

A careful dietary history is also required, as many young athletes have the misconception that dietary manipulations and health foods can improve their performance. Some of these diets may actually be deleterious to the health of the young athlete.

Roller-skating and skateboarding have become even more hazardous since the advent of nylon wheels and more efficient bearings, thus leading to more frequent wrist and forearm injuries. Of those patients injured in one series, over 90 percent wore no protective gear, and most of them were inexperienced. The great majority of the injuries involved the wrist.[20]

In a study of those patients treated for injuries at a "roller disco," it was found that protective gear was not utilized for social reasons.[73] This study also demonstrated that the great majority of injuries involved the wrist. This injury pattern, as well as the lack of use of protective equipment, holds true also for skateboarders. Although the injury rate is higher in inexperienced skateboarders and skaters, surgery is more frequently necessary in the more experienced participant, probably because of the increased complexity and velocity of the maneuvers they perform.

One of the more recent athletic overuse syndromes reported was "break dancing wrist." This was an isolated distal ulnar physeal overuse injury reported following repetitive axial loading and rotation on the dorsiflexed wrist in the adolescent.[27]

Football, in the young patient, leads most frequently to injuries of the least protected areas such as the hands, the wrists, the knees, and the ankles. In one series, which studied 2079 boys in an organized tackle league, 2.3 percent sustained injuries serious enough to miss a game or a practice. Six percent of the total injuries involved the epiphysis. However, the injury rate appeared lower than that predicted for random play.[57]

MISCELLANEOUS CONDITIONS

When a child presents with a painful wrist without antecedent trauma or stigmata of infection, the differential diagnosis must include juvenile rheumatoid arthritis, child abuse, and sympathetic dystrophy.

Juvenile Rheumatoid Arthritis

More than 50 percent of patients with juvenile rheumatoid arthritis (JRA) have involvement of the wrist and hand. The area of swelling may or may not be warm, and the wrist may or may not be painful. One of the earliest clinical findings is loss of full extension of the wrist, which may be present prior to a palpable synovitis or other finding in JRA.[12] There may be monarticular, pauciarticular, or polyarticular involvement.

The ulna is typically short in juvenile rheumatoid arthritis, with concomitant ulnar deviation of the wrist and radial deviation of the metacarpophalangeal joints. There is also more marked loss of flexion at the metacarpophalangeal joint in the child, as opposed to loss of extension in the adult. It is unclear whether the ulnar deviation of the wrist is related to the ulnar shortening[12, 20] (Fig. 27–18).

The erythrocyte sedimentation rate is usually elevated somewhat, with a normal white blood cell count. The wrist aspirate is typically in the inflammatory range but fails to demonstrate bacterial involvement on Gram's stain or culture.

The treatment of choice is medical initially, with synovectomy reserved for only the rare patient with resistant disease that resembles the adult form of rheumatoid arthritis. Conservative treatment and splinting are indicated in the great majority of patients. The extent of involvement and virulence of the disease process vary but should be noted. It is of utmost importance that these patients be evaluated every six to 12 months for uveitis; this is a treatable disorder that may cause blindness if not recognized early.

Child Abuse

Child abuse should be suspected in any child under 18 months who presents with a long-bone fracture, especially if a torsional pattern is noted. Child abuse should also be strongly suspected and social services notified in the child who repeatedly presents with different fractures in varying stages of healing or with inappropriate or changing histories, or both.[18, 28] One must also consider the diagnosis of osteogenesis imperfecta and Menkes's kinky hair syndrome with such a clinical presentation.

Sympathetic Dystrophy

This problem infrequently occurs in the adolescent patient after relatively minor trauma. These patients develop exquisite localized tenderness and hypersensitivity throughout the wrist, arm, and hand. Typically, the discomfort is not well localized or described and cannot be explained on a purely anatomic basis.

Occult pathologic conditions must be excluded first. X-ray and laboratory studies are initially normal, except, possibly, for some patchy periarticular osteoporosis, which is common later in the clinical course. Bone scanning can be most revealing, with patchy periarticular increased uptake.

Treatment consists primarily of honest psychological support and explanation. A short period of immobilization followed by a desensitization program will often provide relief. This approach is much more successful in the child than in the adult. Seldom is sympathetic block or medical management necessary.

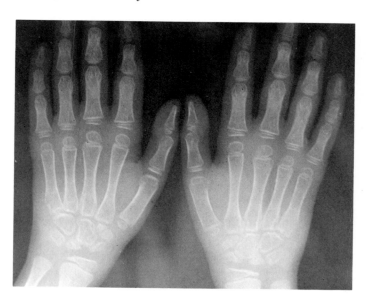

Figure 27–18. Juvenile rheumatoid arthritis. Soft tissue swelling at the interphalangeal joints and decreased size of the proximal carpal row. There are mild periarticular osteoporosis and early erosive changes at the radiocarpal joint.

SUMMARY

The child's wrist is amazingly resistant to many of the traumas sustained by the adult wrist. However, it is important to recognize the many developmental, anatomic, and physiologic variations present in children in order to diagnose abnormalities. The identification and treatment of these problems will allow the patient to enjoy the benefits of a normal wrist at maturity.

Any child presenting with a post-traumatic, tender, swollen wrist should be evaluated thoroughly, both clinically and radiographically. Even with normal radiographs, appropriate immobilization is indicated to prevent long-term, potentially lifelong disability.

References

1. Aitken AP: The end result of the fractured distal radial epiphysis. J Bone Joint Surg 17(2):301–308, 1935.
2. Akbarnia BA, et al: Manifestations of the battered child syndrome. J Bone Joint Surg 56A(6):1159–1166, 1974.
3. Almquist EE, Gordon LH, and Blue AI: Congenital dislocation, radial head. J Bone Joint Surg 51A:1118–1127, 1969.
4. Asher M: Dislocation of the upper extremity in children. Orthop Clin North Am 7(3):583–591, 1976.
5. Bachrach S, Fisher J, and Parks JS: An outbreak of vitamin D deficiency rickets in a susceptible population. Pediatrics 64(6):871–877, 1979.
6. Benton JW: Epiphyseal fracture in sport. Physician Sportsmed 10:62, 1982.
7. Bragdon RA: Fractures of the distal radial epiphysis. Clin Orthop 41:59–63, 1965.
8. Bright R: Operative correction of partial epiphyseal plate closure by osseous bridge resection and silicone rubber implant. J Bone Joint Surg 56A:655–664, 1974.
9. Broudy AS, and Smith RJ: Deformities of the hand and wrist with ulnar deficiency. J Hand Surg 4:304–315, 1979.
10. Cleary JE, and Omer GE: Congenital proximal radioulnar synostosis. Natural history and functional assessment. J Bone Joint Surg 67A(4):539–545, 1985.
11. Compere EL: Growth arrest in long bones as result of fractures that include the epiphysis. JAMA 105(26):2140–2146, 1928.
12. Cranberry WM, and Mangum GL: The hand in the child with juvenile rheumatoid arthritis. J Hand Surg 5:105–113, 1980.
13. Dameron TB: Traumatic dislocation of the distal radioulnar joint. Clin Orthop 83:55–63, 1972.
14. Darnwalla JS: A study of radioulnar movements following fractures of the forearm in children. Clin Orthop 139:114–120, 1979.
15. Davis DR, and Green DP: Forearm fractures in children. Clin Orthop 120:172–183, 1976.
16. Dawe C, Wynne-Davies R, and Fulford GE: Clinical variations in dyschondrostenosis. J Bone Joint Surg 64B:377–381, 1982.
17. Dell PC, and Sheppard JE: Thrombocytopenia, absent radius syndrome. Clin Orthop 162:129–134, 1982.
18. Doyle M, and Downey EF: Trevor's disease of the carpal navicular bone. J Am Osteopath Assoc 83:793–794, 1984.
19. Engber WD, and Keene JS: Irreducible fracture separation of the distal ulnar epiphysis. J Bone Joint Surg 67A:1130–1132, 1985.
20. Ferkel RD, Mai LL, Ullis KC, et al: An analysis of roller skating injuries. Am J Sports Med 10(1):24–30, 1981.
21. Findley TW, Halperin D, and Easton JK: Wrist subluxation in juvenile rheumatoid arthritis: Pathophysiology and management. Arch Phys Med Rehabil 64:69, 1983.
22. Fischer L, Moulin R, Deidier Ch, et al: Luxation postérieure du trapèze et du trapézoïde chez une enfant en fin de croissance, avec fracture de l'apophyse antérieure du trapèze, traitée orthopédiquement. Lyon Méd 12:222:556–559, 1969.
23. Fogel GR, McElfresh EL, Peterson HA, et al: Management of deformities of the forearm in multiple hereditary osteochondromas. J Bone Joint Surg 66A:670–680, 1925.
24. Fumich RM, and Essig GW: Hypervitaminosis A: case report in an adolescent soccer player. Am J Sports Med 11:34–37, 1983.
25. Gandhi RK, Wilson P, Mason-Brown JJ, et al: Spontaneous correction of deformity following fractures of the forearm in children. Br J Surg 50:5, 1962.
26. Gerard FM: Post-traumatic carpal instability in a young child. J Bone Joint Surg 62A:131–133, 1980.
27. Gerber SD, Griffin PP, and Simmons BP: Break dancer's wrist. J Pediatr Orthop 6:98–99, 1986.
28. Graham CE, and Mehta MC: Bilateral congenital carpal fusion in a champion golfer. Clin Orthop 83:70–72, 1972.
29. Green WT, and Mital MA: Congenital radio-ulnar synostosis: surgical treatment. J Bone Joint Surg 61A:738–743, 1979.
30. Greene WB, and Anderson WJ: Simultaneous fracture of the scaphoid and radius in a child. J Pediatr Orthop 2(2):191–194, 1982.
31. Gross R: Child abuse: Are you recognizing it when you see it? Contemp Orthop 2(9)676–678, 1980.
32. Grundy M: Fractures of the carpal scaphoid in children. Br J Surg 56:523–524, 1969.
33. Harle TS, and Stevenson JR: Hereditary symphalangism associated with carpal and tarsal fusion. Radiology 89:91–94, 1967.
34. Hartwig RH, and Louis DS: Multiple carpometacarpal dislocations. J Bone Joint Surg 61A:906–908, 1979.
35. Hensinger RN, Cowell HR, Ramsey PC, et al: Familial dysplasia epiphysealis hemimelica. J Bone Joint Surg 56A:1513–1516, 1974.
36. Jackson MA, and Nelson JD: Etiology and medical management of acute suppurative bone and joint infections in pediatric patients. J Pediatr Orthop 2:313–323, 1982.
37. Karpel JT, and Pedeu VH: Copper deficiency in long-term parenteral nutrition. J Pediatr 80:32–36, 1972.
38. Kettelkamp DB, Campbell CJ, and Bonfiglio M: Dysplasia epiphysealis hemimelica. J Bone Joint Surg 48A:746–766, 1966.

39. Lamb DW: Radial club hand. J Bone Joint Surg 59A:1–13, 1977.
40. Langenskiold A: Surgical treatment of partial closure of the growth plate. J Pediatr Orthop 1(1)3–11, 1981.
41. Lonon WD, Jost LA, Perlman AW, et al: Chronic hypervitaminosis A. Orthop Rev 10(3):93–97, 1981.
42. Lumpkins L, and Oestreich AE: Rickets as an unexpected x-ray finding. J Natl Med Assoc 75(3):255–258, 1983.
43. Manoli A: Irreducible fracture separation of the distal radial epiphysis. J Bone Joint Surg 64A:1095–1096, 1982.
44. Maxted M, and Owen R: Two cases of non-union of carpal scaphoid fractures in children. Injury 13:441–443, 1982.
45. MGindyo BS: Considerations on cases of epiphyseal injury observed at Kenyatta National Hospital. East Afr Med J 431–435, 1979.
46. Mikic Z DJ: Galeazzi fracture dislocations. J Bone Joint Surg 57A:1071–1080, 1975.
47. Mussbichler H: Injuries of the carpal scaphoid in children. Acta Radiol 56:361–368, 1961.
48. Nelson OA, Buchanon JR, and Harrison CS: Distal ulnar growth arrest. J Hand Surg 9A:164–171, 1984.
49. Paterson CR: Vitamin D deficiency rickets simulating child abuse. J Pediatr Orthop 1:423–425, 1981.
50. Pierce DS, Wallace WM, and Herndon CH: Long-term treatment of vitamin D-resistant rickets. J Bone Joint Surg 46A:978–995, 1964.
51. Piero A, Mertos F, Mat T, et al: Transcaphoid perilunate dislocation in a child. Acta Orthop Scand 52:31–34, 1981.
52. Price CT, and Mills WL: Radial lengthening for septic growth arrest. J Pediatr Orthop, 3:88–91, 1983.
53. Pulvertaft RG: Twenty-five years of hand surgery. J Bone Joint Surg 55B:32–55, 1973.
54. Ranawat CS, DeFiore J, and Straub LR: Madelung's deformity. J Bone Joint Surg 57A:772–755, 1975.
55. Rang M: Children's Fractures. 2nd ed. JB Lippincott Co, Philadelphia, 1983.
56. Rockwood CA, Wilkins KE, and King RE: Fractures in Children. JE Lippincott Co, Philadelphia, 1984.
57. Rosen LA, and Clawson DK: Football injuries in the very young athlete. Clin Orthop 69:219–223, 1970.
58. Seal PV, and Morris CA: Brucellosis of the carpus—a case report. J Bone Joint Surg 56B:327–330, 1974.
59. Seimon LP, and Stram RA: Staphylococcal osteomyelitis of the carpal scaphoid. J Pediatr Orthop 4:123–125, 1984.
60. Shapiro F: Ollier's disease, an assessment of angular deformity, shortening, and pathologic fracture in twenty-one patients. J Bone Joint Surg 64A:95–103, 1982.
61. Shapiro F, Simon S, and Glimcher MJ: Hereditary multiple exostosis. J Bone Joint Surg 61A:815–824, 1979.
62. Skerik SK, and Flatt AE: The anatomy of congenital radial dysplasia: its surgical and functional implications. Clin Orthop 66:125–143, 1969.
63. Slater P, and Rubinstein H: Aplasia of interphalangeal joints associated with synostosis of carpal and tarsal bones. Sea View Hosp Bull 7:419–444, 1942.
64. Snook GA, Chrisman OD, Wilson TC, et al: Subluxation of the distal radio-ulnar joint by hyperpronation. J Bone Joint Surg 51A:1315–1323, 1969.
65. Southcott R, and Rosman MA: Non-union of carpal scaphoid fractures in children. J Bone Joint Surg 59B:20–23, 1977.
66. Sterling AP, and Habermann ET: Acute post-traumatic median nerve compression associated with a Salter II fracture dislocation of the wrist. Bull Hosp J Dis Orthop Inst 34(2):167–171, 1973.
67. Szilaggi A, Mendelson J, Portnoy J, et al: Caseating granulomas in chronic osteomyelitis: salmonellosis, tuberculosis, or both? Can Med Assoc J 120:963–965, 1979.
68. Tachdjian MO: Pediatric Orthopaedics. Philadelphia, WB Saunders Co, 1972.
69. Tehranzadeh J, Labosky DA, and Gabriele OF: Ganglion cysts and tear of triangular fibrocartilages of both wrists in a cheerleader. Am J Sports Med 11:357–359, 1983.
70. Teitz CC: Sports medicine concerns in dance and gymnastics. Pediatr Clin North Am 29:1399–1421, 1982.
71. VanHerpe LB: Fractures of the forearm and wrist. Orthop Clin North Am 7:543–556, 1976.
72. Vahvanen V, and Westerlund M: Fracture of the carpal scaphoid in children: a clinical and roentgenological study of 108 cases. Acta Orthop Scand 51:909–913, 1980.
73. Wilkinson A: Injuries incurred at "roller discos." Br Med J 284:1163, 1982.
74. Wiss DA, and Peden VH: Copper deficiency in long-term parenteral nutrition. Orthopaedics 3(10):969–973, 1980.
75. Worland RL, and Dick HM: Transnavicular perilunate dislocations. J Trauma 15(5):407–412, 1975.

PART V

Surgical Options for Common Wrist Conditions

CHAPTER 28

Implant Arthroplasty in the Carpal and Radiocarpal Joints

ALFRED B. SWANSON, M.D.
and GENEVIEVE DE GROOT SWANSON, M.D.

Disabilities of the wrist occur frequently and can develop in rheumatoid arthritis, osteoarthritis, or following fractures and dislocations. Involvement of individual carpal bones and of the intercarpal, radiocarpal, or distal radioulnar joints can occur singly or in combination. The ideal goal of reconstructive procedures in the wrist and carpus is to provide pain relief with reasonable stability, strength, and mobility for assistance in hand adaptations. Proper evaluation of the specific problems presented, including the severity of the disease and the patient's age and functional requirements, is essential in selecting the best treatment from the wide range of available procedures. Treatment recommendations are discussed for the carpal bones (trapezium, scaphoid, lunate) and for the radiocarpal and distal radioulnar joints. These recommendations are based on a classification of severity of disease developed by the senior author. The concepts, indications, surgical techniques, and pitfalls of implant arthroplasty in the wrist and carpus are presented in detail.

Flexible Implant Resection Arthroplasty

The development of medical-grade silicone elastomer implants to be used as an adjunct to resection arthroplasty of the small joints of the extremities has been an ongoing project in our research department since 1962. This study has included considerations of implant durability, host tolerance, and refinements in implant designs and surgical techniques. Recent technical developments include the use of titanium grommets to shield the wrist, metacarpophalangeal, and toe flexible hinge implants from abrasion by sharp bone edges; titanium scaphoid, lunate, thumb convex condylar, and single stem toe implants have been evaluated since 1983 and have now been approved for general use. A metal hemiwrist implant is under current clinical investigation. A separate review of carpal bone implants made of the original silicone material has demonstrated a significant lesser incidence of cystic formation than those cases reconstructed with

404

the high-performance silicone material; therefore, the senior author now prefers the use of the original silicone material for the trapezium implant, the use of titanium for the single stem toe implant, the use of the original silicone material or titanium for the scaphoid, lunate, convex condylar and radial head implants. The use of stem fixation and sutures through silicone implants have been abandoned. It should be noted that the higher-performance silicone elastomers, used in combination with grommets, is the preferred material for flexible hinge implants in the finger, wrist, and toe joints.

THE CARPAL SCAPHOID AND THE LUNATE

A wide variety of procedures are used in the treatment of necrosis, fracture, or fracture dislocation and subluxation of the scaphoid and the lunate, including conservative methods, such as localized bone grafting, excision, or implant replacement and intercarpal fusions, or more radical methods, such as total wrist implant arthroplasty or fusion. The senior author has devised a classification of lunate and scaphoid disorders to help

assist in the selection of the appropriate treatment method based on the stages of severity of disease (Tables 28–1 and 28–2).

Examples of the various treatment methods recommended are illustrated (Figs. 28–1 through 28–12). The procedures for scaphoid and lunate implant arthroplasty are presented in detail.

Carpal Bone Implant Arthroplasty

The carpal bone implants act as articulating spacers to maintain the relationship of the adjacent carpal bones following local resection procedures while preserving wrist mobility and resolving associated intercarpal instability, thereby preventing collapse and settling of the carpus. These implants have essentially the same shapes as their anatomic counterparts, with the concavities being more pronounced to provide greater stability.

Implants can be extremely difficult to stabilize in the carpal bone complex. Ligamentous instability and carpal collapse are frequently associated with pathologic conditions of the scaphoid or the lunate. Total removal of these bones leaves defects in the

Text continued on page 412

Table 28–1. **CLASSIFICATION AND TREATMENT FOR AVASCULAR NECROSIS OF THE LUNATE**

Stage	Pathologic Conditions	Treatment Options
I	Sclerosis of the lunate with Minimal symptoms Normal carpal bone relationships	Splinting and rest Revascularization Ulnar and radial lengthening or shortening
II	Sclerosis of the lunate with cystic changes with Clinical symptoms Normal carpal bone relationships	Lunate implant replacement Ulnar and radial lengthening or shortening
III	Sclerosis, cysts, and fragmentation of the lunate with Scaphoradial angle: 40° to 60° Carpal height collapse: 0 to 5 percent Carpal translation minimal	Lunate implant replacement with or without intercarpal fusions
IV	Sclerosis, cysts, and fragmentation of the lunate with Scaphoradial angle: <70° Carpal height collapse: 5 to 10 percent Carpal translation moderate	Lunate implant replacement with scaphoid stabilization (distal fusion) Intercarpal fusions if early changes are found in contiguous bones
V	Sclerosis, cysts, and fragmentation of the lunate with Scaphoradial angle: >70° Carpal height collapse: >10 percent Carpal translation severe Cystic changes in contiguous bones	Lunate implant replacement and intercarpal fusions Scapholunate implant replacement Wrist arthrodesis Ulnar impingement treatment, as needed
VI	Sclerosis, cysts, and fragmentation of the lunate with Scaphoradial angle: > 70° Carpal height collapse: >15 percent Carpal translation severe Cystic changes in contiguous bones Significant intercarpal and radiocarpal degenerative arthritic changes	Total wrist implant arthroplasty Wrist arthrodesis Ulnar impingement treatment, as needed

Table 28–2. **CLASSIFICATION AND TREATMENT FOR PATHOLOGIC CONDITIONS OF THE SCAPHOID**

Stage	Pathologic Conditions	Treatment Options
I	Acute scaphoid fractures Acute scaphoid fracture-dislocation	Immobilization Open or closed reduction
II	Nonunion of the scaphoid	Bone graft Bone stimulator

III	Avascular necrosis of a fragment with
	    Carpal height collapse: 0 to 5 percent
	    Lunate dorsiflexion minimal (R-L angle: 0° to 10°)
		Partial scaphoid implant replacement
		Scaphoid implant replacement

IV	Comminuted or grossly displaced fracture
	Avascular necrosis with scaphoid degenerative arthritic
	    changes
	Subluxation of scaphoid with degenerative arthritic
	    changes
	Nonunion of scaphoid with cystic changes with
	    Carpal height collapse: 5 to 10 percent
	    Lunate dorsiflexion minimal to moderate (R-L angle:
	        10° to 30°)
	    Mild degenerative arthritic changes of contiguous
	        bones (particularly between lunate and capitate)
		Scaphoid implant replacement with or without
		  intercarpal fusions

V	Stage IV pathology of the scaphoid with
	    Carpal height collapse >10 percent
	    Lunate dorsiflexion moderate to severe (R-L angle
	        >30°)
	    Mild to moderate degenerative arthritic changes of
	        contiguous bones
		Scaphoid implant replacement with intercarpal fusions
		Scapholunate implant replacement
		Proximal row carpectomy
		Fusion of the proximal carpus to the radius
		Hemiarthroplasty

VI	Stage IV pathology of the scaphoid or previous surgery
	  with
	    Carpal height collapse >15 percent
	    Lunate dorsiflexion severe (R-L angle: >30°)
	    Severe intercarpal and radiocarpal degenerative
	        arthritic changes
		Total wrist implant arthroplasty
		Wrist arthrodesis
		Ulnar impingement treatment, as needed

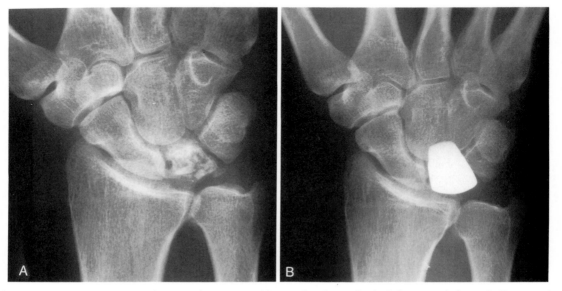

Figure 28–1. A, Preoperative radiogram of a 31-year-old man showing a Grade II lunate pathology. B, Postoperative radiogram showing a metal lunate implant replacement.

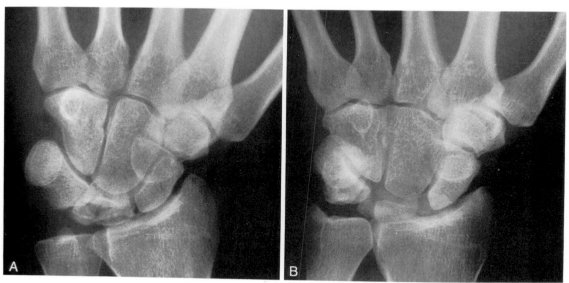

Figure 28–2. *A,* Kienböck's disease, Class III, with cystic changes and fragmentation of the lunate and minimal collapse changes of the carpus (carpal height 0.492, scaphoradial angle 46°) in a 21-year-old man. *B,* Fifteen-year postoperative radiograph. The carpal height is 0.478 and the scaphoradial angle is 52°, demonstrating excellent maintenance of carpal bone structure and stability. The patient is an extremely active man doing heavy work and is completely free of symptoms. (From Swanson AB, de Groot Swanson G, et al: J Hand Surg 10A [Part 2]:1013–1024, 1985.)

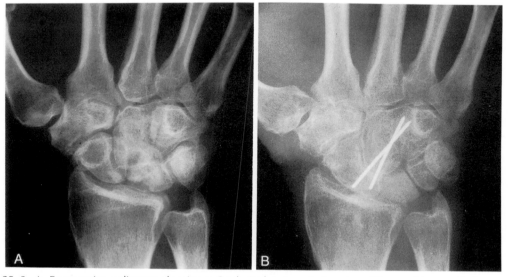

Figure 28–3. *A,* Preoperative radiogram showing a Grade IV lunate pathology in a 50-year-old man. *B,* Postoperative radiogram showing a lunate implant replacement with associated scaphocapitate fusion and bone grafting of cyst in the capitate. Patient has pain-free function and motion.

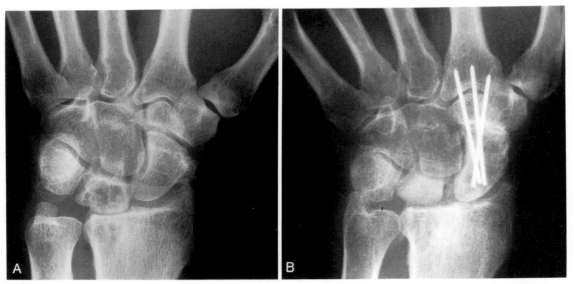

Figure 28–4. *A*, Kienböck's disease, Class IV, showing cystic changes in the lunate and in the adjacent radius in a 40-year old man. Associated rotary subluxation of the scaphoid is noted. An exostosis on the radial aspect of the scaphoid can be seen. *B*, Postoperative view shows excision of the lunate and implant replacement, bone grafting of the cyst in the radius, and corrected rotation of the scaphoid, with distal fusion to the trapezium and trapezoid. Kirschner wires will be removed at a later date. (From Swanson AB, de Groot Swanson G, et al: J Hand Surg 10A [Part 2]:1013–1024, 1985.)

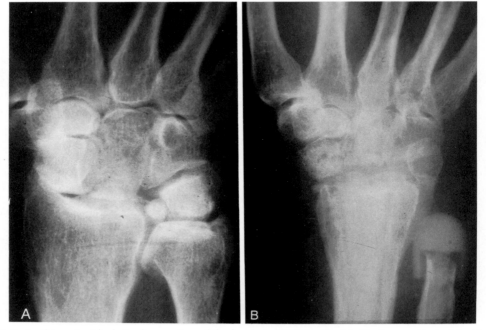

Figure 28–5. *A*, This patient had simple resection of the lunate in 1947 for Kienböck's disease. He had had increasing pain and disability for 10 years, when he was seen in 1982. Note the severe carpal collapse and ulnar translation. *B*, Radiograph shows 2-year follow-up results of a silicone flexible hinge radiocarpal arthroplasty and resection of the ulnar head with ulnar head implant replacement. The patient is relieved of symptoms and has a good, functioning wrist. (From Swanson AB, de Groot Swanson G, et al: J Hand Surg 10A [Part 2]:1013–1024, 1985.)

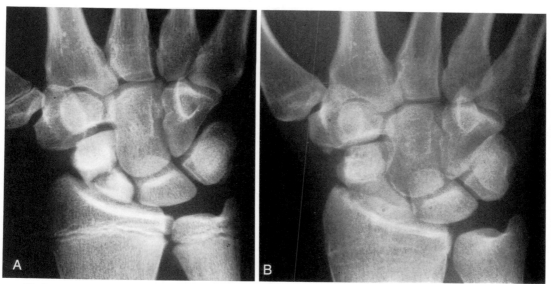

Figure 28–6. *A,* Preoperative radiogram of 16-year-old athlete showing a Stage III scaphoid pathology. *B,* Postoperative radiogram five years after partial silicone implant replacement of the proximal pole of the scaphoid. The patient has a good, pain-free functional result.

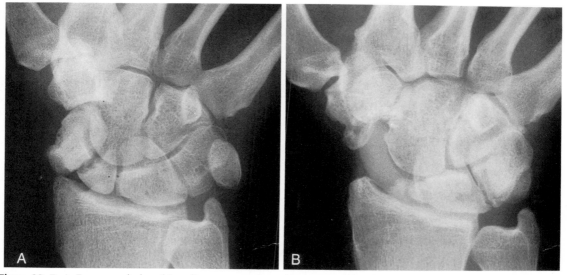

Figure 28–7. *A,* Two years before this radiogram was taken, this 19-year-old male sustained a hyperextension wrist injury while pole-vaulting. The preoperative radiogram shows a scaphoid nonunion, with early degenerative changes between the distal scaphoid fragment and the radial styloid. The wrist has a Stage III involvement, with carpal height of 0.485 and radiolunate angle of 10°. *B,* Postoperative radiograph 16 years after scaphoid implant arthroplasty. The patient is very active and is pain-free, with full functional use of the wrist. The implant remains well positioned, and there have been no cystic changes in the adjacent bones. (*B,* From Swanson AB, de Groot Swanson G, Maupin BK, et al: Scaphoid implant resection arthroplasty: long-term results. J Arthroplasty 1:47–62, 1986, Churchill Livingstone Inc, New York.)

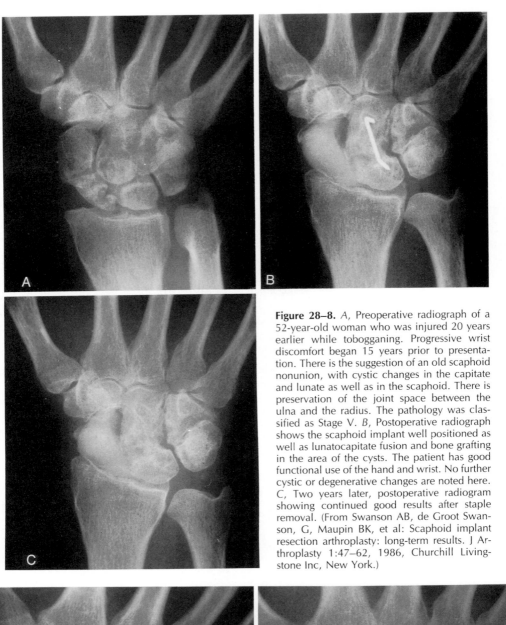

Figure 28–8. *A,* Preoperative radiograph of a 52-year-old woman who was injured 20 years earlier while tobogganing. Progressive wrist discomfort began 15 years prior to presentation. There is the suggestion of an old scaphoid nonunion, with cystic changes in the capitate and lunate as well as in the scaphoid. There is preservation of the joint space between the ulna and the radius. The pathology was classified as Stage V. *B,* Postoperative radiograph shows the scaphoid implant well positioned as well as lunatocapitate fusion and bone grafting in the area of the cysts. The patient has good functional use of the hand and wrist. No further cystic or degenerative changes are noted here. *C,* Two years later, postoperative radiogram showing continued good results after staple removal. (From Swanson AB, de Groot Swanson, G, Maupin BK, et al: Scaphoid implant resection arthroplasty: long-term results. J Arthroplasty 1:47–62, 1986, Churchill Livingstone Inc, New York.)

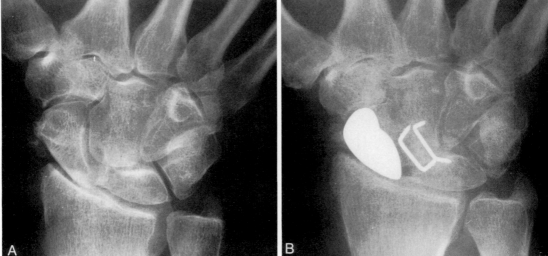

Figure 28–9. *A,* Preoperative radiogram of the wrist of a 66-year-old man, showing a Stage V scaphoid pathology. *B,* Postoperative radiogram showing a metal scaphoid implant replacement and carpal stabilization with a lunocapitate fusion using a bone graft and staple fixation.

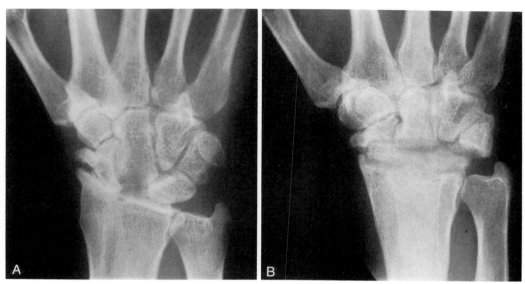

Figure 28–10. *A*, Preoperative radiogram showing a Stage VI scaphoid pathology, with marked carpal height collapse and degenerative changes in the wrist of a 50-year-old man. *B*, Postoperative radiogram three years after silicone flexible hinge wrist implant arthroplasty. The patient has a pain-free wrist with good functional mobility.

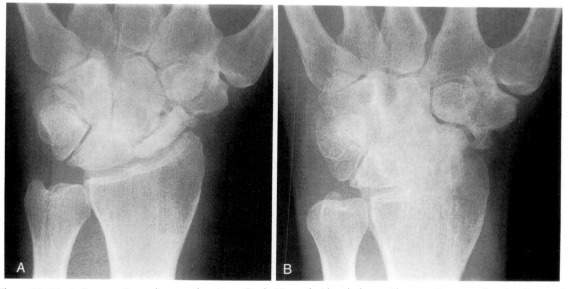

Figure 28–11. *A*, Preoperative radiogram showing a Grade VI scaphoid pathology with severe intercarpal and radiocarpal degenerative changes. *B*, Postoperative radiogram 10 years following a radiocarpal fusion.

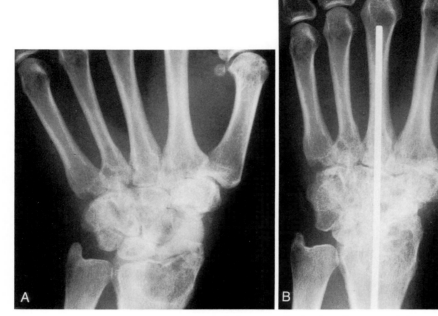

Figure 28–12. *A*, A bricklayer with Stage VI pathology initially developed cystic and degenerative changes and carpal collapse six years after scaphoid replacement with a large implant and Kirschner wire fixation. *B*, Postoperative radiogram showing revision to a wrist fusion with iliac bone graft and an intramedullary wire fixation. The patient is back to work without symptoms. (*B*, From Swanson AB, de Groot Swanson G, Maupin BK, et al: Scaphoid implant resection arthroplasty: long-term results. J Arthroplasty 1:47–62, 1986, Churchill Livingstone Inc, New York.)

palmar ligamentous structures that can further cause implant instability (Fig. 28–13). A subluxated carpal implant is under abnormal shear stress, and if it is also subjected to excessive loading forces across the wrist joint, exaggerated wear of the silicone and eventual failure of the arthroplasty will result. The palmar ligaments should be preserved during carpal bone excision by leaving a small portion of the palmar part of the bone, or they should be repaired if weakened. Associated collapse patterns should be treated at the time of implant arthroplasty, by appropriate intercarpal bone fusions. Carpal bone implant replacement is not indicated in cases of advanced disease; in these cases, wrist implant arthroplasty or fusion is preferred.

LUNATE IMPLANT

Indications

Lunate implant resection arthroplasty can be indicated in the presence of avascular necrosis (Kienböck's disease), localized osteoarthritic changes, and long-standing dislocations. The procedure is contraindicated in cases in which arthritic involvement is not localized to the lunate articulations, if

complete relief of pain is to be expected. In long-standing dislocations or in cases of Kienböck's disease, the normal space for the lunate is markedly decreased, and it may be difficult to fit the implant. Loss of integrity of the capsular structures, owing to a fracture-dislocation or a collapse deformity of the wrist, may be a contraindication to the implant procedure, unless a stable relationship of the carpal bones can be re-established. Associated collapse patterns should be treated at the time of implant arthroplasty by appropriate intercarpal fusions. Pre-existing cysts in contiguous bones should be bone-grafted at the time of the procedure. If severe carpal collapse is present, more extensive procedures may be indicated.

Surgical Procedure

A dorsal longitudinal incision across the radiocarpal area and centered at Lister's tubercle is used to expose the lunate bone. A transverse skin incision may be used in some of the uncomplicated cases, especially in the female. A volar approach is recommended when the lunate bone is dislocated volarly. The superficial sensory branches of the radial and ulnar nerves are carefully preserved. The extensor retinaculum is incised over the extensor pollicis longus tendon, which is mobilized for radial retraction (Fig. 28–14A). The extensor digitorum communis tendons are retracted ulnarly. With the wrist flexed, the dorsocarpal ligament is incised in a T shape and elevated close to bone (Fig. 28–14B). Adequate dissection is necessary to properly identify the capitate, triquetrum, scaphoid, radius, and lunate. Roentgenograms are taken, if necessary, for further anatomic orientation. The lunate is removed piecemeal, and care is taken to avoid injury to the dorsal and palmar carpal ligaments. A thin, bony shell remnant of the lunate is left with the palmar ligaments to assure their important supportive continuity; their integrity must be verified and obtained, if necessary, to prevent palmar subluxation of the implant. If the lunate bone is totally removed, there will be a defect between the two strong bands of the palmar ulnocarpal and radiocarpal ligaments, which are attached on each side of the lunate (Fig. 28–13). A tendon graft or a slip of the flexor carpi radialis tendon can be used if direct reapproximation of these structures is impossible.

The associated bones should be evaluated for the presence of arthritic changes, loss of cartilage, surface irregularities, cystic changes, and collapse patterns. Traction and compression of the hand across the wrist joint can help reveal instability patterns, particularly that of vertical rotation of the scaphoid bone. In the presence of collapse patterns or instability of the carpus, associated limited carpal bone fusions are very important to improve the distribution of forces across the wrist joint and, consequently, across the hand. Rotary subluxation of the scaphoid must be corrected and the carpus stabilized, either by triscaphe or scaphocapitate fusion, using an iliac bone graft. The scaphocapitate fusion is preferred when there are cystic changes in the capitate. A spline type of bone graft, which is keyed into a slot made in the two adjacent bones, is preferred. Firm internal fixation is obtained with staples or Kirschner wires. Any pre-existing cyst is curetted and grafted, preferably with an iliac bone graft.

Selection of the proper implant size is made from the five that are available. The stem of the silicone implant is resected. The stemless titanium implant has holes for suture placement. Implant sizing is started with the smallest one to allow appreciation of the spatial relationships of the implant to the contiguous bones. In long-standing dislocations of the lunate, the space can be greatly decreased, and the smallest implant is used whenever possible. The deep con-

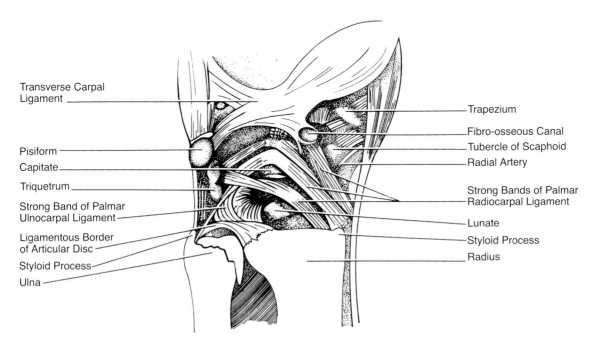

Figure 28–13. Palmar carpal ligaments. Complete excision of carpal bones (trapezium, scaphoid, or lunate) may leave "holes" or defects in palmar carpal ligaments, because they firmly attach to carpal bones. A small shell of bone should be left on the palmar capsule to preserve its continuity. (From Swanson AB, de Groot Swanson G, and Watermeier JJ: J Hand Surg, 6:125–141, 1981.)

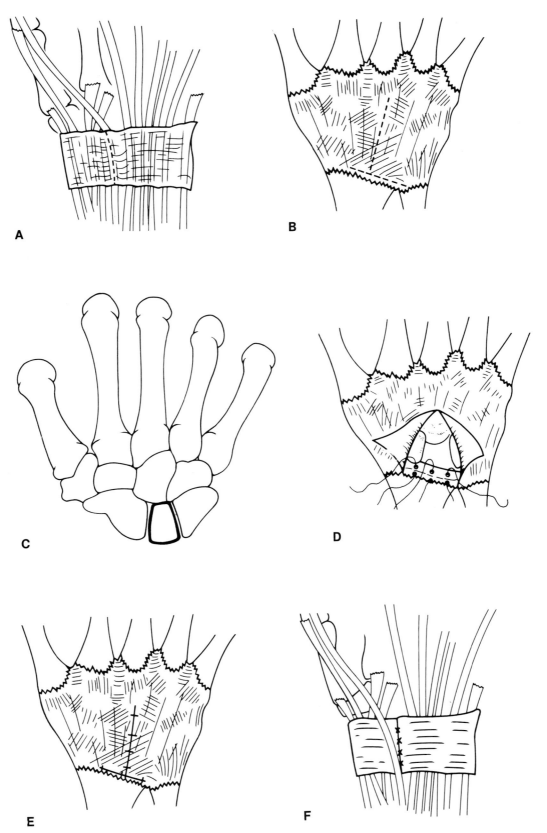

Figure 28–14. *A* through *F*, Lunate implant resection arthroplasty. *C* shows lunate implant in position. See text for description of technique. (From Swanson AB, de Groot Swanson G, et al: J Hand Surg 10A [Part 2]:1013–1024, 1985.)

cavity of the lunate implant straddles the head of the capitate. It is very important not to use an oversized implant, as this causes excessive implant loading, resulting in abrasion particles that can participate in a foreign body reaction.

The silicone implant is not stabilized with sutures (Fig. 28–14C). The titanium implant is stabilized with O–Dacron sutures to the carpal ligaments or to the adjacent carpal bones.

Approximately 1 cm of the posterior sensory branch of the posterior interosseous nerve is resected to provide some sensory denervation of part of the carpal area. The preserved dorsal capsule is firmly sutured, inverting the knots to prevent adherence to overlying tendons (Fig. 28–14D and E). A strip of extensor retinaculum or a strip of extensor carpi radialis longus or brevis tendon can be used to reinforce the dorsal carpal ligaments, if necessary. The stability of the capsular repair should be verified by passive movement of the wrist in all directions. An excessively tight repair could prevent adequate wrist motion; at least 30° of flexion and extension should be obtained. The retinaculum is sutured over the extensor tendons, except for the extensor pollicis longus, which is left free in the subcutaneous tissue (Fig. 28–14F). The wound is closed and drained. A secure voluminous conforming dressing, including anterior and posterior plaster splints, is fashioned.

The extremity is kept elevated for three to five days, and the patient is instructed to move the shoulder and fingers. A short- or long-arm thumb spica cast is applied, depending upon the stability of the carpal bones. If a cast has been applied at surgery, it should be bivalved. Skin sutures are removed after two to three weeks through a window in the cast, which is worn for six to eight weeks and may be tightened or changed, as needed. The rehabilitation program includes isometric gripping exercises for development of the extrinsic and intrinsic muscles of the hand and forearm. Full use of the wrist is usually resumed at 12 weeks, unless an intercarpal fusion was done, which requires a longer immobilization. Postoperative roentgenograms are made to evaluate the position of the implant and the status of the bone.

SCAPHOID IMPLANT

Indications

Scaphoid implant resection arthroplasty can be indicated in the following: (1) acute fractures, either comminuted or grossly displaced; (2) pseudarthrosis of the scaphoid, especially if a small proximal fragment is present; (3) Preiser's disease; (4) avascular necrosis of a fragment; and (5) failures of previous surgery.

The procedure is contraindicated in cases in which arthritic involvement is not localized to the scaphoid articulations if complete relief of pain is to be expected. In long-standing subluxations or in cases of Preiser's disease, the normal amount of space can be markedly decreased, and it may be difficult to fit the implant. If the radial styloid has been removed, there is no provision for lateral stability of the implant. Loss of integrity of the capsular structures, due to a fracture dislocation or collapse deformity of the wrist, may be a contraindication to the implant procedure, unless a stable relationship of the carpal bones can be re-established. Associated collapse patterns should be treated at the time of implant arthroplasty by appropriate intercarpal fusions. Pre-existing cysts in contiguous bones should be bone-grafted at the time of the procedure. If severe carpal collapse is present, more extensive procedures may be indicated.

Surgical Procedure

A 7- to 10-cm dorsoradial longitudinal incision is made across the radiocarpal joint midway between the tip of the styloid and Lister's tubercle. The longitudinal veins and branches of the superficial radial nerve are carefully preserved. The extensor retinaculum is incised over the extensor pollicis longus, which is retracted radially. The extensor retinaculum is elevated from the third compartment radially to expose the second compartment. The extensor carpi radialis longus and brevis are mobilized to their insertion for appropriate retraction. The transverse metacarpal vessels, located immediately under the insertion of the wrist extensors, are protected. The dorsocarpal wrist ligament is incised in a T shape. With the wrist flexed, the dorsal ligament is elevated from the radius by sharp dissection kept close to bone to preserve adequate tissue for reattachment. By retracting the wrist extensor tendons radially, the scapholunate junction and the capitate bone can be identified. By retracting the extensor tendons ulnarly, the distal portion of the scaphoid bone can be visualized, and its articulations with the trapezoid and trapezium, as well as with the radius, can be shown. If necessary, intraoperative radiograms can be obtained to identify the carpal bones. The scaphoid bone is removed piecemeal with a rongeur, avoiding injury to the underlying palmar ligaments and to both dorsal and palmar scapholunate ligaments. A thin, bony shell remnant of the scaphoid is left in the palmar ligament area distal to the radiocapitate ligament and extending up to the trapezium to assure their important supportive continuity. If the scaphoid distal pole is completely removed, there will be a hole left in the palmar supporting structures, through which the implant could protrude (Fig. 28–13).

The associated bones should be evaluated for the presence of arthritic changes, loss of cartilage, surface irregularities, cystic changes, and collapse patterns, as previously described for lunate implant arthroplasty. In the presence of collapse patterns or instability, rotation of the lunate must be corrected and the carpus stabilized by fusion of the lunate to the capitate or to the triquetrum or both, with or without associated fusion of other involved carpal bones. A spline type of bone graft, preferably iliac, is keyed into a slot made in the adjacent bones. Resected bone, if healthy, can also be used. Firm internal fixation is obtained with staples or Kirschner wires. Any pre-existing cyst is curetted and bone-grafted.

Using trial implants, sizing is started with the smallest implant to appreciate its spatial relationships to the contiguous bones. The stem of the scaphoid silicone implant is resected. The stemless titanium implant has holes for suture fixation. Scaphoid implants are available in seven sizes, and, because of mirror-image differences, there are separate models for the right and left hands. It is very important not to use an oversized implant, as this would cause excessive implant loading, resulting in abrasion particles that can participate in a foreign body reaction. The implant is handled with blunt instruments to avoid abrasion or contamination with foreign particles.

The silicone scaphoid implant is not stabilized with sutures. The stemless titanium scaphoid implant is stabilized with O–Dacron sutures to the carpal ligaments or the adjacent carpal bones. Prior to implant insertion, integrity of the palmar ligaments and capsule is determined; if necessary, they are either tightened with sutures or reinforced with a strip of flexor carpi radialis tendon.

Approximately 1 cm of the posterior sensory branch of the posterior interosseous nerve is resected to provide some sensory denervation of part of the carpal area. The method of suturing the dorsal capsule, the extensor retinaculum, and the skin is similar to that described for lunate implant arthroplasty. A strip of extensor retinaculum or a strip of extensor carpi radialis longus or brevis tendon can be used to reinforce the dorsal carpal ligaments, if necessary. A secure conforming dressing, including an anterior and posterior splint, is applied.

The extremity is kept elevated for three to five days, and shoulder and finger movements are encouraged. A long-arm thumb spica cast is applied for four weeks, and a short-arm thumb spica cast is used for an additional four weeks. If a plaster cast is applied at surgery, it should be bivalved. The postoperative care and rehabilitation are similar to those described for lunate implant arthroplasty.

Pitfalls of Lunate and Scaphoid Implant Arthroplasty and Their Prevention

A series of 248 carpal bone silicone implants made of the original silicone material and of high-performance silicone was previously reviewed to evaluate their relationship to degenerative or cystic changes in contiguous carpal bones. The follow-up ranged from 12 to 207 months (average, 56 months). No cystic changes were found in 80 percent of cases and changes were minimal in 12 percent, moderate in 6 percent, and severe in 2 percent. Cystic changes were more frequent around scaphoid implants. Degenerative arthritic changes of the entire hand and wrist equaled cystic changes in 72.5 percent, were greater in 16 percent, and were less severe in 11.5 percent of cystic cases. Association with carpal collapse was noted in 84 percent of cystic cases. Cysts were present in 50 percent of cases in which Kirschner wire fixation was used and in 15 percent of cases in which it was not used. There was a 2.3 percent revision rate, including performance of synovectomy, bone grafting of cysts, selected intercarpal bone fusions, removal or replacement of implant, and wrist implant arthroplasty or fusion (Fig. 28–12). A recent review of the original silicone material implants showed a very significantly lower incidence of cystic changes than in those cases treated with the high-performance silicone implants.

A particle-induced reactive synovitis can occur in the presence of (1) excessive force loading of the implant, with shear stress and implant abrasion due to implant oversize or malposition, carpal collapse, excessive motion and abuse from daily activity; (2) preexisting cysts; (3) Kirschner wire fixation; and (4) evidence of arthritic diasthesis.

To avoid these problems, attention must be paid to the following considerations:

1. Patient selection—In the young, active, or hard-laboring patient, associated procedures in implant arthroplasty, such as limited intercarpal fusion and motion restriction by soft tissue capsular reconstruction, as well as strict postoperative care and instructions, are indicated. Alternative nonimplant procedures such as soft tissue reconstruction or arthrodesis may be considered;

2. Identification of prior disorders—these include preoperative collapse or instability patterns, bone cysts, and arthritis of other intercarpal joints;

3. Meticulous surgical technique;

4. Stabilization of collapse deformities—if there is scaphoid instability in a wrist requiring lunate implant arthroplasty, a scaphotrapeziotrapezoid or a scaphocapitate fusion may be considered (Figs. 28–3 and 28–4). If there is lunate instability in a wrist requiring scaphoid implant arthroplasty, a lunocapitate or lunotriquetral fusion may be considered (Figs. 28–8 and 28–9). Intercarpal fusions are carried out with cancellous bone grafting (preferably of iliac bone) and internal fixation, either with staples or Kirschner wires;

5. Presence of pre-existing subchondral bone cysts—these must be treated at the time of carpal bone implant arthroplasty by curettage and cancellous bone grafting (Figs. 28–3, 28–4, and 28–8). Failure to recognize and treat pre-existing cysts will result in their progression;

6. Implant sizing—if there is inadequate space, an implant should not be used; if used, the implant must not be oversized;

7. Stabilization of the implant—This is obtained chiefly by capsuloligamentous reconstruction. The titanium implant is sutured to the carpal ligaments or to the adjacent bones;

8. Avoidance of the use of Kirschner wires or sutures placed through silicone implants;

9. Plaster cast immobilization for a minimum of six weeks and avoidance of excessive or abusive motion postoperatively.

Revision procedures may be indicated for symptomatic progression of disease to other carpal articulations, for implant subluxation or fracture, or for bone cyst formation. These procedures can include synovectomy of the surrounding tissues, removal or replacement of the implant, curettage of cysts with cancellous bone grafting, selective intercarpal bone fusions, and implant arthroplasty or arthrodesis of the radiocarpal joint. In cases of implant fracture, subluxation, or instability, silicone particulate debris and cystic formation may follow; therefore, in these cases, the implant should be removed, and appropriate corrective surgery should be carried out. Good results have usually followed revisional surgery.

We feel that lunate and scaphoid implant arthroplasties are useful procedures. Longterm good results can be achieved if the pathologic condition is well identified, the severity of disease is not too advanced, and the proper surgical indications and techniques are followed.

THE THUMB BASAL JOINTS

In any reconstructive surgery of the thumb, the entire ray must be considered—its balanced musculotendinous system and the position, mobility, and stability of all three articulations. Each joint may be affected primarily or secondarily by imbalances of the other joints, as seen in the boutonnière and swan-neck deformities.

The problems that develop at the basal joints of the thumb are different in osteoarthritis and in rheumatoid arthritis. Proper evaluation of the location of the arthritic involvement and of the condition and alignment of adjacent bones is essential in selecting the preferred method of treatment. The pathologic condition can involve the trapeziometacarpal joint, with or without involvement of peritrapezial articulations or other carpal bone articulations; this can be present with or without resorption or displacement of adjacent carpal bones. The proper method of treatment must be selected from the following: resection arthroplasty of the trapeziometacarpal joint or of the entire trapezium with or without either a convex or concave condylar implant in the former or a trapezium implant in the latter (Fig. 28–15).

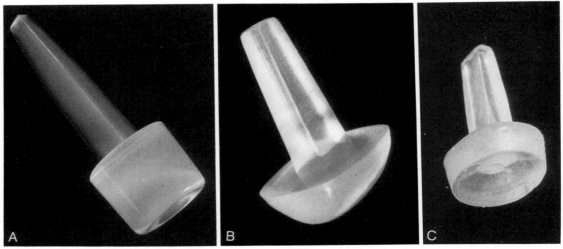

Figure 28–15. Silicone implants for reconstruction of the thumb basal joint. *A,* Trapezium implant; *B,* convex condylar implant; *C,* concave condylar implant.

The use of an implant in resection arthroplasty of the basal joints of the thumb helps maintain the joint space and a smooth articulation to improve joint stability, mobility, relief of pain, and strength. Meticulous capsuloligamentous reconstruction around these implants and correction of any associated deformity of the thumb ray are essential for a good result.

Titanium convex condylar implants for the trapeziometacarpal joint have been evaluated since 1983 and have been approved for general usage. Because of the significantly lower incidence of cystic formation around the original silicone elastomer compared with that in the high-performance silicone, the senior author prefers the use of the original material for trapezium implants without the use of suture fixation; the use of the titanium convex condylar implants for trapeziometacarpal joint reconstruction is preferred in the osteoarthritic joint. Silicone convex or concave implants of the original material or simple resection arthroplasty is preferred for the rheumatoid joint.

Trapezium Implant Arthroplasty

Indications

Trapezium implant resection arthroplasty is indicated when the following conditions are present, whether the disability is due to degenerative or post-traumatic arthritis (e.g., following an old Bennett's fracture) with localized bone changes: (1) localized pain and palpable crepitation during circumduction movements, with axial compression of the thumb (the "grind" test); (2) loss of motion with decreased pinch and grip strength; (3) radiologic evidence of arthritic changes of the trapeziometacarpal, trapezioscaphoid, trapeziotrapezoid, and trapezoid-second metacarpal joints, singly or in combination; and (4) unstable, stiff, or painful distal joints of the thumb, or swan-neck collapse deformity. This procedure is contraindicated when there is severe displacement, resorption, or involvement of contiguous carpal bones.

Surgical Procedure

A 7-cm longitudinal incision centered over the trapezium is made parallel to the extensor pollicis brevis tendon; the incision is then directed proximally and ulnarly to the distal wrist crease. To expose the flexor carpi radialis tendon at the wrist, the incision is curved palmarly and continued proximally, parallel to this tendon (Fig. 28–16A). Branches of the superficial radial nerve are carefully identified and preserved (Fig. 28–16B). Small transverse veins may be ligated; however, longitudinal veins are spared. The retinaculum of the first dorsal compartment is incised longitudinally, and the dissection is carried down between the abductor pollicis longus and the extensor pollicis brevis tendons. The radial artery is exposed and mobilized for proximal retraction; small arterial branches going into the trapeziometacarpal joint are ligated (Fig. 28–16C). The joint capsule is incised longitudinally or in a **T** fashion, and the flaps are carefully incised off the underlying bone to retain all capsular tissue. The trapezioscaphoid and trapeziometacarpal joints are identified, and, with traction on the thumb, further freeing of the dorsal capsular attachments around the trapezium can be done. It is important to keep the dissection close to the bone to avoid injury to the artery, the underlying tendons, or the capsule.

The trapezium is sectioned into pieces and removed piecemeal with a bone-biting rongeur, including its ulnar distal projection, often seen between the first and second metacarpals. Traction on the thumb or distal retraction, with a small two-pronged rake retractor on the base of the metacarpal, will facilitate the exposure. Small flecks of bone are left with the underlying capsule to preserve good palmar capsuloligamentous support; this is especially true on the radial palmar aspect of the trapezium, where it attaches to the transverse carpal ligament and to the underlying thenar muscles (Fig. 28–13). Any osteophytes or irregularities on the distal end of the scaphoid or trapezoid are trimmed. The trapezium should be positively identified to prevent removing portions of adjacent bones. Frequently, a radial shift of the trapezoid has occurred, preventing adequate seating of the implant over the scaphoid facet; a portion of the radial aspect of the trapezoid should be removed to improve this fit.

The base of the metacarpal is brought up into the wound and squared off with a rongeur, leaving most of its cortical and subchondral bone intact. Any osteophytes, especially on its medial portion, should be removed. The intramedullary canal of the metacarpal should be probed first with a thin broach or a small curette to prevent inadvertent perforation through its side wall and consequent extrusion of the implant stem through this defect. Special burs with a small leader point are then used to develop a triangular intramedullary shape, which should be no larger than necessary to receive the implant stem easily.

The appropriate-sized implant should fit the trapeziectomy space, with its collar sitting properly on the metacarpal base and its base well over the distal scaphoid facet to allow full and stable circumduction of the thumb. Test implants are used to select the proper size; of the five available sizes, implant sizes 2 and 3 are most commonly used. The wound must be thoroughly irrigated with saline to remove all debris before inserting the implant.

It is important to secure the implant in place over the scaphoid by reconstruction of the capsuloligamentous structures around the implant. The palmar capsule and ligaments are inspected in the depths of the wound for inadvertent tears or "holes." If present, these should be sutured so that there is firm support by the palmar capsule.

The flexor carpi radialis tendon is exposed at the wrist, its radial third is incised, and a 7- to 8-cm slip is dissected distally to the fibro-osseous canal. The tendon slip is pulled up into the site of the trapeziectomy and further dissected to its insertion on the second metacarpal, which is carefully preserved. Great care should be taken to avoid transverse lacerations of the tendon slip. A small hemostat is passed through the abductor policis brevis muscle to pull the tendon slip under the residual portion of the flexor carpi radialis tendon and then through the abductor pollicis brevis muscle (Fig. 28–16D). The slip is brought anteriorly through the abductor pollicis longus tendon and the lateral portion of the capsular tissues (Fig. 28–16E). It is important that the slip not be pulled too tight, as it may have a tendency to lift the implant from the floor of the wound; this can be prevented by placing the tendon slip under the flexor carpi radialis tendon and suturing it to this tendon and to the palmar capsule. As the radial artery is retracted proximally, three 3–0 Dacron sutures are placed through the preserved capsular reflection off the scaphoid to secure the closure of the radial capsule. If necessary, these sutures are placed through 1-mm drill holes made in the edge of the scaphoid. The tendon slip is then brought over and through the radial capsule to exit through the ulnar capsule. The tendon slip may also be passed through the distal portion of the extensor carpi radialis longus tendon, avoiding the overlying radial artery. After implant insertion, it is pulled out and folded over and across the dorsal capsular repair and sutured in position (Fig. 28–16F). In some cases, sutures may be required in the proximal end of the metacarpal to securely close the distal portion of the capsular repair. The longitudinal dorsal capsular incision is repaired with 3–0 Dacron sutures or other nonabsorbable material, using multiple interrupted sutures and inverting the knots. The abductor pollicis longus is advanced distally on the metacarpal, and the extensor pollicis longus is tenodesed at the ligament repair

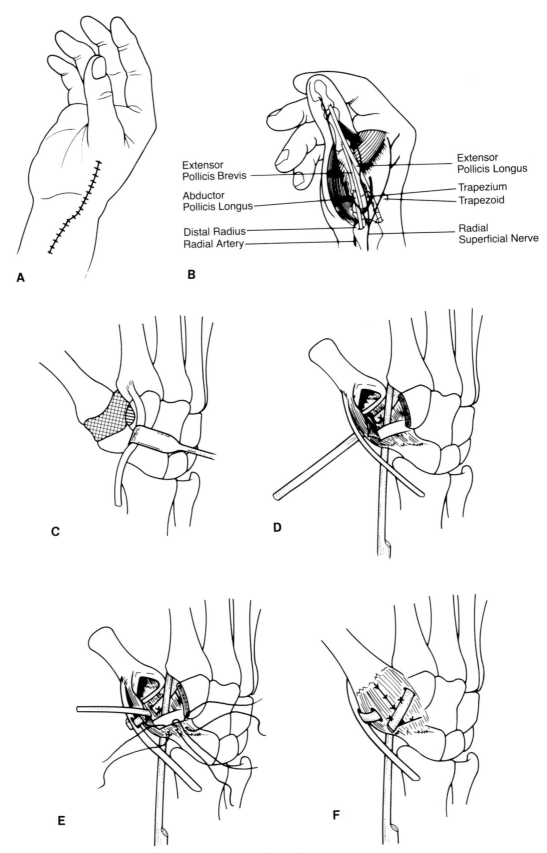

A

B

Extensor
Pollicis Brevis

Abductor
Pollicis Longus

Distal Radius
Radial Artery

Extensor
Pollicis Longus

Trapezium
Trapezoid

Radial
Superficial Nerve

C

D

E

F

Figure 28–16. *See legend on opposite page.*

site. This ligamentous repair provides a firm capsular reinforcement on the palmar, ulnar, radial, and dorsal sides. It is noted again that a portion of the trapezoid bone may have to be removed for proper seating of the implant. The appropriate capsular closure, with or without tendon reinforcement, is carried out after the implant is positioned.

The first dorsal compartment is loosely closed over the abductor pollicis longus and extensor pollicis brevis tendons. Dorsal bowstringing of the extensor pollicis brevis tendon could result in an increased moment arm and could produce hyperextension of the metacarpophalangeal joint of the thumb; however, increasing the moment arm of the abductor pollicis longus tendon has advantages for thumb abduction and can be accomplished by advancing its distal insertion on the metacarpal.

The wound is closed in layers, and small silicone rubber drains are inserted subcutaneously. A secure dressing, including an anterior and posterior plaster splint, is then applied. It is also possible to apply a plaster cast at the end of the operative procedure; the cast should be bivalved and the extremity elevated because of the potential for postoperative swelling. The extremity is kept elevated for two to three days, and the drains are removed in approximately 48 hours. After two to three days, depending on the amount of soft tissue swelling, a short-arm thumb spica type of cast is applied and worn for six weeks; sutures are removed through a window in the cast at three weeks. The patient then starts guarded range of motion exercises, including pinch and grasp activities. A small, 2.5-cm diameter dowel is a good exercise device; it can be grasped in the first web space to improve abduction and to build strength in the hand and forearm (Fig. 28–17).

Trapeziometacarpal Implant Arthroplasty

In rheumatoid arthritis and in certain cases of severe erosive osteoarthritis, destructive changes of the contiguous carpal bones make trapezial implant arthroplasty difficult. Frequently, the trapezium is fused to the scaphoid, or the scaphoid may be absorbed or shifted ulnarly. An intramedullary stemmed convex condylar implant has been designed for use in these situations (Fig. 28–15). The use of tinanium convex condylar implants is now preferred in the osteoarthritic thumb, and the use of the original silicone material implant is preferred in the rheumatoid thumb. A concave condylar implant can be used as an alternative to the convex condylar implant, when there is inadequate trapezial bone stock to allow shaping of this bone to receive the convex implant head. These implants can provide a stable, pain-free, functional thumb joint, although the usual range of motion that can be obtained with the standard trapezial implant cannot be expected.

Surgical Procedure

The surgical approach to the trapeziometacarpal joint is similar to that described for the trapezium implant. The joint capsule is incised longitudinally over the radial side of the trapeziometacarpal joint. Approximately 2 to 4 mm of the base of the metacarpal is resected. The articulating projection of the trapezium to the second metacarpal must also be resected. The distal facet of the trapezium is shaped in a slightly concave contour with a bur and air drill (Fig. 28–18A). A sufficient bone resection must be carried out to provide a joint space of approximately 4 mm and to allow 45° radial abduction of the first metacarpal. To achieve this goal, more bone may be resected from the metacarpal base, or the origin of the adductor pollicis may be released from the third metacarpal through a separate palmar incision, if indicated. The intramedullary canal of the first metacarpal is then prepared in the usual manner. The appropriate-sized implant is selected.

There is usually a radial subluxating tendency in these cases, which can be corrected by a firm capsuloligamentous reconstruction, using a slip of the abductor pollicis longus tendon. A distally based slip of the abductor pollicis longus tendon 8 cm long

---

Figure 28–16. *A* through *F*, Scaphoid resection implant arthroplasty. *F* shows procedure after implant insertion. See text for description of operation. (*A*, Reproduced with permission from Swanson AB, and de Groot Swanson G: Thumb disabilities in rheumatoid arthritis: classification and treatment. In AAOS Symposium on Tendon Surgery in the Hand. St. Louis, 1975, The CV Mosby Co, p 241. *B*, From Swanson AB: *C* through *F*, From Swanson AB, de Groot Swanson, G, and Watermeier JJ: J Hand Surg 6:125–141, 1981.

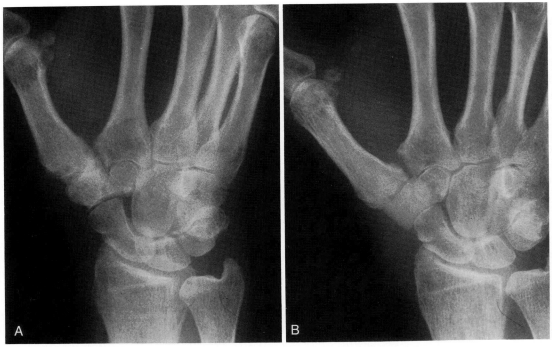

Figure 28–17. *A,* Preoperative x-ray of a 65-year-old woman's right hand shows pantrapezial osteoarthritic changes. Note preservation of the metacarpophalangeal articular surfaces of the thumb. The patient had presented with pain at the basal thumb joints. Examination revealed a 35° flexible hyperextension deformity of the metacarpophalangeal thumb joint, a positive grind test, and adequate lateral stability. *B,* Radiograph shows the implant well seated over the scaphoid two years after surgery. The patient's thumb had remained pain-free, stable, and functional, and she had returned to her job as a beautician.

and 2 mm wide is prepared, preserving its insertion on the radial aspect of the base of the first metacarpal. The slip is looped into the intramedullary canal of the first metacarpal, and the end of the slip is pulled out with a wire loop through a 2- to 3-mm drill hole in the radiodorsal aspect of the metacarpal. A similar hole is made in the trapezium, and the end of the slip is then drawn from inside the trapezium to the outside,

using a wire loop (Fig. 28–18B). The implant is placed in position after a thorough irrigation of the wound. The thumb is then held in 45° abduction as the slip is pulled up tight and securely interwoven to reinforce the capsular closure. The distal end of the slip is passed through or under the insertion of the abductor pollicis longus tendon and sutured to the radial capsular structures (Fig. 28–18C). It can be noted that when the slip

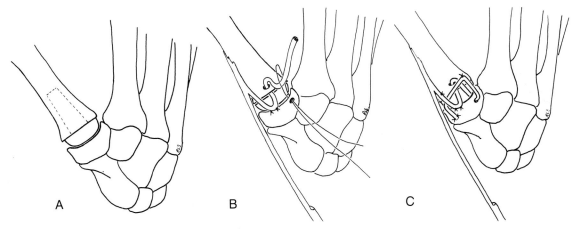

Figure 28–18. *A, B, C,* Surgical technique for trapeziometacarpal implant. See text for description. (From Swanson AB, de Groot Swanson G, and Watermeier JJ: J Hand Surg 6:125–141, 1981.)

is pulled up tight, it draws the metacarpal slightly toward the ulna, providing an excellent checkrein to radial subluxation of the base of the metacarpal. If a secure capsular closure can be achieved with 3–0 Dacron sutures passed through small drill holes in the base of the first metacarpal, reinforcement with a slip of abductor pollicis longus is not always necessary. However, the abductor pollicis longus insertion is always advanced distally. Any associated deformities of the thumb ray must be corrected. The techniques for wound closure, postoperative immobilization, and therapy are similar to those described for trapezium implant arthroplasty (Figs. 28–19 and 28–20). The use of a metal convex condylar implant is now preferred and has been approved for general use (Fig. 28–21).

Special Considerations

Adduction Contracture of the First Metacarpal. If severe and untreated, this condition unbalances the thumb and seriously affects the result of trapezium implant arthroplasty. If the angle of abduction between the first and second metacarpals is not at least 45°, the origin of the adductor pollicis muscle should be released from the third metacarpal through a separate palmar incision.

Hyperextension Deformity of the Metacarpophalangeal Joint. This disorder contributes to the adduction tendency of the metacarpal and prevents proper abduction of the metacarpal and seating of the implant. It should be corrected at the same time that the basal

joint reconstruction is performed. If the metacarpophalangeal joint hyperextends less than 10°, no treatment is necessary, except to apply the postoperative cast so that the metacarpal is abducted and not the proximal phalanx. If the metacarpophalangeal joint hyperextends 10° to 20°, it is pinned in 10° flexion for four to six weeks. If hyperextension of the joint is greater than 20° with nearly normal flexion, good lateral stability, and adequate articular surfaces, a palmar capsulodesis of the metacarpophalangeal joint, as described by the senior author, may be indicated to preserve available flexion and to restrict the hyperextension (Fig. 28–22). Fusion of the metacarpophalangeal joint should be done for hyperextension deformities in which there is no available flexion, or if there is lateral instability due to collateral ligament disruption, or in cases of articular destruction.

Boutonnière Deformity. This deformity of the thumb is usually not associated with arthritis of the basal joints of the type that would require implant arthroplasty. However, when this situation occurs, fusion of the metacarpophalangeal joint and release of the extensor pollicis longus at the distal joint may be performed at the same time as the basal joint reconstruction.

Pitfalls of Thumb Basal Joint Implant Arthroplasty and Their Prevention

The success of this procedure is related to the stability of the arthroplasty, which de-

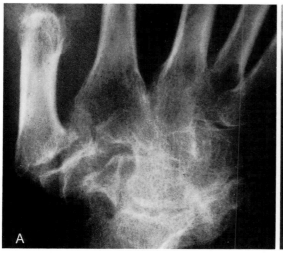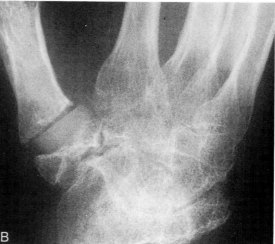

Figure 28–19. *A*, Preoperative radiograph of a rheumatoid thumb showing severe destruction at the trapeziometacarpal joint and at the articulations of the contiguous carpal bones. *B*, Radiograph taken three years after surgery, showing trapeziometacarpal joint arthroplasty with a convex condylar implant. The patient had good pain relief and a functional result. (From Swanson AB, and de Groot Swanson G: Arthroplasty of the thumb basal joints. In Leach RE, Hoaglund FT, and Riseborough EJ (eds): Controversies in Orthopaedic Surgery. Philadelphia, WB Saunders, 1982, p 48.)

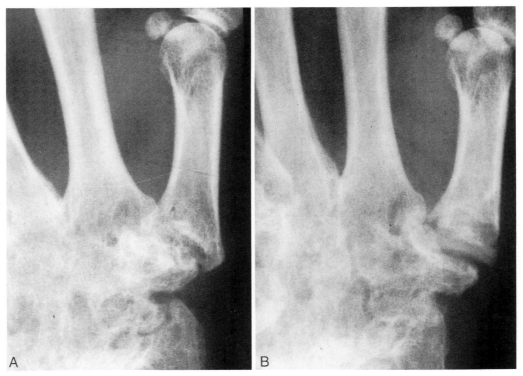

Figure 28–20. *A,* Preoperative radiogram of a rheumatoid thumb showing involvement of the thumb basal joints. *B,* Radiogram taken two years after surgery, showing a concave condylar implant in position.

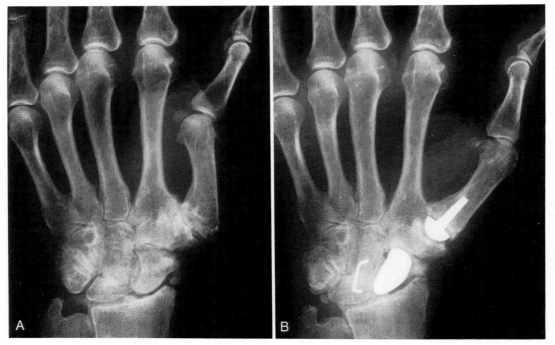

Figure 28–21. *A,* Preoperative radiogram of a patient with osteoarthritis involving the carpometacarpal joint of the thumb, with associated hyperextension deformity of the first metacarpophalangeal joint. There is also arthritis of the scaphoradial and the lunocapitate joints. The cartilage between the lunate and the radius is preserved. *B,* Postoperative radiogram showing a metal convex condylar implant for replacement of the thumb carpometacarpal joint. Hyperextension of the first MP joint was corrected with a capsulodesis procedure. The scaphoid was replaced with a metal implant. Note the bony remnant retained on the palmar surface of the distal scaphoid to preserve ligamentous stability. The lunocapitate joint was fused using a bone graft and staple fixation.

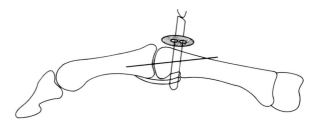

Figure 28–22. Palmar capsulodesis. See text for description of operation. (Reproduced with permission from Swanson AB, and de Groot Swanson G: Thumb disabilities in rheumatoid arthritis: Classification and treatment. AAOS Symposium on Tendon Surgery in the Hand. St. Louis, 1975, The C. V. Mosby Co, p 251).

pends on the proper positioning of the implant over the scaphoid, the correction of collapse deformity of the distal joints of the thumb, and a firm capsuloligamentous repair. Permanent fixation of the implant to the scaphoid is not appropriate because there is decreased movement of the implant at the implant-scaphoid interface and increased stem movement in the intramedullary canal. The use of the Kirschner wire implant transfixation technique for temporary stabilization was abandoned in 1978 because of potential problems of pin-track infection.

Complications can occur that are caused by improper surgical technique. These procedures are technically demanding because of the close association of the branches of the superficial radial nerve and radial artery, which must be carefully protected and preserved at surgery.

A retrospective radiographic study was recently completed of 111 cases of trapezium implant arthroplasty and of 40 cases of trapeziometacarpal implant (condylar) arthroplasty performed by the senior author using implants made of the original material and of the high performance silicone elastomer. All patients had a complete pre-operative and postoperative portfolio, with a minimum of one year's follow-up. There were no infections in our series. The separation of the stem from the implant occurred in 1 of 40 reviewed cases of condylar arthroplasty and in 3 of 111 cases of trapezium implant arthroplasty. Bone remodeling around these implants was excellent in the majority of cases. However, it was noted that cystic and degenerative changes can occur. There was no evidence of cystic changes around 96 trapezium implants (86 percent), and there were minimal changes in 8 cases, moderate changes in 5, and severe changes in 2. The trapezoid and scaphoid were most often affected. There was no evidence of cystic changes around 38 (95 percent) trapeziometacarpal condylar implants, and minimal changes occurred around 1 implant and

moderate changes around 1 implant. The development of cystic and degenerative changes was related to implant instability or subluxation, excessive physical activity, use of Kirschner wires for temporary fixation, and the degree of pre-operative carpal disorders. In case of implant subluxation, excessive motion of the implant stem occurs in the intramedullary canal because of the lack of motion at the implant/scaphoid interface. The intramedullary canal has poor tolerance for this movement, which results in intramedullary synovitis of the thumb metacarpal, as seen in an area of translucency around the stem on radiograph. This "intramedullary sign" is consistent with the early appearance of cystic changes in adjacent carpal bones (Fig. 28–23). A recent separate review of original material implants for the thumb basal joints has shown a significantly lower incidence of cystic changes related to particle-induced synovitis than in cases treated with high-performance silicone elastomer implants.

Implant wear particles can be generated by abnormal or excessive implant motion and can then aggravate existing degenerative or cystic changes. If cystic or degenerative changes are noted, the implant should be removed, and appropriate reconstructive procedures, including bone grafting, should be carried out to convert the treatment to a simple resection arthroplasty.

Important considerations in reconstruction of the thumb basal joints are as follows: (1) There are definite separate indications for the use of the trapezium, convex condylar, and concave condylar implants. The trapezium implant is preferred for cases of pantrapezial arthritis, provided there is integrity of the contiguous carpal bones and a possibility of good seating on the scaphoid facet. The condylar implants are used most often in cases of localized trapeziometacarpal arthritis or when destructive changes of the contiguous carpal bone make trapezium implant arthroplasty difficult, as is often seen in cases of rheumatoid arthritis.

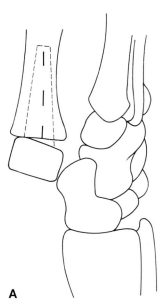

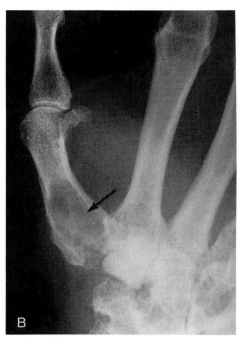

Figure 28–23. *A,* Palmar dislocation of implant due to unrepaired hole in capsule after trapeziectomy. The implant is anterior to the carpus and is angled at the body-stem junction. There is minimal movement of the body of the implant, with most of the movement occurring between stem and intramedullary canal. *B,* Bone resorption is noted (*arrow*), demonstrating the phenomenon of poor tolerance of endosteal bone to this movement pattern. Wear particles can be generated from abrasive forces applied on silicone implants. A secondary foreign body synovitis may lead to bone degeneration and cystic changes. (From Swanson AB, de Groot Swanson G, and Watermeier JJ: J Hand Surg 6:125–141, 1981).

(2) Proper medialization of the trapezium or condylar implants is essential. The scaphoid facet (in the case of trapezium implants) or the trapezial surface (in the case of condylar implants) should be large enough to accept the base of the implant. A partial trapezoidectomy and resection of exostoses at the base of the first metacarpal are important to assure a stable position of the implant over the contiguous bone. (3) The importance of a firm capsuloligamentous reconstruction must be stressed. A slip of flexor carpi radialis tendon is used for trapezium implant arthroplasty. A slip of abductor pollicis longus tendon is used for trapeziometacarpal implant (condylar) arthroplasty. However, if the capsule is adequate in the latter, good stability can be obtained by placing 3–0 Dacron sutures through small drill holes in the base of the first metacarpal. (4) Associated imbalances of the thumb ray, especially hyperextension of the metacarpophalangeal joint and adduction contracture of the first metacarpal, must be corrected at the same time that the basal joint reconstruction is carried out.

We feel that implant reconstruction of the basal thumb joints can provide pain-free,

stable mobility and improved strength. The complications are few and essentially retrievable. The recommended operative procedures are challenging and must be carefully executed to obtain rewarding results.

THE RADIOCARPAL JOINT

The radiocarpal, distal radioulnar, and intercarpal joints can be affected individually or in combination. Synovitis and tendon involvement are common, especially in rheumatoid arthritis. Therefore, selection of the appropriate treatment must depend on the localization and degree of involvement, instability, deformity, arthritic destruction, and the patient's wrist usage requirements. The senior author has devised a classification of wrist pathology based on the localization and severity of disease to help assist in selection of the appropriate treatment (Table 28–3) (Figs. 28–24 through 28–28).

Radiocarpal Joint Implant Arthroplasty

The wrist is the key joint for proper hand function, and disabilities about the wrist can

Table 28–3. **CLASSIFICATION AND TREATMENT FOR WRIST ARTHRITIS***

Stage	Pathologic Conditions	Treatment Options
I	Transient synovitis, pain, and weakness without instability or deformity in Radiocarpal, intercarpal, and distal radioulnar joints; tendons	Physical treatment: Protection, splinting, therapy Medical treatment: Injection of steroids or alkylating agents or both
II	Persistent synovitis, pain, and weakness, without instability or deformity in Radiocarpal, intercarpal, and distal radioulnar joints; tendons	Surgical treatment: Synovectomy Tendons, joints, capsular stabilization of the wrist joint and tendon rebalancing
III	Distal radioulnar deformity and destruction, with a stable radiocarpal joint	Partial or total resection of the distal ulna, with ligament and tendon reconstruction, with or without an ulnar head implant Shortening of the ulna and reconstruction; stability achieved with capsuloligamentous tendon repair
IV	Arthritis limited to a stable radiocarpal joint	Fusion of the proximal row carpus to the radius Hemiarthroplasty of the radiocarpal joint Total joint arthroplasty Treatment of the distal radioulnar joint, as needed
V	Arthritis limited to the radiocarpal joint, with ulnar translation instability	Fusion of the proximal row to the radius Fusion of a segment of the distal ulna to the radius with pseudarthrosis of the proximal ulnar diaphysis with or without an ulnar head implant Hemiarthroplasty—semiconstrained Total joint arthroplasty Treatment of the distal ulna, as needed
VI	Subluxation of the radiocarpal joint Severe intercarpal and radiocarpal arthritic changes Destruction of the proximal carpal row Stiffness of the wrist Tendon balance achievable	Total joint arthroplasty Total joint arthrodesis Treatment of the distal ulna, as needed
VII	Severely unstable wrist Loss of bone in the carpus and distal radius Progressive bone destruction (multilans type) Great physical activity requirements of the patient Tendon balance unachievable	Total joint arthrodesis Treatment of the distal ulna, as needed

*Patients requiring treatment for wrist problems all present with pain and weakness, which may or may not be associated with deformity or instability and tendon defects. In each stage, there may be treatment options, depending not only on the anatomic defect but also on associated defects and patient wrist usage requirements.

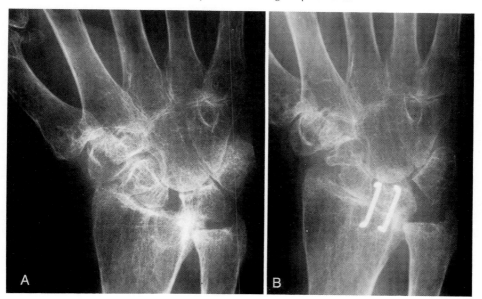

Figure 28–24. *A,* Preoperative radiogram of patient with rheumatoid arthritis, showing collapse deformity of the carpus with ulnar translation and arthritis of the radiocarpal joint (Stage V). *B,* Postoperative radiogram showing relocation of the carpus with fusion of the lunate to the radius. Alternatively, the scaphoid can also be fused to the radius. Useful, pain-free mobility occurs at the midcarpal joints.

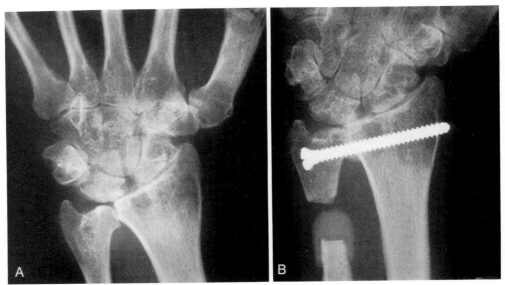

Figure 28–25. *A,* Preoperative radiogram of patient with ulnar translation tendency and minimal arthritic changes (Stage V). *B,* Postoperative result following a synovectomy and a Lauenstein (Suavé-Kapanji) procedure. A silicone cap was used on the ulna at the pseudarthrosis level in this case.

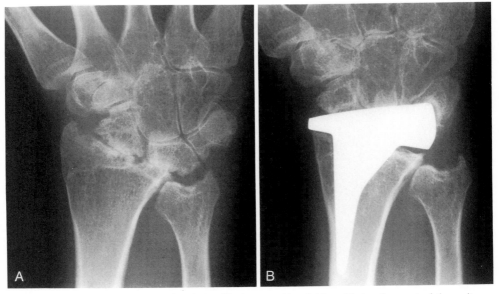

Figure 28–26. *A,* Preoperative radiogram of patient with rheumatoid arthritis, with involvement of the radiocarpal joint and ulnar translation of the carpus. There is minimal involvement of the distal radioulnar joint (Stage V). *B,* Postoperative radiogram showing reconstruction with a semiconstrained metal hemiwrist implant. The proximal carpal row is placed into the deep concavity of the implant.

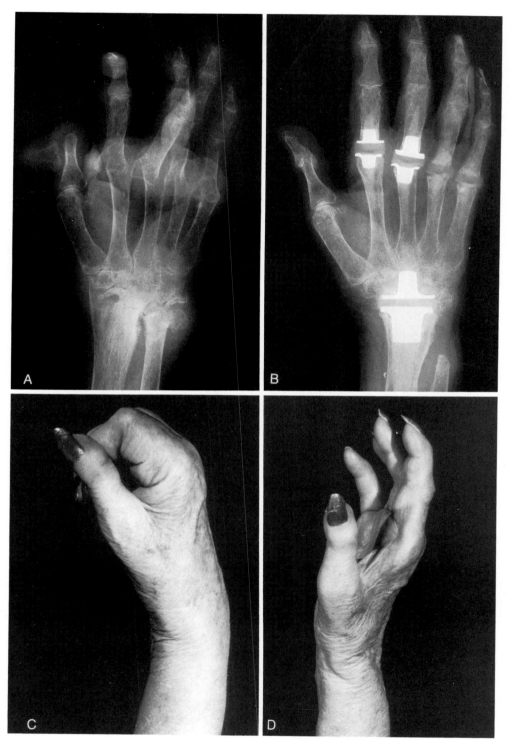

Figure 28–27. *A,* Preoperative radiogram showing severe rheumatoid arthritic involvement of the hand and wrist, with complete destruction of the carpus and distal radioulnar joint (Stage IV). *B,* Reconstruction of the wrist with a silicone flexible hinge implant, using proximal and distal grommets. A resection of the distal ulnar was done. Note the fusion of the distal joint of the thumb and the silicone implant resection arthroplasty of the metacarpophalangeal joints of the index and middle fingers; grommets were used proximally and distally. *C, D,* Good correction of deformities, with a pain free, useful range of motion.

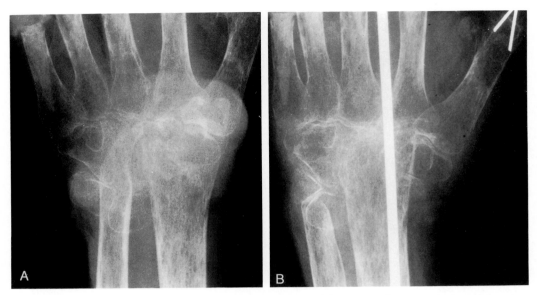

Figure 28–28. *A,* Preoperative radiogram showing severe destruction of the carpus. The patient had multiple wrist tendon ruptures, pain, and instability (Stage VII). *B,* Postoperative radiogram showing wrist fusion with an intramedullary wire fixation.

result in severe functional handicaps. A stable wrist is necessary for proper transmission of forces from the forearm to the digits. However, a mobile wrist is important for positioning the hand.

Flexible hinge implant resection arthroplasty has been used in 301 wrists in our clinic since 1967. The implant has a barrel-shaped midsection, slightly flattened on its dorsal and volar surfaces; the core of the implant contains a Dacron reinforcement to provide axial stability and resistance to rotatory torque. The implant is available in five sizes, in both a standard and wide design of the midsection, to meet the various operative anatomic requirements in the wrist. The wider midsection design is preferred in the authors' clinic because it provides better separation of the joint space and seems to prevent subsidence over time of the implant into the bone.

The implant acts as a flexible hinge to help maintain an adequate joint space and alignment, while supporting the development of a new capsuloligamentous system; it allows vertical and lateral movements through its flexible mid-section and stems. This implant is used with a proximal row resection, which includes a resection of the base of the capitate. The distal implant stem is directed through the capitate into the third metacarpal, and the proximal implant stem is directed into the intramedullary canal of the radius. This positions the implant very well, in respect to the normal flexural area.

It has been demonstrated that the axis of motion of the wrist is at the level of the head of the capitate bone. However, in most of these severely diseased wrists, the normal radiocarpal and intercarpal articular movements have been altered. The flexible hinge has an advantage over rigid implants because its flexibility allows adjustments to the required axis of rotation, with little resistance; because the stems are not fixed, further adjustment can occur, as demonstrated on cinefluorographic studies. Furthermore, this procedure is essentially retrievable; in the event of a fracture, the implant is easily replaced, and if fusion is indicated, this can easily be done with a bone graft.

Observation of the author's own cases over a period of more than 15 years has shown good tolerance of the implant by the host tissues, which is an indication of its biomechanical acceptability. Proper reinforcement of the capsule and balance of the musculotendinous system are very important for obtaining adequate stability, mobility, durability, and biologic tolerance with this method of treatment.

The flexible hinge silicone implants have been generally accepted as a method of small joint arthroplasty and have been used in 500,000 joints in 83 countries. Our studies have shown the radiocarpal hinge implant to fail because of tearing and cutting of the device by sharp bone edges in 16 percent of cases in which a silicone number 372 elastomer implant was used and in 4 percent of cases in which a high-performance silicone elastomer was used. It should be noted that higher-performance silicone elastomer is the preferred material for flexible hinge implants in the finger, wrist, and toe joints.

In an effort to improve durability of the implant and, therefore, of the arthroplasty, we initiated a research project in 1976 to develop an acceptable shielding device to protect the implant from sharp bone edges. Laboratory and animal studies and a three-year human clinical study using eight different materials have shown that a titanium metal bone liner (grommet) appears to be most satisfactory for use in the radiocarpal joint. There have been no fractures of the implant at 109 radiocarpal hinge sites when the metal grommet was used in a series of 58 wrist arthroplasties. There was no evidence of host intolerance.

Indications

A flexible wrist implant arthroplasty is indicated in cases of rheumatoid arthritis, osteoarthritis, or post-traumatic disabilities resulting in (1) instability of the wrist due to subluxation or dislocation of the radiocarpal joint; (2) severe deviation of the wrist, causing musculotendinous imbalance of the digits; (3) stiffness or fusion of the wrist in a nonfunctional position; or (4) stiffness of a wrist, when movement is required for hand function.

Reconstruction of the wrist should be performed before finger joint reconstruction, unless extensor tendon ruptures are present. This procedure is contraindicated in patients with open epiphyses, in those with inadequate skin, bone, or neurovascular system if there is irreparable tendon damage, and in uncooperative individuals. The authors do not recommend this method for patients who perform heavy manual labor.

Surgical Procedure

A straight, longitudinal incision is made over the dorsal wrist with care taken to preserve the superficial sensory nerves. The extensor retinaculum is incised, as shown in Figure 28–29A. Synovectomy of the extensor compartments is performed, with special care taken to remove only the synovium. The dorsal capsuloligamentous structures are carefully preserved for later resuture and are reflected from the underlying radius and carpal bones as a distally based flap (Fig. 28–29B).

A part of the proximal carpal row is usu-

ally absorbed, and the remnants are displaced toward the palm on the radius. Resection of the remaining lunate is carefully done with a rongeur, and the proximal edge of the capitate is squared off. Part of the distal scaphoid and the triquetrum can be retained in some cases. Injury to the underlying tendons and neurovascular structures should be avoided. The end of the radius is squared off to fit against the distal carpal row, which should be left intact because of its importance in maintaining the stability of the metacarpal bones (Fig. 28–29C). The intramedullary canal of the radius is prepared with a broach, curette, or air drill to receive the proximal stem of the implant. The radiocarpal subluxation should be completely reduced. If there is a marked radiocarpal dislocation with soft tissue contracture, it is preferable to shorten the distal radius rather than to remove more of the carpal bones. The distal stem of the implant is inserted through the capitate bone into the intramedullary canal of the third metacarpal. Precise positioning is assured by carefully passing a wire or a very thin broach through the capitate bone and across the base of the metacarpal into the third metacarpal (Fig. 28–29D). A Kirschner wire can be passed into the metacarpal and out through its head to verify the intramedullary orientation. An air drill is used for the final reaming procedure. The distal stem should not be distal to the metaphysis of the third metacarpal and should be shortened as necessary. The proper implant size is determined by the fit of the proximal stem in the radius, using a sizing set. The hand is then centered over the radius. Enough bone should have been removed so that 30° extension and 30° flexion of the wrist can be obtained on passive manipulation. Usually, 1.0 to 1.5 cm of separation between the radius and the carpus is adequate.

Synovectomy and reconstruction of the distal radioulnar joint, with or without the use of an ulnar head implant, are carried out when there is symptomatic involvement of this joint.

When using titanium grommets, further preparation of the distal radius and the base of the capitate is required to allow a precise press-fit of the appropriate-sized grommet. The distal grommet is used on the dorsal surface of the implant and the proximal grommet on its palmar side to protect the implant from sharp bone edges. The grommet size corresponds to the implant size.

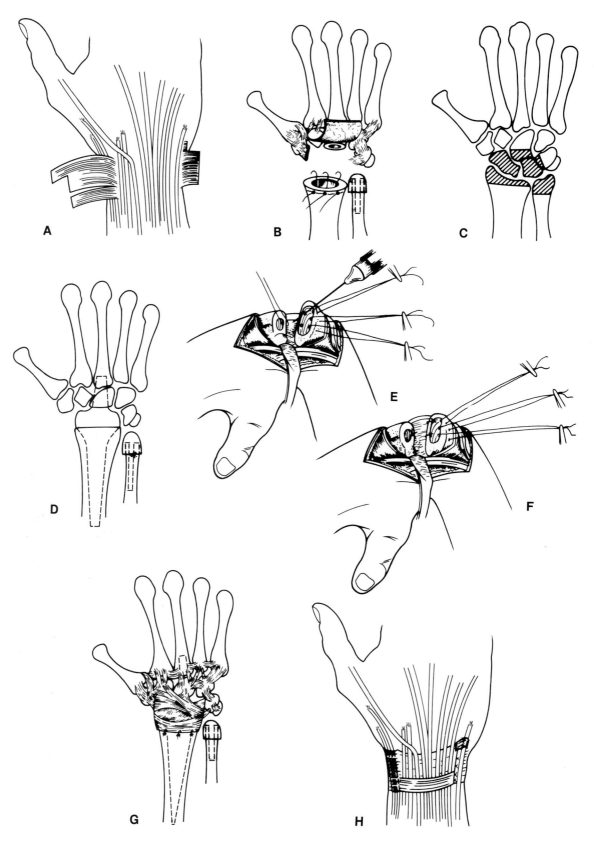

Figure 28–29. *A* through *H,* Surgical procedure for flexible implant arthroplasty of the radiocarpal joint. See text for details. (From Swanson AB, de Groot Swanson G, and Maupin BK: Clin Orthop 187:94–106, 1984.)

The bone ends are smoothened with a diamond bur and slightly grooved laterally to allow perfect seating of the slightly curvilinear grommet shoulder directly on the bone ends to avoid contact with the overlying soft tissues. There should be sufficient bone stock to allow a good press-fit; otherwise rotation of the grommet could occur. The grommets must be accurately centered over the bone ends to avoid impingement on the intramedullary canal on one side, which could cause bone resorption. Final seating is done by gentle pressure or tapping against a curved instrument held against the exposed surface of the grommet, taking care to avoid bending or distorting it. The grommet shoulders should seat directly against resected bone and must not protrude. If too loose, the next larger size is selected. When necessary, a grommet one size larger than that of the flexible implant can be used, but one smaller than that of the implant is never used.

With grommets in place, the sizer is inserted, and joint space and flexion-extension are assessed. The joint space must be adequate to accommodate the implant mid-section. The implant must slide under the distal grommet and not be impinged upon by it. Impingement is usually caused by too narrow a space or by an uncorrected palmar subluxation. If the joint space is too small, the proximal grommet is removed, and it is reseated more deeply to create a larger joint space. The wound is thoroughly irrigated with triple antibiotic solution. The proximal stem of the implant is first inserted into the intramedullary canal of the radius, and the distal stem is then introduced through the capitate into the intramedullary canal of the third metacarpal.

Repair of both the palmar and the dorsal capsuloligamentous structures around the implant is critical to obtain an optimal result. The palmar ligaments are reefed proximally or distally or both, according to where they are loose (Fig. 28–29E and F). The proximal palmar reefing is done with 2–0 Dacron sutures passed through two small drill holes made in the palmar distal edge of the cut end of the radius. The distal palmar reefing is done by passing a suture through a small drill hole made in the cut end of the capitate bone. The dorsal carpal ligament is firmly sutured over the implant with 3–0 Dacron sutures passed through three small drill holes made in the dorsal

cortex of the radius (Fig. 28–29G). The sutures are placed prior to implant insertion.

After implant insertion and closure, the repair should be tested, so that approximately 30° of extension and flexion and 10° of ulnar and radial deviation are possible on passive manipulation. An excessive range of motion may increase the potential for implant failure and does not improve wrist function significantly. Since patients with significant bone loss or loose ligaments can have excessive wrist extension or radial or ulnar deviation, it may be necessary to add sutures to the palmar, radial, and ulnar cortices of the radius to tighten the capsule in these areas. Adequate ligamentous repair is very important for proper function and durability of results.

The previously prepared extensor retinaculum flap is brought down over the wrist joint under the extensor tendon and sutured in place to provide further capsular support (Fig. 28–29H). The pull of the extensor tendons of the wrist joint is then evaluated; the tendons are shortened or transferred, as required, to obtain wrist extension without lateral deviation. The extensor carpi radialis longus may be transferred under the brevis to attach to the third metacarpal by a suture through the bone or interwoven into the distal attachment of the brevis. The extensor tendons of the digits are repaired if necessary. One of the flexor superficialis muscles is often used for tendon transfer to reconstruct ruptured extensor digitorum communis tendons. If isolated extensor tendons are ruptured, side-to-side suture can be performed. Ruptures of the extensor pollicis longus tendon can be repaired by transferring the extensor indicis proprius tendon. The extensor retinaculum flap is placed over the extensor tendons to prevent bowstringing (Fig. 28–29H).

The wound is closed in layers, and silicone sheeting drains are inserted subcutaneously. A voluminous, conforming hand dressing with a palmar splint is applied, with the wrist in neutral position. The extremity is elevated for three to five days by use of an arm sling, with the patient remaining at bed rest. A dorsally well-padded short-arm cast is applied with the wrist in neutral position and is fitted with outriggers that hold rubber-band slings to keep the fingers in extension, if the tendons have been repaired. This is worn for approximately four to six weeks to assure satisfactory stability

Table 28–4. **CLASSIFICATION AND TREATMENT FOR PATHOLOGIC CONDITIONS OF THE DISTAL RADIOULNAR JOINT**

Stage	Pathologic Conditions	Treatment Options
I	Congenital short or long ulna	Osteotomy to shorten or lengthen the ulna
II	Cartilaginous degeneration or derangement Trauma of the triangular fibrocartilage	Joint débridement, with or without ulnar shortening
III	Localized arthritic changes	Partial ulnar resection, with or without capsular reconstruction
IV	Instability, dorsal or volar Traumatic or congenital	Capsuloligamentous reconstruction, with or without angulation osteotomy
V	Disruption of the distal ulna as a result of fracture, tumor, or infection	Resection of the distal ulna with or without angulation osteotomy Capsuloligamentous Reconstruction of distal ulna, rerouting of the extensor carpi ulnaris
VI	Instability with synovitis, with a stable radiocarpal joint	Synovectomy and resection of the distal ulna, with or without silicone capping of the end of the ulna Capsuloligamentous reconstruction of the distal ulna, rerouting of the extensor carpi ulnaris
VII	Instability with synovitis with an unstable radiocarpal joint	As above, with partial or complete radiocarpal fusion Semiconstrained hemiwrist arthroplasty Total wrist arthroplasty
VIII	Severe bone absorption or shortening, with or without instability	No treatment Construct ligament checkrein (ulna to radius), with or without silicone capping of the end of the ulna Fusion of the ulna to the radius

of the wrist. Following cast removal, the patient should begin an active exercise program aimed at achieving 30 to 40 percent normal arc of flexion and extension. If there is a tendency for excessive tightness, some active and passive exercises are prescribed. Therapy includes forearm musculature strength-building exercises. The patient should avoid excessive or abusive activity.

THE DISTAL RADIOULNAR JOINT

Problems at the distal radioulnar joint are common. A classification of selective treatment options was developed by the senior author, based on the nature and severity of the pathologic condition (Table 28–4) (Figs. 28–30 through 28–33).

Implant arthroplasty of the distal radioulnar joint is more specifically described.

Distal Radioulnar Joint Implant Arthroplasty

In 1966 the senior author developed a silicone intramedullary stemmed implant to cap the end of the resected ulna in an effort to preserve the anatomic relationships and physiology of the distal radioulnar joint fol-

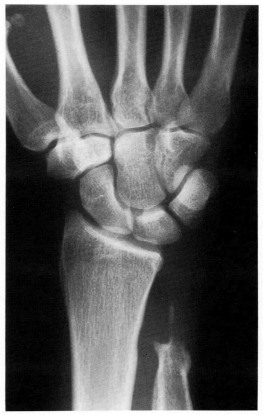

Figure 28–30. Radiogram demonstrating excessive resection of the distal ulna, resulting in a painful and unstable distal radioulnar joint.

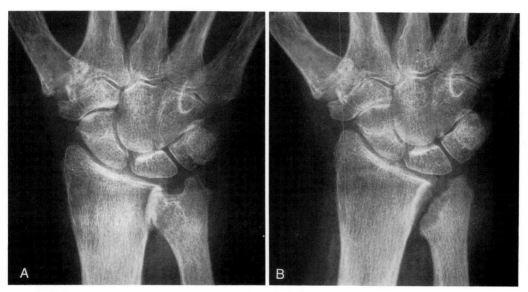

Figure 28–31. *A,* Preoperative radiogram showing painful articulation between the distal ulna and radius in a patient with generalized primary osteoarthritis (Stage III). *B,* Postoperative radiogram showing partial oblique resection of the distal ulna, which provided the patient with good pain relief. Note the carpometacarpal joint arthroplasty, with a silicone convex condylar implant.

Figure 28–32. *A,* Preoperative radiogram showing a congenital palmar subluxation of the distal ulna (Stage IV). *B,* Correction of the deformity, with angulation osteotomy of the ulna.

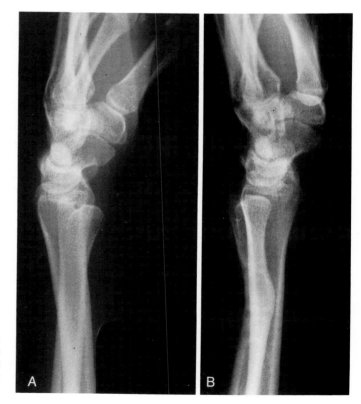

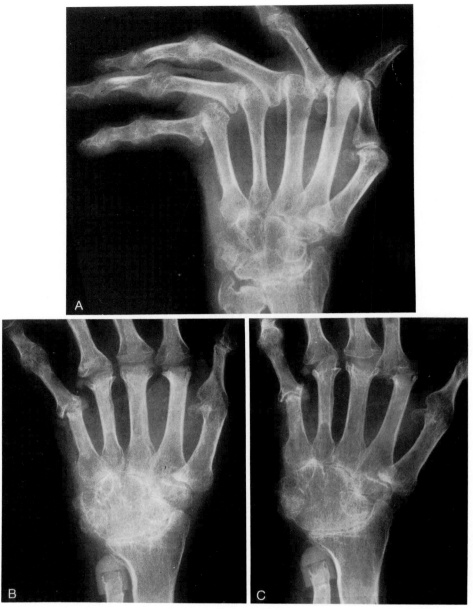

Figure 28–33. *A*, Preoperative radiogram of a patient with rheumatoid arthritis, showing involvement of the hand and wrist. The radiocarpal joint is stable, and the midcarpal joints are fused (Stage V). *B*, Postoperative radiogram taken 11 years later shows spontaneous fusion of the carpus with improved stable radiocarpal joint and implant resection arthroplasty of the distal radioulnar joint. Note the surgical fusion of the first metacarpophalangeal joint and the silicone implant arthroplasties of the second through fifth metacarpals. *C*, Radiogram taken 17 years later shows continued good results at the radiocarpal and distal radioulnar joints. There is radiographic evidence of implant disruption at the level of the metacarpophalangeal joints of the index and middle fingers. The patient, however, continues to present an excellent clinical result.

lowing ulnar head resection. The goal of this procedure is to preserve ulnar length in order to help prevent ulnar carpal shift and to provide greater wrist stability (Fig. 28–30). The ulnar head implant provides a smooth articular surface for the radioulnar and carpoulnar joints and for the overlying

extensor tendons. It decreases the incidence of bone overgrowth of the resected bone end and allows reconstruction of the distal radioulnar joint. The implant is fabricated from HP 100 medical grade silicone elastomer. The stem of the implant has an attached, nonabsorbable, polyester retention

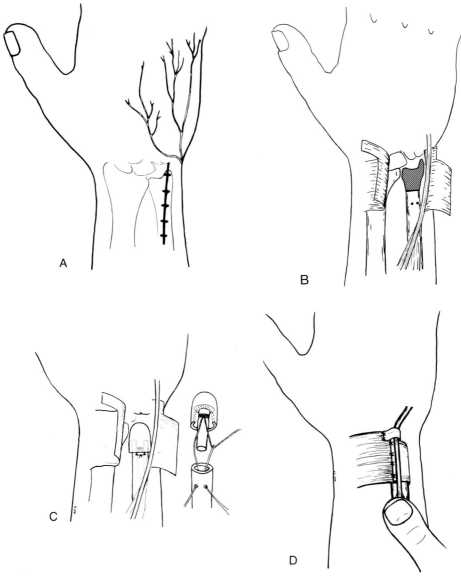

Figure 28–34. *A* through *D*, Technique for ulnar head implant arthroplasty. See text for details.

cord to secure the implant in position at the time of surgery. The last third of the stem is covered with polyester velour to provide fixation of the stem in the intramedullary canal by ingrowth.

Indications

Ulnar head implant replacement arthroplasty may be considered for disabilities of the distal radioulnar joint in rheumatoid, degenerative, and post-traumatic dysfunctions of this joint. Specific indications include pain and weakness of the wrist joint that are not improved by conservative treatment as well as instability of the ulnar head with radiographic evidence of dorsal sublux-

ation and erosive changes. The procedure can also be used to correct sequelae of the failed simple ulnar head resection.

Surgical Procedure

A 6- to 8-cm longitudinal incision centered over the ulnar head is made. The dorsal cutaneous branch of the ulnar nerve is preserved (Fig. 28–34A). The extensor retinaculum of the sixth dorsal compartment is incised as shown in Figure 28–34B. Synovectomy of the dorsal compartments, if indicated, may be carried out at the same time. The extensor carpi ulnaris, which is usually subluxated palmarly off the ulnar head, is retracted. Retractors are placed under the ulnar neck to protect the underlying structures, and the bone is sectioned at the neck with an air drill or motor saw. The periosteum is not stripped off the distal ulna, but muscular attachments on the anterior surface of the ulna are released over the distal 2 cm. The ulnar head and attached synovial sac are removed en bloc, and synovectomy of the joint is completed. The cut edge of the distal ulna and any bone irregularities, especially at the undersurface of the ulna, are smoothed. The intramedullary canal of the ulna is prepared.

An appropriate-sized implant is selected so that the stem will fit snugly into the intramedullary canal and the cuff will fit loosely over the bone. Occasionally, digital extensor tendons are ruptured as a result of the ulnar head irregularities or because of synovitis and must be repaired. The implant is secured to the end of the ulna with the pretied polyester suture to prevent the slight tendency of the implant to extrude from the intramedullary canal in the early postoperative course (Fig. 28–34C). Prior to implant insertion, sutures are placed through the interosseous ligament close to the radioulnar border to secure the preserved capsule over the ulnar head implant; these may be placed through small drill holes in the radius if the local tissues are inadequate. The retinaculum of the sixth dorsal compartment is used as a checkrein ligament to hold the dorsally subluxated ulna in a reduced position and is repaired while an assistant maintains the reduction of the ulna toward the palm (Fig. 28–34D). It is important to release the extensor carpi ulnaris tendon proximally and distally to allow it free excursion. The narrow distal retinacular flap is used to form a pulley around the extensor carpi ulnaris tendon to maintain it over the dorsum of the ulnar head.

The wound is closed and drained in the usual manner. A voluminous, conforming hand dressing, including a plaster palmar splint, is applied with the hand in slight dorsiflexion. On the third postoperative day, the drain is removed, and if there is no swelling, a short-arm cast or a splint is applied in the same position to protect the wrist from excessive activity for three to four weeks. The best immobilization is obtained by using a long-arm cast with the forearm in supination. However, because most rheumatoid arthritis patients are quite inactive, less immobilization is adequate.

References

1. Lichtman DM, Alexander AH, Mack GR, et al: Kienböck's disease—update on silicone replacement arthroplasty. J Hand Surg 7:343–347, 1982.
2. Swanson AB: Silicone rubber implants for replacement of arthritic or destroyed joints in the hand. Surg Clin North Am 48:1113–1127, 1968.
3. Swanson AB: Finger joint replacement by silicone rubber implants and the concept of implant fixation by encapsulation. International Workshop on Artificial Finger Joints. Ann Rheum Dis 28(Suppl):47–55, 1969.
4. Swanson AB: Silicone rubber implants for the replacement of the carpal scaphoid and lunate bones. Orthop Clin North Am 1:299–309, 1970.
5. Swanson AB: Disabling arthritis at the base of the thumb: treatment by resection of the trapezium and flexible (silicone) implant arthroplasty. J Bone Joint Surg 54A:456–471, 1972.
6. Swanson AB: Flexible implant arthroplasty in the hand and extremities. St Louis, CV Mosby Co, 1973.
7. Swanson AB: Reconstructive surgery in the arthritic hand and foot. Ciba Found Symp 31(6), 1979.
8. Swanson AB: A grommet bone liner for flexible implant arthroplasty. Bull Pros Res Rehab Engl Res Devel 18:108–114, 1981.
9. Swanson AB, and de Groot Swanson G: Thumb disabilities in rheumatoid arthritis: classification and treatment. AAOS Symposium on Tendon Surgery in the Hand. St Louis, CV Mosby Co, 1975, pp 233–254.
10. Swanson AB, de Groot Swanson G, and Watermeier JJ: Trapezium implant arthroplasty. J Hand Surg 6:125–141, 1981.
11. Swanson AB, and de Groot Swanson G: Arthroplasty of the thumb basal joints. In Leach RE, Hoaglund FT, and Riseborough EJ (eds): Controversies in Orthopaedic Surgery. Philadelphia, WB Saunders Co, 1982, pp 36–57.
12. Swanson AB, and de Groot Swanson G: Flexible implant arthroplasty of the radiocarpal joint: surgical technique and long-term results. In Inglis A (ed): The American Academy of Orthopaedic Surgeons Symposium on Total Joint Replacement of the Upper Extremity. St Louis, CV Mosby Co, 1982, pp 301–316.
13. Swanson AB, and de Groot Swanson G: Osteoarthritis in the Hand. J Hand Surg 8(5):669–675, 1983.
14. Swanson AB, de Groot Swanson G, and Maupin BK: Flexible implant arthroplasty of the radiocarpal joint—surgical technique and long-term study. Clin Orthop 187:94–106, 1984.
15. Swanson AB, and de Groot Swanson G: Arthroplasty of the thumb basal joints. Clin Orthop 195:151–160, 1985.
16. Swanson AB, Maupin BK, de Groot Swanson G, et al: Lunate implant resection arthroplasty: long-term results. J Hand Surg 10A (Part 2):1013–1024, 1985.
17. Swanson AB, de Groot Swanson G, Maupin BK, et al: Scaphoid implant resection arthroplasty—long-term results. J Arthrop 1:47–62, 1986.
18. Swanson AB, Maupin BK, Page BJ II, de Groot Swanson G, et al: Long-term bone response around carpal bone implants. Presented at the 40th Annual Meeting of the American Society for Surgery of the Hand, Las Vegas 1985.

CHAPTER 29

Total Wrist Arthroplasty: Review of Current Concepts

ROBERT D. BECKENBAUGH, M.D.

HISTORY AND CONCEPTS

The procedure of total wrist arthroplasty refers to the surgical resection of all or a portion of the carpus, removal of the articulating surface of the radius and usually the ulna as well, and replacement with an articulated implant. Conceptually, silicone interpositional arthroplasty accomplishes the same result and is discussed separately in Chapter 28.

The concept of using an articulated nonhinged prosthesis in the wrist was simultaneously developed by Meuli[1] in Switzerland and Volz[2] in Arizona in the early 1970s. With the development of appropriate prosthetic materials and methylmethacrylate bone cement for fixation of components in total hip arthroplasties during the 1960s, these pioneers sought to apply to the wrist the principles learned in the replacement of other joints of the body.

The need for the development of a total wrist replacement became evident as a result of the limited surgical options available in the treatment of destructive wrist arthrosis. Arthrodesis can successfully relieve pain and provide stability to the wrist. However, in patients with rheumatic disease involving the elbows, the shoulder, and the hand, absence of wrist motion further accentuates the overall upper extremity disability. Some patients with noninflammatory wrist disease occasionally have careers with special needs for wrist motion; for example, some professionals in music and some mechanics working in small spaces. Synovectomy in rheumatic disease and proximal row carpectomy in traumatic disease have been procedures

associated with successful relief of pain and restoration of mobility but have had variable predictability and longevity. The goals in developing a total wrist replacement are to provide a mobile, stable, painless wrist with reasonable durability. Experience has shown that the concept is viable, but problems associated with its development have been encountered.

The First Designs

Meuli elected to proceed with a ball and socket trunnion design, whereas Volz developed a dorsovolar tracking model (Fig. 29–1).

The Meuli design allows rotation within the articulation and significant degrees of motion before prosthetic impingement. The prosthesis is thus essentially unconstrained in most degrees of motion, in a biomechanical sense. However, as will be seen, in the functional mode the distal cup firmly encompasses the ball, and if stress is applied to the hand with the wrist held motionless by soft tissue constraints (capsule or muscle), the resultant forces are transmitted to the stems as if the prosthesis were constrained.

The Volz design essentially incorporates a flexion-extension arc of motion but is a "sloppy" fit, allowing slight anteroposterior and radial ulnar translation: a moderate amount of radial ulnar deviation can occur, but only a few degrees of carpal rotation are possible. Thus, whereas the Volz design incorporates a smaller range of intrinsic motion, it is functionally less constrained than the Meuli, owing to the loose contact fit

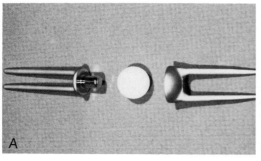

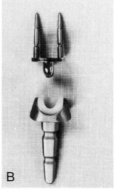

Figure 29–1. A, Meuli prosthesis: Trunnionated ball is added after fixation of components. Distal cupped portion is on the right. B, Volz prosthesis: Polyethylene bearing is press-fit into proximal component. (A, From Beckenbaugh RD, and Linscheid, RL: J Hand Surg 2:337–344, 1977.)

between the proximal and the distal components.

Both designs utilized two-pronged distal components for seating in the medullary canals of the nonmobile index and long metacarpals. The purpose in utilizing both metacarpals was to enhance fixation. Because of the fixed intermetacarpal distance, in some cases this was technically difficult to achieve. The process was facilitated by the Meuli device because of the ability of its stems to be bent with special instruments. The location of fixation in the index and the long metacarpals proved to be biomechanically unsound in many patients, as is discussed.

With the Meuli design, two lengths of polyethylene ball insertions were available to adjust tension as necessary. In both techniques, the distal ends of the radius and the ulna and all of the carpus except the distal portion of the distal row were resected (Fig. 29–2). Both techniques utilized methyl-

methacrylate cement for fixation of the prosthetic stems.

Initial reports of wrist arthroplasties with these prostheses demonstrated satisfactory motion and pain relief. Deformity was occasionally a problem.[2, 3]

PROBLEMS AND DESIGN CHANGES

The major early problem with total wrist arthroplasty was balance. With both prosthetic designs, a significant number of patients developed ulnar deviation deformity and contractures. Analysis of case failures and biomechanical evaluation confirmed that insertion of the distal component within the second and third metacarpals abnormally placed the prosthetic center of rotation too radially[3, 4] (Fig. 29–3), functionally lengthening the ulnar lever arm. Initially, this problem was managed in the Meuli design by bending stems or altering placement to the third and fourth metacarpals or by tendon transfers of the extensor carpi

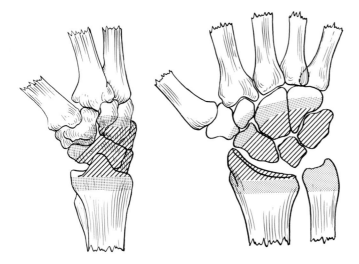

Figure 29–2. Hatched area shows the amount of bone resection needed for insertion of a Meuli prosthesis. Dotted area shows optional bone resection in patients with collapse and dislocation of carpus and ulna. (From Beckenbaugh RD, and Linscheid RL: J Hand Surg 2:337–344, 1977.)

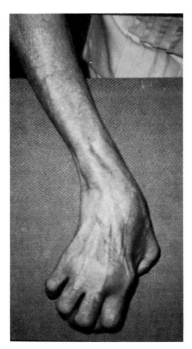

Figure 29–3. Ulnar deviation stance secondary to radial center of rotation in wrist with Meuli prosthesis. (From Beckenbaugh RD, Linscheid RL: J Hand Surg 2:337–344, 1977.)

have occurred in over 50 percent of cases in the author's long-term follow-up study of the Meuli prosthesis; these changes paralleled the findings in early cemented hip designs. Stress shielding refers to the absorption of cortical bone adjacent to the articulating surface of the prosthesis and has been seen with use of both the Meuli and the Volz. It occurs only in the proximal component and comes from absence of stress to the bone adjacent to the cemented proximal stem (Fig. 29–7). Stress shielding is common but rarely reaches the extreme shown in Figure 29–7. Its occurrence implies the need for a more uniform method of fixation of the proximal stem.

Another distressing problem associated with total wrist arthroplasty has been distal component loosening. Unlike total joint loosening at other anatomic locations, in the wrist this complication is rarely associated with significant pain. Rather, it can result in decreasing motion, a tendency toward deformity, and eventual impingement within the carpal canal. With the Meuli design, as the distal component loosens, it tends to migrate volarly into the carpal canal. This

ulnaris to the center of the wrist. Lack of predictability of these measures and loosening of stems in the mobile fourth metacarpal demonstrated the need for prosthetic modification. Meuli modified his stem structure by offsetting the stems on the distal component; Volz and Hamas and the author of this chapter developed single-stemmed centered distal components with offset dorsal volar stems to enhance dorsiflexion[4, 5] (Fig. 29–4). These modifications significantly reduced balance problems in total wrist arthroplasty, but the difficulty in precisely placing single-stemmed components led to persistence of problems in some cases (Figs. 29–5 and 29–6).

In addition to the problems of recurrent deformity, other causes of total wrist arthroplasty failure were eventually encountered.[6] Infections occurred at a rate of less than 2 percent and required prosthetic removal. Dislocations were infrequent and were managed by closed treatment, but those that were associated with deformity usually required revisional surgery.[6]

By far the most significant problem of total wrist arthroplasty has related to stem fixation. Loosening of the distal component and stress shielding of the proximal component

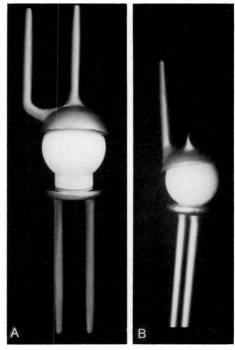

Figure 29–4. *A,* Offset Meuli design. Note the third metacarpal stem centered in the middle of the prosthetic cup. *B,* Single stem Meuli design. Lateral view: Single stem is centered over cup and placed dorsally to enhance extension. (From Beckenbaugh, RD: Mayo Clin Proc 54:513–515, 1979.)

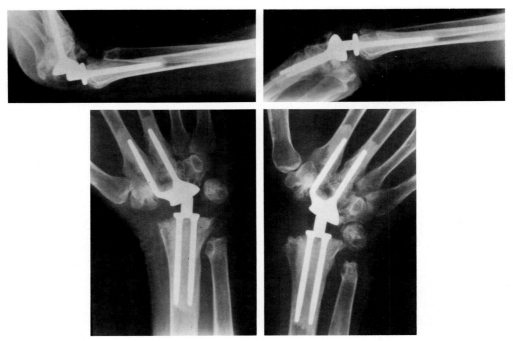

Figure 29–5. Excellent balance and movement, as seen on these motion views one year following Meuli offset total wrist arthroplasty.

may cause symptoms of median neuropathy but more importantly may result in flexor tendon attritional ruptures at the edge of the prosthesis (Fig. 29–8). The loosening of the Meuli distal component has reached 50 percent in our series and is felt to occur because of the close fit between the proximal ball and the distal cup. Functional wrist activi-

ERRORS IN SINGLE STEM

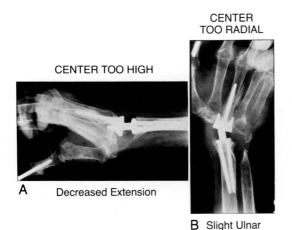

CENTER TOO RADIAL

CENTER TOO HIGH

A Decreased Extension

B Slight Ulnar
Position

Figure 29–6. Malpositioned single stem wrist arthroplasty. *A,* Dorsally positioned stem results in decreased dorsiflexion. *B,* Radially positioned stem results in increased ulnar deviation.

ties, such as pushing open a door, pushing up from a chair, or even moderate lifting, place great stress on the prosthetic stems. Since the wrist is fixed in position by the capsule and musculotendinous units in the dorsiflexed position, the force of the proximal stem and ball is transmitted directly and completely to the inferior portion of the cup, producing angular forces on the distal stems, and loosening occurs. In the Volz design, the "sloppiness" of the fit plus the slight subluxation of the component possibly dampens this force, and loosening occurs much less frequently.[7, 8] The presence of this phenomenon with the ball and socket design has led the author to believe that it is an unsatisfactory configuration for total wrist arthroplasty. The problem is experienced less frequently with the Volz design, but with the low contact area and loose bone fit, there is greater potential for wear problems and polyethylene deformity. Painless clicking and a slight sense of instability are also occasionally associated with use of the Volz prosthesis, owing to the loose fit.

SALVAGE

Fortunately, salvage following failed total wrist arthroplasty has always been possible. Conversion to arthrodesis may be achieved with the addition of iliac bone graft. Occa-

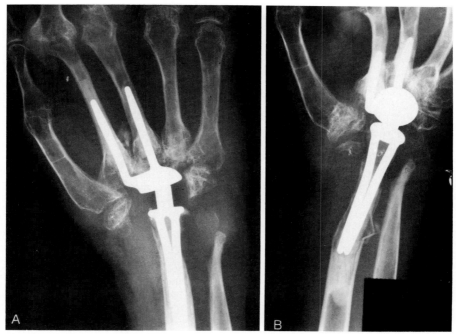

Figure 29–7. Stress shielding. *A*, Three months postoperative view of Meuli prosthesis. Note that proximal cortex extends to the base of the prosthesis. *B*, One year later, the distal cortex has resorbed; all fixation is proximal and the radius has fractured. This is an extreme example of this phenomenon.

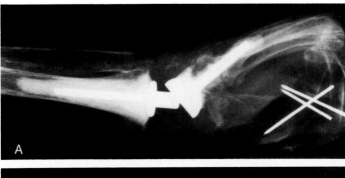

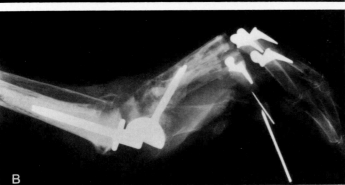

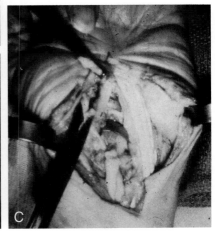

Figure 29–8. *A, B,* Immediate postoperative six-year follow-up x-rays. The distal cup has loosened and migrated into the carpal canal. *C,* The instrument holds the ruptured end of a flexor tendon, which is the result of attrition over the cup of the prosthesis.

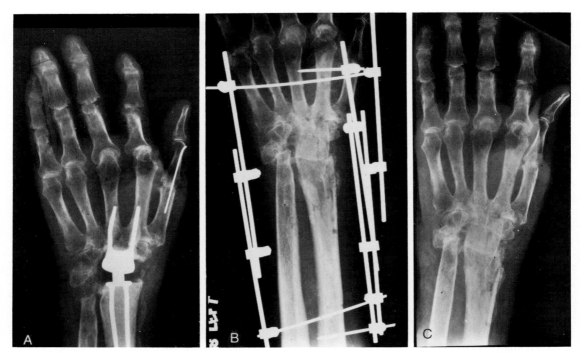

Figure 29–9. *A,* X-ray taken three months after operation in a patient with infection. *B,* The prosthesis has been removed, an iliac graft has been inserted, and stabilization has been accomplished with external fixation. *C,* Three months after grafting the arthrodesis is solid. A cast may be used in lieu of fixation. (From Cooney WP III, Beckenbaugh RD, and Linscheid RL: Clin Orthop 187:121–128, 1984.)

sionally, resectional arthroplasty with or without Silastic interposition is indicated. Arthrodesis is achieved by removal of the prosthesis and insertion of the bone graft in the space formerly occupied by the arthroplasty (Fig. 29–9). To remove the prosthesis, it is generally easiest to split the dorsal cortex of the radius and the metacarpals with an osteotome. The medullary canals are then opened like a book, and the component and its cement mantle are disimpacted. The cortices then close elastically and graft insertion is permitted. As an alternative, the cement may be slowly removed with an osteotome and drills. If grafting is not performed, casting for four months will generally result in a stable and painless wrist pseudarthrosis, although with significant shortening.

Future Considerations

The very excellent early results of total wrist arthroplasty and salvageability of failures have prompted continued attempts to achieve a more satisfactory implant. Several designs have been developed with various parameters of stability and balance, but results have not been clearly superior to the current Volz design. The author has developed a semiconstrained, intrinsically balanced prosthesis that has shown considerable promise in its four years of use (Fig. 29–10). The prosthesis consists of an ellipsoidal, biaxial articulating surface, oriented along the axis of the normal, articulating wrist. Stems are offset and curved distally to enhance press-fit seating and intrinsic

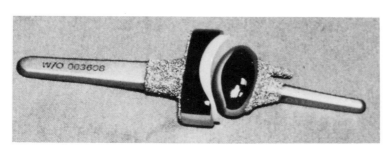

Figure 29–10. New wrist prosthesis design. The periarticular surfaces have a porous coating to enhance fixation and possibly eliminate the need for cement.

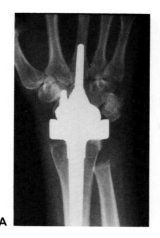 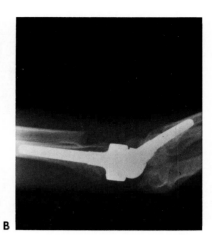

Figure 29–11. *A, B,* Ellipsoidal wrist prosthesis inserted without bone cement.

A **B**

balance. Figures 29–11A and B depict the prosthetic positioning in a rheumatoid patient, in which cement was not utilized. To date, the biaxial design has provided an increased sense of wrist "normality" to patients. It is hoped that the larger contact area, the improved stem design, and the unconstrained but stable articulating surfaces of this new prosthesis will increase the longevity and predictability of total wrist arthroplasty.

SUMMARY AND CONCLUSIONS

Since the inception of total wrist arthroplasty in the early 1970s, much has been learned. Wrist replacement appears to be clinically viable and preferable to arthrodesis, in view of the early functional results, with outcomes of the "best" wrist arthroplasties being far superior to the traditional alternatives of arthrodesis and biologic arthroplasty. Contraindications to the use of the procedure have been an unacceptable loosening rate and difficulties in achieving proper balance. The latter problem has been satisfactorily corrected with progressive de-

sign improvement, but prosthetic longevity and security of fixation have not yet been delineated. Upon failure, a satisfactory salvage is possible; this fact provides impetus to the continued efforts at achieving a mobile, stable, and durable wrist implant.

References

1. Meuli HC: Reconstructive surgery of the wrist joint. Hand 4:88–90, 1972.
2. Volz RG: The development of a total wrist arthroplasty. Clin Orthop 116:209, 1976.
3. Beckenbaugh RD, and Linscheid RL: Total wrist arthroplasty: preliminary report. J Hand Surg 2:337–344, 1977.
4. Hamas RS: A quantitative approach to total wrist arthroplasty: development of a "precentered" total wrist prosthesis. Orthopedics 2:245, 1979.
5. Beckenbaugh RD: Total joint arthroplasty: the wrist. Mayo Clin Proc 54:513–515, 1979.
6. Cooney WP, III, Beckenbaugh RD, and Linscheid RL: Total wrist arthroplasty. Problems with implant failures. Clin Orthop 187:121–128, 1984.
7. Volz RG: Total wrist arthroplasty. A clinical review. Clin Orthop 187:112–120, 1984.
8. Dennis DA, Ferlic DC, and Clayton ML: Volz total wrist arthroplasty in rheumatoid arthritis: a long-term review. Presented at the Annual Meeting of the ASSH, New Orleans, January, 1986.

CHAPTER 30

Wrist Fusions: Intercarpal and Radiocarpal

PAUL FELDON, M.D.

INTERCARPAL (LIMITED) WRIST FUSION

Fusions of wrist joints have been performed for many conditions that cause painful, unstable, or arthritic intercarpal or radiocarpal joints. Complete wrist fusion is a time-honored, predictable, and reliable salvage procedure for these conditions. It provides a stable, pain-free wrist, preserves forearm rotation, and provides reasonable upper extremity function as long as forearm rotation and elbow and shoulder motion are preserved.

However, in many patients, the pathologic disorder causing symptoms is confined to only one or several of the joints making up the wrist unit. In these cases, it is reasonable to attempt to provide a stable and pain-free wrist, while preserving some wrist motion. Even significant loss of motion will still allow functional use of the wrist. Brumfield[4] demonstrated that functional use of the wrist required a range of 45° (15° palmar flexion and 30° dorsiflexion). Palmer,[28] using more sophisticated measuring techniques, demonstrated that even less range of motion was sufficient for most normal daily activities (30° extension, 5° flexion, 10° radial deviation, and 15° ulnar deviation). Thus, limited wrist fusions that preserve some wrist motion have considerable appeal in the treatment of localized problems of the wrist unit. Rozing[30] showed in an experimental cadaver study that fusion of the radioscaphoid or radioscapholunate joints resulted in preservation of 40 percent of flexion and extension and 61 percent of radioulnar deviation. In this study, fusion of the midcarpal joint (scaphoid-capitate-lunate) resulted in preservation of 59 percent of flexion and exten-

sion and 91 percent of radioulnar deviation. Most authors have reported at least a 50 percent preservation of wrist range of motion in their series of intercarpal fusions, and some have reported considerably higher percentages.*

Radiolunate and radioscaphoid fusions result in greater loss of wrist motion.[22, 33, 44] Although limited intercarpal arthrodeses have been used for treatment of scaphoid nonunions and localized arthritides for many years, it has been only recently that such procedures have been advocated for conditions such as carpal instability, Kienböck's disease, or as an adjunct to Silastic implant arthroplasty of the carpus (see Chapter 28). Since Watson[45] published a study of his experience with intercarpal fusions in 1980, the use of various combinations of intercarpal fusions has become more frequent. The success rate and the predictability of limited wrist fusions in these conditions have been varied, and the long-term effects of such fusions remain unknown. Watson[47] has reported no significant long-term effects of various combinations of limited wrist fusions for as long as almost 12 years. As more experience with these fusions is gained and reported, their indications, effectiveness, predictability, and durability will become clearer. At present, the treatment of some wrist conditions by partial arthrodesis remains controversial.

Indications

There are several general indications for limited wrist arthrodesis.

---

*References 1, 16, 17, 41, 44, 45, 47, 50.

446

NONUNITED FRACTURES OF THE SCAPHOID

Limited wrist arthrodeses were first described for the treatment of this condition.[36] Although scaphocapitate fusion may still be a treatment alternative in long-standing symptomatic scaphoid nonunion with preservation of the radioscaphoid joint, bone grafting, electrical stimulation or both remain the first procedures of choice. The natural course of untreated scaphoid nonunions[13, 14, 32, 42, 43, 46] results in radioscaphoid arthritis, progressive carpal collapse or both, which require treatment either by a more extensive intercarpal fusion, by scaphoid implant arthroplasty supplemented by an intercarpal fusion, or by total wrist fusion.

LOCALIZED ARTHRITIS OF THE CARPUS

Arthritis limited to one or several of the carpal articulations can be treated by limited carpal fusion. Osteoarthritis involving the scaphoid, the trapezium, and the trapezoid joints is perhaps the most common condition in which intercarpal fusion should be considered. Limited arthrodesis of the involved joints is an excellent procedure, particularly if there is already some loss of wrist motion.[10, 33, 50]

Intercarpal and radiocarpal fusions for wrist involvement in rheumatoid arthritis have been performed with increasing frequency. They are useful in arresting carpal translocation and in preserving motion when only a portion of the wrist joint has been destroyed.[3, 22, 26, 38, 39]

Localized arthritis from sepsis may also be amenable to treatment by limited wrist fusion, either intercarpal or radiocarpal.

CARPAL INSTABILITY

The carpus is intrinsically unstable. Its stability is provided by the shape and contact of the individual carpal bones and by the intrinsic and extrinsic wrist ligaments. Loss of ligamentous support can result in varying degrees of carpal instability, which may cause symptoms of pain and clicking in the wrist and may lead to progressive degenerative arthritis of the carpus. This instability can occur at the scapholunate joint, the lunotriquetral joint, or the midcarpal joints. The diagnosis of these instabilities is straightforward in so-called *static instability*, in which the collapse pattern is present at all times and therefore is apparent on radiographs of the wrist. The use of inter-

carpal fusions with reasonable functional results in the treatment of these instability patterns has been reported by several authors.*

Dynamic carpal instability occurs when the ligamentous supporting structures of the carpus have been less severely damaged, and the instability does not occur until stress or load is applied to the wrist. The unloaded wrist appears normal on standard radiographs, and stress views or cineradiographs may or may not show the instability pattern. Accurate diagnosis is difficult but is critical in determining the appropriate treatment, particularly if intercarpal fusion is being considered. The predictability of outcome after intercarpal fusion for dynamic instability is less than that for the static instabilities. All nonoperative treatment options should be exhausted before an intercarpal fusion is considered for correction of dynamic instability. An error in determining the site of the instability may lead to the incorrect choice of specific intercarpal fusion and, therefore, failure to correct the instability. In this case, the patient's symptoms will persist, and extension of the fusion may be necessary.[20, 49]

ADJUNCT TO SILASTIC CARPAL IMPLANTS

Silastic implants have a limited ability to bear load without deforming to some extent. Progressive deformation of these implants, particularly of the lunate, and the recent reports of silicone synovitis associated with Silastic wrist implants[35] have led to the recommendation that both scaphoid and lunate Silastic carpal implants be supported with a limited intercarpal fusion performed at the same time that the implant is inserted.[37] Scaphocapitate fusion is usually selected when a lunate implant is performed. Although a scaphoid-trapezium-trapezoid fusion would work as well, this fusion is more difficult to perform through the midline wrist incision usually used for the implant procedure. A fusion of the capitate to the lunate is the procedure of choice when a scaphoid implant is performed.

KIENBÖCK'S DISEASE

Partial carpal fusion is an alternative salvage procedure for advanced Kienböck's disease.[14]

Chuinard[7] advocated the fusion of the cap-

---

*References 1, 9, 16, 18, 29, 41, 43–45, 47.

itate to the hamate in Kienböck's disease. He postulated that this fusion would prevent progressive proximal migration of the capitate as the avascular lunate bone collapsed. Watson[48] has advocated scaphoid-trapezium-trapezoid fusion for Kienböck's disease, on the basis that this fusion will provide a load-bearing column radial to the capitate-lunate axis, thereby decreasing the load borne by the lunate and preventing progressive carpal collapse. Such treatment for Kienböck's disease has the disadvantage of limiting wrist motion. Trumble[40] has shown significant reduction in lunate compression during wrist loading after scaphoid-trapezium-trapezoid fusion but not after capitate-hamate fusion.

SALVAGE SURGERY FOR PARTIAL CARPAL BONE LOSS

Partial loss of carpal bone stock may occur from high impact injuries such as motor vehicle accidents or gunshot wounds, following tumor resection, and as the result of avascular necrosis of bones such as the scaphoid in Preiser's disease or following scaphoid fracture with proximal pole nonunion. Salvage of partial wrist function and prevention of progressive carpal collapse and degenerative arthritis may be possible if a limited carpal fusion is performed; for example, fusion of the scaphoid to the capitate and excision of the proximal pole of the scaphoid for a nonunited fracture.[38, 41] Campbell[6] has described the use of inlay grafts about the wrist following bone resection in tumor surgery.

Limited wrist fusion has also been described for stabilization in cases of flail wrist following radial nerve palsy and for loss of wrist control in cerebral palsy.[33]

General Considerations in Intercarpal Fusions

The interest in limited wrist fusion has increased dramatically over the past decade. However, the results obtained by various groups have not been consistent, and the long-term results remain unknown. It has been accepted that limited wrist fusion in certain conditions can stabilize the wrist, relieve pain, and arrest or prevent progressive loss of carpal height. However, patients being considered for intercarpal fusion should be made aware of the limitations of the procedure, the tradeoff of loss of wrist

motion to obtain stability and pain relief, the long period of rehabilitation necessary before the final result has been obtained, and the fact that the long-term effects of these procedures are unknown.

Proper patient selection is important when considering intercarpal fusion for dynamic instabilities, as these conditions are much more difficult to diagnose and, in my experience, respond less predictably to intercarpal fusion than do static instabilities or arthritic conditions. I caution my patients with dynamic instability that more than one surgical procedure may be necessary.

TRIAL PERCUTANEOUS PIN FIXATION OF THE WRIST

Because diagnosis and localization of dynamic instabilities are difficult and because an intercarpal fusion is likely to fail if either of these is incorrect, I have added examination of the wrist using the image intensifier for "real-time" cineradiography and temporary pin stabilization of the carpus as initial procedures before a recommendation for intercarpal arthrodesis is made in patients with suspected dynamic wrist instability.

Temporary pin fixation is done in the operating room under intravenous regional anesthesia. For the first 15 minutes or so after the block has been administered, the patient retains muscular control and can actively move the wrist, make a fist, and so forth. Motions that reproduce the click can be studied under the image intensifier and recorded on videotape. Pins are inserted percutaneously under image intensifier control. The click and instability should be eliminated if the appropriate carpal bones have been stabilized. This allows the simulation of an intercarpal fusion. If the click persists, other carpal bones can be incorporated, or different combinations of carpal bones can be tried. At the conclusion of the procedure, the carpus should be stable on stress testing, and the click should be absent. Measurement of wrist motion after pin insertion allows estimation of the final wrist range of motion for any given carpal fusion. Occasionally, an unsuspected problem such as distal radioulnar joint stability or triangular fibrocartilage damage can be detected with this method (Fig. 30–1).

After the procedure has been completed, the pins are cut short beneath the skin level, the puncture wounds are dressed with Band-Aids, and the drapes removed. The patient

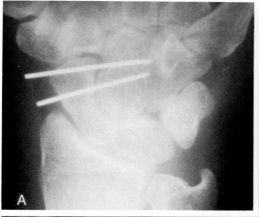

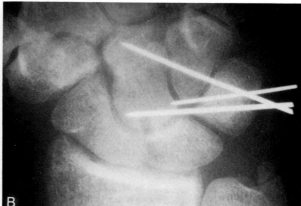

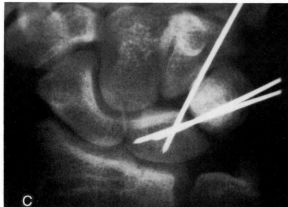

Figure 30–1. *A,* Temporary pin stabilization of the scaphoid bone in a 25-year-old woman who had chronic wrist pain after a fall. Standard x-ray examination of the wrist and wrist arthrograms showed no abnormalities. A painful click occurred during stress testing of the scaphoid. The wrist click was eliminated after the scaphoid was pinned to the capitate. The patient was asymptomatic after the trial scaphoid pinning and remained so after stabilization by scaphoid-capitate fusion. *B,* A 33-year-old mechanic had wrist pain on the ulnar side after an impact injury of the wrist that occurred when a wrench that he was using slipped. The diagnosis of midcarpal instability was made on the basis of his clinical examination. Both the click and the pain were eliminated after trial pinning of the lunate-triquetrum-hamate joints. The patient has remained asymptomatic and has returned to work after midcarpal fusion. Note the avulsion fracture from the tip of the styloid process of the ulna. *C,* A 25-year-old warehouseman had chronic wrist pain and a painful "clunk" with wrist motion after an intra-articular fracture of the radius and an ulnar styloid fracture. His clinical examination was consistent with wrist instability on the ulnar side. The wrist arthrogram showed a dye leak between the lunate and the triquetrum. Trial pin fixation of the lunotriquetral joint did not stabilize the carpus, and midcarpal subluxation could be reproduced under the fluoroscope with the triquetrum-lunate pins in place. The carpus was stable after addition of a pin inserted through the hamate into the lunate. The patient remained minimally symptomatic until the pins were removed two weeks later, after which the symptomatic instability recurred.

is allowed to see the amount of wrist motion that is possible after pinning. A volar splint or cast is applied.

Patients in whom the instability has been corrected (i.e., pinned) note dramatic relief of their wrist pain, although they may have some discomfort from the intra-articular bleeding and joint irritation for one to two days after the procedure. Limited periods of wrist motion and use are allowed only under supervision. Unlimited use without external immobilization is not allowed, as this increases the risk of pin breakage.

I am able to recommend intercarpal fusion with more confidence in patients with dynamic instability on clinical criteria, who have symptomatic relief after trial pin fixation.

The pins are removed under local anesthesia in the office seven to 10 days after insertion. Usually, the prepinning symptoms

recur following pin removal. Patients who receive no relief have the pins removed, and further evaluation or nonoperative treatment or both are recommended.

This protocol has provided a useful diagnostic tool in patients with difficult wrist problems. The risks and potential complications of the procedure are few. They include possible complications from the use of intravenous regional anesthetic, possible pin tract infection, and all of the usual risks associated with the use of percutaneous pins, as described in the section on internal fixation later in this chapter.

Specific Limited Wrist Fusions

SCAPHOID-LUNATE

Although this would seem to be the most logical intercarpal fusion to consider in scapholunate dissociation, it has not been advocated widely. Hastings[16] reported his experience with this procedure in 1984. Watson[41] specficially recommends against this combination, both because it is difficult to obtain union of these bones and because, even if union is obtained, he feels that there may be inadequate bone volume at the fusion site to carry the load imposed at the junction of the lunate and the scaphoid during wrist use. My own results in two cases were disappointing, both patients requiring extension of their fusions to obtain union. Others have had satisfactory clinical results when bone union at the fusion site was obtained.[31]

SCAPHOID-TRAPEZIUM-TRAPEZOID (STT)

This fusion was reported by Sutro[36] in 1946 for the treatment of a nonunited scaphoid fracture and in 1967 by Peterson and Lipscomb[29] for rotatory subluxation of the scaphoid. It was popularized by Watson's report[45] in 1980. Several authors have reported their experience with this fusion since that time.[9, 18] The kinematics of the wrist following STT fusion have been studied by Kleinman.[17] He has shown that the capitate moves with the STT fusion mass. The ulnar carpus is not affected by the fusion because a plane of motion develops between the scaphoid and the lunate. This disruption of the scapholunate link preserves the normal kinematics of the hamate and the triquetrum. Wrist motion following STT fusion is therefore a combination of motion between the scaphoid and the lunate and radiocarpal motion.

Watson[47] has reported a series of STT fusions with follow-up studies averaging nearly four years. He describes preservation of 55° (73 percent) wrist extension, 68° (84 percent) wrist flexion, 12° radial deviation, 28° ulnar deviation, and 31 kg (90 percent) of grip strength. He reports no degenerative changes of adjacent joints in patients followed as long as 11 years and nine months.

The indications for STT fusion include both static and dynamic scaphoid instability (Fig. 30–2) without the presence of radioscaphoid arthritis and in localized degenerative arthritis of the STT joints. Its use in the treatment of Kienböck's disease has also been reported as a means to unload force transmission across the lunate (Chapters 23 and 28).[48]

SCAPHOID-CAPITATE

This combination is an alternative to scaphoid-trapezium-trapezoid fusion, and its indications are similar. It results in more restriction of wrist motion but is easier to perform through a longitudinal, midline excision. A broad surface contact area is available for fusion. I have been satisfied with this fusion in patients with scapholunate dissociation. It is used in conjunction with lunate implant to diminish the compressive load on the implant, to transmit load across the wrist, and to prevent carpal collapse (Fig. 30–3). It also has been used as a salvage procedure for nonunion of proximal pole fractures of the scaphoid with avascular necrosis of the nonunited fragment.

SCAPHOID-CAPITATE-LUNATE

This fusion includes the midcarpal joint and therefore can be used for treatment of midcarpal instability or scapholunate dissociation with significant dorsiflexion instability of the lunate. Its use in late Kienböck's disease and in diffuse intercarpal arthritis with preservation of the radiocarpal joints has also been described.[14, 39] As with all midcarpal fusions, it limits wrist motion considerably.

CAPITATE-LUNATE

This fusion is used for stabilization of the midcarpal joint, particularly when a scaphoid implant is to be inserted for radioscaphoid arthritis (Fig. 30–4). Other indications are degenerative arthritis limited to this joint, fractures of the lunate, and Kienböck's disease.[41]

LUNATE-TRIQUETRUM

This fusion has been advocated by Alexander and Lichtman[1] for symptomatic ulnar-sided instabilities secondary to lunotriquetral dissociation (see Chapter 20). It reproduces the most common of the congenital carpal coalitions, which are usually asymptomatic.[34] Taleisnik[38, 39] has suggested this fusion for static volar collapse (VISI) deformities (Fig. 30–5A).

LUNATE-CAPITATE-HAMATE-TRIQUETRUM

This fusion, often referred to as the "four-corner" fusion, can be used for both midcarpal and lunotriquetral instabilities. It does not cause significantly more loss of wrist

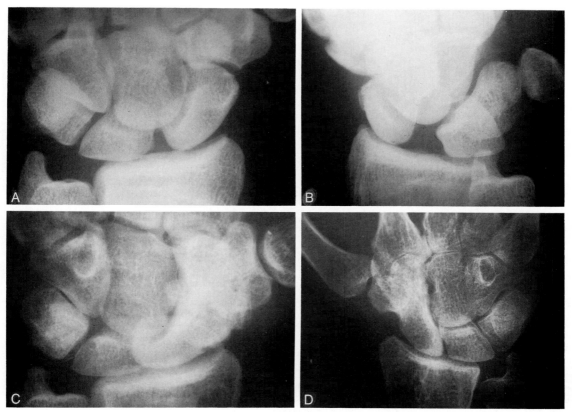

Figure 30–2. *A*, A 27-year-old firefighter with a symptomatic scapholunate dissociation that prevented him from working. *B*, The extent of the dissociation is seen on the oblique view of the wrist. *C*, Treatment by scaphoid-trapezium-trapezoid fusion stabilized the scaphoid and eliminated his pain. He was able to return to his regular work five months following surgery. At that time his grip strength was 80 lb (90 percent of that of the contralateral side). Wrist flexion was 55°, extension was 55°, ulnar deviation was 28°, and radial deviation 10°. *D*, A 26-year-old secretary was treated for dynamic scaphoid instability by scaphoid-trapezium-trapezoid (STT) fusion. The scapoid was "over-reduced", locking it into an excessively horizontal position. Although the patient's symptoms were alleviated and she was able to return to work, radial deviation of the wrist was limited. Watson has described over-reduction of the scaphoid as one of the most common errors made during STT fusion.

motion than a capitolunate fusion alone. It provides very wide surfaces for bone union and results in a stable carpus (Fig. 30–5B).

TRIQUETRUM-HAMATE

This fusion stabilizes the midcarpus and is indicated for midcarpal instability or degenerative changes between these two bones (see Chapter 20). The presence of instability of this joint is difficult to ascertain at the time of surgery. It is one of the most mobile joints in the carpus, its dorsal stabilizing ligaments are thin, and arthrotomy of the joint increases its laxity. Alexander and Lichtman[1, 20] recommend pinning the joint at the time of surgery to confirm the diagnosis and to assure that the instability has been corrected prior to preparing the joint for fusion. They have described recurrent

but less severe clicks that occur postoperatively, as well as pain over the hamate hook or degenerative changes of the pisotriquetral joint or both. My experience has been similar, and I have had to resect one hamate hook and remove several pisiform bones in cases in which these conditions occurred following triquetrohamate fusions. For these reasons I prefer the "four-corner" fusion for significant ulnar or midcarpal instability (Fig. 30–6).

PANCARPAL

I have used pancarpal fusion in patients with multiple areas of intercarpal arthritis or in patients with instability not corrected by a more localized fusion. All motion occurs at the radiocarpal joint, resulting in significant loss of wrist motion. In my series, most

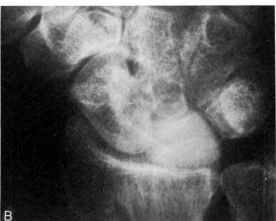

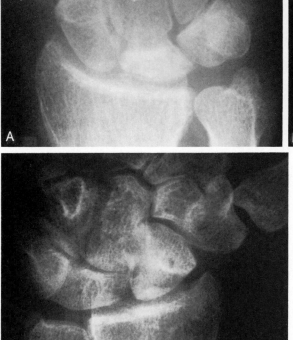

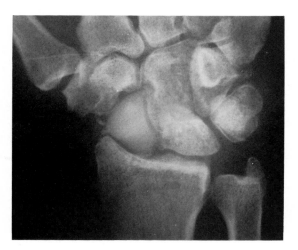

Figure 30–3. A 50-year-old man with advanced Kienböck's disease with painful, limited wrist motion and loss of grip strength. *A,* The pre-operative x-ray shows the sclerotic and collapsed lunate. *B,* The postoperative x-ray after Silastic lunate replacement and scaphocapitate fusion. Nine months after surgery, the patient was asymptomatic, with the exception of occasional aching wrist pain after strenuous work. Grip strength was 95 lb (76 percent of that of the contralateral side). Wrist flexion was 30°, wrist extension was 50°, ulnar deviation was 20°, and radial deviation was 10°. *C,* A 30-year-old truck driver underwent scaphoid-capitate fusion for symptomatic scaphoid instability. He was able to return to work as a truck driver. At one year, his grip strength was 40 lb (67 percent of that of the contralateral side). Wrist flexion was 75°, wrist extension was 55°, ulnar deviation was 30°, and radial deviation was 10°.

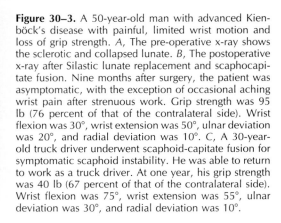

Figure 30–4. Capitate-lunate fusion to support axial wrist loading after replacement of the scaphoid bone with a Silastic implant. (Courtesy of Lewis Millender, M.D.)

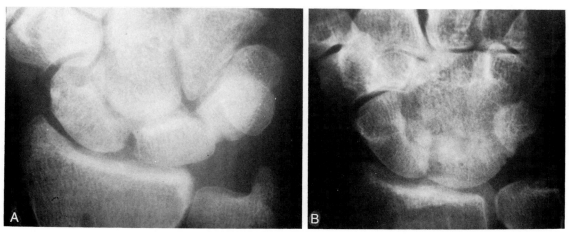

Figure 30–5. *A,* Lunate-triquetrum fusion in a 37-year-old firefighter who injured his wrist in a fall, after which he had signs and symptoms of triquetrum instability. Five months after surgery, his grip strength was 70 lb (64 percent of the contralateral side). Wrist flexion was 50°, wrist extension was 50°, ulnar deviation was 15°, and radial deviation was 20°. *B,* A 24-year-old woman was treated by lunate-capitate-hamate-triquetrum ("four-corner") fusion for midcarpal instability. Nine months after surgery, her grip was 35 lb (54 percent of the contralateral side). She had intermittent aching pain after prolonged use of the wrist. Wrist flexion was 30°, wrist extension was 50°, ulnar deviation was 10°, and radial deviation was 10°.

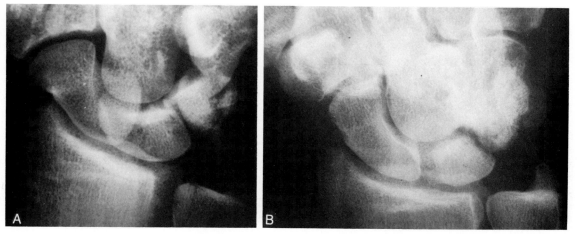

Figure 30–6. *A,* An 18-year-old student fell from a rooftop, sustaining a closed fracture dislocation of his triquetrum among other extremity and abdominal injuries. He was treated by open reduction and primary triquetrum-hamate fusion. *B,* Nine months after treatment, his wrist was asymptomatic. His grip strength was 85 lb (85 percent of that of the contralateral side). Wrist flexion was 56°, wrist extension was 75°, ulnar deviation was 20°, and radial deviation was 15°.

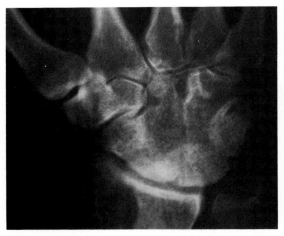

Figure 30–7. A 28-year-old man sustained a wrist injury when the bit of a large post-hole boring machine became bound in concrete, resulting in sudden rotatory stress. He underwent a pancarpal fusion for complex wrist instability. He was able to return to work as a house painter six months after the fusion. Grip strength was 95 lb (76 percent of that of the contralateral side). Wrist flexion was 15°, wrist extension was 40°, ulnar deviation was 10°, and radial deviation was 10°.

wrists with pancarpal fusions have been stable and pain-free, with patients able to return to doing work requiring strenuous use of the hands. There may be a residual click during radial and ulnar deviation as the fixed scapholunate unit slides over the ridges in the radius that separate the scaphoid fossa from the lunate fossa (Fig. 30–7).

RADIOSCAPHOID

This fusion can be used when there is extensive localized arthritis of the articulation between the radius and the scaphoid. This combination will allow wrist motion only through the midcarpal joints and results in significant loss of motion. It can be combined with radiolunate arthrodesis if the lunate-radius articulation is involved (Fig. 30–8).

RADIOLUNATE

This fusion has been proposed by Taleisnik[39] for lunate instability with either dorsal or volar instability patterns when strong grip is required. The other indications include post-traumatic degenerative disease involving the radiocarpal joints (destruction of the articular surfaces of the radius or the proximal articular surfaces of the scaphoid and lunate or both, with preservation of the midcarpal articular surfaces) and rheumatoid arthritis with localized degenerative changes of the radiolunate articulation or ulnar translocation of the carpus (see Chapter 24).[26, 39] Fusion of the proximal row or of the scaphoid or the lunate individually to the distal articular suface of the radius allows motion, albeit limited, of the wrist through the midcarpal joints. In my series, this has provided a stable wrist with minimal pain, but with restriction of wrist motion to between 25

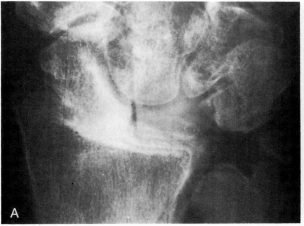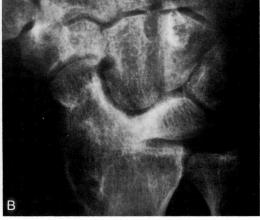

Figure 30–8. *A,* A 37-year-old salesman with advanced radiocarpal arthritis three years after a fall onto his outstretched hand while skiing. A fusion of the scaphoid to the radius and a replacement of the arthritic lunate bone with a Silastic implant were performed. Ten months after this procedure, he had no pain, and was able to use his hand and wrist for all of his normal daily activities including sports. Grip strength was 75 lb (65 percent of that of the contralateral side). Wrist flexion was 15°, wrist extension was 35°, ulnar deviation was 10°, and radial deviation was 15°. *B,* A 38-year-old attorney had a radius-scaphoid-lunate fusion for advanced radioscaphoid arthritis 10 years after a traumatic scapholunate dissociation. One year after fusion, his grip strength was 120 lb (86 percent of the contralateral side). Wrist flexion was zero, wrist extension was 30°, ulnar deviation was 10°, and radial deviation was 10°. He had no wrist pain but had difficulty adusting to the loss of wrist flexion.

and 33 percent of normal. The technique of limited wrist fusion in rheumatoid arthritis is discussed in Chapter 25.

Intercarpal Fusion—Technique

SURGICAL EXPOSURE

I prefer a longitudinal incision for all intercarpal fusions other than the scaphoid-trapezium-trapezoid. A slightly curved incision (convex side toward the radius) matches the normal slight ulnar deviation stance of the hand and, in my opinion, is more pleasing esthetically than a straight longitudinal incision. The incision need not be greater than 2 to 3 inches in length. This provides excellent exposure of most of the carpus as well as access to the distal radius for obtaining bone graft (Fig. 30–9).

Transverse incisions heal with a less conspicuous scar, but they limit exposure and increase the risk of damage to the superficial sensory nerves. It is difficult to extend or incorporate a transverse scar into the incision necessary for revisional surgery.

The extensor tendons must be retracted to expose the dorsal wrist capsule. The extensor retinaculum is divided through the midportion of the fourth dorsal extensor compartment. The vertical septi of the retinaculum between compartments three through five are divided. This allows the extensor tendons to be retracted to either side. Care must be taken to identify and protect the extensor pollicis longus tendon as it crosses the second compartment tendons distal to Lister's tubercle. Alternatively, the dorsal wrist capsule may be exposed by making a longitudinal incision carried down through periosteum between the third and fourth dorsal compartments. The entire fourth retinacular compartment can be mobilized as a unit by subperiosteal dissection.[21] This avoids exposing the individual finger extensors and preserves the restraining function of the retinaculum. The capsule is exposed by retracting the extensor pollicis longus tendon radially and the fourth compartment ulnarly.

The terminal branch of the posterior interosseous (radial) nerve lies in the floor of the fourth compartment. The wrist may be partially denervated by dividing this nerve, as described by Buck-Gramcko[5] for rheumatoid wrist disease and by Dellon[12] for chronic wrist pain.

The capsule may be opened with a longitudinal capsulotomy or with a T or "cross" capsular incision, depending on how much

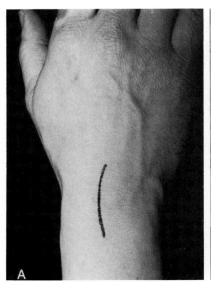
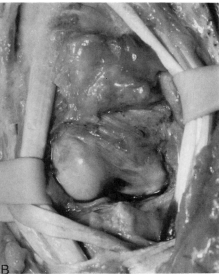

Figure 30–9. *A*, The author's preferred incision for access to the wrist for intercarpal fusion (other than STT: it is difficult to reach the STT joints through this incision) and for total wrist fusion. A slight curve is used for esthetic reasons, although a straight incision is equally effective for exposure. The incision may be moved slightly to the radial side or to the ulnar side of the midline in order to enhance exposure on one side or the other of the carpus. *B*, Using a longitudinal incision, skin flaps have been retracted, the fourth dorsal compartment incised, retinacular flaps and extensor tendons retracted, and the wrist capsule incised to expose the carpus. The proximal pole of the scaphoid bone is seen on the left (rotated vertically), and the chronically stretched scapholunate interosseous ligament and the lunate are seen to the right of the scaphoid.

of the carpus must be visualized. I prefer a U-shaped capsular incision, based either radially or ulnarly. This allows a large flap of capsule to be placed over the mid-portion of the carpus following fusion, providing a smooth bed for the extensor tendons without a longitudinal suture line, while affording excellent exposure. Loose closure may be obtained by tacking back the corners of flap.

The triangular fibrocartilage complex or distal radioulnar joint or both can be explored by mobilizing the tendons of the fifth and sixth compartments and by extending the capsular incision or elevating another small flap of capsule if the patient's symptoms or clinical findings are suggestive of damage in these areas or if the arthrographic results are positive.

Tight closure of the capsule is not necessary and is probably not desirable. Maximum wrist motion following intercarpal fusion is obtained if the wrist motion limits are determined by the bone constraints and are not compounded by capsular fibrosis. Tight closure combined with normal scar contracture and prolonged immobilization may produce more restriction in motion than the theoretical limits imposed by any given bone fusion; therefore, I close the capsule loosely with several absorbable sutures. The capsule should provide a smooth bed for extensor tendons but should not limit wrist motion unless a capsulodesis effect is desired for a specific reason.

PREPARATION OF THE CARPUS FOR FUSION

Exploration of the wrist prior to fusion is of critical importance. The presence of synovitis, capsular tears, cartilage erosion, and/or interosseous ligament damage can alert the surgeon to unsuspected intercarpal problems and may allow or even dictate an alternative procedure to the one planned preoperatively. For example, the presence of radioscaphoid arthritis precludes performing a scaphoid-trapezium-trapezoid fusion.

After the fusion to be performed has been selected, careful alignment of the carpus to restore or maintain proper position of individual carpal bones is important. The scaphoid should be aligned so that its proximal articular surface, when reduced, is concentric with the scaphoid fossa of the radius but not over-reduced so that the bone is too horizontal. Reduction of the scaphoid so that the scapholunate angle is less than the nor-

mal 45° limits radial deviation more than is necessary and may not provide concentric reduction of the proximal pole. Over-reduction of the scaphoid is probably the most common error committed when performing a scaphoid-trapezium-trapezoid fusion. The specific technique used for scaphoid-trapezium-trapezoid fusion as described by Watson[45] is shown in Figure 30–10.

I attempt to correct the alignment of the lunate if there is volar or dorsal tilt of this bone. A K wire introduced vertically into the body of the lunate can be used as a handle to correct rotation. It is removed after the lunate is secured with a horizontal K wire to another of the carpal bones. In wrists with mild to moderate lunate rotation, the dorsal surface of the lunate can be decorticated to promote adherence of the capsule to the bone. The resulting "capsulodesis" supplements lunate stability. Midcarpal fusion may be required to correct severe lunate rotation. Correction of lunate rotation keeps the lunate reduced concentrically in the lunate fossa of the radius and provides a more normal contour of the entire articular surface of the proximal carpal row.

The overall dimensions of the carpus should be preserved as the carpal bones are prepared for fusion.[44, 45] If I am concerned about maintaining alignment or carpal dimension or both, I pin the carpus in the position desired for intercarpal fusion prior to removal of articular cartilage and subchondral bone. The wrist is held in neutral position by the assistant. The carpal bones are reduced and fixed with one or two transversely oriented K wires. Articular cartilage and subchondral bone are removed by working around the pin or pins, which prevent the carpal bones from migrating. If a pin remains undamaged and solidly fixed, it is retained and used as one of the pins in the final fixation of the fusion. If it is damaged by the osteotome or saw, it is replaced after the final pins used for internal fixation are inserted. The difficulty in working around the pin or pins is offset by the ease in maintaining proper carpal alignment. This technique may become less useful as the surgeon gains experience with limited wrist fusion techniques.

CARTILAGE REMOVAL AND BONE PREPARATION

An osteotome, rongeur, or "micro" sagittal saw is used to remove articular cartilage and

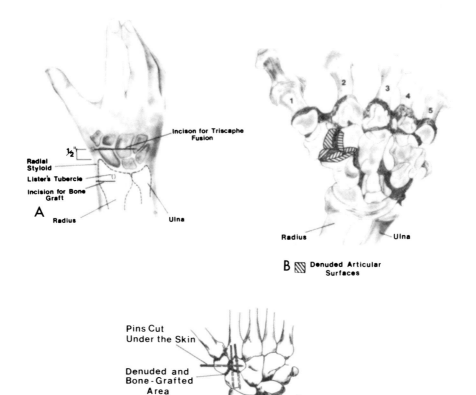

Figure 30–10. The technique of scaphoid-trapezium-trapezoid intercarpal fusion as described by Watson. (From Watson HK and Ryu J: Orthop Clin North Am 15:337–353, 1984.)

subchondral bone. Standard high-speed power burs should not be used, as the heat generated may cause thermal necrosis of the bone, which may interfere with primary bone healing. The only nonunions in my series of intercarpal fusions have occurred after the use of burs to remove articular cartilage. The Midas Rex system has been used to prepare fusion sites without adverse effect,[25] although I have no personal experience with this method. If using the Midas, extreme care must be taken to protect adjacent structures and soft tissues.

The subchondral bone should be removed or softened by "fish-scaling" to expose cancellous bone in order to maximize the potential for primary bone healing and joint fusion. This can be accomplished with the sagittal saw, rongeur, or osteotome, or by making multiple perforations in the subchondral plate, using the sharp point of a 0.045-in diameter K wire driven by a high-

speed drill after the articular cartilage has been removed with a rongeur or a curette.

INTERNAL FIXATION

K wires (0.045-in diameter) are used for internal fixation. They are inserted easily and can usually be removed without undue difficulty in the physician's office under local infiltration anesthesia. I prefer to cut the pins below the skin level, leaving them long enough so that they can be palpated in the subcutaneous tissue but not so long that they tent the skin. If they are left too long, they may be impinged by the postoperative dressing or cast, causing skin irritation and pain. If a pin erodes through the skin, it is removed as soon as possible to minimize the possibility of a pin tract infection. However, if the pins are cut too short, they may be difficult to palpate after healing has occurred, and removal in the physician's office may be difficult if not impossible. It is safer and less frustrating to remove such buried pins in the operating room under optimal conditions, using adequate anesthesia, with a C-arm image intensifier available to aid in localization of the pin.

I have no personal experience with the use of Herbert screws for the internal fixation of intercarpal fusion. The mechanical advantages of fixation with such a device are attractive. The screws can be inserted without the use of the jig (i.e., freehand) and can be left in place after union has occurred.

Complications

The use of K wires for internal fixation is not without problems. These include arterial puncture, nerve impingement, tendon impingement, and pin breakage, as well as the difficulty in pin removal previously discussed.

Arterial Puncture. Occasionally puncture of the radial artery occurs, manifested by large amounts of bright red blood escaping from the pin site. In this case, the pin is removed and pressure is applied to the bleeding site. In my experience, the bleeding has stopped without permanent damage to the artery or distal circulation.

Nerve Impingement. Impingement of a superficial sensory nerve by the pin is possible. This is manifested by intense pain in a localized area after the patient recovers from the anesthetic. The pin should be removed as soon as possible, taking care to protect the involved nerve from further damage. Transient paresthesias or numbness or both in the distribution of the affected nerve usually occur and resolve slowly over several weeks.

Tendon Impingement. Tendon impingement is manifested by pain in a localized area accompanying wrist, thumb, or finger motion. Again, should this occur, the pin is removed as soon as possible to avoid tendon attrition. On several occasions in my experience, steroid injection of the first dorsal compartment has been necessary for relief of semiacute or chronic tenosynovitis, which I have attributed to scarring and bleeding resulting from violation of the tendon sheath by the pin. This can be minimized by careful pin insertion technique, with palpation of the subcutaneous structures prior to insertion of the pin.

The wrist should be moved through its range of motion to be sure that the pins do not impinge on the radiocarpal joint before they are cut short. Pins should not be placed across the radiocarpal joint when an intercarpal fusion is performed. Preservation of radiocarpal joint motion acts as a safety valve to decrease stress at the intercarpal fusion site.

Bone Graft

The distal metaphysis of the radius provides an excellent source of bone graft for most limited carpal fusions and is an alternative to the iliac crest as a bone donor site.[23] A corticocancellous graft can be harvested by removing a cortical window from the dorsal metaphyseal area after the periosteum has been reflected. Access to the metaphysis is possible by retracting the extensor tendons in the proximal portion of a longitudinal wound, or through a separate transverse incision over the metaphysis. If a transverse incision is used, the interval between the tendons of the first and second compartments or between the second and third compartments is opened to expose the dorsal cortex of the radius. A cortical window is removed with osteotomes or a small sagittal saw. Cancellous bone is harvested with curettes. The cortical window is usually used as a strut at the fusion site and is not replaced. Care is taken not to penetrate the subchondral bone and the articular surface of the distal radius.

If a large bone defect is present or if the distal radius has been used previously as a bone graft donor site, sufficient bone may not be available from the distal radius. In these cases, iliac bone graft should be used. If there is any question about the amount of bone available from the distal radius, patient permission should be obtained in advance for an iliac bone graft.

Drains

I do not use drains routinely in intercarpal fusions in young, healthy patients with normal skin and subcutaneous tissue. I do use drains in wrist procedures on rheumatoid patients because of their atrophic skin and minimal subcutaneous tissue over the wrist. If used, the drain should be placed in the subcutaneous space dorsal to the repaired extensor retinaculum. The drain is removed on the first or second postoperative day.

Dressing and Postoperative Management

A bulky compressive dressing is applied with the wrist held in neutral position by a volar plaster splint. It is my preference to leave the fingers free so that early postoperative motion can be started. Occasionally the fingers must be supported for several days to minimize postoperative pain. Watson[45] suggests the use of a volar splint to prevent use of the hand for gripping, which adds compressive load to the fusion site. I prefer to start finger motion on the first postoperative day, but I do warn my patients about the potential adverse effect of grip on bone healing at the fusion site. I use a sugar-tong splint for one to two weeks, followed by a short-arm cast (with a thumb spica if the fusion includes the radial side of the carpus). The cast is extended as proximally as possible on the forearm, without causing impingement of the antecubital fossa when the elbow is flexed.

The retained K wires are removed between six and eight weeks postoperatively if radiographs show satisfactory progress toward bone union. External support with a short-arm cast or a short-arm thumb-spica cast is continued for eight to 10 weeks, until there is evidence of bone union on radiographs. Others recommend the use of a long-arm cast for several weeks after surgery.[39, 45] I find that it is helpful to use a removable splint for two to three weeks after the solid cast is discontinued, to wean the patient away from the use of external support.

REHABILITATION

After discontinuing solid external immobilization, a gentle range-of-motion exercise program is started. Care must be taken to avoid forced wrist motion by the patient or by the therapist. I emphasize progressive grip strengthening rather than motion for the first several months after surgery. Wrist motion increases steadily over six to nine months postoperatively. Vigorous attempts to regain motion early can cause an exacerbation of wrist pain. Anti-inflammatory medication is helpful in some patients during the first few weeks of therapy.

A gradual increase in wrist motion over nine to twelve months can be expected as new planes of motion develop around the fusion site and as the wrist capsule stretches.[17, 47]

Intercarpal (Limited) Wrist Fusion—Summary

Limited wrist fusion is a reasonable alternative to total wrist fusion or implant ar-
throplasty in static instabilities of the wrist, localized arthritis of the carpus, and loss of carpal bone stock from fracture or avascular necrosis. Intercarpal fusion is a valuable adjunct to carpal implant arthroplasty and has a role in the treatment of Kienböck's disease. Relief of the symptomatic dynamic instability can be obtained with this technique, but the correct diagnosis and localization of the site of instability are critical in obtaining satisfactory results.

Careful attention must be given to carpal alignment, surgical technique, and postoperative management. Unsatisfactory results may be salvaged by extension of the intercarpal fusion, conversion to wrist fusion, or, in some cases, the use of Silastic implants.

RADIOCARPAL (TOTAL) WRIST FUSION

Wrist fusion is the salvage procedure of choice for a variety of conditions, including arthritis, infection, tumor, loss of wrist motor function, and failure of other wrist procedures such as arthroplasty and limited wrist fusion. Fortunately, the upper extremity functions well with a stable and painless wrist that does not move, as long as the forearm, elbow, and shoulder joints have relatively well preserved function and are able to position the hand in space. Most patients adapt rapidly to wrist fusion, particularly when their pain is relieved and the hand is aligned with the axis of the forearm. While some of my patients have objected to or resisted the recommendation of wrist fusion, the same patients are the most ardent advocates of fusion after the procedure has been performed, their pain has resolved, and they realize that their loss of function is not as great as they had anticipated. One young woman who refused wrist fusion for several years was so pleased with her result after fusion that she offered to organize a patients' "wrist support group." A preoperative trial of wrist immobilization in a light short-arm cast to simulate wrist fusion may be helpful in some cases. Patients can be reassured that the procedure is reliable and predictable in outcome.

Indications

The indications for total wrist fusion include *pain* (with or without loss of motion) or *instability* or both from post-traumatic degenerative joint disease following intra-articular fracture of the radius or carpal bones; *degenerative changes* from chronic loss of ligamentous support resulting from destruction by rheumatoid arthritis, infection, or tumor; *loss of motor control* of the wrist with resultant wrist deformity, which interferes with function and occurs as the result of polio or acquired hemiplegia, either flaccid or spastic.[6, 11, 24, 39]

Dick[11] lists the following as situations in which wrist fusion is contraindicated: the presence of open epiphyseal plates; in quadriparetics, when wrist motion is required for the performance of tendon transfers or for modified grasp and transfer techniques; in patients with major sensory deprivation in the hand.

Position for Wrist Fusion

The position in which the wrist should be fused is controversial. The recommendations by different authors range from neutral to 30° wrist extension, with zero to 10° ulnar deviation. If bilateral fusions are indicated, neutral or slight extension has been recommended for one wrist and neutral or even palmar flexion up to 30° in the other wrist to facilitate toilet and hygiene functions.[11, 39] Milford[24] prefers 10° to 20° extension, with the third metacarpal and the radius aligned. Dick[11] prefers 15° to 20° wrist extension for most wrist fusions but recommends the neutral position in patients with wrist deformity secondary to spastic hemiplegia. In bilateral wrist fusions, he suggests that the dominant wrist be fused in 20° extension and the nondominant side in neutral extension.

Haddad and Riordan[15] recommend that the wrist be fused with both slight dorsiflexion and ulnar deviation, in such a way that the shaft of the second metacarpal is aligned with the distal end of the radius.

My preferred position for unilateral wrist fusions is 10° extension and 5° ulnar deviation. It is my opinion that this position provides the best compromise between function and cosmesis. For bilateral wrist fusions, I prefer that the dominant wrist be fused in the position described above, with the nondominant wrist in neutral extension.

Inclusion of Carpometacarpal Joints in Wrist Fusion

Haddad and Riordan[15] recommend that the second and third carpometacarpal joints be included in the fusion to prevent painful motion from developing at these joints after wrist fusion. In my experience, this has occurred only in patients performing very heavy labor or in those using the hand-wrist-forearm unit for repetitive or strenuous activities or both, or in patients with previous injuries of the carpometacarpal joints. This has been the observation of my colleagues as well.[25, 31] Therefore, I now recommend including the second and third carpometacarpal joints in the fusion in patients whose employment or avocations will stress the carpometacarpal joints after the wrist has been fused. I do not incorporate these joints in fusions in patients who have only light or moderate use requirements of the extremity or in those who have rheumatoid arthritis.

Radiocarpal Wrist Fusion— Technique

Many wrist fusion techniques have been described in the literature.[2, 6, 11, 15, 19, 24, 27] Most of these use the dorsal approach to expose the radiocarpal joints. Articular cartilage is removed from the joints to be fused, bone graft either from the iliac crest or from the dorsal or intramedullary areas of the distal radius or both is added, and some form of internal fixation is inserted to maintain the wrist in the desired position.

Haddad and Riordan[15] describe a radial approach to the wrist, a block resection of the radiocarpal, intercarpal, and second and third carpometacarpal joints, and an insertion of a contoured iliac crest strut graft. This method does not disturb the extensor tendons, does not enter the distal radioulnar joint, does not add bone bulk around the wrist, and derives some stability from the corticocancellous strut graft. However, care must be taken to avoid damaging the branches of the superficial radial nerve.

Various types of internal fixation devices have been used to stabilize the wrist fusion until bone union occurs. Rods,[27] staples,[2] and compression plates[19] have all been advocated. Of these, I am least inclined to use dorsal compression plates, except in special circumstances. These impose bulk on the dorsum of the wrist, which may interfere with gliding of the extensor tendon, make dorsal soft tissue closure more difficult, and increase pressure on the dorsal skin postoperatively. In addition, the plate must be removed through a long incision, which requires dissection of the extensor tendons and the retinaculum and cannot be performed under local anesthesia or as an office procedure.

My preferred technique of wrist fusion is a modification of that described by Millender and Nalebuff[27] for the rheumatoid wrist. In their method, the carpus is exposed as described in the previous section on intercarpal fusions. The incision and dissection are extended slightly more proximally to expose the articular surface of the distal radius. The articular cartilage is removed from the distal radius, the proximal and middle carpal rows and, if necessary, from the carpometacarpal joints of the second and third metacarpals. Bleeding cancellous bone is exposed using rongeurs or osteotomes. High-speed burs are not used because of the risk of thermal bone necrosis. Enough bone is removed from the proximal row to allow correction of any wrist deformity. Bone graft from either the distal radius, distal ulna (if this is resected at the same time), or the iliac crest is packed between the carpal bones after internal fixation has been obtained. If the distal radioulnar joint is involved, it should be attended to at the time of wrist fusion by distal ulna resection and soft tissue stabilization, by hemiresection of the distal ulna, or by one of the variations of distal-ulna-to-radius fusion, with creation of a proximal pseudarthrosis to allow forearm rotation, such as the Lauenstein procedure.

In the technique described by Millender and Nalebuff,[27] a large Steinmann pin is used for internal fixation. The medullary canal of the radius is perforated with an awl to create a channel for the Steinmann pin. The largest pin that fits the medullary canal of the radius is selected. The diameter of this pin varies from $\frac{1}{8}$ to $\frac{1}{16}$ in. The pin is drilled or tapped through the carpus from proximal to distal to exit between the second and third or between the third and fourth metacarpals, depending on the alignment between the carpus and the radius. The proximal pin end is then inserted into the radius and tapped proximally with a mallet into the medullary canal of the radius. It is countersunk approximately 2 cm proximal to the level of the metacarpophalangeal joints. Staples or K wires are used to supplement the internal fixation if necessary. In the rheumatoid patient with loss of bone stock, the pin is introduced into the third metacarpal bone to augment stability.

The length of the pin must be determined carefully to avoid migration postoperatively of a pin that is too short. If the pin is too long, it may become impacted in the proximal portion of the radius, or perforate or split the radius as it is driven proximally. Usually, the medullary canal of the radius is "sounded" with the pin selected prior to final insertion. This allows accurate determination of proper pin length. If there is any question about the position of the pin, intraoperative radiographs should be obtained.

This method dictates that the wrist be positioned very close to neutral flexion/extension. The position of the wrist cannot be altered after the rod has been inserted. The single rod, even though large in diameter, does not provide secure rotatory stability of the carpus to the distal radius.

I use a modification of the technique described above for wrist fusions in both rheumatoid and nonrheumatoid patients. The wrist is prepared as described above. Rather than use a single, large Steinmann pin, I use two relatively thin pins (5/64- to 7/64-in diameter), which are inserted through the second and third web spaces between the metacarpal bones, across the carpus, and into the medullary canal of the radius. This results in a "stacked-pin" effect in the radius, which provides rotational stability as well as anteroposterior and lateral stability without the need for supplementary internal fixation (Fig. 30–11). The pins are thin enough to be bent after insertion into the radius, allowing final correction and adjustment of the wrist position. Thus, if slightly more dorsification is desired after the rods are in place, the wrist is gently manipulated into the correct position. The use of thinner pins minimizes the potential for compression of the intrinsic muscles of the hand (interossei) by a large rod, which may result in fibrosis and secondary intrinsic contracture. Care must be taken to insert the pins through the dorsal portion of the web space to avoid damage to the neurovascular structures in the palm. I have found it useful to make a small cortical window in the distal radius. This allows the pins to be guided into the medullary canal of the radius under direct vision. Additional cancellous bone graft may be harvested from the distal radius as well. The pins are cut short beneath the skin in the web spaces and are removed after solid bone union has occurred, usually between four and six months postoperatively. The pins have been left in situ for as long

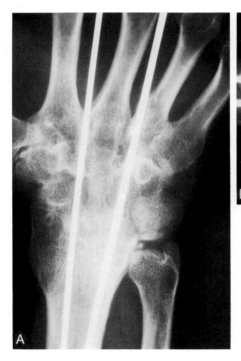

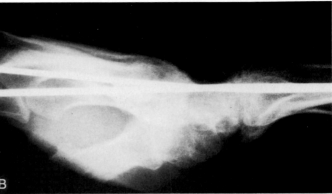

Figure 30–11. *A, B,* Two views of total wrist fusion using iliac crest bone graft and dual intermetacarpal-intramedullary rod internal fixation for post-traumatic arthritis of the wrist. Note wrist fusion position in slight dorsiflexion and slight ulnar deviation.

as four years without adverse effect. The pins can be removed under local anesthesia. A vertical incision in the web space is made and the pin end is grasped with a small, sterile, needle-nose Vise-grip.

Solid union has been obtained in 15 consecutive patients in my experience using this method over the past five years. The majority of these patients were nonrheumatoid, although the method has been used successfully in rheumatoid patients, even when carpal bone stock has been minimal. The advantages of this method include ease of hardware insertion and removal, the ability to adjust the position of the wrist at the time of surgery in both the anteroposterior and lateral planes, and stable fixation even with suboptimal bone stock. Postoperatively, the need for only a short-arm cast allows early forearm motion.

POSTOPERATIVE CARE

The postoperative care following total wrist fusion is very similar to that described in the preceding sections for intercarpal fusions. I prefer to use drains routinely after wrist fusion because of the large surface of bleeding, cancellous bone that is exposed during the procedure. Most authors describe the use of long-arm postoperative immobilization following total wrist fusion. How-

ever, I still prefer to use sugar-tong splints for the first seven to 10 days, followed by short-arm cast immobilization if the internal fixation utilized provides satisfactory rotatory stability. Short-arm cast immobilization facilitates early motion of the elbow and shoulder as well as the forearm and is much easier for patients to tolerate, particularly those with rheumatoid arthritis.

COMPLICATIONS OF WRIST FUSION

The complications following wrist fusion were reviewed by Clendenin and Green.[8] The most frequent complication in their series was pseudarthrosis. Other complications occurred rarely but included deep wound infection, superficial skin necrosis, transient median nerve or superficial radial nerve compression, and fracture of the healed fusion. One case of Steinmann pin migration caused flexor tendon impingement and mechanical block to metacarpophalangeal joint flexion.

I have had several patients with transient sensory neuropathies of the median nerve following wrist fusion. These have all resolved, most within several days of the procedure. I have seen no superficial skin necrosis since using a straight or slightly curved longitudinal skin incision. Skin necrosis occurred occasionally when zig-zag or

S-shaped incisions were used. Two patients developed intrinsic contractures affecting metacarpophalangeal joint motion (i.e., loss of extension) after large-diameter Steinmann pins were placed between the metacarpals. This complication has not occurred since small-diameter pins or rods have been used.

Radiocarpal (Total) Wrist Fusion—Summary

Total wrist fusion remains the single most predictable and reliable surgical procedure for treating wrist problems, regardless of their cause. It is tolerated very well by most patients and results in a stable and painless wrist that permits strenuous use. Most patients are able to return to their regular occupations, even though some modifications in the use of the extremity may be necessary; however, mechanics and others who must position their hands in tight or cramped spaces (e.g., behind engines) have difficulty. Sports activities that require wrist motion are also more difficult. Many of my patients have been able to modify the use of their extremities after wrist fusion so that they are still able to enjoy their chosen sports and avocations. According to the American Medical Association's Guide to the Evaluation of Impairment, total wrist fusion in "neutral" position results in a 30 percent loss of upper extremity function.

Total wrist fusion should be considered as an excellent option in the surgical treatment of wrist disease.

References

1. Alexander CE, and Lichtman DM: Ulnar carpal instabilities. Orthop Clin North Am 15:307–320, 1984.
2. Benkeddache Y, Gottesman H, and Fourrier P: Multiple stapling for wrist arthrodesis in the nonrheumatoid patient. J Hand Surg 9A:256–260, 1984.
3. Bertheussen K: Partial carpal arthrodesis as treatment of local degenerative changes in wrist joints. Acta Orthop Scand 52:629–631, 1981.
4. Brumfield RH, and Champoux JA: Biomechanical study of normal functional wrist motion. Clin Orthop 187:23–25, 1984.
5. Buck-Gramcko D: Denervation of the wrist joint. J Hand Surg 2:54–61, 1977.
6. Campbell CJ, and Koekarn T: Total and subtotal arthrodesis of the wrist. J Bone Joint Surg 46A:1520–1533, 1964.
7. Chuinard RG, and Zeman SC: Kienböck's disease: an analysis and rationale for treatment by capitate-hamate fusion. Orthop Trans 4:18, 1980.
8. Clendenin MB, and Green DP: Arthrodesis of the wrist—complications and their management. J Hand Surg 6:253–257, 1981.
9. Cooney WP: Intercarpal fusions. J Hand Surg 9A:601, 1984.
10. Crosby EB, Linsheid RL, and Dobyns JH: Scapho-trapezial trapezoidal arthrosis. J Hand Surg 3:233–234, 1978.
11. Dick HM: Wrist and intercarpal arthrodesis. In Green DP (ed): Operative Hand Surgery. New York, Churchill Livingstone Inc, 1982.
12. Dellon AL: Partial dorsal wrist denervation: resection of the distal posterior interosseous nerve. J Hand Surg 10A:527–533, 1985.
13. Gordon LH, and King D: Partial wrist arthrodesis for old ununited fractures of the carpal navicular. Am J Surg 102:460, 1961.
14. Graner O, Lopes EI, Carvalho BC, et al: Arthrodesis of the carpal bones in the treatment of Kienböck's disease, painful ununited fractures of the navicular and lunate bones with avascular necrosis, and old fractures-dislocations of carpal bones. J Bone Joint Surg 48A:767–774, 1966.
15. Haddad RJ, and Riordan DC: Arthrodesis of the wrist. J Bone Joint Surg 49A:950–954, 1967.
16. Hastings DE, and Silver RL: Intercarpal arthrodesis in the management of chronic carpal instability after trauma. J Hand Surg 9A:834–840, 1984.
17. Kleinman WB: Carpal kinematics following scapho-trapezio-trapezoid arthrodesis. Presented at the Annual Meeting, American Society for Surgery of the Hand, 1986.
18. Kleinman WB, Steichen JB, and Strickland JW: Management of chronic rotatory subluxation of the scaphoid by scapho-trapezio-trapezoid arthrodesis. J Hand Surg 7:125–136, 1982.
19. Larsson S: Compression arthrodesis of the wrist. Clin Orthop 99:146–153, 1974.
20. Lichtman DM, Schneider JR, Swafford AR, et al: Ulnar midcarpal instability—clinical and laboratory analysis. J Hand Surg 6:515–523, 1981.
21. Linscheid RL: Correspondence Newsletter, American Society for Surgery of the Hand. July 11, 1985.
22. Linscheid RL, and Dobyns JH: Radiolunate arthrodesis. J Hand Surg 10A:821–829, 1985.
23. McGrath MH, and Watson HK: Late results with local bone graft donor sites in hand surgery. J Hand Surg 6:234–237, 1981.
24. Milford L: The Hand. St Louis, CV Mosby Co, 1982.
25. Nalebuff EA: Personal communication, 1986.
26. Nalebuff EA, and Garrod KJ: Present approach to the severely involved rheumatoid wrist. Orthop Clin North Am 15:369–380, 1984.
27. Millender LH, and Nalebuff EA: Arthrodesis of the rheumatoid wrist: an evaluation of sixty patients and a description of a different surgical technique. J Bone Joint Surg 55A:1026–1034, 1973.
28. Palmer AK, et al: Functional wrist motion: a biomechanical study. J Hand Surg 10A:39–46, 1985.
29. Peterson HA, and Lipscomb PR: Intercarpal arthrodesis. Arch Surg 95:127–134, 1967.
30. Rozing PM, and Kauer JMG: Partial arthrodesis of the wrist: investigation in cadavers. Acta Orthop Scand 55:66–68, 1984.
31. Ruby LK: Personal communication, 1986.
32. Ruby LK, Stinson J, and Belsky MR: The natural history of scaphoid nonunion. J Bone Joint Surg 67A:428–432, 1985.
33. Schwartz S: Localized fusion at the wrist joint. J Bone Joint Surg 49A:1591–1596, 1967.

34. Simmons BP, and McKenzie WD: Symptomatic carpal coalition. J Hand Surg 10A:190–193, 1985.

35. Smith RJ, Atkinson RE, and Jupiter JB: Silicone synovitis of the wrist. J Hand Surg 10A:47–60, 1985.

36. Sutro CJ: Treatment of nonunion of the carpal navicular bone. Surgery 20:536, 1946.

37. Swanson AB, et al: Lunate implant resection arthroplasty: long-term results. J Hand Surg 10A:1013–1024, 1985.

38. Taleisnik J: Subtotal arthrodeses of the wrist joint. Clin Orthop 187:81–88, 1984.

39. Taleisnik J: The Wrist. New York, Churchill Livingstone Inc, 1985.

40. Trumble T, Glisson RR, Seaber AV, et al: A biomechanical comparison of the methods for treating Kienböck's disease. J Hand Surg 11A:88–93, 1986.

41. Watson HK: Limited wrist arthrodesis. Clin Orthop 149:126–136, 1980.

42. Watson HK, and Ballet FL: The SLAC wrist: scapholunate advanced collapse pattern of degenerative arthritis. J Hand Surg 9A:358–365, 1984.

43. Watson HK, and Brenner LH: Degenerative disorders of the wrist. J Hand Surg 10A:1002–1006, 1985.

44. Watson HK, Goodman ML, and Johnson TR: Limited wrist arthrodesis. Part II: Intercarpal and radiocarpal combinations. J Hand Surg 6:223–233, 1981.

45. Watson HK, and Hempton RF: Limited wrist arthrodesis. Part I: The triscaphoid joint. J Hand Surg 5:320–327, 1980.

46. Watson HK, and Ryu J: Degenerative disorders of the carpus. Orthop Clin North Am 15:337–353, 1984.

47. Watson KH, Ryu J, and Akelman E: Limited triscaphoid arthrodesis for rotatory subluxation of the scaphoid. J Bone Joint Surg 68A:345–349, 1986.

48. Watson HK, Ryu J, and DiBella A: An approach to Kienböck's disease: triscaphe arthrodesis. J Hand Surg 10A:179–187, 1985.

49. Weber ER: Concepts governing the rotational shift of the intercalated segment of the carpus. Orthop Clin North Am 15:193–207, 1984.

50. Zemel NP, et al: Operative treatment for isolated scaphotrapezial-trapezoidal arthritis. J Hand Surg 10A:436, 1985.

Index

Note: Page numbers in *italics* indicate illustrations; page numbers followed by "t" indicate tables.